The Metabolic Syndrome

CONTEMPORARY ENDOCRINOLOGY

P. Michael Conn, SERIES EDITOR

THE METABOLIC SYNDROME

EPIDEMIOLOGY, CLINICAL TREATMENT, AND UNDERLYING MECHANISMS

Edited by

BARBARA CALEEN HANSEN, PhD

Professor of Internal Medicine and Pediatrics
Director, Obesity, Diabetes, and Aging Research Center
University of South Florida College of Medicine, Tampa, FL

GEORGE A. BRAY, MD

Boyd Professor, Pennington Biomedical Research Center
Louisiana State University, Baton Rouge, LA

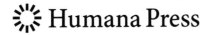 Humana Press

© 2008 Humana Press, a part of Springer Science+Business Media, LLC
999 Riverview Drive, Suite 208
Totowa, New Jersey 07512

humanapress.com

Cover design by Nancy K. Fallatt

Cover illustrations: (Top, left) Scanning electron micrograph of a large raised lesion on the aortic artch of a 9-month-old cp/cp rat (Fig. 3A, Chapter 8; see complete caption on p. 143 and discussion on p. 141. (Right) Scanning electron micrograph of a large intimal lesion in a human coronary artery (Fig. 4A, Chapter 8; see complete caption on p. 144 and discussion on p. 143). (Bottom) Swollen adipocytes in the pancreas (Fig. 1, Chapter 12; see complete caption and discussion on p. 222).

This publication is printed on acid-free paper. ∞

ANSI Z39.48-1984 (American Standards Institute) Permanence of Paper for Printed Library Materials.

For additional copies, pricing for bulk purchases, and/or information about other Humana titles, contact Humana at the above address or at any of the following numbers: Tel.: 973-256-1699; Fax: 973-256-8341; or visit our Website: www.humanapress.com

10 9 8 7 6 5 4 3 2 1

e-ISBN: 978-1-60327-116-5

Library of Congress Control Number: 2007931648

PREFACE

In the United States, 40 to 45% of those over 60 years of age have the *metabolic syndrome* (1,2,3), and this percentage, based on estimates of the increasing prevalence of excess body weight and the more comprehensive diagnostic criteria for the syndrome, is likely to exceed 60% in newer survey analyses. Children and adolescents, too, are being affected by the metabolic syndrome, in parallel with the increasing prevalence of overweight in young people, now estimated to include 16% of those age 6 to 19 years. Clinicians see with increasing frequency that routine office visits demonstrate the metabolic syndrome, a constellation of discrete but closely related metabolic disturbances indicative of increased risk for (or presence of) cardiovascular disease and/or diabetes. All estimates suggest the increasing impact of the metabolic syndrome on mortality and morbidity (4).

Our aim in developing this new synthesis and analysis of the metabolic syndrome has been to bring together the viewpoints of the epidemiologists, the physiologists, the molecular biologists/biochemists, and the clinicians toward understanding the current state of knowledge of both the causes and the consequences of the metabolic syndrome. These writers aim to stimulate new thinking concerning underlying mechanisms and to encourage heightened efforts to develop new therapeutics, potentially targeting uniquely intersecting pathways or points of intervention. This book is an extended call to action to slow or halt the rising tide of the metabolic syndrome (5).

The metabolic syndrome, including the links among its features, its underlying causes, and its recognized clinical importance, provides the framework for this book, which considers the current status of both basic and clinical science. This is part of a series initiated by G. Reaven and A. Laws (eds.), with *Insulin Resistance: The Metabolic Syndrome X* (Humana Press, 1999). By design, it builds upon two other prior volumes: E. Shafrir and B.C. Hansen (eds.), *Insulin Resistance and Insulin Resistance Syndrome* (United Kingdom: Harwood Academic Publishing, 2002), and B.C. Hansen, J.A. Saye, and L.P. Wennogle (eds.), *The Metabolic Syndrome X: Convergence of Insulin Resistance, Glucose Intolerance, Hypertension, Obesity and Dyslipidemias—Searching for the Underlying Defects* (*Annals of New York Academy of Sciences*, New York, NY, 1999). During these eight years, many of the concepts of the metabolic syndrome have been examined, tested, and strengthened, and, while the basic parameters remain, our thinking about this syndrome and its treatment has undergone considerable refinement.

Major progress has been made in understanding the importance of this syndrome, and in recognizing it as a clinical diagnosis through its inclusion, in 2001, as a new (ICD-9-CM) code (277.7) termed the *dysmetabolic syndrome*.

The interrelationships between metabolic syndrome features and the utility of a metabolic syndrome diagnosis are debated by several authors, with the current but limited conclusion concerning treatment that the best approach may be to treat ". . . individually and aggressively all cardiovascular disease risk factors, . . ." and to treat all collectively as therapeutic agents and new developments allow. Acceptance of risk factor clustering (obesity, hyperglycemia, elevated triglycerides and low HDL cholesterol levels, hypertension) is shared by all authors, although their perspectives vary widely on the interpretation of this undisputed fact. Both obesity and insulin resistance are frequently named as underlying or predisposing features of the metabolic syndrome; however, multiple metabolic disturbances have now been identified as early markers and potential contributors to the underlying pathology, including inflammatory cytokines and adipokines, endothelial dysfunction, tissue-specific defects in insulin action and signaling, oxidative stress, ectopic lipid deposition, and disordered neuroregulation.

Beyond the basic features of the metabolic syndrome lies a sophisticated array of pathway alterations, for example, in the complex profiling of the dyslipidemia, together with its multi-organ sources of disturbances.

While the first line of treatment, sometimes referred to as *lifestyle modifications*, including diet to produce weight reduction and reduce adiposity and exercise as a general health modifier, remains, more aggressive attention to medically modifying the specific features of the metabolic syndrome toward healthier levels is broadly supported by the authors.

Metabolic syndrome today is one of our most challenging health problems and one with an extraordinary need for early intervention and prevention to slow or halt its progression. Only through an understanding of the science underlying this syndrome can successful interventions be developed and implemented. The editors welcome your input and dialog as together we advance the field of metabolic syndrome and its prevention/treatment.

ACKNOWLEDGMENTS

This volume could not have been put together without the help of a number of people. First and foremost, we want to thank Rosemary Peternel, who has provided invaluable help in assembling all of the pieces, providing initial editorial work, and keeping us in touch with the authors. To the authors, we express our gratitude for their thoughtful contributions and their outstanding expertise. Their efforts are sure to facilitate a better understanding of the metabolic syndrome. We also wish to thank the publishers for their fine efforts to bring it all together. We thank our spouses, Dr. Kenneth D. Hansen and Mitzi Bray, for their support in all of our academic efforts. Thanks to all!

Barbara Caleen Hansen, PhD
George A. Bray, MD

REFERENCES

1. Ford ES, Giles WH, Dietz WH. Prevalence of the metabolic syndrome among U.S. adults: Findings from the third National Health and Nutrition Examination Survey. *JAMA* 2002; 287(3):356–359.
2. Duncan GE, Li SM, Zhou XH. Prevalence and trends of a metabolic syndrome phenotype among U.S. adolescents, 1999–2000. *Diabetes Care* 2004; 27(10):2438–2443.
3. Ford ES, Giles WH, Mokdad AH. Increasing prevalence of the metabolic syndrome among U.S. adults. *Diabetes Care* 2004; 27(10):2444–2449.
4. Malik S et al. Impact of the metabolic syndrome on mortality from coronary heart disease, cardiovascular disease, and all causes in United States adults. *Circulation* 2004; 110(10):1245–1250.
5. International Diabetes Federation. Diabetes and cardiovascular disease: A time to act. http://www.idf.org/webdata/docs/DiabetesandCVD.pdf, 2001.

CONTENTS

CONTRIBUTORS

CHRISTIAN X. ANDERSSON, MD, *Assistant Researcher, Lundberg Laboratory for Diabetes Research, Sahlgrenska University Hospital at Göteborg University, Göteborg, Sweden*

ALAIN BARON, MD, PhD, *Senior Vice President of Clinical Research, Amylin Pharmaceuticals, San Diego, CA*

GEORGE A. BRAY, MD, *Boyd Professor, Pennington Biomedical Research Center, Louisiana State University, Baton Rouge, LA*

TINA J. CHAHIL, MD, *Columbia University School of Medicine, New York, NY*

ANNE CLARK, *Reader in Diabetic Medicine, Churchill Hospital's Oxford Centre for Diabetes, Endocrinology, and Metabolism, Oxford, UK*

G.J. COONEY, *Kraegen Research Group, Garvan Institute of Medical Research, St. Vincent's Hospital, Sydney, New South Wales, Australia*

ROBERT V. FARESE, MD, *Director of the Division of Endocrinology and Metabolism, University of South Florida and James A. Haley Veterans Hospital, Tampa, FL*

EARL S. FORD, MD, MPH, *Senior Scientist, Centers for Disease Control, Atlanta, GA*

STUART M. FURLER, PhD, *Senior Research Officer of Kraegen Research Group, Garvan Institute of Medical Research, St. Vincent's Hospital, Sydney, New South Wales, Australia*

HENRY N. GINSBERG, MD, *Professor of Medicine, Columbia University School of Medicine, New York, NY*

ANN HAMMARSTEDT, MD, *Assistant Researcher, Lundberg Laboratory for Diabetes Research, Sahlgrenska University Hospital at Göteborg University, Göteborg, Sweden*

BARBARA CALEEN HANSEN, PhD, *Professor of Internal Medicine and Pediatrics, Director, Obesity, Diabetes, and Aging Research Center, University of South Florida College of Medicine, Tampa, FL*

JENS JUUL HOLST, MD, *Professor of Medical Physiology, The Panum Institute of the University of Copenhagen, Copenhagen, Denmark*

PER-ANDERS JANSSON, MD, *Physician, Lundberg Laboratory for Diabetes Research, Sahlgrenska University Hospital at Göteborg University, Göteborg, Sweden*

FILIP KRAG KNOP, MD, *Professor, Department of Internal Medicine of Gentofte Hospital, University of Copenhagen, Hellerup, Denmark*

E.W. KRAEGEN, PhD, *Professor and Head of Diabetes Group, Garvan Institute of Medical Research, St. Vincent's Hospital, Sydney, New South Wales, Australia*

LEWIS LANDSBERG, MD, *Dean and Vice President of Medical Affairs in the College of Medicine, Northwestern University, Evanston, IL*

SIMIN LIU, MD, MPH, MS, ScD, *Professor of Medicine and Epidemiology, Harvard Medical School and School of Public Health, Boston, MA*

JoAnn E. Manson, MD, Dr.PH, *Professor and Chief of Preventive Medicine, Brigham and Women's Hospital, Boston, MA*

Kieren J. Mather, MD, FRCPC, *Assistant Professor, Indiana University School of Medicine, Indianapolis, IN*

James B. Meigs, MD, MPH, *Senior Scientist, Department of Medicine, Massachusetts General Hospital, Boston, MA*

Jenni Moffitt, *Churchill Hospital's Oxford Centre for Diabetes, Endocrinology, and Metabolism, Oxford, UK*

Rosemary Peternel, *Writer and Coordinator, Baltimore, MD*

Katherine Pinnick, *Churchill Hospital's Oxford Centre for Diabetes, Endocrinology, and Metabolism, Oxford, UK*

Spencer D. Proctor, PhD, *Assistant Professor of Nutrition, University of Alberta, Edmonton, Alberta, Canada*

Susan Pye, *University of Ottawa Health Research Institute, Ottawa, Ontario, Canada*

Michael J. Quon, MD, PhD, *Chief of the Diabetes Unit, National Institute of Health's National Center for Complementary and Alternative Medicine, Bethesda, MD*

Jerry Radziuk, MD, PhD, *Director of Diabetes Research and Professor of Medicine, University of Ottawa Health Research Institute, Ottawa, Ontario, Canada*

Gerald M. Reaven, MD, *Professor Emeritus, Stanford University Medical Center, Stanford, CA*

Gissette Reyes, MD, *Columbia University School of Medicine, New York, NY*

James C. Russell, PhD, *Professor Emeritus, University of Alberta Metabolic and Cardiovascular Diseases Laboratory, Edmonton, Alberta, Canada*

Farhina Sayyed, *Churchill Hospital's Oxford Centre for Diabetes, Endocrinology, and Metabolism, Oxford, UK*

Ulf Smith, MD, *Professor of Internal Medicine, Lundberg Laboratory for Diabetes Research, Sahlgrenska University Hospital at Göteborg University, Göteborg, Sweden*

Yiqing Song, MD, ScD, *The Channing Laboratory, Brigham and Women's Hospital, Boston, MA*

Lianne van de Laar, *Churchill Hospital's Oxford Centre for Diabetes, Endocrinology, and Metabolism, Oxford, UK*

Morris F. White, PhD, *Investigator and Professor of Pediatrics, Division of Endocrinology, Harvard University, Boston, MA*

Jiming M. Ye, PhD, *Senior Research Officer of Kraegen Research Group, Garvan Institute of Medical Research, Sydney, New South Wales, Australia*

Jack F. Youngren, PhD, *Associate Research Biochemist, Mt. Zion Medical Center at the University of California San Francisco, San Francisco, CA*

Color Plates

Color Plates follow p. 372.

Figure 14.5. Islet histology of *IRS2*$^{+/-}$::*Pten*$^{+/-}$ intercross mice. Representative islet histology of pancreas sections from 3-month-old (left panels) and 6–8-month-old (right panels) mice immunostained with antibodies against insulin (green) and glucagon (red) photographed with a 5× or 20× objective. Scale bars: 500 μm. Islet morphometric analysis of *IRS2*$^{+/-}$::*Pten*$^{+/-}$ intercross mice at 6–8 months of age. Islet size calculated by mean cross-sectional area of multicelled islets reported as microns ×10^3/islet. Results are expressed as mean ±SEM of at least 5 mice per group. (See discussion on p. 263.)

Figure 14.6. A diagram showing the putative specificity between IRS1 and IRS2 signaling in hepatic regulation of gene expression through the phosphorylation and cytosolic translocation of FOXO1 and FOXA2. Nuclear FOXO1 largely mediates gluconeogenesis, whereas nuclear FOXA2 promotes fatty acid oxidation and inhibits synthesis. Since FOXA2 might be targeted for phosphorylation through IRS1 and IRS2 signaling, it might be coupled more tightly than FOXO1 to insulin stimulation under certain conditions. This imbalanced coupling can result in the characteristic gluconeogenesis and fatty acid synthesis that occurs in type 2 diabetes. (See discussion on p. 265.)

Figure 14.7. Schematic diagram of feedback inhibition of insulin signaling mediated by serine phosphorylation of IRS1. Various kinases in the insulin signaling cascade are implicated in this feedback mechanism, including PKB, mTOR, S6K, and ERK. Other kinases activated by heterologous signals are also involved. (See discussion on p. 266.)

Figure 14.8. A diagram describing the intersection of glucagon-like peptide-1 (GLP1) signaling and insulin/IGF signaling. GLP1 strongly activates the cAMP→CREB signaling cascade in β-cells, which promotes the expression of various genes, including IRS2. Since IRS2 is important for activation of various pathways that promote β-cell function, some of the long-term effects of GLP1 can be mediated through IRS2 expression. IRS-2 function is also a target of proinflammatory cytokines, so IRS2 can integrate many of the conflicting signals that reach β-cell. (See discussion on p. 268.)

Figure 18.3. Effects of insulin on metabolic pathways in the liver. Inhibitory effects on enzyme activities or substrate concentrations are indicated with (–) and stimulatory effects with (+). Primary effects are indicated by circles and secondary effects by boxes. Effects on new enzyme synthesis are preceded by an "S". (See discussion on p. 353.)

Figure 18.4. Summary of insulin effects on the components of principal glucose fluxes during meal absorption, and their impairment in type 2 diabetes. (See discussion on p. 355.)

Figure 18.5. Schematic illustrating some of the interactions between glucose and lipid metabolism, and demonstrating that increased glucose production will increase both FFA and liver lipid deposition, which in turn will accelerate gluconeogenesis. (See discussion on p. 357.)

1

Metabolic Syndrome— Past and Future

An Introduction to the Features of This Book

Barbara Caleen Hansen, Rosemary Peternel, and George A. Bray

CONTENTS

BACKGROUND
NATURAL HISTORY
CHAPTER SUMMARIES

BACKGROUND

This volume is a review by clinicians and researchers of the broad spectrum of research on the *metabolic syndrome* and its underlying disturbed pathways. It provides insights useful in understanding some of the features and processes in the development of diabetes and cardiovascular disease. Although there are differences of opinion about the value of the metabolic syndrome, it has one important aspect: It focuses attention on clinical considerations related to diabetes and heart disease.

The present volume is divided into three parts: The first part covers the epidemiological and clinical treatment perspectives; the second part is a discussion of endothelial function, inflammation, and dyslipidemia—features central to insulin resistance and vascular disease, including the contributions of C-reactive protein and adipocytes/ adipose tissue; and the third part explores insulin secretion and action and their underlying mechanisms, involving pancreatic islet pathophysiology, glucagonsrelated peptides, the insulin receptor signaling cascade, deposition of fat in muscle, alterations in atypical protein kinase-C (APK-C), and the role of the liver.

There are also pointers for future research directions, for improved diagnostic criteria, and for recognition of important pathways that will allow for better treatment alternatives and understanding of micro- and macrophysiological processes. As expected with a cross-disciplinary book of this type, some chapters cover topics that appear in other chapters providing different perspectives on the same problem. Several themes are reinforced throughout this volume: First, multiple, simultaneous treatment strategies

From: *Contemporary Endocrinology: The Metabolic Syndrome: Epidemiology, Clinical Treatment, and Underlying Mechanisms*
Edited by: B.C. Hansen and G.A. Bray © Humana Press, Totowa, NJ

are needed to improve individual risk factors and the pathophysiology they represent; second, changes in behavioral lifestyle are needed, including reducing obesity, smoking and alcohol use, improving diet, and increasing daily exercise; and third, drugs targeting peroxisome proliferator–activated receptors, as well as other multifunctional drugs, hold promise for overall improved health status and reduction or prevention of the metabolic syndrome.

NATURAL HISTORY

The metabolic syndrome can be considered as a clustering of several risk factors, including hypertension, dyslipidemia, impaired glucose tolerance, and central adiposity. The recognition of this clustering has evolved over almost 90 years. According to Panteleimon Sarafidis' and Peter Nilsson's historical account of the origins of the metabolic syndrome, during World War I, two Austrian physicians, Karl Hitzenberger and Martin Richter-Quittner, identified a link between hypertension and diabetes (1). Furthermore, they identify Eskil Kylin and Gregorio Maranon, respectively a Swede and a Spaniard, who published similar findings in this period (1). Another discovery that Sarafidis and Nilsson refer to is H.P. Himsworth's distinguishing between insulin-resistant and insulin-sensitive diabetics in 1936—suggesting a common pathophysiological background linking metabolic risk factors (1). During the 1940s, M.J. Albrink and J.W. Meigs associated obesity with hyperglycemia and dyslipidemia, as reported by Sarafidis and Nilsson (1). Also during the 1940s, Jean Vague described the male fat distribution and its consequences (2–6). The link between the syndrome features and cardiovascular disease was made as early as the 1960s by Welborn and by Camus, the latter coining the term *trisyndrome métabolique* (7–9).

Nutrition and lifestyles were implicated during the 1960s, and fatty acids were identified as contributing to diabetes and insulin resistance. Advances in the 1970s and early 1980s expanded our understanding of the link of these to coronary heart disease, even in the absence of diabetes, and linked the metabolic risk factors to atherosclerosis (10–12). In 1988, G.M. Reaven grouped several metabolic disorders together as *syndrome X* and proposed that insulin resistance was the underlying event explaining dyslipidemia, high blood pressure, and diabetes (13), and this characterization was further examined by DeFronzo and Ferranini in 1991 (14). These factors were then observed to be influenced by both genetic and environmental factors. Many other names were proposed for this syndrome (15–19), including the *plurimetabolic syndrome* (1988) (20), the *deadly quartet* (1989) (21), *syndrome X plus* (1991) (22), *metabolic syndrome X* (13), the *metabolic syndrome* (23), the *insulin resistance syndrome* (1991) (14), the *cardiovascular disease risk factor cluster* (1992) (24), and *diabesity* (1993) (25); however, from the mid-1990s onward, the term *metabolic syndrome* has been most used. Since the underlying mechanisms are not yet known, the insulin resistance syndrome (the secondary contender for a syndrome title), which implies cause, has been less used.

Over the past 10 years, the definition of the metabolic syndrome has been hotly debated, and debate continues on even whether there is or is not such a syndrome (26). (Also, see Reaven, Chapter 2 in this volume.) The organization-endorsed definitions began with the World Health Organization proposal of 1998 (27), and this was followed in 1999 by an insulin resistance–focused definition by the European Group for the Study of Insulin Resistance (28). An important step was the 2001 proposal by the National Cholesterol Education Program Adult Treatment Panel (NCEP ATP) III report, which aimed to make the clinical diagnosis of the metabolic syndrome more user friendly (29). This was followed by a more flexible definition from the American Association of Clinical Endocrinologists in 2003 (30). Today, the most common definitions are the (WHO version, revised) International Diabetes Federation definition of 2005 (31) and the revised NCEP ATP definition of 2005 (32).

The prevalence of the metabolic syndrome based on the National Health and Nutrition Examination Survey (NHANES 2001–02) has been estimated at 36.8% according to the NCEP ATP definition and 39.9% according to the International Diabetes Federation (IDF) definition (33). An estimated 12 million adults greater than or equal to 40 years of age have diagnosed and undiagnosed diabetes, of whom most have metabolic syndrome (69.9% for whites, 64.8% for blacks, and 62.4% for Mexican Americans) (34), and some estimates suggest that as many as 90% of persons with established type 2 diabetes have the metabolic syndrome. An estimated 41 million people aged 40–74 years have pre-diabetes (raised blood glucose levels insufficiently high enough to be called diabetes) (34).

Analysis of data from the NHANES 1999–2002 demonstrates racial differences in the prevalence of components of the metabolic syndrome among diabetics and nondiabetics (34). Kidney disease and neuropathy are co-morbidities associated with diabetes and components of the metabolic syndrome. Treatment of high blood pressure has been shown to delay the progression to renal disease (35). Analysis of NHANES data indicates that about a third of diabetics are undiagnosed, of whom a significant proportion have signs of nephropathy and peripheral neuropathy. Prevalence estimates of multiple cardiac risk factors for U.S. adults with and without diabetes and heart disease are high enough to demonstrate the extensiveness of metabolic syndrome components as a public health issue (36).

Medical providers have an obligation to treat modifiable risk factors, including obesity (37), in patients with and without full-blown diabetes. Several studies indicate that aggressive use of lifestyle modification as well as pharmacotherapy can reduce the conversion of individuals with prediabetes to diabetes. Early treatment and delaying the onset of stroke, heart attack, and full-blown diabetes has important implications for the rise in U.S. health-care spending. Over the past 15 years, spending has been found to be related to rising rates of treated disease prevalence, which is related to the doubling of obesity and clinical changes related to cardiovascular risk factors (38).

CHAPTER SUMMARIES

In Part I, Chapter 2 by Gerald Reaven discusses the interrelationships between the metabolic syndrome and the diseases it predicts, where the best approach is to treat "... individually and aggressively all cardiovascular disease risk factors ...." In Chapter 3, James Meigs accepts that the statistical occurrence of risk factor clustering (obesity, hyperglycemia, elevated triglycerides and low HDL cholesterol levels, and hypertension) may reflect the underlying roles of plasma-free fatty acids, systemic inflammation, adiponectin, and endothelial dysfunction and he suggests that treatment with dietary interventions, lifestyle changes, and insulin-sensitizing drugs may reduce these risks. George Bray in Chapter 4 focuses on the role of weight reduction in improving all components of the metabolic syndrome. He finds that removal of visceral fat by lipectomy improves lipids or blood pressure and that growth hormone, testosterone, cortisol, and dehydroepiandosterone all have independent effects on visceral tissue.

The complexity of prospective measurement of insulin resistance using the "gold standard methods" is highlighted by Earl Ford et al. in Chapter 5. They suggest that there is some tentative support for recognizing insulin resistance as an independent risk factor for cardiovascular disease. In Chapter 6, Lewis Landsberg focuses on the sympatho-adrenal system as a physiological response to obesity and insulin resistance. There are "significant causal factors in the pathogenesis of major clinical manifestations," whereby the sympathetic nervous system (SNS) activity is increased in metabolic syndrome. The *hows* and *whys* of insulin stimulation of the SNS lead to a discussion of diet, fasting, sleep disturbances, the "metabolic economy of the obese state," and interrelationships between metabolic parameters such as blood pressure and dyslipidemia. He argues that despite the paucity of controlled studies, treatment should focus on lowering blood pressure; lifestyle modifications, including weight loss; restriction of salt intake, calories, and alcohol; and pharmacological agents.

In Part II, Chapter 7, Kieren Mather and Alain Baron et al. address the relationships between insulin resistance and endothelial dysfunction and the molecular mechanisms of insulin signaling in the vasculature. Attention is directed to the well-established importance of the interacting roles of nitric oxide and endothelin in the vessel wall and insulin's overall actions on carbohydrate metabolism. A promising research direction leading to new beneficial therapeutic approaches to metabolic syndrome and related disorders is examination of "hormonal factors associated with obesity, insulin resistance, and endothelial dysfunction, including adipokines and inflammatory markers and mediators." In Chapter 8, James C. Russell and Spencer D. Proctor review a rodent model, the Kolesky rat, which displays both micro- and macrovascular pathology in the pre-diabetic state as well as marked insulin resistance. JoAnn Manson et al. in Chapter 9 accept the construct that it is difficult to "tease out the causes and consequences among highly intercorrelated biological variables," and note that determining whether it is more efficacious to treat individual components of the metabolic syndrome or to treat the entire syndrome is unknown. An additional question is raised about the value of incorporating the C-reactive protein measurement. In cross-sectional epidemiological research, particularly for women, it may be a key indicator of cardiovascular and metabolic risk. For clinicians, the reasonable response is to evaluate and treat individual and traditional risk factors.

Ulf Smith et al. in Chapter 10 review the action of inflammatory markers such as C-reactive protein and serum amyloid A, and adipose tissue dysregulation in insulin signaling. Notwithstanding the other benefits of improved insulin sensitivity, thiazolidinediones are thought "to improve insulin sensitivity of adipose tissue by recruiting new and more insulin-sensitive adipocytes and to drive the terminal differentiation of preexisting adipocytes." In Chapter 11, Henry Ginsberg et al. review the epidemiological and physiological associations between dyslipidemia and insulin resistance. He notes that defects present in the fasting state are exaggerated in insulin resistance states, and that improving the body's energy balance is key to improving insulin sensitivity.

In the examination of underlying mechanisms associated with the metabolic syndrome, Anne Clark et al. in Chapter 12 (Part III) lead off by identifying the metabolic syndrome as a "complex of interrelated metabolic imbalances, . . . including . . . abnormal insulin secretion, . . . especially . . . in obesity the hypersecretion of insulin associated with increased insulin resistance." The reference to "disturbances" and their impact on pancreatic islet function is the main topic of this chapter on obesity and the pathology of pancreatic islets, where the formation of "fibrils between the basement membrane and islet beta cells . . . ultimately . . . contribute[s] to an irreversible loss of insulin secretory capacity." With an emphasis on other features of obesity, Jens Holst and Filip Krag Knop in Chapter 13 focus on the actions of glucagon-like peptides (GLP) and report on treatment findings showing beneficial effects of GLP-1 infusions and analog treatments on normalizing fasting blood glucose concentrations in patients with type 2 diabetes and improving blood lipids, reducing body weight, and increasing beta cell secretion and insulin sensitivity.

Morris White in Chapter 14 relates findings from animal studies on the role of tyrosine phosphorylation of *insulin receptor substrate-1* or its homologs IRS2 or other scaffold proteins in mediating many of the metabolic effects of insulin. One suggested treatment for diabetes and related metabolic disorders is targeting the increased IRS2 expression in beta cells or other tissues. Jack Youngren in Chapter 15 focuses on insulin signaling pathways with reference to mouse models. The discussion focuses on the functions of insulin receptors, the structural aspects of insulin resistance, the insulin receptor gene, mechanisms of tyrosine kinase activity, and the contributions of obesity, diet, physical activity, and diabetes to insulin resistance. This review of human and animal studies indicates that "insulin resistance signaling capacity is a relatively labile parameter than can be modulated by physiological, hormonal, or biochemical factors." In Chapter 16, E.W. Kraegen et al. discuss oxidative capacity as a possible mechanism for enhancing insulin sensitivity, based on the hypothesis that "oversupply and/or accumulation of lipid in muscle and liver leads to changes in metabolism . . . that account for insulin resistance seen in . . . metabolic syndrome and type 2 diabetes."

Chapter 17, by Robert Farese, and Chapter 18, by Jerry Radziuk and S. Pye, offer insight respectively into two defective insulin signaling molecules. Atypical protein kinase C (aPKC) and protein kinase B (PKB/Akt) in the muscle and liver are discussed in Chapter 17. In Chapter 18, the focus is on glucose metabolism in the liver and hepatic insulin action. It is noted that there are a lack of data on insulin signaling defects in human livers of obese and diabetic humans, and there remains a need for therapeutic intervention to "improve aPKC and PKB activation in muscle, inhibit aPKC and aPKC-dependent processes in the liver, and improve PKB activation in the liver."

In the final chapter, Chapter 19, Barbara Hansen concludes with an analysis of the controversies surrounding the *clinical* and *research* definitions of the metabolic syndrome, and introduces a new factor, the *chronomics* of the syndrome, for further study.

REFERENCES

1. Sarafidis PA, Nilsson PM. The metabolic syndrome: a glance at its history. *J Hypertens* 2006; 24(4):621–626.
2. Vague J, Vague P, Jubelin J. A 35-year follow-up of diabetogenic obesity. *Int J Obes* 1987; 11(suppl 2):38.

3. Vague J. *La differentiation sexuelle: Facteur determinant des formes de l'obesite.* See http://www.obesityresearch.org/cgi/reprint/10/1/14.pdf. *Presse Med* 1947; 55:339–341.
4. Vague J. *La differenciation sexuelle humaine: Ses incidences en pathologie.* Masson, Paris, 1953; reprinted in http://www.blackwell-synergy.com/links/doi/10.1111/j.1467–3010.2004.00403.x/enhancedabs/WHO (World Health Organization1999 Report, p. 386).
5. Vague J. The degree of masculine differentiation of obesities: A factor determining predisposition to diabetes, atherosclerosis, gout, and uric calculous disease. *Am J Clin Nutr* 1956; 4(1):20–34.
6. Vague J et al. Forms of obesity and metabolic disorders. *Verh Dtsch Ges Inn Med* 1987; 93:448–462.
7. Camus JP. Gout, diabetes, hyperlipemia: A metabolic trisyndrome. *Rev Rhum Mal Osteoartic* 1966; 33(1):10–14.
8. Welborn TA et al. Serum-insulin in essential hypertension and in peripheral vascular disease. *Lancet* 1966; 1(7451):1336–1337.
9. Welborn TA, Wearne K. Coronary heart disease incidence and cardiovascular mortality in Busselton with reference to glucose and insulin concentrations. *Diabetes Care* 1979; 2(2):154–160.
10. Modan M et al. Hyperinsulinemia: A link between hypertension obesity and glucose intolerance. *J Clin Invest* 1985; 75(3):809–817.
11. Modan M et al. Elevated serum uric acid: A facet of hyperinsulinaemia. *Diabetologia* 1987; 30(9):713–718.
12. Pyorala K. Relationship of glucose tolerance and plasma insulin to the incidence of coronary heart disease: Results from two population studies in Finland. *Diabetes Care* 1979; 2(2):131–141.
13. Reaven GM. Banting lecture 1988: Role of insulin resistance in human disease. *Diabetes* 1988; 37(12):1595–1607.
14. DeFronzo RA, Ferrannini E. Insulin resistance: A multifaceted syndrome responsible for NIDDM, obesity, hypertension, dyslipidemia, and atherosclerotic cardiovascular disease. *Diabetes Care* 1991; 14(3):173–194.
15. Florez H et al. Women relatives of Hispanic patients with type 2 diabetes are more prone to exhibit metabolic disturbances. *Invest Clin* 1999; 40(2):127–142.
16. Foster DW. Insulin resistance: A secret killer? *N Engl J Med* 1989; 320(11):733–734.
17. Hayashi H et al. Contribution of a missense mutation (Trp64Arg) in beta3-adrenergic receptor gene to multiple risk factors in Japanese men with hyperuricemia. *Endocr J* 1998; 45(6):779–784.
18. Lempiainen P et al. Insulin resistance syndrome predicts coronary heart disease events in elderly non-diabetic men. *Circulation* 1999; 100(2):123–128.
19. Liese AD et al. Association of serum uric acid with all-cause and cardiovascular disease mortality and incident myocardial infarction in the MONICA Augsburg cohort: World Health Organization Monitoring Trends and Determinants in Cardiovascular Diseases. *Epidemiology* 1999; 10(4):391–397.
20. Crepaldi G, Nosadini R. Diabetic cardiopathy: Is it a real entity? *Diabetes Metab Rev* 1988; 4(3):273–288.
21. Kaplan NM. The deadly quartet: Upper-body obesity, glucose intolerance, hypertriglyceridemia, and hypertension. *Arch Intern Med* 1989; 149(7):1514–1520.
22. Zimmet P. The epidemiology of diabetes mellitus and related conditions. In: *The Diabetes Annual/6*, Alberti K, Krall LP (eds.), 1991, Elsevier, Amsterdam.
23. Eriksson J, Taimela S, Koivisto VA. Exercise and the metabolic syndrome. *Diabetologia* 1997; 40(2):125–135.
24. Scott R et al. Will acarbose improve the metabolic abnormalities of insulin-resistant type 2 diabetes mellitus? *Diabetes Research and Clinical Practice* 1999, March; 43(Issue 3):179–185.
25. Shafrir E. Animal models of syndrome X. *Current Topics in Diabetes Research* 1993; 12: 165–181.
26. Kahn R et al. The metabolic syndrome: Time for a critical appraisal—joint statement from the American Diabetes Association and the European Association for the Study of Diabetes. *Diabetes Care* 2005; 28(9):2289–2304.
27. Alberti KG, Zimmet PZ. Definition, diagnosis and classification of diabetes mellitus and its complications. Part 1: Diagnosis and classification of diabetes mellitus provisional report of a WHO consultation. *Diabet Med* 1998; 15(7):539–553.
28. Balkau B, Charles MA. Comment on the provisional report from the WHO consultation: European Group for the Study of Insulin Resistance (EGIR). *Diabet Med* 1999; 16(5):442–443.

29. Executive Summary of the Third Report of the National Cholesterol Education Program (NCEP) Expert Panel on Detection, Evaluation, and Treatment of High Blood Cholesterol in Adults (Adult Treatment Panel III). *JAMA* 2001; 285(19):2486–2497.
30. Einhorn D et al. American College of Endocrinology position statement on the insulin resistance syndrome. *Endocr Pract* 2003; 9(3):237–252.
31. Federation ID. The IDF Consensus Worldwide Definition of Metabolic Syndrome, April 14, 2005, http://www.idf.org/webdata/docs/IDF_Metasyndrome_definition.pdf.
32. Grundy SM et al. Diagnosis and management of the metabolic syndrome: An American Heart Association/National Heart, Lung, and Blood Institute Scientific Statement. *Circulation* 2005; 112(17):2735–2752.
33. Hollenbeak CS et al. Predicting the prevalence of cardiometabolic risk factors when clinical data are limited. *Value Health* 2007; 10(suppl 1):S4–S11.
34. Lin SX, Pi-Sunyer EX. Prevalence of the metabolic syndrome among US middle-aged and older adults with and without diabetes: A preliminary analysis of the NHANES 1999–2002 data. *Ethn Dis* 2007; 17(1):35–39.
35. Barri YM. Hypertension and kidney disease: A deadly connection. *Curr Cardiol Rep* 2006; 8(6):411–417.
36. Koopman RJ et al. Evidence of nephropathy and peripheral neuropathy in US adults with undiagnosed diabetes. *Ann Fam Med* 2006; 4(5):427–432.
37. Tjepkema M. Adult obesity. *Health Rep* 2006; 17(3):9–25.
38. Thorpe KE, Florence CS, Joski P. Which medical conditions account for the rise in health care spending? *Health Aff (Millwood)* 2004; Suppl Web Exclusives:W4–437–445.

I

EPIDEMIOLOGY AND CLINICAL TREATMENT: ISSUES IN DEFINING AND TREATING THE METABOLIC SYNDROME

2

Metabolic Syndrome
To Be or Not to Be?

Gerald M. Reaven

CONTENTS

INTRODUCTION

Two separate statements published in the autumn of 2005 expressed diametrically opposed views as to the clinical utility of "diagnosing" the metabolic syndrome (MetS). On the one hand (1), the American Heart Association (AHA) and the National Heart, Lung, and Blood Institute (NHLBI) firmly endorsed the need to establish such a diagnostic category, and, with some minor modifications, utilized the approach outlined by the report of the Adult Treatment Panel III (ATP III) (2). On the other hand, the American Diabetes Association (ADA) and the European Association for the Study of Diabetes (EASD) simultaneously issued a joint statement sharply critical of the notion of the clinical utility of making a "diagnosis" of the MetS (3).

One difficulty in coming to grips with this budding controversy is that multiple approaches to diagnosing the MetS now exist, and although the name may be the same, and the components quite similar, the conceptual constructs underlying the multiple definitions are quite different. Consequently, one goal of this chapter will be to examine the implications of the biological/philosophical basis of the various definitions of the MetS.

Published versions of the MetS also differ considerably as to their view of the association between the various criteria proposed to make this diagnosis. Thus, it seems important to examine the relationship between the common components of the various

From: *Contemporary Endocrinology: The Metabolic Syndrome: Epidemiology, Clinical Treatment, and Underlying Mechanisms*
Edited by: B.C. Hansen and G.A. Bray © Humana Press, Totowa, NJ

definitions of the MetS, as well as their link to cardiovascular disease (CVD). For example, is there a biological connection that links the individual diagnostic criteria of the MetS to each other, and, if so, is the relationship hierarchical in nature? Conversely, are the individual components simply CVD risk factors that have no physiological relationship with each other (i.e., they cluster together for no discernible reason)? A discussion of these issues is the second goal of this chapter.

Finally, there is much more unanimity concerning the relationship between the individual components and specific clinical syndromes than there is as to whether it is useful to make a diagnosis of the MetS, or the best way to accomplish that goal. For example, there is little or no argument as how to diagnose type 2 diabetes or essential hypertension. Thus, the third goal of this chapter is to examine the concept that there is clinical utility in making a diagnosis of the MetS. Specifically, does a diagnosis of the MetS provide more clinical information concerning CVD risk than the presence of any one of its components? More important, is it possible that failure to make a diagnosis of the MetS in patients with known CVD risks results in less effective therapeutic efforts?

Finally, it would be disingenuous if I did not make known the fact that I have published previous articles (4–6) indicating my skepticism as to either the pedagogical or clinical utility of making a diagnosis of the MetS. Consequently, since the readers have been forewarned, they should be forearmed.

IT'S A BIRD! IT'S A PLANE! IT'S THE METABOLIC SYNDROME!

The World Health Organization (WHO) was the first major organization to propose a set of clinical criteria for the MetS, formalized and published (7) in a 1998 document entitled, "Definition, Diagnosis and Classification of Diabetes Mellitus and its Complications." The primary purpose of this report was to update the classification and diagnostic criteria of diabetes mellitus. In this context, the WHO Consultation Group designated the MetS as a special classification for individuals with, or with the potential for developing, type 2 diabetes: manifested by having impaired glucose tolerance (IGT), impaired fasting glucose (IFG), or insulin resistance by hyperinsulinemic, euglycemic clamp. The Consultation Group felt that once these individuals developed certain "CVD risk components" they became a unique entity and qualified as having the MetS. Aside from glucose tolerance status and/or insulin resistance, risk components deemed useful to identify individuals with the MetS included obesity, dyslipidemia, hypertension, and microalbuminuria. It was the view of the WHO Consultation Group that each component conveyed increased CVD risk, but as a combination became more "powerful." Therefore, the primary goal of recognizing an individual as having the MetS was to identify persons at heightened risk for CVD. Secondarily, by design, the diagnosis also helped identify individuals with high risk for diabetes if they did not already have it. Table 2.1 displays the criteria proposed by the WHO by which to make a diagnosis of the MetS.

The ATP III, representing the National Cholesterol Education Program (NCEP), published their initial definition of the MetS in 2001 (2). As indicated in the ATP III document, its primary purpose was somewhat different from that of the WHO report in that its focus was not on diabetes, but instead to update clinical guidelines for cholesterol testing and management. In addition, a major thrust of this third report by the

Table 2.1
WHO Definition of the Metabolic Syndrome

Must have one of the following (glucose concentration given in mmol/L (mg/dL)):
- Diabetes mellitus
  o Fasting plasma glucose ≥7 (126) or 2-hr post-glucose load ≥11.1 (200)
- Impaired glucose tolerance
  o Fasting plasma glucose <7 (126) and 2-hr post-glucose load ≥7.8 (140) and <11.1 (200)
- Impaired fasting glucose
  o Fasting plasma glucose ≥6.1 (110) and <7 (126) and (if measured) 2-hr post-glucose load <7.8 (140)
- Insulin resistance
  o Glucose uptake below lowest quartile for background population under investigation under hyperinsulinemic, euglycemic conditions

Plus any two of the following:
- Waist:hip ratio >0.9 in men, >0.85 in women; and/or BMI >30 kg/m^2
- Triglycerides ≥1.7 mmol/L (150 mg/dL); and/or HDL-C <0.9 mmol/L (35 mg/dL) in men, <1.0 mmol/L (39 mg/dL) in women
- Blood pressure ≥140/90 mmHg (revised from ≥160/90)
- Microalbuminuria (urinary albumin excretion rate ≥20 µg/min or albumin:creatinine ratio ≥30 mg/g)

NCEP was to "focus on primary prevention in persons with multiple risk factors." With these goals in mind, the ATP III introduced the MetS as "multiple, interrelated factors that raise CVD risk." The panel believed that the MetS increased CVD risk at any given low-density lipoprotein cholesterol (LDL-C) concentration, and should be a secondary target of therapy in cholesterol management. Similar to the WHO, the ATP III goal for establishing criteria for the MetS was to identify individuals at special risk for CVD, and to institute intensified lifestyle changes to mitigate these risks. In contrast to the WHO, the ATP III did not consider direct evidence of insulin resistance necessary to make a diagnosis of the MetS.

Although both the WHO and ATP III considered the MetS as conveying high risk for CVD, they viewed the underlying concept of the MetS somewhat differently. The WHO introduced the MetS in the context of classifying diabetes mellitus and impaired glucose regulation. They believed that having the MetS syndrome elevated the CVD risk profile of individuals who had diabetes, or who were at risk for diabetes, and that these individuals should be classified separately. This point of view has the potential of resulting in two separate diagnostic categories of patients with type 2 diabetes: those with, or without, the MetS. The ATP III agreed that having the MetS enhanced CVD risk, but in keeping with their organizational focus, they viewed the MetS, not in terms of diabetes, but as a special risk factor for CVD that was additive to other known risk factors. However, the fundamental goal of the two organizations was similar: a more effective way to prevent CVD in high-risk individuals.

The ATP III criteria for diagnosing the MetS appear in Table 2.2, and although there are many similarities, fundamental differences exist between the WHO and ATP III definitions. The most prominent difference is that the ATP III does not identify any one essential criterion, but proposes that an individual meeting any three of the five criteria

Table 2.2
ATP III Definition of the Metabolic Syndrome

Any three of the following:
- Fasting glucose   ≥6.1 mmol/L (110 mg/dL)
- Waist circumference
  ○ Men   >102 cm (40 in)
  ○ Women   >88 cm (35 in)
- Triglycerides   ≥1.7 mmol/L (150 mg/dL)
- HDL-C
  ○ Men   <1.036 mmol/L (40 mg/dL)
  ○ Women   <1.295 mmol/L (50 mg/dL)
- Blood pressure   ≥130/85 mmHg

in Table 2.2 has the MetS. Thus, not only is the presence of insulin resistance no longer required to make a diagnosis of the MetS, a person can be identified as having the ATP III version without any evidence of abnormal glucose tolerance. The two definitions also contain minor differences in the actual values needed to have an "abnormal" plasma triglyceride (TG) or high-density lipoprotein cholesterol (HDL-C) concentration or blood pressure. However, there are two more substantive differences between the two organizations in that the ATP III no longer lists microalbuminuria as one of the possible diagnostic criteria, and abdominal obesity, as assessed by measuring waist circumference (WC), is the only acceptable index of excess adiposity.

The International Diabetes Federation (IDF) is the most recent group to propose criteria with which to diagnose the MetS, and Table 2.3 lists the specific components they have chosen for this purpose (8). The IDF definition is similar to that of the WHO in that they have identified one essential criterion with which to make a diagnosis of the MetS. However, in contrast to the need to demonstrate the presence of glucose intoler-

Table 2.3
IDF Definition of the Metabolic Syndrome

In order for a person to be diagnosed with the metabolic syndrome, he or she must have:

- **Central obesity** (defined as a waist circumference ≥94 cm for Europid men and ≥80 cm for Europid women, with ethnicity-specific values for other groups)

plus any two of the following four factors:

1. Raised TG level: ≥150 mg/dL (i.7 mmol/L), or specific treatment for this abnormality.
2. Reduced HDL cholesterol: <40 mg/dL (1.03 mmol/L) in males and <50 mg/dL (1.29 mmol/L) in females, or specific treatment for this lipid abnormality.
3. Raised blood pressure: systolic BP ≥130 or diastolic BP ≥85 mmHg, or treatment of previously diagnosed hypertension.
4. Raised fasting glucose (FPG) ≥100 mg/dL (5.6 mmol/L), or previously diagnosed type 2 diabetes. If FPG is above the values stated above, an oral glucose tolerance test is strongly recommended but is not necessary to define presence of the syndrome.

ance and/or insulin resistance, the diagnostic criterion that must be fulfilled is abdominal obesity as determined by measuring WC.

Inspection of Tables 2.1–2.3 demonstrates that the individual components of the various definitions of the MetS do not differ a great deal, but the superficial similarities should not serve to obscure fundamental differences among them. The most obvious difference is a conceptual one, involving the pathophysiological relationship between the individual diagnostic criteria. Thus, in the case of the ATP III version, the five criteria represent separate, but apparently equal CVD risks, and an abnormality in any three of them suffices to make a diagnosis of the MetS. In contrast, a diagnosis of the MetS with either the WHO or IDF version relies on a hierarchal ordering of the criteria, and in both instances, one essential ingredient must be satisfied: glucose intolerance and/or insulin resistance in the case of the WHO, whereas an abnormal WC must be present to satisfy IDF criteria for the MetS.

The second substantive difference involves the role of excess adiposity in the diagnosis of the MetS, specifically the clinical utility of assessing overall obesity, as measured by body mass index (BMI), versus abdominal obesity, quantified by WC or the ratio of waist/hip girth (WHR). Thus, excess adiposity, one of several supplemental criteria in the WHO definition, measured as either BMI or WHR, remains a criterion with the ATP III definition, but can only be met by having an abnormal WC, whereas in the IDF version WC has become the essential criterion with which to diagnose the MetS. The implication of these two fundamental areas of disparity among the various definitions of the MetS deserves careful consideration.

WHAT IS THE RELATIONSHIP AMONG THE METABOLIC SYNDROME DIAGNOSTIC CRITERIA: CASUAL OR CAUSAL?

In its recent statement, the AHA/NHLBI (1) indicates that the most widely recognized of the metabolic risk factors underlying the MetS are an "atherogenic dyslipidemia, elevated blood pressure, and elevated plasma glucose." They further point out that "individuals with these characteristics commonly manifest a prothrombotic and proinflammatory state." Although acknowledging that these changes represent "a grouping of ASCVD risk factors," the cluster identified "probably has more than one cause." This point of view is different from that expressed by either the WHO (7) or IDF (8) versions of the MetS, in that the former considers evidence of insulin resistance essential to make this diagnosis, whereas the IDF states that an increase in WC is the necessary ingredient.

It is difficult to disagree with the conclusion of the AHA/NHLBI that the cluster of abnormalities that make up the MetS "probably has more than one cause." In fact it is obvious that there are multiple examples of why this is the case. For example, Ahrens and associates (9) indicated that there were at least two divergent causes of increase in plasma triglyceride (TG) concentration: one related to the amount of carbohydrate ingested (CHO-induced lipemia) and the other to the quantity of fat consumed (fat-induced lipemia). However, they further pointed out that CHO-induced lipemia was by far the most common finding.

Returning to the AHA/NHLBI version of the MetS, do the authors believe that their "grouping of ASCVD risk factors" is coincidental? Alternatively, is it possible that a *common* physiological event greatly increases the likelihood that an individual will develop the changes that make up their definition of the MetS? The proposed answer to this rhetorical question is that the abnormalities that comprise all three versions of the MetS do not "cluster" together by accident, and that a defect in insulin action plays a fundamental role in the development of the CVD risk factors that comprise all versions of the MetS. The evidence in support of the formulation follows.

Glucose Intolerance

The prevalence of some degree of abnormal glucose tolerance and/or type 2 diabetes—one of the criteria in all three definitions of the MetS—is the abnormality most closely related to insulin resistance. Indeed, more than 60 years ago, in 1939, Himsworth and Kerr (10) challenged the conventional wisdom that "all cases of human diabetes could be explained by deficiency of insulin." Instead, they suggested that "a state of diabetes might result from inefficient action of insulin as well as from a lack of insulin," and stated, "the diminished ability of the tissues to utilize glucose is referable either to a deficiency of insulin or to insensitivity to insulin, although it is possible that both factors may operate simultaneously." In the same vein, in 1949, Himsworth concluded by indicating that "we should accustom ourselves to the idea that a primary deficiency of insulin is only one, and then not the commonest, cause of the diabetes syndrome" (11).

The prescience of Himsworth's observations is borne out by the fact that we now know that resistance to insulin-mediated glucose disposal is present in the great majority of individuals with type 2 diabetes (12–16). It is also clear that insulin resistance (or hyperinsulinemia as a surrogate estimate of insulin resistance) is a powerful and independent predictor of the development of type 2 diabetes (17–21). Finally, the greater the degree of insulin resistance, the higher the plasma insulin response to oral glucose is in individuals with normal oral glucose tolerance (22). Parenthetically, although insulin resistance was highly predictive of the magnitude of hyperglycemia following a glucose load in glucose-tolerant individuals, there was no relationship between excess adiposity and glucose response in these same individuals. Thus, there is an enormous amount of evidence documenting a very close relationship between insulin resistance and abnormal elevations in plasma glucose concentrations.

Finally, it should be emphasized that nondiabetic individuals with relatively minor degrees of glucose tolerance also have higher blood pressures, and the dyslipidemic changes—a high TG and a low HDL-C concentration—that comprise the remaining metabolic criteria of all three definitions of the MetS (23–26).

Dyslipidemia

It has been known for approximately 40 years that there is a highly significant relationship among insulin resistance, *compensatory* hyperinsulinemia, and hypertriglyceridemia (27,28). It is now apparent that the link between insulin resistance/hyperinsulinemia and dyslipidemia is a much broader one, and not limited to an increase in plasma TG concentrations. Thus, although the various definitions of the MetS have selected the combination of a high plasma TG and a low HDL-C concentration as diagnostic criteria, it is clear that these changes are also associated with a decrease in low-density lipoprotein (LDL) particle size (small, dense LDL) and the postprandial accumulation of TG-rich remnant lipoproteins (29). Not only are all of these changes

Table 2.4
Relationship Between Insulin Resistance and Plasma Triglyceride Concentration

---

A. Triglyceride concentration (69–546 mg/dL)*
IMGU $\rightarrow$ Insulin conc ($r = 0.74$) $\rightarrow$ VLDL-TG secretion rate ($r = 0.74$) $\rightarrow$ TG conc
($r = 0.88$)
B. Triglyceride concentration (33–174 mg/dL)**
IMGU $\rightarrow$ Insulin conc ($r = 0.81$) $\rightarrow$ VLDL-TG secretion rate ($r = 0.68$) $\rightarrow$ TG conc
($r = 0.87$)

---

*Based on data in ref. 28.
**Based on data in ref. 40.
IMGU = insulin-mediated glucose uptake as quantified by the insulin suppression test; VLDL = very low density lipoprotein; TG = triglyceride; conc = concentration.

significantly associated with insulin resistance/hyperinsulinemia (27–33), *each one* has been shown to increase the risk of CVD (34–39).

Plasma TG Concentration

The schema outlined in Table 2.4 is based on the results in two published studies (28,40). Table 2.4A depicts the relationship among insulin resistance, plasma insulin response, hepatic very-low-density (VLDL)–TG synthesis and secretion, and plasma TG concentrations in nondiabetic individuals (28) whose baseline plasma TG concentrations range from 69 to 546 mg/dL, whereas Table 2.4B describes the same relationships in individuals with plasma TG concentrations <175 mg/dL (40). These findings provide the experimental basis for the conclusion that the major cause of elevated plasma TG concentration in nondiabetic individuals is an increase in hepatic VLDL-TG secretion rate, secondary to insulin resistance and the resultant hyperinsulinemia.

Although there is widespread agreement as to the validity of the relationships (outlined above), controversy remains concerning the causal relationships among insulin resistance, compensatory hyperinsulinemia, hepatic VLDL-TG secretion, and plasma TG concentration. One view is that resistance to insulin regulation in muscle and adipose tissue leads to higher ambient levels of both insulin and FFA, and these two changes stimulate hepatic VLDL-TG secretion, leading to the increase in plasma TG concentration in insulin-resistant individuals (27,28,40,41). Alternatively, it is argued that hypertriglyceridemia occurs in insulin-resistant, nondiabetic individuals because the normal ability of insulin to inhibit hepatic VLDL-TG secretion is diminished (42). Irrespective of which of these alternatives is correct, there is no disagreement with the conclusion that hypertriglyceridemia is a characteristic finding in insulin-resistant individuals.

Postprandial Lipemia

The higher the fasting TG concentration, the greater will be the postprandial accumulation of TG-rich lipoproteins (VLDL, chylomicron remnants, and VLDL remnants) in nondiabetic individuals (43). In addition to the relationship between fasting TG concentration and postprandial lipemia, the daylong increase in TG-rich lipoproteins in nondiabetic individuals is significantly correlated with the magnitude of their insulin resistance/compensatory hyperinsulinemia (32,33,44). Although the postprandial elevation of TG-rich lipoproteins is related to the fasting TG concentration, it can also be demonstrated that postprandial lipemia is enhanced when insulin resistant/ hyperinsulinemic individuals are matched for degree of fasting hypertriglyceridemia with an insulin-sensitive population (45). These observations suggest that increases in postprandial lipemia are highly correlated to insulin resistance, directly by decreasing the removal from plasma of TG-rich lipoproteins by mechanisms not clearly defined, and indirectly by virtue of the role played by insulin resistance and compensatory hyperinsulinemia in stimulating hepatic VLDL-TG secretion and increasing fasting plasma TG concentration.

HDL CHOLESTEROL

Increases in plasma VLDL-TG concentration are usually associated with low HDL-C concentrations, and it appears that insulin resistance/compensatory hyperinsulinemia are independently associated with both of these changes (30). In part, this is likely due to the transfer, catalyzed by cholesteryl ester transfer protein, of cholesterol from HDL to VLDL (46); the higher the VLDL pool size, the greater the transfer rate from HDL to VLDL, and the lower the ensuing HDL-C concentration. There is also evidence that the fractional catabolic rate (FCR) of apoprotein A-I is increased in patients with primary hypertriglyceridemia (47), hypertension (48), and type 2 diabetes (49). In type 2 diabetes, it has been shown that the greater the degree of hyperinsulinemia, the lower the HDL-C concentration (49). It has also been demonstrated in nondiabetic individuals that the higher the apoprotein A-I FCR, the lower the HDL-C concentration (50), and that these changes are associated with increases in plasma insulin concentrations. Thus, it is likely that insulin resistance and hyperinsulinemia contribute to a low HDL-C concentration indirectly by being responsible for the increase in VLDL pool size, and directly by increasing the FCR of apoprotein A-I.

LDL PARTICLE DIAMETER

Analysis of LDL particle size distribution (35) has identified multiple distinct LDL subclasses, and it appears that LDL in most individuals can be characterized by either a predominance of larger LDL (diameter > 255 Å, pattern A) or of smaller LDL (<255 Å, pattern B). Individuals with pattern B have higher plasma TG and lower HDL-C concentrations. Not surprisingly, healthy volunteers with small, dense LDL particles (pattern B) are relatively insulin resistant, glucose intolerant, hyperinsulinemic, hypertensive, and hypertriglyceridemic, with decreases in HDL-C concentration (31).

ATHEROGENIC LIPOPROTEINS AND INSULIN RESISTANCE

In summary, the lipoprotein abnormalities that are part of all three definitions of the MetS are more likely to occur in insulin resistant/hyperinsulinemic individuals. However, not all individuals with these abnormalities are insulin resistant. A high fasting plasma TG concentration and hyperchylomicronemia can occur (9,43) in individuals who have a fundamental defect in the catabolism of TG-rich lipoproteins (fat-induced lipemia). Similarly, a low HDL-C concentration can exist as a familial defect in lipoprotein metabolism (51), independent of any change in insulin sensitivity. Furthermore, not all insulin-resistant individuals will develop the atherogenic lipoprotein profile associated with the defect in insulin action. On the other hand, if the question becomes what fundamental physiological abnormality can account for the atherogenic lipoprotein profile discussed above that occurs in combination with an elevated plasma glucose concentration and blood pressure, the sole contender is insulin resistance/hyperinsulinemia.

Blood Pressure

The blood pressure criteria suggested by the WHO for diagnosing the MetS have been lowered by both the ATP III and the IDF. However, since the objective basis of the values chosen by either organization is not clear, it is difficult to know which set of blood pressure criteria will be more useful. More importantly, the blood pressure link between insulin resistance on one hand, and CVD on the other, is more complicated than that of any of the criteria selected by the ATP III and the WHO. However, the following three sets of observations provide strong evidence linking insulin resistance/ hyperinsulinemia to essential hypertension. First, patients with essential hypertension, as a group, are insulin resistant and hyperinsulinemic (52–54). Second, normotensive first-degree relatives of patients with essential hypertension are relatively insulin resistant and hyperinsulinemic as compared to a matched control group without a family history of hypertension (55–57). Finally, hyperinsulinemia, as a surrogate estimate of insulin resistance, has been shown in population-based studies to predict the eventual development of essential hypertension (58–61). These data provide substantial support that insulin resistance/hyperinsulinemia plays a role in the pathogenesis of essential hypertension.

On the other hand, since probably no more than 50% of patients with essential hypertension are insulin resistant (62), it is obvious that patients can have an elevated blood pressure and not be insulin resistant/hyperinsulinemic. However, although only approximately half the patients with essential hypertension are likely to be insulin resistant/hyperinsulinemic, this subset has the other components of the various definitions of the MetS that render them at greatest CVD risk. For example, patients with essential hypertension and electrocardiographic evidence of myocardial ischemia are insulin resistant, somewhat glucose intolerant, and hyperinsulinemic, with a high TG and low HDL-C as compared to either a normotensive control group or patients with essential hypertension whose electrocardiograms are entirely normal (63). The link between the dyslipidemia present in insulin resistant/hyperinsulinemic patients with essential hypertension and CVD is consistent with findings from the Copenhagen Male Study (64), in which 2,906 participants were divided into three groups based on their fasting plasma TG and HDL-C concentrations. Men whose plasma TG and HDL-C concentrations were in the upper third or lower third, respectively, of the whole population, were assigned to the high TG–low HDL-C group, whereas a low TG–high HDL-C group was composed of those individuals whose plasma TG and HDL-C concentrations were in the lower third and upper third, respectively, of the study population for these two lipid measurements. The intermediate group consisted of those participants whose lipid values did not qualify them for either of the two extreme groups. The results of this prospective study indicated that CVD risk was not increased in patients with hypertension in the absence of a high TG and low HDL-C, and that the group at greatest risk was those with a high blood pressure and a high TG and low HDL-C.

In summary, (1) insulin resistant/hyperinsulinemic individuals are more likely to develop essential hypertension; (2) hypertension is a well-recognized CVD risk factor; and (3) patients with essential hypertension *and* a high TG and a low HDL-C are at greatest CVD risk. Patients with essential hypertension are more likely to be insulin resistant/hyperinsulinemic with a high TG and low HDL-C concentration than they are to have type 2 diabetes, IGT, or IFG. Since clinicians will not be performing clamp studies, a dyslipidemic patient with essential hypertension frequently may not qualify for the metabolic syndrome by WHO criteria. Fortunately, failure to accomplish the goal for which these criteria were introduced (i.e., identifying insulin-resistant individuals at greatest CVD risk) should not prevent any thoughtful clinician from treating both the elevated blood pressure and the accompanying dyslipidemia in an effective manner.

Insulin Resistance and Procoagulant and Proinflammatory Factors

All three definitions of the MetS comment on the fact that the cluster of components that make up the diagnostic category are also associated with a procoagulant and/or proinflammatory state. Although measures of the latter changes have not been elevated to become diagnostic criteria, there is no doubt that both of these changes are closely associated with insulin resistance. The association between insulin resistance/hyperinsulinemia, elevated concentrations of plasminogen activator inhibitor-1 (PAI-1), and CVD have been known for some time (65–67). Of greater relevance to this review are the data in Table 2.5 showing that PAI-1 concentration in a group of apparently healthy individuals was significantly correlated with the degree of insulin resistance (as quantified by SSPG concentration during the insulin suppression test), and fasting

Table 2.5
Simple and Partial Correlations Among PAI-1 and Other Relevant Variables in
Normotensive Volunteers

Variable	Simple Correlation		Partial Correlation	
	R	P	R	p
Age (years)	−0.42	0.02	—	—
BMI (kg/m≤)	0.39	0.03	—	—
Waist/hip (WHR)	0.15	0.49	−0.004	0.98
MAP (mmHg)	−0.06	0.77	−0.06	0.76
SSPG (mg/dL)	0.62	<0.001	0.56	<0.001
Fasting plasma insulin (μU/mL)	0.65	<0.001	0.58	<0.001
Triglyceride (mg/dL)	0.32	0.07	0.39	<0.05
HDL cholesterol (mg/dL)	−0.69	<0.001	−0.65	<0.001
LDL cholesterol (mg/dL)	0.22	0.23	0.29	0.13

Partial correlations were calculated after adjustment for age and BMI.

MAP = mean arterial pressure; WHR = waist to hip ratio; SSPG = the steady-state plasma glucose concentration (SSPG) during the last 30 min of a 180-min infusion of octreotide (0.27 μg/m^2/min), insulin (32 mU/m^2/min), and glucose (267 mg/m^2/min).

Since the steady-state plasma insulin concentrations are comparable in all individuals, and the glucose infusion rate is identical, the resultant SSPG concentration provides a direct measure of the ability of insulin to mediate the disposal of a given glucose load (i.e., the higher the SSPG, the more insulin resistant the individual).

Source: Reprinted from ref. 67 with permission of the journal and the authors.

plasma insulin, TG, and HDL-C concentrations (67). Thus, variations in PAI-1 concentrations cluster with insulin resistance/compensatory hyperinsulinemia, and the dyslipidemia characteristic of the defect in insulin action.

The proinflammatory factor currently attracting the most attention as indicating increased CVD risk is C-reactive protein (CRP), but there is a much longer history of a relationship between an increase in white blood count (WBC) and heart disease. Indeed, data from the Women's Health Initiative Observational Study suggest that a high WBC was comparable in magnitude as a predictor of CVD risk to increases in CRP concentration (68). Evidence published several years ago (69) of a relationship between WBC and insulin resistance/compensatory hyperinsulinemia indicated that the WBC in apparently healthy individuals was significantly correlated with degree of insulin resistance ($r = 0.50$, $p > 0.001$), the magnitude ($p < 0.001$) of the plasma glucose ($r = 0.48$) and insulin responses ($r = 0.50$) to an oral glucose challenge, and higher TG ($r = 0.37$) and lower HDL-C ($r = -0.38$) concentrations ($p > 0.005$).

These observations provide evidence that the additional CVD risk factors considered to be present in patients diagnosed as having the MetS are significantly related to both insulin resistance/hyperinsulinemia as well as the other components of the MetS. As such, they provide additional evidence indicating that insulin resistance/ hyperinsulinemia offers the only coherent explanation to account for how all of these individual variables cluster together in apparently healthy individuals, and increase the risk of CVD.

EXCESS ADIPOSITY, INSULIN RESISTANCE, CVD, AND THE METS

The use of an index of excess adiposity as a criterion with which to diagnose the MetS is qualitatively different from any of the other components listed in Tables 2.1–2.3. Dyslipidemia (a high TG and low HDL-C concentration), hyperglycemia, and hypertension are independent factors that directly increase risk of CVD (34,36,37,70,71). The relationship between excess adiposity and CVD risk is not the same. At the simplest level, there are substantial numbers of overweight/obese individuals who do not display the components used to make a diagnosis of the MetS (72,73). Being overweight/obese simply increases the probability that an individual will become glucose intolerant, dyslipidemic, and hypertensive, and the linchpin between excess adiposity and the remaining components of the various definitions of the MetS is largely a consequence of the adverse effect of being overweight/obese on insulin sensitivity (72–74). This point of view is consistent with the results of the recent study of Ninomiya et al. (75), showing that abdominal obesity, as defined by the ATP III, was the only one of their five variables not statistically associated with the development of either CVD or stroke in an analysis of the NHANES III data. The authors suggested that this finding "may reflect an indirect effect of high WC through other components of the syndrome." Consequently, this section will examine the relationship between excess adiposity, insulin resistance, and the diagnosis of the MetS.

Obesity and Insulin-Mediated Glucose Uptake (IMGU)

The most insightful study of the relationship between obesity and IMGU is the report from the European Group for the Study of Insulin Resistance (76). Based on the results of euglycemic, hyperinsulinemic clamp studies in 1,146 nondiabetic, normotensive volunteers, these investigators concluded that only ~25% of the obese volunteers were insulin resistant by the criteria they used. Parenthetically, these authors also pointed out that differences in WC were unrelated to insulin sensitivity after adjustments for age, gender, and BMI.

We have published results similar to those of the European Group for the Study of Insulin Resistance, finding that the differences in degree of obesity account for approximately one-third of the variability of IMGU in apparently healthy individuals (72,73). Furthermore, these estimates did not take into account that overweight individuals tend to be more sedentary, and the more physically fit an individual, the more insulin sensitive (77). Indeed, in a bi-ethnic study involving nondiabetic Pima Indians and individuals of European ancestry, it was shown that differences in degree of physical fitness are approximately as powerful as variations in adiposity in modulation of IMGU (78). Thus, the heavier an individual the more likely they are to be insulin resistant, but although differences in adiposity are an important modulator of insulin action, it is only *one* of the variables determining whether an individual is sufficiently insulin resistant to develop an adverse clinical outcome.

WC versus BMI as Predictors of IMGU

Measurements of BMI and WC in approximately 15,000 participants in the National Health and Nutrition Examination Survey (NHANES) indicated that the correlation coefficient between the two indexes of obesity was greater than 0.9 irrespective of the age, gender, and ethnicity of groups evaluated (79). Given this degree of correlation between BMI and WC, it is not immediately obvious why WC is considered to be a more useful index of metabolic abnormality associated with excess adiposity than is BMI. It is even less clear why it is considered to be the essential diagnostic criterion in the IDF version of the MetS (Table 2.3).

Figure 2.1 displays the results of a study in which IMGU was quantified with the Insulin Suppression Test (IST) in 208 apparently healthy individuals, and the relationship between these values and measurements of BMI and WC determined (80). The IST (12,13,16,22,28,30–32,40,44,53,54,56,63,67,69,72,73,77) is based on determining the steady-state plasma glucose (SSPG) and insulin (SSPI) concentrations during the last 30 minutes of a 180-minute infusion of octreotide (0.27 µg/m^2/min), insulin (32 mU/m^2/min), and glucose (267 mg/m^2/min). Since the SSPI concentrations are comparable in all individuals, and the glucose infusion rate is identical, the resultant SSPG concentration provides a direct measure of the ability of insulin to mediate the uptake of a given glucose load (IMGU); that is, the higher the SSPG, the more insulin resistant the individual. The results in men (upper two panels) and women (lower two panels) are shown separately. The fact that the correlation coefficient relationships (r-values) between the two indexes of obesity and the SSPG concentration are essentially identical was not surprising in light of the NHANES data (79). However, it was surprising, and of considerable interest, to find that the magnitude of the correlation between the two indexes of adiposity and the measure of IMGU was much greater in men (r-value ~0.7) than in women (r-value ~0.5). Consistent with the results of the NHANES study described above, BMI and WC were also highly correlated (r-value = 0.9). Since there is substantial evidence that the relationship between IMGU and overall obesity (BMI)

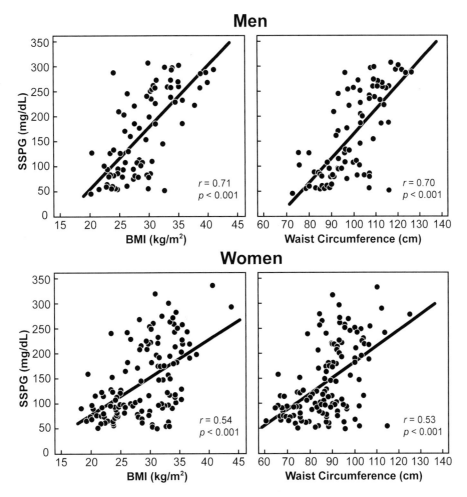

Figure 2.1. Relationship between degree of insulin resistance (SSPG concentration*) and BMI or waist circumference in 208 apparently healthy volunteers. (Reprinted from ref. 80 with permission of the journal and the authors.)

*SSPG = the steady-state plasma glucose concentration (SSPG) during the last 30 min of a 180-min infusion of octreotide ($0.27\ \mu g/m^2/min$), insulin ($32\ mU/m^2/min$), and glucose ($267\ mg/m^2/min$). Since the steady-state plasma insulin concentrations are comparable in all individuals, and the glucose infusion rate is identical, the resultant SSPG concentration provides a direct measure of the ability of insulin to mediate the disposal of a given glucose load (i.e., the higher the SSPG, the more insulin resistant the individual).

is no different from that between IMGU and abdominal obesity (WC), it seems that either index of adiposity is equally predictive of differences in insulin action.

Relationship Among Adiposity, Insulin Resistance, and CVD Risk

Rates of IMGU vary by more than sixfold in apparently healthy individuals, and the distribution of these values is continuous (81). Consequently, there is no objective way to select cut points that define individuals as being either insulin resistant or insulin sensitive. Obviously, this complicates any discussion of the relationship among excess

Table 2.6
Distribution of Body Mass Index (kg/m^2) According to Degree of Insulin Resistance
(number and percent)

BMI (kg/m^2)	Most Insulin-Sensitive Third	Intermediate Third	Most Insulin-Resistant Third
<25.0	109 (70%)	75 (48%)	24 (15%)
25.0–29.9	39 (25%)	54 (35%)	75 (48%)
30.0–34.9	7 (5%)	26 (17%)	56 (36%)
Total	155	155	155

Source: Reprinted from ref. 85 with permission of the journal and the authors.

adiposity, insulin resistance, and CVD. However, there are prospective studies that can serve as the basis for a more or less reasonable approach to address this issue. For example, if the magnitude of the insulin response to oral glucose is used as a surrogate marker of insulin resistance, 25% of an apparently healthy population with the highest insulin concentrations is at statistically significant increased risk to develop CVD (82). Based on the results of two studies in which the IST (a specific measure of IMGU) was used at baseline, the third of the population with the greatest defect in IMGU (the highest SSPG concentrations) was at significantly greater risk to develop CVD (83,84). Thus, for the purposes of this discussion, the third of the population at large with the highest SSPG concentrations will be operationally defined as being insulin resistant (IR), and those with SSPG concentrations in the lower third will be considered to be insulin sensitive (IS).

PREVALENCE OF INSULIN RESISTANCE AS A FUNCTION OF BMI

The results shown in Table 2.6 come from a study of 465 apparently healthy individuals, divided into tertiles of IMGU based on their BMI (85). Although the majority of normal-weight individuals (BMI < 25.0 kg/m^2) are in the most IS third (70%), 30% of the most IS individuals are either overweight/obese. Furthermore, approximately two-thirds of those in the IR third were either normal weight or overweight, and only approximately one-third of the most IR individuals were actually obese (BMI 30–35 kg/m^2). These data provide further evidence that, in general, the heavier the individuals, the more likely they are to be insulin resistant, but that obesity does not necessarily equal insulin resistance.

INTERACTION AMONG BMI, INSULIN ACTION, AND CVD RISK FACTORS

Figure 2.2 illustrates the results of applying the operational definitions of IR and IS to 314 healthy, nondiabetic individuals (72). Each panel displays the best-fit line describing the relationship among BMI and a series of CVD risk factors following the separation of the population into thirds on the basis of their SSPG concentration. Results in the two left panels indicate that the greater the BMI, the higher the total (upper left) and LDL-C (lower left) concentrations, but that these relationship do not vary as a function of degree of insulin resistance. In contrast, results in the middle panels of Figure 2.2 demonstrate that the relationship between BMI and plasma (upper middle) and HDL-C (lower middle) concentrations are quite different in IR as compared to IS

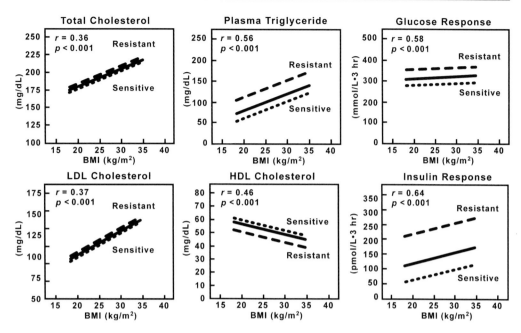

Figure 2.2. Relationship between BMI and SSPG* tertile and several cardiovascular disease risk factors. (Reprinted from ref. 72 with permission of the journal and the authors.)
*SSPG = the steady-state plasma glucose (SSPG) concentration during the last 30 min of a 180-min infusion of octreotide (0.27 μg/m²/min), insulin (32 mU/m²/min), and glucose (267 mg/m²/min). Since the steady-state plasma insulin concentrations are comparable in all individuals, and the glucose infusion rate is identical, the resultant SSPG concentration provides a direct measure of the ability of insulin to mediate the disposal of a given glucose load (i.e., the higher the SSPG, the more insulin resistant the individual).

individuals; at any given BMI, the plasma concentrations of TG are higher and HDL-C lower in IR as compared to IS individuals. Finally, the results in the right panels of Figure 2.2 highlight the untoward impact of being insulin resistant on the total integrated plasma glucose (upper right) and insulin (lower right) responses to a 75 g oral glucose challenge. In addition to documenting the enormous impact that being insulin resistant has on the plasma insulin response to oral glucose, the results in Figure 2.2 also emphasize that the plasma glucose response to oral glucose is relatively well maintained despite increasing degrees of both obesity and insulin resistance. These latter comparisons emphasize the extraordinary ability of compensatory hyperinsulinemia to prevent gross decompensation of glucose homeostasis in insulin-resistant individuals.

OBESITY DOES NOT NECESSARILY TRANSLATE INTO INCREASED CVD RISK

If insulin resistance/hyperinsulinemia increases CVD risk at any given BMI, and not all overweight/obese persons are insulin resistant, it seems clear that excess adiposity, per se, does not necessarily increase CVD risk. One way to look at this issue is to evaluate CVD risk factors in obese individuals selected to be either insulin resistant (IR) or insulin sensitive (IS) with the IST as defined above. The results in Figure 2.3 compare daylong glucose, insulin, and free fatty acid (FFA) concentrations in response to breakfast and lunch in 20 IR and 18 IS obese individuals, matched for age, gender, BMI, and WC (86). In addition to having daylong increase in plasma glucose, insulin,

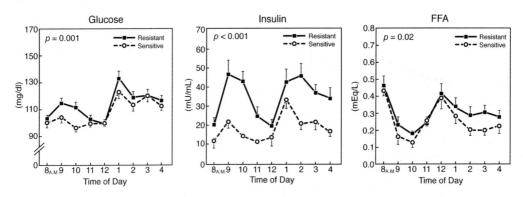

Figure 2.3. Comparison of daylong plasma glucose, insulin, and free fatty acid (FFA) concentrations in insulin-resistant and insulin-sensitive obese individuals. Test meals were consumed at 8 A.M. and noon, and blood drawn before and at hourly intervals after the meals. (Reprinted from ref. 86 with permission of the journal and the authors.)

and FFA concentrations, the C-reactive protein concentrations were also significantly higher in the IR subjects (0.39 ± 0.08 vs. 0.12 ± 0.03 mg/dL, $p < 0.005$).

WC IS NOT THE SAME AS VISCERAL OBESITY

Based on the experimental data summarized in the previous section, it can be concluded that measurements of BMI and WC are highly correlated, and associated with a specific measure of IMGU to an identical degree, and that CVD risk factors are increased primarily in those overweight/obese individuals who are also insulin resistant. It is apparent that this formulation is at odds with the views of the ATP III (1,2) and IDF (8) that abdominal obesity is the ultimate villain. A possible explanation for this discrepant view of the central role (pun intended) of abdominal obesity in the genesis of insulin resistance and its consequences is that measurements of WC provide only a surrogate estimate of visceral obesity, and it is visceral obesity that is responsible for the manifestations of the MetS that increase CVD.

Visceral Obesity and Insulin Resistance

Table 2.7 presents the results of 19 studies (22 comparisons) attempting to define the relative magnitude of the relationship between IMGU and various estimates of adiposity, including visceral obesity (VF), in nondiabetic subjects (87–105). The studies are listed in chronological order, and several inclusion criteria were used to construct the table. In the first place, imaging techniques had to be used to determine the magnitude of the various fat depots. Second, IMGU had to be quantified with specific methods, and studies using surrogate estimates were not included. In addition, the actual experimental data had to be available prior to the use of arbitrary "adjustments" or multiple regression analysis. For example, following an "adjustment" for the relationship between differences in total body fat and IMGU, it is not clear how much one learns from now discerning a relationship between IMGU and VF. Finally, the omission of any study that satisfied these two simple criteria was inadvertent, and no information was deliberately excluded. However, given the number of studies included, and the diversity in the experimental populations represented, it is unlikely that the inclusion of additional reports would substantially alter the interpretation of these data. It should also be realized that space constraints prohibit a thoughtful discussion of possible differences in the imaging techniques used in individual studies, and the same considerations apply to the specific methods used to quantify IMGU. Finally, given the diversity of the participants enrolled in these studies, as well as the differences in experimental techniques used, it will not be possible to discuss each one thoroughly. Instead, an effort will be made to draw the general conclusions that seem to be both consistent with the data and most relevant to the issue at hand.

First, perhaps the simplest conclusion to be drawn from the results in Table 2.7 is that correlation coefficients (r-values) between visceral fat (VF) and IMGU are usually less than 0.6 and certainly no greater than the r-value between IMGU and either BMI or WC seen in Figure 2.1. Indeed, r-values between IMGU and VF varied from 0.4 to 0.6 in 17 of the 22 measurements in Table 2.7, with differences in VF accounting for approximately 25% of the variability in IMGU in most instances.

Second, although the relationship between BMI and IMGU was analyzed in only four studies (89,97,101,103), the correlation coefficients were comparable in these instances to the values between VF and IMGU. More comparisons were made between the relationships of IMGU with VF as contrasted to total fat (TF), and it appears that either estimate of adiposity provided r-values of similar magnitude. If anything, the

Table 2.7
Correlation Coefficients (r-values) Between IMGU and Body Fat Distribution

Ref No.	Population	VF	SF	TF	BMI
87	39 men	−0.51	−0.62	−0.61	
88	60 subjects	−0.50	−0.50	−0.57	
89	26 OB subjects	−0.56		−0.54	−0.55
90	54 subjects	−0.52	−0.61	−0.58	
91	20 S. Asian men	−0.59	−0.54	−0.56	
92	47 men	−0.61	−0.53		
93	27 postM women	−0.39	−0.43	−0.30	
94	44 OB postM women	−0.40	−0.17		
95	68 Cau children	−0.59	−0.70	−0.68	
	51 AA children	−0.43	−0.47	−0.52	
96	55 postM women	−0.49	−0.43		
97	48 subjects	−0.58	−0.41		−0.52
98	24 subjects	−0.55	−0.47	−0.61	
99	89 Ob males	−0.41			
100	40 Ob preM women	−0.34	−0.06		
101	174 subjects	−0.69	−0.57		−0.63
102	32 Hispanic children	−0.44	−0.46	−0.46	
103	39 men	−0.71			−0.56
104	44 AA men	−0.57	−0.57		
	35 AA women	−0.50	−0.67		
105	11 Thai women	−0.60	−0.47	−0.38	
	11 Thai men	−0.54	−0.45	−0.80	

IMGU = measurement of insulin-mediated glucose uptake; OB = obese; postM = postmenopausal; Cau = Caucasian; AA = African American; preM = premenopausal.

relationship of TF with IMGU was somewhat greater in 8 of the 12 comparisons (87,88,90,95,98,102,105).

However, the emphasis in the studies listed in Table 2.7 was a comparison of the relationship between IMGU and subcutaneous abdominal fat (SF) with that between IMGU and VF. As before, the magnitude of the relationship with IMGU was reasonably comparable with either fat depot, but in this case there were two examples in which the values were quite discrepant (94,100). In both of these, the study population consisted of obese women, and whether this accounts for the somewhat discrepant results cannot be determined. On the other hand, in the remaining 17 available comparisons, the *r*-values between IMGU with VF or SF did not vary a great deal, being somewhat higher with VF 8 times (91,92,96–98,101,105), higher with SF 7 times (87,90,93,95,102,104), and identical on two occasions (88,104).

Given the information in Table 2.7, it is not easy to understand the basis for the conventional wisdom that visceral obesity has a uniquely adverse effect on IMGU. One of the explanations may be the widespread use of multiple regression analysis to decide which variable is an *independent* predictor of an outcome, in this case IMGU. Although this approach can provide useful information, it is well recognized that it presents problems when very closely related variables are entered into the model being used. Since all measures of adiposity are highly correlated, there is no clear biological significance of the results of a multivariate analysis indicating that only one of them is an independent predictor of IMGU. However, it is clear from the data in Table 2.7 that there is hardly overwhelming experimental support for the notion of a uniquely close relationship between VF and IMGU, in contrast to the relationship among IMGU and BMI, WC, SF, or TF. Indeed, this conclusion should not be too surprising in view of the results of a study showing that "independent of age and sex, the combination of BMI and WC explained a greater variance in nonabdominal, abdominal, subcutaneous and visceral fat than either BMI or WC alone" (106).

Visceral Fat and Adverse Clinical Outcomes

Although the data presented in Figure 2.2 and Table 2.7 do not identify a uniquely close relationship between either WC or VF and IMGU, measurements of abdominal obesity might still be the most effective way to identify individuals at increased risk of developing clinical syndromes related to insulin resistance. For example, many studies have been published emphasizing the relationship between abdominal obesity in general, or VF specifically, as predicting the development of the clinical syndromes related to insulin resistance (107–112). On the other hand, there are also publications that come to a somewhat different conclusion. For example, in Pima Indians, increases in visceral obesity did not correlate with decreases in IMGU (113), and BMI was the estimate of adiposity with the highest hazard ratio in the prediction of type 2 diabetes (114). Furthermore, adding WC to this study's model did not improve its predictive ability. In a prospective study of Mexican Americans (115), Haffner and colleagues reported somewhat similar results, illustrating that those individuals with the highest baseline plasma glucose and insulin values were most likely to develop type 2 diabetes, independently of differences in age, BMI, or central obesity. In addition, a prospective study in a predominantly Caucasian population concluded that "both overall and abdominal adiposity strongly and independently predict risk of type 2 diabetes" (116). It has also been shown in studies of several ethnic groups that BMI is more strongly associated with blood pressure than is abdominal obesity (117–119). Finally, the clustering of dyslipidemia, hyperuricemia, diabetes, and hypertension described in both whites and African Americans was most strongly related to insulin concentration, although the magnitude decreased when adjusted for differences in BMI and abdominal obesity (120). In this latter instance, it was concluded that all three variables (insulin concentration, abdominal girth, and BMI) contributed to the adverse consequences related to insulin resistance. Thus, although WC may be a powerful predictor of clinical outcomes linked to insulin resistance, there is also considerable evidence that overall obesity, as estimated by BMI, not only contributes to insulin resistance, but also increases the likelihood that an individual will develop the clinical syndromes associated with the defect in insulin action.

IS THERE CLINICAL UTILITY IN DIAGNOSING THE METS?

Although the specific approaches to diagnose the MetS vary from version to version (Tables 2.1–2.3), the components listed in each of them are remarkably similar in that they are significantly associated with insulin resistance and increased CVD risk. It also seems reasonable that the more of these abnormalities that exist in an individual, the greater will be the risk of CVD. On the other hand, once the values of these measurements are known, how much clinical benefit is there in knowing whether the number of arbitrary criteria exceeded qualifies an individual as having the MetS? It seems to me that the answer to this rhetorical question is "not much," and the following brief examples explain the basis of my view.

All three versions of the MetS include type 2 diabetes as one of the diagnostic criteria. It is well recognized that patients with type 2 diabetes are at increased risk of CVD, and, in addition to being hyperglycemic, are often dyslipidemic, hypertensive, with a procoagulant and proinflammatory state. Furthermore, there are clinical guidelines (121) outlining the appropriate treatment paradigms for patients with type 2 diabetes. Once this diagnosis is made, the clinical problem is how best to control the hyperglycemia appropriately and effectively address all remaining CVD risk factors, not deciding whether the MetS is present.

Rather than continue to describe a series of situations that question the clinical utility of diagnosing the MetS, it might be more informative to explore the clinical implications of *not* identifying patients at increased CVD risk who *do not* meet the requisite diagnostic criteria. Perhaps the simplest way to address this issue is to consider how the same individual is classified by the three versions of the MetS. The patient in question is a man, of European ancestry, with a WC of 93 cm, with an elevated blood pressure (145/95 mm/Hg), associated with a high TG (155 mg/dL) and a low HDL-C (30 mg/dL) concentration. However, since his fasting plasma glucose concentration is only 103 mg/dL, he does not meet the diagnostic criteria for the MetS by WHO criteria unless his physician is willing to perform either an oral glucose tolerance test or a euglycemic, hyperinsulinemic clamp study. Should the lack of a positive diagnosis of the MetS adversely affect the treatment plan for this patient? Would it make any substantive difference in the treatment if the patient's fasting plasma glucose concentration had been 111 mg/dL? Alternatively, what if a second physician is willing to measure the patient's glucose level 120 minutes after a 75 g oral glucose challenge, and it turns out to be 145 mg/dL. The patient would now have the MetS. Would this additional information make any substantive difference in the treatment program? I hope not! The patient has hypertension and the dyslipidemia characteristic of insulin resistance and there are well-established algorithms for treating both abnormalities. Parenthetically, approximately one-third of apparently healthy, insulin-resistant individuals have neither IFG nor IGT (122).

In contrast to the WHO version of the MetS, the patient described would meet ATP III criteria for this diagnosis, even if his fasting plasma glucose concentration was only 98 mg/dL. However, this would not be the case if his plasma TG concentration were 145 mg/dL, rather than 155 mg/dL. Is there any doubt that a hypertensive patient with a low HDL-C concentration is at increased CVD risk? Would use of ATP III criteria lead to a different treatment approach to a patient with hypertension and a low HDL-C concentration if his fasting plasma glucose and TG concentrations were 98 mg/dL and 145 mg/dL, as compared to 103 mg/dL and 155 mg/dL? If not, what is the clinical utility of making, or not making, this diagnosis?

Finally, since this patient did not meet the essential criterion of abdominal obesity (his WC was only 93 cm), he does not have the MetS by the IDF definition, and this is true despite the presence of hypertension (145/95 mmHg), a high TG (155 mg/dL) and low HDL-C (30 mg/dL) concentration, and IFG (103 mg/dL). Clearly, this proto-typical patient is at considerable increased CVD risk, despite not having the IDF version of the MetS. Would his clinical status be any different if he now satisfied the essential criterion of abdominal obesity (WC = 95 cm)? Clearly, neither the CVD risk nor the appropriate therapeutic approach has changed because the abdominal girth has increased by 2 cm!

The values of WC needed to diagnose the MetS shown in Table 2.3 are specific for "Europids," and the IDF indicates that these values should vary with ethnicity. The requirement of ethnic-specific criteria for abdominal obesity raises additional questions concerning the clinical utility of the IDF criteria. As defined by the IDF, a normotensive man of Japanese ancestry will have the MetS if he has a WC of 88 cm, and moderately increased fasting plasma concentrations of glucose (103 mg/dL) and TG (155 mg/dL). In contrast, a Chinese man with the same WC will not have the IDF version of the MetS, even if he is hypertensive (145/95 mmHg), frankly diabetic (fasting plasma glucose concentration = 150 mg/dL), with a plasma TG concentration of 220 mg/dL. Is there any doubt that the Chinese patient is at greater CVD risk, even though he does not have the IDF version of the MetS?

The examples discussed above were chosen purposefully to question the clinical utility of making a diagnosis of the MetS, irrespective of what organization's definition is used. It is obvious that it would be possible to continue almost indefinitely to describe clinical findings in individuals who had the MetS by one or another of the three versions whose CVD risk was less than persons who did not meet the diagnostic criteria. The point of this exercise is to emphasize that the specific components of the various defini-tions of the MetS are CVD risk factors, and should be recognized as such, but there is not a great deal to be gained by deciding whether any particular combination of them merits diagnosis of the MetS. This point of view is consistent with recent findings based on the Framingham database (123), in which the authors used the ATP III criteria for the MetS, and concluded that "clusters of 3 traits do not substantially increase risk for outcomes over risk associated with clusters of 2 traits." They further pointed out that these findings are "consistent with the hypothesis that even a modest degree of risk clustering reflects a global underlying insulin-resistant pathophysiology, and individual risk factors may contribute marginally to risk associated with the insulin-resistant phenotype."

CONCLUSION

The ability of insulin to simulate glucose disposal varies six- to eightfold in apparently healthy individuals (81). Approximately one-third of the most insulin-resistant of these individuals are at greatly increased risk to develop a number of abnormalities and clinical syndromes, only one of which is CVD (83,84). Approximately 50% of this extraordinary degree of variability in insulin action can be attributed to differences in degree of adiposity (25%) and level of physical fitness (25%), with the remaining 50% most likely related to genetic differences (78). Despite being composed of almost identical components, the three versions of the MetS differ profoundly in the philosophical basis underlying their approach to making a positive diagnosis. In this review, a number of issues have been raised that question the pedagogical utility of classifying an individual as having the MetS. Finally, it seems to me most reasonable to forget about making a clinical diagnosis of the MetS, irrespective of which version seems most appealing, and adhere to the following clinical advice from the joint report of the ADA and EASD (3):

• "Providers should avoid labeling patients with the term metabolic syndrome."
• "Adults with any major CVD risk factor should be evaluated for the presence of other CVD risk factors."
• "All CVD risk factors should be individually and aggressively treated."

If these goals are achieved, it will end (1) the need to make a diagnosis of the MetS; (2) the controversy over the best definition of the MetS; and (3) the confusion as to the clinical approach to patients who, although they are at increased CVD risk, do not qualify for a diagnosis of the MetS.

REFERENCES

1. Grundy SM, Cleeman JI, Daniels SR et al. Diagnosis and management of the metabolic syndrome: An American Heart Association/Heart, Lung, and Blood Institute Scientific Statement. *Circulation* 2005; 112:2735–2752.
2. Executive Summary of Third Report of the National Cholesterol Education Program (NCEP) Expert Panel on Detection, Evaluation, and Treatment of High Blood Cholesterol in Adults (Adult Treatment Panel III). *JAMA* 2001; 285:2486–2497.
3. Kahn R, Buse J, Ferrannini E, Stern M. The metabolic syndrome: Time for a critical appraisal. Joint statement from the American Diabetes Association and the European Association for the Study of Diabetes. *Diabetes Care* 2005; 28:2289–2304.
4. Kim SH, Reaven GM. The metabolic syndrome: One step forward, two steps back. *Diabetes Vasc Dis Res* 2004; 1:68–76.
5. Reaven G. The metabolic syndrome or the insulin resistance syndrome?: Different names, different concepts, and different goals. *Endocrinol Metab Clin North Am* 2004; 33:283–303.
6. Reaven GM. The metabolic syndrome: Requiescat in pace. *Clin Chem* 2005; 51:931–938.
7. Alberti KG, Zimmet PZ. Definition, diagnosis and classification of diabetes mellitus and its complications. Part 1: Diagnosis and classification of diabetes mellitus provisional report of a WHO consultation. *Diabet Med* 1998; 15:539–553.
8. The IDF consensus worldwide definition of the metabolic syndrome. Available at: www.idf.org. Part 1: Worldwide definition for use in clinical practice.

9. Ahrens EH Jr, Hirsch J, Oette K, Farquhar JW, Stein Y. Carbohydrate-induced and fat-induced lipemia. *Trans Med Soc Lond* 1961; 74:134–46.
10. Himsworth HP, Kerr RB. Insulin-sensitive and insulin-insensitive types of diabetes mellitus. *Clinical Science* 1939; 4:119–152.
11. Himsworth HP. The syndrome of diabetes mellitus and its causes. *Lancet* 1949; 1:465–473.
12. Shen S-W, Reaven GM, Farquhar JW. Comparison of impedance to insulin mediated glucose uptake in normal and diabetic subjects. *J Clin Invest* 1970; 49:2151–2160.
13. Ginsberg H, Kimmerling G, Olefsky JM, Reaven GM. Demonstration of insulin resistance in untreated adult onset diabetic subjects with fasting hyperglycemia. *J Clin Invest* 1975; 55:454–461.
14. DeFronzo R, Deibert D, Hendler R, Felig P, Soman V. Insulin sensitivity and insulin binding to monocytes in maturity-onset diabetes. *J Clin Invest* 1979; 63:939–946.
15. Kolterman OG, Gray RS et al. Receptor and postreceptor defects contribute to the insulin resistance in non-insulin-dependent diabetes mellitus. *J Clin Invest* 1981; 68:957–969.
16. Reaven GM. Insulin resistance in non-insulin-dependent diabetes mellitus: Does it exist and can it be measured? *Am J Med* 1983; 74:3–17.
17. Sicree RA, Zimmet PZ, King HOM, Coventry JS. Plasma insulin response among Nauruans: Prediction of deterioration in glucose tolerance over 6 yr. *Diabetes* 1987; 36:179–186.
18. Saad MF, Pettit DJ, Mott DM, Knowler WC, Nelson, RG, Bennett, PH. Sequential changes in serum insulin concentration during development of non-insulin-dependent diabetes. *Lancet* 1989; 1:1356–1359.
19. Haffner SM, Stern MP, Mitchell BD, Hazua HP, Patterson JK. Incidence of type II diabetes in Mexican Americans predicted by fasting insulin and glucose levels, obesity and body-fat distribution. *Diabetes* 1990; 39:283–288.
20. Warram JH, Martin BC, Krolewski AS, Soeldner JS, Kahn CR. Slow glucose removal rate and hyperinsulinemia precede the development of type II diabetes in the offspring of the diabetic parents. *Ann Intern Med* 1990; 113:909–912.
21. Lillioja S, Mott DM, Spraul M et al. Insulin resistance and insulin secretory dysfunction as precursors of non-insulin-dependent diabetes mellitus. *N Engl J Med* 1993; 329:1988–1992.
22. Reaven GM, Brand RJ, Chen Y-D, Mathur AK, Goldfine I. Insulin resistance and insulin secretion are determinants of oral glucose tolerance in normal individuals. *Diabetes* 1993; 42:1324–1332.
23. Zavaroni I, Dall'Aglio E, Bonora E, Alpi O, Passeri M, Reaven GM. Evidence that multiple risk factors for coronary artery disease exist in persons with abnormal glucose tolerance. *Am J Med* 1987; 83:609–612.
24. Reaven G. Role of insulin resistance in human disease. *Diabetes* 1988; 37:1595–1607.
25. Zavaroni I, Bonora E, Pagliara M et al. Risk factors for coronary artery disease in healthy persons with hyperinsulinemia and normal glucose tolerance. *N Engl J Med* 1989; 320:702–706.
26. Haffner SM, Stern MP, Hazuda HP, Mitchell BD, Patterson JK. Cardiovascular risk factors in confirmed prediabetic individuals: Does the clock for coronary heart disease start ticking before the onset of clinical diabetes? *JAMA* 1990; 263:2893–2898.
27. Reaven GM, Lerner RL, Stern MP et al. Role of insulin in endogenous hypertriglyceridemia. *J Clin Invest* 1967; 46:1756–1767.
28. Olefsky JM, Farquhar JW, Reaven GM. Reappraisal of the role of insulin in hypertriglyceridemia. *Am J Med* 1974; 57:551–560.
29. Reaven GM. The insulin resistance syndrome. *Curr Atheroscler Rep* 2003; 5:364–371.
30. Laws A, Reaven GM. Evidence for an independent relationship between insulin resistance and fasting plasma HDL-cholesterol, triglyceride and insulin concentrations. *J Int Med* 1992; 231:25–30.
31. Reaven GM, Chen Y-DI, Jeppesen J et al. Insulin resistance and hyperinsulinemia in individuals with small, dense, low density lipoprotein particles. *J Clin Invest* 1993; 92:141–146.
32. Jeppesen J, Hollenbeck CB, Zhou M-Y et al. Relation between insulin resistance, hyperinsulinemia, postheparin plasma lipoprotein lipase activity, and postprandial lipemia. *Arterioscler Thromb Vasc Biol* 1995; 15:320–324.
33. Abbasi F, McLaughlin T, Lamendola C et al. Fasting remnant lipoprotein cholesterol and triglyceride concentrations are elevated in nondiabetic, insulin-resistant, female volunteers. *J Clin Endocrinol Metab* 1999; 84:3903–3906.
34. Castelli WP, Doyle JT, Gordon T et al. HDL cholesterol and other lipids in coronary heart disease. *Circulation* 1977; 55:767–772.

35. Austin MA, Breslow JL, Hennekens CH et al. Low-density lipoprotein subclass patterns and risk of myocardial infarction. *JAMA* 1988; 260:1917–1921.
36. Manninen V, Tenkanen L, Koskinen P et al. Joint effects of serum triglyceride and LDL cholesterol and HDL cholesterol concentrations on coronary heart disease risk in the Helsinki heart study: Implications for treatment. *Circulation* 1992; 85:37–45.
37. Assmann G, Schulte H. Relation of high-density lipoprotein cholesterol and triglycerides to incidence of atherosclerotic coronary artery disease (the PROCAM experience). *Am J Cardiol* 1992; 70:733–737.
38. Patsch JR, Miesenbock G, Hopferwieser T et al. Relation of triglyceride metabolism and coronary artery disease: studies in the postprandial state. *Arterioscler Thromb* 1992; 12:1336–1345.
39. Karpe F, Bard JM, Steiner G et al. HDLs and alimentary lipemia: studies in men with previous myocardial infarction at young age. *Arterioscler Thromb* 1993; 13:11–22.
40. Tobey TA, Greenfield M, Kraemer F et al. Relationship between insulin resistance, insulin secretion, very low density lipoprotein kinetics, and plasma triglyceride levels in normotriglyceridemic man. *Metabolism* 1981; 30:165–171.
41. Reaven GM, Greenfield MS. Diabetic hypertriglyceridemia: Evidence for three clinical syndromes. *Diabetes* 1981; 30(suppl 2):66.
42. Lewis GF. Fatty acid regulation of very low density lipoprotein production. *Curr Opin Lipidol* 1997; 8:146–153.
43. Steiner G. Lipoprotein lipase in fat-induced hyperlipemia. *N Engl J Med* 1968; 279:70–74.
44. Kim, H-S, Abbasi F, Lamendola C, Mclaughlin, T, Reaven GM. Effect of insulin resistance on postprandial elevations of remnant lipoprotein concentrations in postmenopausal women. *Am J Clin Nut* 2001; 74:592–595.
45. Chen Y-DI, Swami S, Skowronski R et al. Differences in postprandial lipemia between patients with normal glucose tolerance and noninsulin-dependent diabetes mellitus. *J Clin Endocrinol Metab* 1993; 76:172–177.
46. Swenson TL. The role of the cholesteryl ester transfer protein in lipoprotein metabolism. *Diabetes Metab Rev* 1991; 7:139–153.
47. Fidge N, Nestel P, Toshitsugu I et al. Turnover of apoproteins A-I and A-II of high density lipoprotein and the relationship to other lipoproteins in normal and hyperlipidemic individuals. *Metabolism* 1980; 29:643–653.
48. Chen Y-DI, Sheu WH-H, Swislocki ALM et al. High density lipoprotein turnover in patients with hypertension. *Hypertension* 1991; 17:386–393.
49. Golay A, Zech L, Shi M-Z et al. High density lipoprotein (HDL) metabolism in noninsulin-dependent diabetes mellitus: Measurement of HDL turnover using tritiated HDL. *J Clin Endocrinol Metab* 1987; 65:512–518.
50. Brinton EA, Eisenberg S, Breslow JL. Human HDL cholesterol levels are determined by apoA-I fractional catabolic rate, which correlates inversely with estimates of HDL particle size: Effects of gender, hepatic and lipoprotein lipases, triglyceride and insulin levels and body fat distribution. *Arterioscler Thromb* 1994; 14:707–720.
51. Frohlich J, Westerlund J, Sparkd D, Pritchard PH. Familial hypoalphalipoproteinemias. *Clin Invest Med* 1990; 13:202–210.
52. Ferrannini E, Buzzigoli G, Bonadona R. Insulin resistance in essential hypertension. *N Engl J Med* 1987; 317:350–357.
53. Shen D-C, Shieh S-M, Fuh M, Wu D-A, Chen Y-DI, Reaven GM. Resistance to insulin-stimulated glucose uptake in patients with hypertension. *J Clin Endocrinol Metab* 1988; 66:580–583.
54. Swislocki ALM, Hoffman BB, Reaven GM. Insulin resistance, glucose intolerance and hyperinsulinemia in patients with hypertension. *Am J Hypertens* 1989; 2:419–423.
55. Ferrari P, Weidmann P, Shaw S et al. Altered insulin sensitivity, hyperinsulinemia and dyslipidemia in individuals with a hypertensive parent. *Am J Med* 1991; 91:589–596.
56. Facchini F, Chen Y-DI, Clinkingbeard C, Jeppesen J, Reaven GM. Insulin resistance, hyperinsulinemia, and dyslipidemia in nonobese individuals with a family history of hypertension. *Am J Hypertens* 1992; 5:694–699.
57. Allemann Y, Horber FF, Colombo M et al. Insulin sensitivity and body fat distribution in normotensive offspring of hypertensive parents. *Lancet* 1993; 341:327–331.
58. Skarfors ET, Lithell HO, Selinus I. Risk factors for the development of hypertension: A 10-year longitudinal study in middle-aged men. *J Hypertension* 1991; 9:217–223.

59. Lissner L, Bengtsson C, Lapidus L, Kristjansson K, Wedel H. Fasting insulin in relation to subsequent blood pressure changes and hypertension in women. *Hypertension* 1992; 20:797–801.
60. Taittonen L, Uhari M, Nuutinen M, Turtinen J, Pokka T, Akerblom HK. Insulin and blood pressure among healthy children. *Am J Hypertens* 1996; 9:193–199.
61. Raitakari OT, Porkka KVK, Rönnemaa T et al. The role of insulin in clustering of serum lipids and blood pressure in children and adolescents. *Diabetologia* 1995; 38:1042–1050.
62. Zavaroni I, Mazza S, Dall'Aglio E, Gasparini P, Passeri M, Reaven GM. Prevalence of hyperinsulinaemia in patients with high blood pressure. *J Intern Med* 1992; 231:235–240.
63. Sheuh WH-H, Jeng C-Y, Shieh S-M et al. Insulin resistance and abnormal electrocardiograms in patients with high blood pressure. *Am J Hypertens* 1992; 5:444–448.
64. Jeppesen J, Hein HO, Suadicani P, Gynterberg F. Low triglycerides-high high-density lipoprotein cholesterol and risk of ischemic heart disease. *Arch Int Med* 2001; 16(3):361–366.
65. Hamsten A, Wiman B, Defaire U, Blomback M. Increased plasma level of a rapid inhibitor of tissue plasminogen activator in young survivors of myocardial infarction. *N Engl J Med* 1985; 313:1557–1563.
66. Juhan-Vague I, Alessi MC, Vague P. Increased plasma plasminogen activator inhibitor 1 levels: A possible link between insulin resistance and atherothrombosis. *Diabetologia* 1991; 34(7):457–462.
67. Abbasi F, McLaughlin T, Lamendola C, Lipinska I, Tofler G, Reaven GM. Comparison of plasminogen activator inhibitor-1 concentration in insulin-resistant versus insulin-sensitive healthy women. *Arterioscler Thromb Vasc Biol* 1999; 19:2818–2821.
68. Margolis KL, Manson JF, Greenland P et al. Leukocyte count as a predictor of cardiovascular events and mortality in postmenopausal women: The Women's Health Initiative Observational Study. *Arch Int Med* 2005; 165:500–508.
69. Facchinii F, Hollenbeck CB, Chen YN, Chen Y-DI, Reaven GM. Demonstration of a relationship between white blood cell count, insulin resistance, and several risk factors for coronary heart disease in women. *J Int Med* 1992; 232:267–272.
70. The Seventh Report of the Joint National Committee on Prevention, Detection, Evaluation, and Treatment of High Blood Pressure: The JNC report. *JAMA* 2003; 289:2560–2572.
71. Pyörälä K. Relationship of glucose tolerance and plasma insulin to the incidence of coronary heart disease: Results from two population studies in Finland. *Diabetes Care* 1979; 2:131–141.
72. Abbasi F, Brown BWB, Lamendola C, McLaughlin T, Reaven GM. Relationship between obesity, insulin resistance, and coronary heart disease. *J Amer Coll Card* 2002; 40:937–943.
73. McLaughlin T, Abbasi F, Cheal K, Chu J, Lamendola C, Reaven GM. Use of metabolic markers to identify overweight individuals who are insulin resistant. *Ann Intern Med* 2003; 139:802–809.
74. Reaven GM. All obese individuals are not created equal: Insulin resistance is the major determinant of cardiovascular disease in overweight/obese individuals. *Diabetes Vasc Dis Res* 2005; 2:105–112.
75. Ninomiya JK, L'Italien G, Criqui MH, Whyte JL, Gamst A, Chen R. Association of the metabolic syndrome with history of myocardial infarction and stroke in the Third National Health and Nutrition Examination Survey. *Circulation* 2004; 109:42–46.
76. Ferrannini E, Natali A, Bell P, Cavallo-Perin, Lalic N, Mingrone G. Insulin resistance and hypersecretion in obesity. *J Clin Invest* 1997; 100:1166–1173.
77. Rosenthal M, Haskell WL, Solomon R, Widstrom A, and Reaven GM. Demonstration of a relationship between level of physical training and insulin-stimulated glucose utilization in normal humans. *Diabetes* 1983; 32:408–411.
78. Bogardus C, Lillioja S, Mott DM, Hollenbeck C, Reaven GM. Relationship between degree of obesity and *in vivo* insulin action in man. *Am J Physiol* 1985; (Endocrinol Metab 11) 248:E286–E291.
79. Ford ES, Mokdad AH, Giles WH. Trends in waist circumference among U.S. adults. *Obesity Research* 2003; 11:1223–1231.
80. Farin HMF, Abbasi F, Reaven GM. Body mass index and waist circumference correlate to the same degree with insulin-mediated glucose uptake. *Metabolsim* 2005; 54:1323–1328.
81. Yeni-Komshian H, Carantoni M, Abbasi F, Reaven, GM. Relationship.between several surrogate estimates of insulin resistance and quantification of insulin-mediated glucose disposal in 490 healthy, nondiabetic volunteers. *Diabetes Care* 2000; 23:71–175.
82. Zavaroni I, Bonini L, Gasparini P et al. Hyperinsulinemia in a normal population as a predictor of non-insulin-dependent diabetes mellitus, hypertension, and coronary heart disease: The Barilla factory revisited. *Metabolism* 1999; 48:989–994.

83. Yip J, Facchini FS, Reaven GM. Resistance to insulin-mediated glucose disposal as a predictor of cardiovascular disease. *J Clin Endocrinol Metab* 1998; 83:2773–2776.

84. Facchini FS, Hua N, Abbasi F, Reaven GM. Insulin resistance as a predictor of age-related diseases. *J Clin Endocrinol Metab* 2001; 86:3574–3578.

85. McLaughlin T, Allison G, Abbasi F, Lamendola C, Reaven G. Prevalence of insulin resistance and associated cardiovascular disease risk factors among normal weight, overweight, and obese individuals. *Metabolism* 2004; 53:495–499.

86. McLaughlin T, Abbasi F, Lamendola C et al. Differentiation between obesity and insulin resistance in the association with C-reactive protein. *Circulation* 2002; 106:2908–2912.

87. Abate N, Garg A, Peshock RM, Stray-Gunderson J, Grundy S. Relationships of generalized and regional adiposity to insulin sensitivity in man. *J Clin Invest* 1995; 96:88–98.

88. Cefalu WT, Wang ZQ, Werbgel S et al. Contribution of visceral fat to the insulin resistance of aging. *Metabolism* 1995; 44:954–959.

89. Macor C, Ruggeri A, Mazzonetto P, Federspil G, Cobelli C, Veiiot R. Visceral adipose tissue impairs insulin secretion and sensitivity, but not energy expenditure in obesity. *Metabolism* 1997; 46:123–129.

90. Goodpaster BH, Thaete JA, Simoneau JA, Kelley DE. Subcutaneous abdominal fat and thigh muscle composition predict insulin sensitivity independently of visceral fat. *Diabetes* 1997; 46:1579–1585.

91. Banerji MA, Faridi N, Atluri R, Chaiken RL, Lebovitz HE. Body composition, visceral fat, leptin and insulin resistance in Asian Indian Men. *J Clin Endocrinol Metab* 1999; 84:137–144.

92. Kelley DE, Thaete FL. Troost F, Huwe T, Goodpaster BH. Subdivisions of subcutaneous abdominal tissue and insulin resistance. *Am J Physiol Endocrinol Metab* 2000; 278:E941–E948.

93. Sites CK, Calles-Escandon J, Brochu M, Butterfield M, Ashikaga T, Poehlman ET. Relation of regional fat distribution to insulin sensitivity in postmenopausal women. *Fertil Sterl* 2000; 73:61–65.

94. Brochu M, Starling RD, Tchernof A, Mathews DE, Garcia-Rubi E, Poehlman ET. Visceral adipose tissue is an independent correlate of glucose disposal in older postmenopausal women. *J Clin Endocrinol Metab* 2001; 85:2378–2384.

95. Goran M, Bergman RN, Gower BA. Influence of total vs. visceral fat on insulin action and secretion in African American and white children. *Obes Res* 2001; 9(8):423–431.

96. Rendell M, Hulthen UL, Tornquist C, Groop L, Mattiason I. Relationship between abdominal fat compartments and glucose and lipid metabolism in early postmenopausal women. *J Clin Endocrinol Metab* 2001; 86:744–749.

97. Purnell JQ, Kahn SE, Schwartz RS, and Brunzell JD. Relationship of insulin sensitivity and apoB levels to intra-abdominal fat in subjects with combined hyperlipidemia. *Arterioscler Thromb Vasc Biol* 2001; 21:567–572.

98. Raji A, Seeley EW, Arky RA, Simonson DC. Body fat distribution and insulin resistance in healthy Asian Indians and Caucasians. *J Clin Endocrinol Metab* 2001; 86:5366–5371.

99. Ross R, Aru J, Freman J, Hudson R, Janssen I. Abdominal obesity and insulin resistance in obese men. *Am J Physiol Endocrinol Metab* 2002; 282:E657–E663.

100. Ross R, Freeman J, Hudson R, Janssen I. Abdominal obesity, muscle composition and insulin resistant in premenopausal women. *J Clin Endocrinol Metab* 2002; 87:5044–5051.

101. Cnop M, Landchild MJ, Vidal J et al. The concurrent accumulation of intra-abdominal and subcutaneous fat explains the association between insulin resistance and plasma leptin concentrations. *Diabetes* 2002; 51:1005–1015.

102. Cruz ML, Bergman RN, Goran MI. Unique effect of visceral fat on insulin sensitivity in obese Hispanic children with a family history of type 2 diabetes. *Diabetes Care* 2002; 25:1631–1636.

103. Gan SK, Krikeos AD, Poynten AM et al. Insulin action, regional fat, and myocyte lipid: Altered relationships with increased adiposity. *Obes Res* 2003; 11:1295–1305.

104. Tulloch-Reid MK, Hanson RL, Sebring NG et al. Both subcutaneous and visceral adipose tissues correlate highly with insulin resistance in African Americans. *Obes Res* 2004; 12(8):1352–1359.

105. Rattarasarn C, Leelawattan R, Soonthornpun S, Setasuban W, Thamprasit A. Gender differences of regional abdominal fat distribution and their relationships with insulin sensitivity in healthy and glucose-intolerant Thais. *J Clin Endocrinol Metab* 2004; 89:6266–6270.

106. Janssen I, Heymsfield SB, Allison DB, Kotler DP, Ross R. Body mass index and waist circumference independently contribute to the prediction of nonabdominal, abdominal, subcutaneous, and visceral fat. *Am J Clin Nutr* 2002; 75:683–688.

107. Kissebah AH, Vydelingum N, Murray R et al. Relation of body fat distribution to metabolic compli-
     cations of obesity. *J Clin Endocrinol Metab* 1982; 54:254–260.
108. Sparrow D, Borkan GA, Gerzof SG, Wisniewski C, Silbert CK. Relationship of fat distribution to
     glucose tolerance: Results of computed tomography in male participants of the Normative Aging
     Study. *Diabetes* 1986; 35:411–415.
109. Bjorntorp P. Adipose distribution, plasma insulin, and cardiovascular disease. *Diabete Metab* 1987;
     13:381–385.
110. Despres JP, Nadeau A, Tremblay A, Ferland M, Lupien PJ. Role of deep abdominal fat in the asso-
     ciation between regional adipose tissue distribution and glucose tolerance in obese women. *Diabetes*
     1989; 38:304–309.
111. Pouliot MC, Despres JP, Nadeau A et al. Visceral obesity in men: Associations with glucose toler-
     ance, plasma insulin, and lipoprotein levels. *Diabetes* 1992; 41:826–834.
112. Kissebah AH, Krakower GR. Regional adiposity and morbidity. *Physiological Reviews* 1994;
     74:761–811.
113. Gautier JF, Milner MR, Elam E, Chen K, Ravussin E, Pratley RE. Visceral adipose tissue is not
     increased in Pima Indians compared with equally obese Caucasians and is not related to insulin action
     or secretion. *Diabetologia* 1999; 42:28–34.
114. Tulloch-Reid MK, Williams DE, Looker HC, Hanson RL, Knowler WC. Do measures of body fat
     distribution provide information on the risk of type 2 diabetes in addition to measures of general
     obesity? *Diabetes Care* 2003; 26:2556–2561.
115. Haffner SM, Stern MP, Mitchell BD, Hazuda HP, Patterson JK. Incidence of type II diabetes in
     Mexican Americans predicted by fasting insulin and glucose levels, obesity, and body fat distribution.
     Diabetes 1990; 39:283–299.
116. Wang Y, Rimm EB, Stampfer MJ, Willett WC, Hu FB. Comparison of abdominal adiposity and
     overall obesity in predicting risk of type 2 diabetes among men. *Am J Clin Nutr* 2005; 81:555–
     563.
117. Seidell JC, Cigolini M, Deslypere JP, Charzewska J, Ellsinger BM, Cruz A. Body fat distribution in
     relation to serum lipids and blood pressure in 38-year-old European men: The European fat distribu-
     tion study. *Atherosclerosis* 1991; 86:251–260.
118. Folsom AR, Li Y, Pao X et al. Body mass, fat distribution and cardiovascular risk factors in a lean
     population of south China. *J Clin Epidemiol* 1994; 47:173–181.
119. Sakurai Y, Kono S, Shinchi K et al. Relation of waist-hip ratio to glucose tolerance, blood pressure,
     and serum lipids in middle-aged Japanese males. *Int J Obes* 1995; 19:632–637.
120. Schmidt MI, Duncan BB, Watson RL, Sharrett AR, Brancati FL, Heiss G. A metabolic syndrome in
     whites and African-Americans. *Diabetes Care* 1996; 19:414–418.
121. Standards of medical care in diabetes. *Diabetes Care* 2004; 27(suppl 1):S15–35.
122. Tuan C-Y, Abbasi F, Lamendola C, McLaughlin T, Reaven G. Usefulness of plasma glucose and
     insulin concentrations in identifying patients with insulin resistance. *Am J Cardiol* 2003;
     92:606–610.
123. Wilson PWF, D'Agostino RB, Parise H, Sullivan L, Meigs JB. The metabolic syndrome as a precur-
     sor of cardiovascular disease and type 2 diabetes. *Circulation* 2005; 112:3066–3072.

3

The Role of Obesity in Insulin Resistance
Epidemiological and Metabolic Aspects

James B. Meigs

CONTENTS

OVERVIEW
METABOLIC SYNDROME AND OBESITY
THE ROLE OF OBESITY IN RISK FACTOR CLUSTERING AND
   METABOLIC SYNDROME
MECHANISMS FOR RISK FACTOR CLUSTERING ASSOCIATED
   WITH OBESITY
TREATMENT OPTIONS TO REDUCE RISK FACTOR CLUSTERING
   ASSOCIATED WITH OBESITY
CONCLUSIONS

OVERVIEW

Obesity is a rapidly growing health problem in the United States. In 2000, about 20% of U.S. adults self-reported a body mass index (BMI) exceeding 30 kg/m^2, a 61% increase in obesity since 1991 (1). This underestimates the real prevalence when body mass index is determined from direct measurements rather than self-report. More than half (56%) reported being at least overweight (BMI ≥ 25 kg/m^2), up from 45% in 1991. Lifetime risk for overweight during the 1990s was approximately 50% for overweight and 25% for obesity in a representative U.S. sample (2). Obesity confers substantial excess risk for morbidity and mortality from a variety of associated conditions, especially type 2 diabetes and atherosclerotic cardiovascular disease (CVD) (3–5). Although overall body fatness, as measured by BMI, is clearly associated with mortality and complications of obesity (6), fat distribution, especially central fatness as measured by

Dr. Meigs is supported by an American Diabetes Association Career Development Award, has received research support from Aventis-Sanofi, Glaxo-Smith-Kline, Novartis, Pfizer, and Wyeth, and has served on safety monitoring or advisory boards for GSK, Lilly, Pfizer, and Merck.

From: *Contemporary Endocrinology: The Metabolic Syndrome: Epidemiology, Clinical Treatment, and Underlying Mechanisms*
Edited by: B.C. Hansen and G.A. Bray © Humana Press, Totowa, NJ

a large waist circumference, may be a more powerful correlate of risk associated with obesity, especially for type 2 diabetes and CVD (7–9).

Obesity confers metabolic risk at least in part through its association with common diabetes and CVD risk factors, including hyperglycemia, hypertension, and dyslipidemia characterized by low levels of HDL cholesterol and elevated levels of triglycerides. This clustering of metabolic risk factors has been called the *metabolic syndrome* (10). Obesity is also strongly associated with tissue resistance to effects of insulin (11). Insulin resistance in turn is a key risk factor for development of diabetes and may also be an independent risk factor for CVD (12–15; see also Chapter 5 in this volume). Despite their observed association, until recently the mechanisms linking obesity with risk factor clustering and insulin resistance have remained obscure. Recent data linking excess adiposity with abnormal fatty acid flux and secretion of inflammatory mediators and novel adipocyte-derived hormones (adipokines) point to mechanisms whereby obesity causes or contributes systemic metabolic risk. In this chapter, we will review the concept of risk factor clustering and its association with obesity; the roles of free fatty acids, inflammatory mediators, adipokines, and endothelial dysfunction in obesity-related insulin resistance; and provide an overview of treatment strategies to reduce metabolic risk associated with obesity.

METABOLIC SYNDROME AND OBESITY

Metabolic syndrome refers to the phenomenon of risk factor clustering—an aggregation of metabolic traits occurring in the same individual with frequencies greater than expected by chance, and presumably reflecting a unifying underlying pathophysiology. Traits that cluster include elevated glucose, triglyceride and blood pressure levels, and/or low HDL cholesterol levels. Clustering most commonly occurs in the setting of obesity (particularly central obesity) as well as a sedentary lifestyle (16).

It has long been recognized that type 2 diabetes and cardiovascular disease (CVD) share many risk factors in common, and that their co-occurrence is probably linked to insulin resistance and obesity (12,17). The concept of trait clustering and shared risk for type 2 diabetes and CVD has been codified into formal criteria for metabolic syndrome. As of 2005, there are five different proposed criteria for metabolic syndrome (10,18–21). The most commonly used definition is that of the National Cholesterol Education Program's Third Adult Treatment Panel (ATP3), where a person is affected if he or she has any three or more of the following five traits: fasting plasma glucose (FPG) $\geq$5.6 mmol/l; waist circumference >102 cm (in men) or >88 cm (in women); fasting triglycerides $\geq$1.7 mmol/l; HDL-C < 1.0 mmol/l (in men) or <1.16 mmol/l (in women); or treatment for lipid disorders, or blood pressure $\geq$130/85 mmHg (or treatment for hypertension) (10). In this chapter, the term *metabolic syndrome* refers to the ATP3 criteria unless otherwise specified.

The metabolic syndrome is common, thought to affect about 25% of U.S. adults aged 20–79 (22). The prevalence of metabolic syndrome is also highly correlated with increasing fatness. In U.S. national survey data, the prevalence of metabolic syndrome increased in a graded fashion from 0.9–3.0% at BMI 18.5–20.9 kg/m^2 to 9.6–22.5% at BMI 25.0–26.9 kg/m^2, such that even upper normal-weight and slightly overweight people had a relatively high prevalence of risk factor clustering (23). Metabolic syndrome is also increasingly common. For instance, in the community-based Framingham

Study, the prevalence of the ATP3 metabolic syndrome in the early 1990s was 13–21% in women and men aged an average of 50 years; later in the 1990s, the prevalence was 24-34% (24). In national survey data, the prevalence of metabolic syndrome has increased about 15% from the early 1990s to the late 1990s, but the cross-sectional design of this analysis probably underestimates the true change in prevalence over time (25).

THE ROLE OF OBESITY IN RISK FACTOR CLUSTERING AND METABOLIC SYNDROME

The major traits of the metabolic syndrome are themselves quite common (especially obesity, measured either as an elevated BMI or a large waist circumference), and could co-occur in some subjects independent of any underlying unifying physiology (26). However, population studies have shown that clusters of two or three or more of obesity, central obesity, hyperglycemia, elevated triglyceride or low HDL cholesterol levels, or hypertension occur from 2- to over 1,000-fold more commonly than would be expected by chance alone (16,27,28). For instance, in the Framingham Offspring Study, clusters of three or more abnormally elevated metabolic traits occurred at twice the rate that would be expected if they co-occurred by chance alone (16). These studies provide strong statistical evidence for risk factor clustering. Clustering appears to be a real phenomenon. The next question is: What underlies clustering?

In many studies, baseline obesity (either high BMI or large waist circumference) and weight gain were major contributors to risk factor clustering. For instance, in the Framingham Study, weight gain of 2.25 kg over 16 years of observation, adjusted for age and baseline BMI, was associated with a significant 19% (men) to 37% (women) increase in risk factor clustering (16). Conversely, weight loss of 2.25 kg was associated with a 4–46% ($p < 0.001$) decrease in risk factor clustering.

In the Atherosclerosis Risk in Communities (ARIC) study, obesity was a stronger risk factor for the occurrence of clusters of risk factors than for the occurrence of isolated disorders (29). In this analysis, 12,340 Insulin Resistance Atherosclerosis Study (ARIC) subjects were followed three years for development of none to any of three occurrences of diabetes, hypertension, or dyslipidemia. Baseline elevated BMI or large waist–hip ratio (WHR) increased the relative risk for single disorders by 1.4- to 1.6-fold and the risk for two or more disorders by 2.6- to 3.3-fold; the relative risk for two or more versus single disorders was 1.8 (WHR) to 2.2 (BMI), suggesting that obesity is twice as likely to lead to risk factor clusters as to isolated metabolic disorders. In ARIC, fasting hyperinsulinemia also increased risk for isolated disorders by 1.4-fold and for two or more disorders by 3-fold. Although fasting hyperinsulinemia and insulin resistance are highly correlated with increasing obesity (11), in ARIC the association of fasting hyperinsulinemia with risk factor clustering was independent and additive to that of obesity. For instance, fasting hyperinsulinemia and a high BMI increased risk for isolated disorders by 2.1-fold and for two or more disorders by 5.3-fold. Large waist circumference and fasting hyperinsulinemia also showed a similar additive risk effect. These data suggest that both obesity and insulin resistance are independent determinants of risk factor clustering.

Fat distribution may be at least as important as overall fatness in determining risk factor clustering. Many studies use waist circumference as an index of central fatness.

In the IRAS study, a large waist circumference was the key predictor of incident ATP3 metabolic syndrome; of 714 subjects free of metabolic syndrome at baseline, 139 developed metabolic syndrome over 5 years of observation (30). Of these, 43% of women with a large waist circumference (≥89 cm) and 46% of men (≥102 cm) developed metabolic syndrome. These proportions were far larger than proportions accounted for by any other metabolic syndrome trait, insulin resistance (assessed by a frequently sampled intravenous glucose tolerance test to generate the insulin sensitivity index (S_i)), or several other usual diabetes risk factors.

Fat imaging using CT or MRI provides more accurate data on fat distribution than measurement of waist circumference. Fat imaging data support a role of central fat in the pathogenesis of risk factor clustering. Carr and colleagues measured S_i and intraabdominal fat (IAF, assessed with single-slice computed tomography scan at the level of the umbilicus) and subcutaneous fat (SCF) areas in 218 healthy individuals across a broad range of BMI (18–47 kg/m^2) (31). In multivariate models, S_i, IAF, and SCF were all independently associated with ATP3 metabolic syndrome, providing additional support for roles of both obesity and insulin resistance in risk factor clustering. However, only IAF was consistently, independently associated with all five of the metabolic syndrome criteria. Data on volumetric measures of SCF and IAF from over 1,000 Framingham Heart Study Offspring further support a key role of central fat determining risk factor clustering (32). Increasing quartiles of both SCF and IAF were strongly correlated with BMI, waist circumference, fasting plasma glucose, systolic and diastolic blood pressure, HDL cholesterol (inverse correlation), and triglycerides. After adjustment for BMI, IAF but not SCF remained correlated with risk factors. Both SCF and IAF were associated with an increased prevalence of ATP3 metabolic syndrome, but the association with SCF was weakened by adjustment for BMI. For IAF, the BMI-adjusted odds ratio for metabolic syndrome was 2.9 (95% CI 1.7–4.8) for women and 2.3 for men (95% CI 1.4–3.9). These data demonstrate that both SCF and IAF are highly correlated with metabolic risk factors, but that only IAF is a correlate of risk factor clustering after accounting for overall body fatness.

Current data are consistent with the hypothesized role of central fat as a unique, pathogenic fat depot, and in aggregate, the data provide strong support for the primacy of obesity and weight gain in the development of risk factor clustering. Insulin resistance also appears to play a major, independent role. However, accounting for correlated insulin resistance diminishes but does not eliminate the association of obesity with risk factor clustering. This suggests that obesity confers risk for risk factor clustering partially through insulin resistance but also via mechanisms separate from insulin resistance. These mechanisms are now being elucidated.

MECHANISMS FOR RISK FACTOR CLUSTERING ASSOCIATED WITH OBESITY

Several mechanisms may account for the associations among obesity, insulin resistance, and risk factor clustering. Central to these mechanisms appears to be disordered crosstalk between adipose tissue and insulin target tissues (primarily pancreatic beta cells, skeletal muscle, and liver). This crosstalk is mediated by a number of molecules that are secreted by adipose tissue and act via autocrine, paracrine, or endocrine mechanisms to modulate insulin sensitivity (33,34). Altered free fatty acid flux, elevated levels of inflammatory cytokines and adipocyte-secreted hormones (adipokines), and endo-thelial dysfunction are correlated with each other and with obesity and insulin resis-tance. Although consistent direct evidence is still forthcoming, there is abundant and intriguing indirect evidence that risk factor clustering may be a direct consequence of dysregulated adipocyte signaling via or in addition to endothelial dysfunction in skeletal muscle and other microvascular beds.

Plasma free fatty acids (FFAs) are the primary oxidative fuel for liver and resting skeletal muscle (35). Plasma FFA levels are a function of their rate of appearance from adipose tissue (lipolysis) and their rate of disappearance from plasma, either by oxida-tion and/or by reesterification to TG (lipogenesis). Recent studies suggest that when positive energy balance exceeds the "fat-buffering capacity," fatty acid spillover from adipose to nonadipose tissue induces insulin resistance, β-cell dysfunction, and whole-body glucose metabolism (36–40). FFAs may directly antagonize insulin action (41), may induce local insulin resistance via ectopic fat deposition in liver and skeletal muscle (36,42), or may mediate insulin resistance via subclinical inflammation. FFAs are potent physiological inducers of TNF-α production in adipocytes (43). TNF-α may mediate insulin resistance by increasing FFA oxidation (in a positive feedback loop), stimulation of other cytokines (e.g., IL6), directly inhibiting GLUT4, or impairing glucose-stimulated insulin release by β-cells. FFAs also induce endothelial dysfunction (44), at least in part via impaired endothelial nitric-oxide synthase (eNOS)-mediated vasodilata-tion (45–48). Prolonged FFA exposure blunts insulin-mediated increases in whole-leg blood flow, and abolishes insulin-induced increases in nitric oxide flux, leading to substantial declines in peripheral glucose uptake (49).

Obesity is also associated with a heightened state of subclinical *systemic inflamma-tion*. Adipocytes, or leukocytes infiltrating excess adipose tissue, are the source of several cytokines upregulating the innate immune response (50–52). Inflammatory cytokines secreted by adipose tissue appear to exert an endocrine effect conferring insulin resistance in liver, skeletal muscle, and vascular endothelial tissue, and may be a key factor linking obesity, insulin resistance, and risk factor clustering. In particular, elevated production of tumor necrosis factor–alpha (TNF-α) and interleukin-6 (IL-6) associated with obesity generates an acute-phase response with increased hepatic pro-duction of C-reactive protein (CRP), the classic marker of low-grade systemic inflam-mation. Adipose tissue is a major source of endogenous TNF-α production, with elevated levels reflecting both upregulated adipocyte signaling and systemic inflamma-tion (53–55). TNF-α may induce insulin resistance via induction of other cytokines, increased free fatty-acid oxidation and turnover, induction of cellular adhesion mole-cules indicating endothelial dysfunction, and impairment of whole-body glucose and lipid metabolism via these indirect effects as well as direct inhibitory effects on glucose transporter protein GLUT4, insulin receptor substrates, or glucose-stimulated insulin release by pancreatic β-cells (43,54–62). IL-6 serves, in part, an anti-inflammatory role, modulating the production of TNF-α and downregulating the immune response (63). IL-6 is also the principal stimulus of CRP production by the liver (64). As much as 30% of circulating IL-6 in healthy humans may arise from subcutaneous adipose tissue (65).

Elevated CRP levels are the downstream result of upregulated TNF-α and IL6 activ-ity. CRP and other inflammatory markers are strongly correlated in cross-sectional studies with obesity, insulin resistance, glucose intolerance, and vascular disease

(50,66–78). Longitudinal analyses confirm that inflammation is a precursor to both CVD and type 2 diabetes, more directly suggesting that inflammation plays an important role in risk factor clustering and its consequences (79–88). In experimental data in rodents, anti-inflammatory salicylate treatment improves insulin sensitivity (89,90), and in humans, anti-inflammatory therapy may prevent diabetes (91). However, it appears that inflammation does not fully account for the adverse effects of excess adiposity, because in most studies BMI or waist circumference remain independently associated with risk of vascular dysfunction or diabetes even after accounting for elevated inflammatory markers (68,87,88,92–94). It is likely that abnormal adipokine regulation is an additional factor associated with obesity that both mediates the inflammatory response as well as directly confers risk for insulin resistance and risk factor clustering.

Adiponectin is one of the several known *adipokines* for which there is the best evidence for association with insulin resistance and risk factor clustering. Adiponectin is a protein exclusively synthesized and secreted by adipose tissue. Adiponectin is thought to play a role in the adaptation of metabolic fluxes to the amount of stored energy (34). Adiponectin has diverse physiological actions that, taken together, are likely to prevent or reverse risk factor clustering. Adiponectin levels are inversely associated with total fat mass, central fat distribution, and levels of insulin and glucose (95–97), such that higher levels of adiponectin are beneficial. Adiponectin levels increase after weight loss, after insulin sensitization with PPAR-γ activators, or after treatment with rimonabant, a selective cannabinoid-1 receptor (CB1) antagonist (95,98–101). Adiponectin may reduce insulin resistance in skeletal muscle (and perhaps other tissues) by modulating intracellular fat storage or by facilitating increased FFA oxidation and disposal (102–104). Adiponectin may also diminish risk factor clustering via its anti-inflammatory and anti-atherogenic properties (105–108). Adiponectin can reduce the induction of TNF-α and inhibit TNF-α-induced monocyte adhesion (97). Intravenous administration of recombinant adiponectin in rodents with insulin resistance restores normal insulin sensitivity (109). Adiponectin circulates in humans as a variably sized multimer; high-molecular-weight adiponectin may be the most bioactive form, especially from the perspective of insulin sensitization (110,111). Finally, data are emerging linking hypoadiponectinemia with increased risk of outcomes associated with risk factor clustering. In several populations, subjects with lower adiponectin levels were more likely to develop type 2 DM, independent of obesity (112–114), and in one recent study, low adiponectin levels predicted development of CVD (115).

Resistin is another adipokine that plays a role in regulation of metabolic flux and may contribute to risk factor clustering associated with obesity, at least in rodents (34,116,117). Circulating levels of resistin are markedly increased in obese, insulin-resistant mice, and are decreased by treatment with insulin-sensitizing PPAR-γ activators (118). In rodents, resistin may increase insulin resistance by directly inhibiting insulin action (119,120). In humans, the role of resistin related to obesity and risk factor clustering remains uncertain (121). Although human fat tissue produces resistin, its exact cellular source remains unclear (122–124). In addition, data addressing the association of elevated resistin levels with obesity, insulin resistance, or diabetes are quite inconsistent, with some studies suggesting positive associations (125–127), and other studies showing no association (128–130). For example, in one recent study of 177 nondiabetic subjects classified into categories of BMI (less than vs. equal to or greater than 27.5 kg/m^2) and insulin sensitivity (S_I) less than versus equal to or greater than

7×10^{-5} min^{-1} (pmol/l)$^{-1}$, resistin levels did not differ between the lean/insulin-sensitive, lean/insulin-resistant, and obese/insulin-resistant groups. Resistin was positively correlated with BMI, subcutaneous fat area (quantified by CT scan), but not with S_I, intraabdominal fat area, or with the number of metabolic syndrome traits (131). This well-done study casts doubt on the role of resistin mediating human insulin resistance or risk factor clustering. Resistin belongs to a class of molecules associated with inflammation, suggesting that, to the extent that elevated levels influence insulin resistance and its consequences, these effects may be mediated through resistin's potential inflammatory effects (118,127). For instance, in a couple of cross-sectional analyses, plasma resistin concentration was positively associated with levels of CRP, vascular cell adhesion molecules, and von Willebrand factor (127,132). There are no current data addressing the association of resistin with CVD, but in one study, resistin was shown to promote endothelial cell activation and upregulate adhesion molecule production, perhaps contributing to endothelial dysfunction and via this mechanism contributing to risk factor clustering associated with obesity (133).

Endothelial dysfunction, marked by impaired brachial artery flow-mediated dilation or elevated levels of cellular adhesion molecules, PAI-1-1, or von Willebrand factor, has been associated with insulin resistance and risk of diabetes or CVD, and may play a role in risk factor clustering associated with these conditions (93,134–137). Arteriolar endothelial dysfunction could contribute to insulin resistance and lead to diabetes, while conduit arterial endothelial dysfunction leads to clinical CVD (134,138,139). Endothelial dysfunction as an antecedent of type 2 diabetes is becoming fairly well established (88,93,135–137,140–148). Evidence that endothelial dysfunction is a precursor to both CVD and type 2 diabetes suggests a central role for endothelial dysfunction in insulin resistance and risk factor clustering associated with obesity.

Endothelial dysfunction may act indirectly to induce insulin resistance via inflammation, as TNF-α, IL-6, and CRP stimulate endothelial production of adhesion molecules, themselves mediators of reduced insulin delivery and enhanced insulin resistance (64). Endothelial dysfunction may also directly affect insulin resistance and risk factor clustering, as elevated plasma levels of biomarkers of endothelial dysfunction are modestly correlated with impaired endothelium-dependent vasodilatation in forearm skin or the brachial artery (135,149), as well as being highly correlated with insulin resistance (50,145,150). In one recent study of postmenopausal women, each one-unit decrease in flow-mediated vasodilatation of the brachial artery was associated with a significant 32% increase in the four-year relative risk for incident diabetes, even after adjustment for most major diabetes risk factors (147). The mechanism for endothelial dysfunction inducing insulin resistance is related in part to impaired endothelium-dependent vasomotion in the arteriolar microcirculation, which may limit insulin-mediated capillary recruitment and redistribution of skeletal muscle blood flow from nonnutritive to nutritive flow routes, diminishing insulin delivery to insulin-sensitive muscle tissue (138,151–153). In one recent experimental study of 15 men with type 2 diabetes randomized in a crossover design to a 30-minute intrafemoral infusion of sodium nitroprusside or verapamil, augmentation of nitric oxide–mediated endothelial function with sodium nitroprusside increased skeletal muscle glucose uptake independent of muscle blood flow and plasma insulin levels, providing direct evidence of the ability of enhanced endothelial function to increase skeletal muscle glucose uptake (154). In addition, altered endothelial permeability also may impair insulin delivery to the interstitium, where insulin levels appear to be a rate-limiting step determining insulin effectiveness (155). Endothelial dysfunction also may act through genetically mediated impairment of endothelium-dependent nitric oxide–mediated vasodilatation (156–158). Treatment data in humans also support a role for endothelial dysfunction contributing to risk factor clustering. Therapy with drugs having beneficial effects on endothelial function (including thiazolidinediones, metformin, renin-angiotensin-system-acting agents, and HMG CoA reductase inhibitors) improves insulin sensitivity and can reduce risk of diabetes and, in some cases, CVD (159–165). All these data consider fat tissue to exert a systemic, endocrine effect on insulin resistance and vascular function. Recently, the intriguing possibility that perivascular fat, which is associated with central fat but does not necessarily produce a low-grade acute phase response, may play a role in influencing endothelial dysfunction, insulin action, and risk factor clustering through locally mediated "vasocrine" signaling (166). Tests of this hypothesis in humans remain to be conducted.

TREATMENT OPTIONS TO REDUCE RISK FACTOR CLUSTERING ASSOCIATED WITH OBESITY

Therapeutic lifestyle change (TLC) that focuses on obesity and physical inactivity to reduce diabetes and CVD risk has an emerging evidence base supporting specific recommendations to reduce risk factor clustering. There are emerging data on drug therapies that influence risk factor clustering, but lack of evidence for direct beneficial outcomes makes specific drug therapy recommendations premature at this time.

Several lines of evidence suggest that *TLC*, through improved physical activity and fitness, weight control, and healthy dietary habits, can prevent or ameliorate risk factor clustering or its consequences. Observational data demonstrate a strong dose-response relationship between physical fitness and reduced incidence of metabolic syndrome, and suggest that increased physical fitness could prevent mortality associated with risk factor clustering (167,168). Similar observations have been made with respect to physical activity and fitness and risk of type 2 diabetes (169) or CVD (170,171) implying that reversal of physical inactivity may be a key treatment for preventing the ultimate complications of risk factor clustering associated with obesity.

Recent dietary intervention studies have specifically addressed treatment and prevention of risk factor clustering. Italian men and women with ATP3 metabolic syndrome randomized to a Mediterranean-style diet (foods rich in mono- and polyunsaturated fat, fiber, a low ratio of omega-6 to omega-3 fatty acids) lost more weight than those randomized to an ad-lib diet, but even after accounting for this difference the Mediterranean diet was associated with a 39% reduction in the prevalence of metabolic syndrome (98). In addition, the Mediterranean diet was associated with significant reductions in levels of inflammatory markers and improved indexes of endothelial function. As with physical fitness, Mediterranean-style diets may be beneficial for prevention of type 2 diabetes or CVD as well as metabolic syndrome (172,173), pointing to dietary change as a key treatment for preventing the complications of risk factor clustering. Another recent trial showed that the DASH diet (reduced calories and increased consumption of fruit, vegetables, low-fat dairy, and whole grains and reduced saturated fat, total fat, and cholesterol, and restricted to 2,400 mg sodium) beneficially lowered adverse metabolic trait levels (174). Other studies have shown that diets high in dietary fiber and low in simple sugars are associated with a lower prevalence of insulin resistance and metabolic syndrome (175). These diets may act by reducing inflammatory stimuli contributing to risk factor clustering (176).

Global benefits on risk factor clustering of TLC that combines physical activity and dietary treatment have been suggested by two type 2 diabetes prevention trials. Post-hoc analysis of the Diabetes Prevention Program (DPP) showed that, at baseline, 47% of enrollees did not have metabolic syndrome, and in these subjects, structured TLC was associated with a 41% reduction in the incidence of metabolic syndrome compared with the placebo group (177). Among DPP subjects with metabolic syndrome at baseline, TLC was associated with a small but significant decrease in the prevalence of the syndrome. Similar benefits were suggested by results from the Finnish Diabetes Study (FDS) (178). These data strongly support recommendations for TLC to prevent risk factor clustering and its complications.

Discussion of *drug therapies* for metabolic syndrome might be straightforward if there were agreement on its underlying pathophysiology, and if there were evidence that treatment of the syndrome per se produces equivalent or better outcomes than treatment to lower levels of the syndrome's component risk factors. There is a strong evidence base for treatment of the component traits common in risk factor clustering, especially hypertension, hyperlipidemia, and glucose intolerance, to prevent diabetes or CVD (179–181). Nonetheless, drug therapies one might consider specifically for metabolic syndrome target endothelial dysfunction (as discussed above), insulin resistance, and the newly discovered endocannabinoid system.

Metformin and thiazolidinediones (TZDs) are insulin-sensitizing drugs. In the DPP, metformin therapy was associated with a 17% reduction in incident metabolic syndrome compared to the placebo group (177), as well as a 31% reduction in the incidence of type 2 diabetes (181). In a post-hoc analysis of the UK Prospective Diabetes Study, metformin significantly reduced risk of CVD death in obese diabetics by 42% (182). TZDs lower blood glucose in type 2 diabetes, improve levels of many CVD risk factors associated with metabolic syndrome (including HDL-C and triglycerides) as well as markers of inflammation, oxidative stress, and endothelial dysfunction (183–187), and may prevent CVD in diabetes (188,189). However, TLC promotes weight loss and improves insulin sensitivity to a greater degree than TZDs (190), emphasizing the value and preference for TLC over insulin sensitization as current, evidence-based therapy to reduce risk factor clustering.

Rimonabant, a cannabinoid CB-1 receptor blocker currently in clinical development, is a promising new therapy for risk factor clustering. Rimonabant acts in the endocannabinoid system to reduce food intake and body weight and increase blood adiponectin levels. The potential benefits of rimonabant have been shown in the RIO-Europe and RIO–North America (obese subjects) and RIO-Lipid (obese subjects with dyslipidemia) trials (101,191,192). In these trials, as compared with placebo, 20 mg per day of rimonabant was associated with a significant weight loss (about 6 kg), reduction in waist circumference (about 5 cm), an increase in HDL cholesterol (about 9%), a reduction in triglycerides (about 12%), and an increase in plasma adiponectin levels (about 50%). The rise in adiponectin was partly independent of weight loss alone. In RIO-Lipid, about 50% of the participants had ATP3 metabolic syndrome. The prevalence of metabolic syndrome at study end in subjects in the rimonabant-20-mg-per-day arm was 26%, compared with 45% in the placebo arm. Reduced prevalence of metabolic syndrome was attributed mainly to the reduction in waist circumference and the increase in HDL cholesterol levels. These data suggest that rimonabant may be uniquely useful for treatment of risk factor clustering, but greater experience with the drug is required, especially with respect to hard outcomes and drug safety.

CONCLUSIONS

Obesity is a rapidly growing health problem, conferring substantial excess risk for morbidity and mortality, especially from type 2 diabetes and CVD. Obesity, especially visceral obesity, confers metabolic risk at least in part through its association with insulin resistance and risk factor clustering or the metabolic syndrome. Mechanisms underlying risk factor clustering associated with obesity include insulin resistance driven by abnormal fatty acid flux and actions of inflammatory cytokines and adipokines. Although the exact nature of these relationships is still being elucidated, solid evidence now exists that TLC comprised of healthy eating habits and regular physical activity will improve insulin resistance and prevent development of risk factor clustering and its morbid complications.

REFERENCES

1. Mokdad AH, Bowman BA, Ford ES, Vinicor F, Marks JS, Koplan JP. The continuing epidemics of obesity and diabetes in the United States. *JAMA* 2001; 286:1195–1200.
2. Vasan RS, Pencina MJ, Cobain M, Freiberg MS, D'Agostino RB. Estimated risks for developing obesity in the Framingham Heart Study. *Ann Intern Med* 2005; 143:473–480.
3. Mokdad AH, Serdula MK, Dietz WH, Bowman BA, Marks JS, Koplan JP. The spread of the obesity epidemic in the United States, 1991–1998. *JAMA* 1999; 282:1519–1522.
4. Willett WC, Dietz WH, Colditz GA. Guidelines for healthy weight. *N Engl J Med* 1999; 341:427–434.
5. Haslam DW, James WP. Obesity. *Lancet* 2005; 366:1197–1209.
6. Manson JE, Skerrett PJ, Greenland P, VanItallie TB. The escalating pandemics of obesity and sedentary lifestyle: A call to action for clinicians. *Arch Intern Med* 2004; 164:249–258.
7. Rexrode KM, Buring JE, Manson JE. Abdominal and total adiposity and risk of coronary heart disease in men. *Int J Obes Relat Metab Disord* 2001; 25:1047–1056.
8. Rexrode KM, Carey VJ, Hennekens CH, Walters EE, Colditz GA, Stampfer MJ, Willett WC, Manson JE. Abdominal adiposity and coronary heart disease in women. *JAMA 1998;* 280:1843–1848.
9. Wei M, Gaskill SP, Haffner SM, Stern MP. Waist circumference as the best predictor of noninsulin dependent diabetes mellitus (NIDDM) compared to body mass index, waist/hip ratio and other anthropometric measurements in Mexican Americans: A 7-year prospective study. *Obes Res* 1997; 5:16–23.
10. Grundy SM, Cleeman JI, Daniels SR, Donato KA, Eckel RH, Franklin BA, Gordon DJ, Krauss RM, Savage PJ, Smith SC Jr, Spertus JA, Costa F. Diagnosis and management of the metabolic syndrome: An American Heart Association/National Heart, Lung, and Blood Institute Scientific Statement. *Circulation*, 2005.
11. Ferrannini E, Natali A, Bell P, Cavallo-Perin P, Lalic N, Mingrone G. Insulin resistance and hypersecretion in obesity: European Group for the Study of Insulin Resistance (EGIR). *J Clin Invest* 1997; 100:1166–1173.
12. Reaven GM. Role of insulin resistance in human disease. *Diabetes* 1988; 37:1595–1607.
13. Rutter MK, Meigs JB, Sullivan LM, D'Agostino RB Sr, Wilson PW. Insulin resistance, the metabolic syndrome, and incident cardiovascular events in the Framingham Offspring Study. *Diabetes* 2005; 54:3252–3257.
14. Despres J-P, Lamarche B, Mauriege P, Cantin B, Dagenais GR, Moorjani S, Lupien P-J. Hyperinsulinemia as an independent risk factor for ischemic heart disease. *N Engl J Med* 1996; 334:952–957.

15. Bonora E, Tessari R, Micciolo R, Zenere M, Targher G, Padovani R, Falezza G, Muggeo M. Intimal-medial thickness of the carotid artery in nondiabetic and NIDDM patients: Relationship with insulin resistance. *Diabetes Care* 1997; 20:627–631.
16. Wilson PWF, Kannel WB, Silbershatz H, D'Agostino RB. Clustering of metabolic factors and coronary heart disease. *Archives of Internal Medicine* 1999; 159:1104–1109.
17. Haffner SM, Valdez RA, Hazuda HP, Mitchell BD, Morales PA, Stern MP. Prospective analysis of the insulin resistance syndrome (syndrome X). *Diabetes* 1992; 41:715–722.
18. Alberti KG, Zimmet P, Shaw J. The metabolic syndrome: A new worldwide definition. *Lancet* 2005; 366:1059–1062.
19. Balkau B, Charles MA. Comment on the provisional report from the WHO consultation: European Group for the Study of Insulin Resistance (EGIR). *Diabet Med* 1999; 16:442–443.
20. Alberti KG, Zimmet PZ. Definition, diagnosis and classification of diabetes mellitus and its complications. Part 1: Diagnosis and classification of diabetes mellitus provisional report of a WHO consultation. *Diabet Med* 1998; 15:539–553.
21. Einhorn D, Reaven GM, Cobin RH, Ford E, Ganda OP, Handelsman Y, Hellman R, Jellinger PS, Kendall D, Krauss RM, Neufeld ND, Petak SM, Rodbard HW, Seibel JA, Smith DA, Wilson PW. American College of Endocrinology position statement on the insulin resistance syndrome. *Endocr Pract* 2003; 9:237–252.
22. Ford ES, Giles WH, Dietz WH. Prevalence of the metabolic syndrome among US adults: Findings from the third National Health and Nutrition Examination Survey. *JAMA* 2002; 287:356–359.
23. St-Onge MP, Janssen I, Heymsfield SB. Metabolic syndrome in normal-weight Americans: New definition of the metabolically obese, normal-weight individual. *Diabetes Care* 2004; 27:2222–2228.
24. Wilson PWF, D'Agostino Sr RB, Parise H, Sullivan L, Meigs JB. The metabolic syndrome as a precursor of cardiovascular disease and type 2 diabetes mellitus. *Circulation* 2005; 112:3066–3072.
25. Ford ES, Giles WH, Mokdad AH. Increasing prevalence of the metabolic syndrome among U.S. adults. *Diabetes Care* 2004; 27:2444–2449.
26. Yarnell JW, Patterson CC, Bainton D, Sweetnam PM. Is metabolic syndrome a discrete entity in the general population? Evidence from the Caerphilly and Speedwell population studies. *Heart* 1998; 79:248–252.
27. Schmidt MI, Watson RL, Duncan BB, Metcalf P, Brancati FL, Sharrett AR, Davis CE, Heiss G. Clustering of dyslipidemia, hyperuricemia, diabetes, and hypertension and its association with fasting insulin and central and overall obesity in a general population. *Metabolism* 1996; 45:699–706.
28. Bonora E, Kiechl S, Willeit J, Oberhollenzer F, Egger G, Targher G, Alberiche M, Bonadonna RC, Muggeo M. Prevalence of insulin resistance in metabolic disorders. *Diabetes* 1998; 47:1643–1649.
29. Liese AD, Mayer-Davis EJ, Tyroler HA, Davis CE, Keil U, Duncan BB, Heiss G. Development of the multiple metabolic syndrome in the ARIC cohort—joint contribution of insulin, BMI, and WHR: Atherosclerosis risk in communities. *Ann Epidemiol* 7:407–416, 1997.
30. Palaniappan L, Carnethon MR, Wang Y, Hanley AJ, Fortmann SP, Haffner SM, Wagenknecht L. Predictors of the incident metabolic syndrome in adults: The Insulin Resistance Atherosclerosis Study. *Diabetes Care* 2004; 27:788–793.
31. Carr DB, Utzschneider KM, Hull RL, Kodama K, Retzlaff BM, Brunzell JD, Shofer JB, Fish BE, Knopp RH, Kahn SE. Intra-abdominal fat is a major determinant of the National Cholesterol Education Program Adult Treatment Panel III criteria for the metabolic syndrome. *Diabetes* 2004; 53:2087–2094.
32. Fox CS, Massaro JM, Hoffmann U, Horvat PM, Vasan RS, Meigs JB, O'Donnell CJ. Volumetric assessment of visceral and subcutaneous adipose tissue compartments and association with metabolic risk factors: The Framingham Heart Study. *Circulation* 2006; 113.
33. Abel ED, Peroni O, Kim JK, Kim YB, Boss O, Hadro E, Minnemann T, Shulman GI, Kahn BB. Adipose-selective targeting of the GLUT4 gene impairs insulin action in muscle and liver. *Nature* 2001; 409:729–733.
34. Saltiel AR. You are what you secrete. *Nat Med* 2001; 7:887–888.
35. Boden G, Shulman GI. Free fatty acids in obesity and type 2 diabetes: Defining their role in the development of insulin resistance and beta-cell dysfunction. *Eur J Clin Invest* 2002; 32(suppl 3):14–23.
36. Frayn KN. Adipose tissue and the insulin resistance syndrome. *Proc Nutr Soc* 2001; 60:375–380.

37. Unger RH, Zhou YT. Lipotoxicity of beta-cells in obesity and in other causes of fatty acid spillover. *Diabetes* 2001; 50(suppl 1):S118–121.
38. Boden G. Role of fatty acids in the pathogenesis of insulin resistance and NIDDM. *Diabetes* 1997; 46:3–10.
39. Paolisso G, Gualdiero P, Manzella D, Rizzo MR, Tagliamonte MR, Gambardella A, Verza M, Gentile S, Varricchio M, D'Onofrio F. Association of fasting plasma free fatty acid concentration and frequency of ventricular premature complexes in nonischemic non-insulin-dependent diabetic patients. *American Journal of Cardiology* 1997; 80:932–937.
40. Baldeweg SE, Golay A, Natali A, Balkau B, Del Prato S, Coppack SW. Insulin resistance, lipid and fatty acid concentrations in 867 healthy Europeans: European Group for the Study of Insulin Resistance (EGIR). *Eur J Clin Invest* 2000; 30:45–52.
41. Roden M, Price TB, Perseghin G, Petersen KF, Rothman DL, Cline GW, Shulman GI. Mechanism of free fatty acid-induced insulin resistance in humans. *J Clin Invest* 1996; 97:2859–2865.
42. Shulman GI. Cellular mechanisms of insulin resistance. *J Clin Invest* 2000; 106:171–176.
43. Hotamisligil GS, Spiegelman BM. TNF-alpha: A key component of obesity-diabetes link. *Diabetes* 1994; 43:1271–1278.
44. Paolisso G, Rizzo MR, Mazziotti G, Tagliamonte MR, Gambardella A, Rotondi M, Carella C, Giugliano D, Varricchio M, D'Onofrio F. Advancing age and insulin resistance: Role of plasma tumor necrosis factor-alpha. *American Journal of Physiology* 1998; 38:E294–E299.
45. Steinberg HO, Tarshoby M, Monestel R, Hook G, Cronin J, Johnson A, Bayazeed B, Baron AD. Elevated circulating free fatty acid levels impair endothelium-dependent vasodilation. *J Clin Invest* 1997; 100:1230–1239.
46. Balletshofer BM, Rittig K, Volk A, Maerker E, Jacob S, Rett K, Haring H. Impaired non-esterified fatty acid suppression is associated with endothelial dysfunction in insulin resistant subjects. *Horm Metab Res* 2001; 33:428–431.
47. Steinberg HO, Paradisi G, Hook G, Crowder K, Cronin J, Baron AD. Free fatty acid elevation impairs insulin-mediated vasodilation and nitric oxide production. *Diabetes* 2000; 49:1231–1238.
48. Lind L, Fugmann A, Branth S, Vessby B, Millgard J, Berne C, Lithell H. The impairment in endothelial function induced by non-esterified fatty acids can be reversed by insulin. *Clin Sci (Lond)* 2000; 99:169–174.
49. Steinberg HO, Baron AD. Vascular function, insulin resistance and fatty acids. *Diabetologia* 2002; 45:623–634.
50. Yudkin JS, Stehouwer CDA, Emis JJ, Coppack SW. C-reactive protein in healthy subjects—associations with obesity, insulin resistance and endothelial dysfunction: A potential role for cytokines originating from adipose tissue? *Arteriosclerosis, Thrombosis and Vascular Biology* 1999; 19:972–978.
51. Weisberg SP, McCann D, Desai M, Rosenbaum M, Leibel RL, Ferrante AW Jr. Obesity is associated with macrophage accumulation in adipose tissue. *J Clin Invest* 2003; 112:1796–1808.
52. Xu H, Barnes GT, Yang Q, Tan G, Yang D, Chou CJ, Sole J, Nichols A, Ross JS, Tartaglia LA, Chen H. Chronic inflammation in fat plays a crucial role in the development of obesity-related insulin resistance. *J Clin Invest* 2003; 112:1821–1830.
53. Hotamisligil GS, Shargill NS, Spiegelman BM. Adipose expression of tumor necrosis factor-alpha: Direct role in obesity-linked insulin resistance. *Science* 1993; 259:87–91.
54. Hotamisligil GS, Arner P, Caro JF, Atkinson RL, Spiegelman BM. Increased adipose expression of tumor necrosis factor-alpha in human obesity and insulin resistance. *J Clin Invest* 1995; 95:2409–2415.
55. Saghizadeh M, Ong JM, Garvey WT, Henry RR, Kern PA. The expression of TNF-alpha by human muscle: Relationship to insulin resistance. *J Clin Invest* 1996; 97:1111–1116.
56. Mantzoros CS, Moschos S, Avramopoulos I, Kaklamani V, Liolios A, Doulgerakis DE, Griveas I, Katsilambros N, Flier JS. Leptin concentrations in relation to body mass index and the tumor necrosis factor-alpha system in humans. *J Clin Endocrinol & Metab* 1997; 82:3408–3413.
57. Katsuki A, Sumida Y, Murashima S, Murata K, Takarada Y, Ito K, Fujii M, Tsuchihashi K, Goto H, Nakatani K, Yano Y. Serum levels of tumor necrosis factor-alpha are increased in obese patients with noninsulin-dependent diabetes mellitus. *J Clin Endocrinol & Metab* 1998; 83:859–862.
58. Zinman B, Hanley AJ, Harris SB, Kwan J, Fantus IG. Circulating tumor necrosis factor-alpha concentrations in a native Canadian population with high rates of type 2 diabetes mellitus. *J Clin Endocrinol & Metab* 1999; 84:272–278.

59. Lofgren P, van Harmelen V, Reynisdottir S, Naslund E, Ryden M, Rossner S, Arner P. Secretion of tumor necrosis factor-alpha shows a strong relationship to insulin-stimulated glucose transport in human adipose tissue. *Diabetes* 2000; 49:688–692.
60. Nilsson J, Jovinge S, Niemann A, Reneland R, Lithell H. Relation between plasma tumor necrosis factor-alpha and insulin sensitivity in elderly men with non-insulin-dependent diabetes mellitus. *Arteriosclerosis, Thrombosis, and Vascular Biology* 1998; 18:1199–1202.
61. Desfaits A, Serri O, Renier G. Normalization of plasma lipid peroxides, monocyte adhesion, and tumor necrosis factor-alpha production in NIDDM patients after gliclazide treatment. *Diabetes Care* 1998; 21:487–493.
62. Winkler G, Salamon F, Salamon D, Speer G, Simon K, Cseh K. Elevated serum tumor necrosis factor-alpha levels contribute to the insulin resistance in type II (non-insulin-dependent) diabetes and in obesity. *Diabetologia* 1998; 41:860–861.
63. Wheeler AP, Bernard GR. Treating patients with severe sepsis. *N Engl J Med* 1999; 340:207–214.
64. Gabay C, Kushner I. Acute-phase proteins and other systemic responses to inflammation. *N Engl J Med* 1999; 340:448–454.
65. Mohamed-Ali V, Goodrick S, Rawesh A, Katz DR, Miles JM, Yudkin JS, Klein S, Coppack SW. Subcutaneous adipose tissue releases interleukin-6, but not tumor necrosis factor-alpha, in vivo. *J Clin Endocrinol & Metab* 1997; 82:4196–4200.
66. Visser M, Bouter LM, McQuillan GM, Wener MH, Harris TB. Elevated c-reactive protein levels in overweight and obese adults. *JAMA* 1999; 282(22):2131–2135.
67. Ford ES. Body mass index, diabetes and c-reactive protein among U.S. adults. *Diabetes Care* 1999; 22(12):1971–1977.
68. Hak AE, Stehouwer CD, Bots ML, Polderman KH, Schalkwijk CG, Westendorp IC, Hofman A, Witteman JC. Associations of c-reactive protein with measures of obesity, insulin resistance, and subclinical atherosclerosis in healthy, middle-aged women. *Arteriosclerosis, Thrombosis and Vascular Biology* 1999; 19:1986–1991.
69. Frohlich M, Imhof A, Berg G, Hutchinson WL, Pepys MB, Boeing H, Muche R, Brenner H, Koenig W. Association between C-reactive protein and features of the metabolic syndrome: A population-based study. *Diabetes Care* 2000; 23:1835–1839.
70. Festa A, D'Agostino Jr R, Williams K, Karter AJ, Mayer-Davis EJ, Tracy RP, Haffner SM. The relation of body fat mass and distribution to markers of chronic inflammation. *Int J Obes Relat Metab Disord* 2001; 25:1407–1415.
71. Festa A, D'Agostino R, Howard G, Mykkanen L, Tracy RP, Haffner SM. Inflammation and micro-albuminuria in nondiabetic and type 2 diabetic subjects: The Insulin Resistance Atherosclerosis Study. *Kidney Int* 2000; 58:1703–1710.
72. Festa A, D'Agostino R, Jr., Howard G, Mykkanen L, Tracy RP, Haffner SM. Chronic subclinical inflammation as part of the insulin resistance syndrome: The Insulin Resistance Atherosclerosis Study (IRAS). *Circulation* 2000; 102:42–47.
73. Pannacciulli N, Cantatore FP, Minenna A, Bellacicco M, Giorgino R, De Pergola G. C-reactive protein is independently associated with total body fat, central fat, and insulin resistance in adult women. *Int J Obes Relat Metab Disord* 2001; 25:1416–1420.
74. Wu T, Dorn JP, Donahue RP, Sempos CT, Trevisan M. Associations of serum C-reactive protein with fasting insulin, glucose, and glycosylated hemoglobin: The Third National Health and Nutrition Examination Survey, 1988–1994. *Am J Epidemiol* 2002; 155:65–71.
75. Pickup JC, Mattock MB, Chusney GD, Burt D. NIDDM as a disease of the innate immune system: Association of acute-phase reactants and interleukin-6 with metabolic syndrome X. *Diabetologia* 1997; 40:1286–1292.
76. Grau AJ, Buggle F, Becher H, Werle E, Hacke W. The association of leukocyte count, fibrinogen, and c-reactive protein with vascular disease risk factors and ischemic vascular diseases. *Thrombosis Research* 1996; 82:245–255.
77. McMillan DE. Increased levels of acute-phase serum proteins in diabetes. *Metabolism* 1989; 38:1042–1046.
78. Vozarova B, Weyer C, Hanson K, Tatarranni PA, Bogardus C, Pratley RE. Circulating interleukin-6 in relation to adiposity, insulin action, and insulin secretion. *Obes Res* 2001; 9:414–417.
79. Ross R. Atherosclerosis: An inflammatory disease. *N Engl J Med* 1999; 340:115–126.

80. Pai JK, Pischon T, Ma J, Manson JE, Hankinson SE, Joshipura K, Curhan GC, Rifai N, Cannuscio CC, Stampfer MJ, Rimm EB. Inflammatory markers and the risk of coronary heart disease in men and women. *N Engl J Med* 2004; 351:2599–2610.
81. Ridker PM. Clinical application of C-reactive protein for cardiovascular disease detection and prevention. *Circulation* 2003; 107:363–369.
82. Pradhan AD, Manson JE, Rifai N, Buring JE, Ridker PM. C-reactive protein, interleukin 6, and risk of developing type 2 diabetes mellitus. *JAMA* 2001; 286:327–334.
83. Barzilay JI, Abraham L, Heckbert SR, Cushman M, Kuller LH, Resnick HE, Tracy RP. The relation of markers of inflammation to the development of glucose disorders in the elderly: The Cardiovascular Health Study. *Diabetes* 2001; 50:2384–2389.
84. Schmidt MI, Duncan BB, Sharrett AR, Lindberg G, Savage PJ, Offenbacher S, Azambuja MI, Tracy RP, Heiss G. Markers of inflammation and prediction of diabetes mellitus in adults (Atherosclerosis Risk in Communities study): A cohort study. *Lancet* 1999; 353:1649–1652.
85. Wei M, Gibbons LW, Mitchell TL, Kampert JB, Blair SN. White blood cell count as a novel predictor of type 2 diabetes. *Diabetes* 1998; 47:0101.
86. Lindsay RS, Krakoff J, Hanson RL, Bennett PH, Knowler WC. Gamma globulin levels predict type 2 diabetes in the Pima Indian population. *Diabetes* 2001; 50:1598–1603.
87. Hu FB, Meigs JB, Li TY, Rifai N, Manson JE. Inflammatory markers and risk of developing type 2 diabetes in women. *Diabetes* 2004; 53:693–700.
88. Festa A, D'Agostino R, Jr., Tracy RP, Haffner SM. Elevated levels of acute-phase proteins and plasminogen activator inhibitor-1 predict the development of type 2 diabetes: The insulin resistance atherosclerosis study. *Diabetes* 2002; 51:1131–1137.
89. Yuan M, Konstantopoulos N, Lee J, Hansen L, Li ZW, Karin M, Shoelson SE. Reversal of obesity- and diet-induced insulin resistance with salicylates or targeted disruption of Ikkbeta. *Science* 2001; 293:1673–1677.
90. Kim JK, Kim YJ, Fillmore JJ, Chen Y, Moore I, Lee J, Yuan M, Li ZW, Karin M, Perret P, Shoelson SE, Shulman GI. Prevention of fat-induced insulin resistance by salicylate. *J Clin Invest* 2001; 108:437–446.
91. Reid J, MacDougall AI, Andrews MM. Aspirin and diabetes mellitus. *Brit Med J* 1957; 2:1071–1074.
92. Weyer C, Bogardus C, Mott DM, Pratley RE. The natural history of insulin secretory dysfunction and insulin resistance in the pathogenesis of type 2 diabetes mellitus. *J Clin Invest* 1999; 104:787–794.
93. Meigs JB, Wilson PWF, Tofler GH, Fox CS, Nathan DM, D'Agostino Sr. RB, O'Donnell CJ. Markers of endothelial dysfunction predict incident type 2 diabetes. *Diabetes* 2005; 54(suppl 1):A90.
94. Wexler DJ, Hu FB, Manson JE, Rifai N, Meigs JB. Mediating effects of inflammatory biomarkers on insulin resistance associated with obesity. *Obes Res* 2005; 13:1772–1783.
95. Arita Y, Kihara S, Ouchi N, Takahashi M, Maeda K, Miyagawa J, Hotta K, Shimomura I, Nakamura T, Miyaoka K, Kuriyama H, Nishida M, Yamashita S, Okubo K, Matsubara K, Muraguchi M, Ohmoto Y, Funahashi T, Matsuzawa Y. Paradoxical decrease of an adipose-specific protein, adiponectin, in obesity. *Biochem Biophys Res Commun* 1999; 257:79–83.
96. Weyer C, Funahashi T, Tanaka S, Hotta K, Matsuzawa Y, Pratley RE, Tataranni PA. Hypoadiponectinemia in obesity and type 2 diabetes: Close association with insulin resistance and hyperinsulinemia. *J Clin Endocrinol Metab* 2001; 86:1930–1935.
97. Havel PJ. Control of energy homeostasis and insulin action by adipocyte hormones: Leptin, acylation stimulating protein, and adiponectin. *Curr Opin Lipidol* 2002; 13:51–59.
98. Esposito K, Marfella R, Ciotola M, Di Palo C, Giugliano F, Giugliano G, D'Armiento M, D'Andrea F, Giugliano D. Effect of a Mediterranean-style diet on endothelial dysfunction and markers of vascular inflammation in the metabolic syndrome: A randomized trial. *JAMA* 2004; 292:1440–1446.
99. Yang WS, Jeng CY, Wu TJ, Tanaka S, Funahashi T, Matsuzawa Y, Wang JP, Chen CL, Tai TY, Chuang LM. Synthetic peroxisome proliferator-activated receptor-gamma agonist, rosiglitazone, increases plasma levels of adiponectin in type 2 diabetic patients. *Diabetes Care* 2002; 25:376–380.
100. Yang WS, Lee WJ, Funahashi T, Tanaka S, Matsuzawa Y, Chao CL, Chen CL, Tai TY, Chuang LM. Weight reduction increases plasma levels of an adipose-derived anti-inflammatory protein, adiponectin. *J Clin Endocrinol Metab* 2001; 86:3815–3819.

101. Despres JP, Golay A, Sjostrom L. Effects of rimonabant on metabolic risk factors in overweight patients with dyslipidemia. *N Engl J Med* 2005; 353:2121–2134.

102. Fruebis J, Tsao TS, Javorschi S, Ebbets-Reed D, Erickson MR, Yen FT, Bihain BE, Lodish HF. Proteolytic cleavage product of 30-kDa adipocyte complement-related protein increases fatty acid oxidation in muscle and causes weight loss in mice. *Proc Natl Acad Sci USA* 2001; 98:2005–2010.

103. Yamauchi T, Kamon J, Minokoshi Y, Ito Y, Waki H, Uchida S, Yamashita S, Noda M, Kita S, Ueki K, Eto K, Akanuma Y, Froguel P, Foufelle F, Ferre P, Carling D, Kimura S, Nagai R, Kahn BB, Kadowaki T. Adiponectin stimulates glucose utilization and fatty-acid oxidation by activating AMP-activated protein kinase. *Nat Med* 2002; 8:1288–1295.

104. Hara K, Yamauchi T, Kadowaki T. Adiponectin: An adipokine linking adipocytes and type 2 diabetes in humans. *Curr Diab Rep* 2005; 5:136–140.

105. Scherer PE, Williams S, Fogliano M, Baldini G, Lodish HF. A novel serum protein similar to C1q, produced exclusively in adipocytes. *J Biol Chem* 1995; 270:26746–26749.

106. Ouchi N, Kihara S, Arita Y, Maeda K, Kuriyama H, Okamoto Y, Hotta K, Nishida M, Takahashi M, Nakamura T, Yamashita S, Funahashi T, Matsuzawa Y. Novel modulator for endothelial adhesion molecules: Adipocyte-derived plasma protein adiponectin. *Circulation* 1999; 100:2473–2476.

107. Ouchi N, Kihara S, Arita Y, Okamoto Y, Maeda K, Kuriyama H, Hotta K, Nishida M, Takahashi M, Muraguchi M, Ohmoto Y, Nakamura T, Yamashita S, Funahashi T, Matsuzawa Y. Adiponectin, an adipocyte-derived plasma protein, inhibits endothelial NF-kappaB signaling through a cAMP-dependent pathway. *Circulation* 2000; 102:1296–1301.

108. Ouchi N, Kihara S, Arita Y, Nishida M, Matsuyama A, Okamoto Y, Ishigami M, Kuriyama H, Kishida K, Nishizawa H, Hotta K, Muraguchi M, Ohmoto Y, Yamashita S, Funahashi T, Matsuzawa Y. Adipocyte-derived plasma protein, adiponectin, suppresses lipid accumulation and class A scavenger receptor expression in human monocyte-derived macrophages. *Circulation* 2001; 103:1057–1063.

109. Yamauchi T, Kamon J, Waki H, Terauchi Y, Kubota N, Hara K, Mori Y, Ide T, Murakami K, Tsuboyama-Kasaoka N, Ezaki O, Akanuma Y, Gavrilova O, Vinson C, Reitman ML, Kagechika H, Shudo K, Yoda M, Nakano Y, Tobe K, Nagai R, Kimura S, Tomita M, Froguel P, Kadowaki T. The fat-derived hormone adiponectin reverses insulin resistance associated with both lipoatrophy and obesity. *Nat Med* 2001; 7:941–946.

110. Lam KS, Xu A. Adiponectin: Protection of the endothelium. *Curr Diab Rep* 2005; 5:254–259.

111. Lara-Castro C, Luo N, Wallace P, Klein RL, Garvey WT. Adiponectin multimeric complexes and the metabolic syndrome trait cluster. *Diabetes* 2006; 55:249–259.

112. Lindsay RS, Funahashi T, Hanson RL, Matsuzawa Y, Tanaka S, Tataranni PA, Knowler WC, Krakoff J. Adiponectin and development of type 2 diabetes in the Pima Indian population. *Lancet* 2002; 360:57–58.

113. Spranger J, Kroke A, Mohlig M, Bergmann MM, Ristow M, Boeing H, Pfeiffer AF. Adiponectin and protection against type 2 diabetes mellitus. *Lancet* 2003; 361:226–228.

114. Daimon M, Oizumi T, Saitoh T, Kameda W, Hirata A, Yamaguchi H, Ohnuma H, Igarashi M, Tominaga M, Kato T. Decreased serum levels of adiponectin are a risk factor for the progression to type 2 diabetes in the Japanese Population: The Funagata study. *Diabetes Care* 2003; 26:2015–2020.

115. Pischon T, Girman CJ, Hotamisligil GS, Rifai N, Hu FB, Rimm EB. Plasma adiponectin levels and risk of myocardial infarction in men. *JAMA* 2004; 291:1730–1737.

116. Steppan CM, Bailey ST, Bhat S, Brown EJ, Banerjee RR, Wright CM, Patel HR, Ahima RS, Lazar MA. The hormone resistin links obesity to diabetes. *Nature* 2001; 409:307–312.

117. Steppan CM, Lazar MA. Resistin and obesity-associated insulin resistance. *Trends Endocrinol Metab* 2002; 13:18–23.

118. Banerjee RR, Lazar MA. Resistin: Molecular history and prognosis. *J Mol Med* 2003; 81:218–226.

119. Ukkola O. Resistin: A mediator of obesity-associated insulin resistance or an innocent bystander? *Eur J Endocrinol* 2002; 147:571–574.

120. Shuldiner AR, Yang R, Gong DW. Resistin, obesity and insulin resistance: The emerging role of the adipocyte as an endocrine organ. *N Engl J Med* 2001; 345:1345–1346.

121. Savage DB, Sewter CP, Klenk ES, Segal DG, Vidal-Puig A, Considine RV, O'Rahilly S. Resistin/Fizz3 expression in relation to obesity and peroxisome proliferator-activated receptor-gamma action in humans. *Diabetes* 2001; 50:2199–2202.

122. Nagaev I, Smith U. Insulin resistance and type 2 diabetes are not related to resistin expression in human fat cells or skeletal muscle. *Biochem Biophys Res Commun* 2001; 285:561–564.

123. Fain JN, Cheema PS, Bahouth SW, Lloyd Hiler M. Resistin release by human adipose tissue explants in primary culture. *Biochem Biophys Res Commun* 2003; 300:674–678.
124. McTernan CL, McTernan PG, Harte AL, Levick PL, Barnett AH, Kumar S. Resistin, central obesity, and type 2 diabetes. *Lancet* 2002; 359:46–47.
125. Azuma K, Katsukawa F, Oguchi S, Murata M, Yamazaki H, Shimada A, Saruta T. Correlation between serum resistin level and adiposity in obese individuals. *Obes Res* 2003; 11:997–1001.
126. Silha JV, Krsek M, Skrha JV, Sucharda P, Nyomba BL, Murphy LJ. Plasma resistin, adiponectin and leptin levels in lean and obese subjects: Correlations with insulin resistance. *Eur J Endocrinol* 2003; 149:331–335.
127. McTernan PG, Fisher FM, Valsamakis G, Chetty R, Harte A, McTernan CL, Clark PM, Smith SA, Barnett AH, Kumar S. Resistin and type 2 diabetes: Regulation of resistin expression by insulin and rosiglitazone and the effects of recombinant resistin on lipid and glucose metabolism in human differentiated adipocytes. *J Clin Endocrinol Metab* 2003; 88:6098–6106.
128. Degawa-Yamauchi M, Bovenkerk JE, Juliar BE, Watson W, Kerr K, Jones R, Zhu Q, Considine RV. Serum resistin (FIZZ3) protein is increased in obese humans. *J Clin Endocrinol Metab* 2003; 88:5452–5455.
129. Fehmann HC, Heyn J. Plasma resistin levels in patients with type 1 and type 2 diabetes mellitus and in healthy controls. *Horm Metab Res* 2002; 34:671–673.
130. Lee JH, Chan JL, Yiannakouris N, Kontogianni M, Estrada E, Seip R, Orlova C, Mantzoros CS. Circulating resistin levels are not associated with obesity or insulin resistance in humans and are not regulated by fasting or leptin administration: Cross-sectional and interventional studies in normal, insulin-resistant, and diabetic subjects. *J Clin Endocrinol Metab* 2003; 88:4848–4856.
131. Utzschneider KM, Carr DB, Tong J, Wallace TM, Hull RL, Zraika S, Xiao Q, Mistry JS, Retzlaff BM, Knopp RH, Kahn SE. Resistin is not associated with insulin sensitivity or the metabolic syndrome in humans. *Diabetologia* 2005; 48:2330–2333.
132. Shetty GK, Economides PA, Horton ES, Mantzoros CS, Veves A. Circulating adiponectin and resistin levels in relation to metabolic factors, inflammatory markers, and vascular reactivity in diabetic patients and subjects at risk for diabetes. *Diabetes Care* 2004; 27:2450–2457.
133. Verma S, Buchanan MR, Anderson TJ. Endothelial function testing as a biomarker of vascular disease. *Circulation* 2003; 108:2054–2059.
134. Pinkney JH, Stehouwer CD, Coppack SW, Yudkin JS. Endothelial dysfunction: Cause of the insulin resistance syndrome. *Diabetes* 1997; 46 Suppl 2:S9–13.
135. Caballero AE, Arora S, Saouaf R, Lim SC, Smakowski P, Park JY, King GL, LoGerfo FW, Horton ES, Veves A. Microvascular and macrovascular reactivity is reduced in subjects at risk for type 2 diabetes. *Diabetes* 1999; 48:1856–1862.
136. Meigs JB, Hu FB, Rifai N, Manson JE. Biomarkers of endothelial dysfunction and risk of type 2 diabetes mellitus. *JAMA* 2004; 291:1978–1986.
137. Meigs JB, O'Donnell C J, Tofler GH, Benjamin EJ, Fox CS, Lipinska I, Nathan DM, Sullivan LM, D'Agostino RB, Wilson PW. Hemostatic markers of endothelial dysfunction and risk of incident type 2 diabetes: The Framingham Offspring Study. *Diabetes* 2006; 55:530–537.
138. Clark MG, Wallis MG, Barrett EJ, Vincent MA, Richards SM, Clerk LH, Rattigan S. Blood flow and muscle metabolism: A focus on insulin action. *Am J Physiol Endocrinol Metab* 2003; 284: E241–258.
139. Lerman A, Zeiher AM. Endothelial function: Cardiac events. *Circulation* 2005; 111:363–368.
140. Stehouwer CD, Nauta JJ, Zeldenrust GC, Hackeng WH, Donker AJ, den Ottolander GJ. Urinary albumin excretion, cardiovascular disease, and endothelial dysfunction in non-insulin-dependent diabetes mellitus. *Lancet* 1992; 340:319–323.
141. Hogikyan RV, Galecki AT, Pitt B, Halter JB, Greene DA, Supiano MA. Specific impairment of endothelium-dependent vasodilation in subjects with type 2 diabetes independent of obesity. *J Clin Endocrinol & Metab* 1998; 83:1946–1952.
142. Meigs JB, Mittleman MA, Nathan DM, Tofler GH, Singer DE, Murphy-Sheehy PM, Lipinska I, D'Agostino RB, Wilson PWF. Hyperinsulinemia, hyperglycemia, and impaired hemostasis: The Framingham Offspring Study. *JAMA* 2000; 283:221–228.
143. Vehkavaara S, Seppala-Lindroos A, Westerbacka J, Groop P-H, Yki-Jarvinen H. In vivo endothelial dysfunction characterizes patients with impaired fasting glucose. *Diabetes Care* 1999; 22:2055–2060.

144. Balletshofer BM, Rittig K, Enderle MD, Volk A, Maerker E, Jacob S, Matthaei S, Rett K, Haring HU. Endothelial dysfunction is detectable in young normotensive first-degree relatives of subjects with type 2 diabetes in association with insulin resistance. *Circulation* 2000; 101:1780–1784.

145. Weyer C, Yudkin JS, Stehouwer CD, Schalkwijk CG, Pratley RE, Tataranni PA. Humoral markers of inflammation and endothelial dysfunction in relation to adiposity and in vivo insulin action in Pima Indians. *Atherosclerosis* 2002; 161:233–242.

146. Wong TY, Klein R, Sharrett AR, Schmidt MI, Pankow JS, Couper DJ, Klein BE, Hubbard LD, Duncan BB. Retinal arteriolar narrowing and risk of diabetes mellitus in middle-aged persons. *JAMA* 2002; 287:2528–2533.

147. Rossi R, Cioni E, Nuzzo A, Origliani G, Modena MG. Endothelial-dependent vasodilation and incidence of type 2 diabetes in a population of healthy postmenopausal women. *Diabetes Care* 2005; 28:702–707.

148. Kanaya AM, Wassel Fyr C, Vittinghoff E, Harris TB, Park SW, Goodpaster BH, Tylavsky F, Cummings SR. Adipocytokines and incident diabetes mellitus in older adults: The independent effect of plasminogen activator inhibitor 1. *Arch Intern Med* 2006; 166:350–356.

149. Holmlund A, Hulthe J, Millgard J, Sarabi M, Kahan T, Lind L. Soluble intercellular adhesion molecule-1 is related to endothelial vasodilatory function in healthy individuals. *Atherosclerosis* 2002; 165:271–276.

150. Agewall S. Insulin sensitivity and haemostatic factors in men at high and low cardiovascular risk: The Risk Factor Intervention Study Group. *J Intern Med* 1999; 246:489–495.

151. Baron AD. Cardiovascular actions of insulin in humans: Implications for insulin sensitivity and vascular tone. In: *Anonymous Insulin Resistance,* Ferrannini E (ed.), Bailliere Tindall, London, 1994, pp. 961–985.

152. Bonadonna RC, Saccomani MP, Del Prato S, Bonora E, DeFronzo RA, Cobelli C. Role of tissue-specific blood flow and tissue recruitment in insulin-mediated glucose uptake of human skeletal muscle. *Circulation* 1998; 98:234–241.

153. Serne EH, RG IJ, Gans RO, Nijveldt R, De Vries G, Evertz R, Donker AJ, Stehouwer CD. Direct evidence for insulin-induced capillary recruitment in skin of healthy subjects during physiological hyperinsulinemia. *Diabetes* 2002; 51:1515–1522.

154. Henstridge DC, Kingwell BA, Formosa MF, Drew BG, McConell GK, Duffy SJ. Effects of the nitric oxide donor, sodium nitroprusside, on resting leg glucose uptake in patients with type 2 diabetes. *Diabetologia* 2005; 48:2602–2608.

155. Miles PD, Levisetti M, Reichart D, Khoursheed M, Moossa AR, Olefsky JM. Kinetics of insulin action in vivo: Identification of rate-limiting steps. *Diabetes* 1995; 44:947–953.

156. Duplain H, Burcelin R, Sartori C, Cook S, Egli M, Lepori M, Vollenweider P, Pedrazzini T, Nicod P, Thorens B, Scherrer U. Insulin resistance, hyperlipidemia, and hypertension in mice lacking endothelial nitric oxide synthase. *Circulation* 2001; 104:342–345.

157. Perreault M, Marette A. Targeted disruption of inducible nitric oxide synthase protects against obesity-linked insulin resistance in muscle. *Nat Med* 2001; 7:1138–1143.

158. Monti LD, Barlassina C, Citterio L, Galluccio E, Berzuini C, Setola E, Valsecchi G, Lucotti P, Pozza G, Bernardinelli L, Casari G, Piatti P. Endothelial nitric oxide synthase polymorphisms are associated with type 2 diabetes and the insulin resistance syndrome. *Diabetes* 2003; 52:1270–1275.

159. Mather KJ, Verma S, Anderson TJ. Improved endothelial function with metformin in type 2 diabetes mellitus. *J Am Coll Cardiol* 2001; 37:1344–1350.

160. Pistrosch F, Passauer J, Fischer S, Fuecker K, Hanefeld M, Gross P. In type 2 diabetes, rosiglitazone therapy for insulin resistance ameliorates endothelial dysfunction independent of glucose control. *Diabetes Care* 2004; 27:484–490.

161. Diabetes Prevention Program: Prevention of type 2 diabetes with Troglitazone in the Diabetes Prevention Program. *Diabetes* 2005; 54:1150–1156.

162. Tan KC, Chow WS, Tam SC, Ai VH, Lam CH, Lam KS. Atorvastatin lowers C-reactive protein and improves endothelium-dependent vasodilation in type 2 diabetes mellitus. *J Clin Endocrinol Metab* 2002; 87:563–568.

163. O'Driscoll G, Green D, Maiorana A, Stanton K, Colreavy F, Taylor R. Improvement in endothelial function by angiotensin-converting enzyme inhibition in non-insulin-dependent diabetes mellitus. *J Am Coll Cardiol* 1999; 33:1506–1511.

164. Freeman DJ, Norrie J, Sattar N, Neely RD, Cobbe SM, Ford I, Isles C, Lorimer AR, Macfarlane PW, McKillop JH, Packard CJ, Shepherd J, Gaw A. Pravastatin and the development of diabetes mellitus: Evidence for a protective treatment effect in the West of Scotland Coronary Prevention Study. *Circulation* 2001; 103:357–362.

165. Yusuf S, Gerstein H, Hoogwerf B, Pogue J, Bosch J, Wolffenbuttel BH, Zinman B. Ramipril and the development of diabetes. *JAMA* 2001; 286:1882-1885.

166. Yudkin JS, Eringa E, Stehouwer CD. "Vasocrine" signalling from perivascular fat: A mechanism linking insulin resistance to vascular disease. *Lancet* 2005; 365:1817–1820.

167. LaMonte MJ, Barlow CE, Jurca R, Kampert JB, Church TS, Blair SN. Cardiorespiratory fitness is inversely associated with the incidence of metabolic syndrome: A prospective study of men and women. *Circulation* 2005; 112:505–512.

168. Katzmarzyk PT, Church TS, Janssen I, Ross R, Blair SN. Metabolic syndrome, obesity, and mortality: Impact of cardiorespiratory fitness. *Diabetes Care* 2005; 28:391–397.

169. Wei M, Gibbons LW, MItchell TL, Kampert JB, Lee CD, Blair SN. The association between cardiorespiratory fitness and impaired fasting glucose and type 2 diabetes in men. *Ann Int Med* 1999; 130:89–96.

170. Blair SN, Kampert JB, Kohl HW, 3rd, Barlow CE, Macera CA, Paffenbarger RS Jr, Gibbons LW. Influences of cardiorespiratory fitness and other precursors on cardiovascular disease and all-cause mortality in men and women. *JAMA* 1996; 276:205–210.

171. Sesso HD, Paffenbarger RS Jr, Lee IM. Physical activity and coronary heart disease in men: The Harvard Alumni Health Study. *Circulation* 2000; 102:975-980.

172. Hu FB, Manson JE, Stampfer MJ, Colditz G, Liu S, Solomon CG, Willett WC. Diet, lifestyle, and the risk of type 2 diabetes mellitus in women. *N Engl J Med* 2001; 345:790–797.

173. Kris-Etherton P, Eckel RH, Howard BV, St Jeor S, Bazzarre TL. AHA Science Advisory—Lyon Diet Heart Study: Benefits of a Mediterranean-style, National Cholesterol Education Program/ American Heart Association step I dietary pattern on cardiovascular disease. *Circulation* 2001; 103:1823–1825.

174. Azadbakht L, Mirmiran P, Esmaillzadeh A, Azizi T, Azizi F. Beneficial effects of a dietary approach to stop hypertension eating plan on features of the metabolic syndrome. *Diabetes Care* 2005; 28:2823–2831.

175. McKeown NM, Meigs JB, Liu S, Saltzman E, Wilson PW, Jacques PF. Carbohydrate nutrition, insulin resistance, and the prevalence of the metabolic syndrome in the Framingham Offspring Cohort. *Diabetes Care* 2004; 27:538–546.

176. Schulze MB, Hoffmann K, Manson JE, Willett WC, Meigs JB, Weikert C, Heidemann C, Colditz GA, Hu FB. Dietary pattern, inflammation, and incidence of type 2 diabetes in women. *Am J Clin Nutr* 2005; 82:675–684; quiz 714-675.

177. Orchard TJ, Temprosa M, Goldberg R, Haffner S, Ratner R, Marcovina S, Fowler S. The effect of metformin and intensive lifestyle intervention on the metabolic syndrome: The Diabetes Prevention Program randomized trial. *Ann Intern Med* 2005; 142:611–619.

178. Ilanne-Parikka P, Eriksson JG, Lindstrom J, Hamalainen H, Keinanen-Kiukaanniemi S, Laakso M, Louheranta A, Mannelin M, Rastas M, Salminen V, Aunola S, Sundvall J, Valle T, Lahtela J, Uusitupa M, Tuomilehto J. Prevalence of the metabolic syndrome and its components: Findings from a Finnish general population sample and the Diabetes Prevention Study cohort. *Diabetes Care* 2004; 27:2135–2140.

179. Chobanian AV, Bakris GL, Black HR, Cushman WC, Green LA, Izzo JL, Jr., Jones DW, Materson BJ, Oparil S, Wright JT, Jr., Roccella EJ. The seventh report of the Joint National Committee on Prevention, Detection, Evaluation, and Treatment of High Blood Pressure: The JNC 7 report. *JAMA* 2003; 289:2560–2572.

180. National Cholesterol Education Program: Executive summary of the third report of the National Cholesterol Education Program (NCEP) Expert Panel on Detection, Evaluation, and Treatment of High Blood Cholesterol in Adults (Adult Treatment Panel III). *JAMA* 2001; 285:2486–2497.

181. Knowler WC, Barrett-Connor E, Fowler SE, Hamman RF, Lachin JM, Walker EA, Nathan DM. Reduction in the incidence of type 2 diabetes with lifestyle intervention or metformin. *N Engl J Med* 2002; 346:393–403.

182. UK Prospective Diabetes Study Group: Effect of intensive blood-glucose control with metformin on complications in overweight patients with type 2 diabetes (UKPDS 34): UK Prospective Diabetes Study (UKPDS) Group. *Lancet* 1998; 352:854–865.

183. Davidson MB. Is treatment of insulin resistance beneficial independent of glycemia? *Diabetes Care* 2003; 26:3184–3186.
184. Yki-Jarvinen H. Thiazolidinediones. *N Engl J Med* 2004; 351:1106–1118.
185. Chiquette E, Ramirez G, Defronzo R. A meta-analysis comparing the effect of thiazolidinediones on cardiovascular risk factors. *Arch Intern Med* 2004; 164:2097–2104.
186. Haffner SM, Greenberg AS, Weston WM, Chen H, Williams K, Freed MI. Effect of rosiglitazone treatment on nontraditional markers of cardiovascular disease in patients with type 2 diabetes mellitus. *Circulation* 2002; 106:679–684.
187. Natali A, Baldeweg S, Toschi E, Capaldo B, Barbaro D, Gastaldelli A, Yudkin JS, Ferrannini E. Vascular effects of improving metabolic control with metformin or rosiglitazone in type 2 diabetes. *Diabetes Care* 2004; 27:1349–1357.
188. Sidhu JS, Kaposzta Z, Markus HS, Kaski JC. Effect of rosiglitazone on common carotid intima-media thickness progression in coronary artery disease patients without diabetes mellitus. *Arterioscler Thromb Vasc Biol* 2004; 24:930–934.
189. Dormandy JA, Charbonnel B, Eckland DJ, Erdmann E, Massi-Benedetti M, Moules IK, Skene AM, Tan MH, Lefebvre PJ, Murray GD, Standl E, Wilcox RG, Wilhelmsen L, Betteridge J, Birkeland K, Golay A, Heine RJ, Koranyi L, Laakso M, Mokan M, Norkus A, Pirags V, Podar T, Scheen A, Scherbaum W, Schernthaner G, Schmitz O, Skrha J, Smith U, Taton J. Secondary prevention of macrovascular events in patients with type 2 diabetes in the PROactive Study (PROspective pioglitAzone Clinical Trial in macroVascular Events): A randomised controlled trial. *Lancet* 2005; 366:1279–1289.
190. Shadid S, Jensen MD. Effects of pioglitazone versus diet and exercise on metabolic health and fat distribution in upper body obesity. *Diabetes Care* 2003; 26:3148–3152.
191. Van Gaal LF, Rissanen AM, Scheen AJ, Ziegler O, Rossner S. Effects of the cannabinoid-1 receptor blocker rimonabant on weight reduction and cardiovascular risk factors in overweight patients: One-year experience from the RIO-Europe study. *Lancet* 2005; 365:1389–1397.
192. Pi-Sunyer FX, Aronne LJ, Heshmati HM, Devin J, Rosenstock J. Effect of rimonabant, a cannabinoid-1 receptor blocker, on weight and cardiometabolic risk factors in overweight or obese patients: RIO-North America—a randomized controlled trial. *JAMA* 2006; 295:761–775.

4 Treatment of the Metabolic Syndrome with Weight Loss, Exercise, Hormones, and Surgery

George A. Bray

CONTENTS

ABSTRACT

Weight reduction improves all components of the metabolic syndrome. This is seen with calorie-reduced diets as well as weight-loss Mediterranean-type diets. Exercise is also an effective strategy, but less so than diets usually because the weight loss is less. Sibutramine, xenical, and rimonabant are effective strategies to lower body weight and improve the metabolic syndrome. Surgery is more effective than the other strategies for reducing body weight and has significant effects on the components of the metabolic syndrome. Simply removing fat, however, is not enough to improve the features of the metabolic syndrome. Removal of subcutaneous fat by liposuction does not improve lipids or blood pressure, whereas removal of visceral fat by lipectomy does. Central adiposity can be attenuated independently of total body fat. Growth hormone, testosterone, cortisol, and dehydroepiandrosterone all have independent effects on visceral adipose tissue.

INTRODUCTION

The metabolic syndrome is a collection of physical signs and laboratory measurements that often cluster together with central adiposity and insulin resistance. The more of these diagnostic features that are present, the higher the predictive power for development of future diabetes or cardiovascular disease. The observation that increasing the number of risk factors increases the prediction of cardiovascular disease has been made

From: *Contemporary Endocrinology: The Metabolic Syndrome: Epidemiology, Clinical Treatment, and Underlying Mechanisms*
Edited by: B.C. Hansen and G.A. Bray © Humana Press, Totowa, NJ

many times before (1–3). Among the constellation of factors that comprise the metabolic syndrome, the value of this syndrome in predicting either heart disease or diabetes depends on which factors are present. When impaired fasting glucose is present, the risk of diabetes is significantly increased. This should not be surprising because impaired fasting glucose has long been known to be a predictor of diabetes and part of the progression toward diabetes. Similarly when hypertension or atherogenic dyslipidemia (i.e., low HDL-cholesterol or high triglylcerides) are present, the prediction of cardiovascular disease is significantly increased.

Because diagnosis of the metabolic syndrome using the criteria proposed by either the National Cholesterol Education Program Adult Treatment Panel III or the International Diabetes Federation is clinically feasible, the syndrome has value in alerting physicians to potential cardiovascular disease or diabetes. A recent detailed critique of the metabolic syndrome concludes that the compilation of factors is not better than the individual factors at predicting disease (4). Nonetheless, in my opinion, the constellation remains clinically useful in helping physicians focus on important risk factors.

There is a large amount of data showing that weight loss will improve all of the components of the metabolic syndrome. However, it is also clear that weight loss is difficult to achieve and sustain and is often deemed inadequate. The question thus arises as to whether it might not be better to treat the components of the metabolic syndrome rather than trying to induce significant loss of weight and loss of visceral fat. We will evaluate this question by examining the effects of weight loss on individual components of the ATP-III defined syndrome. I will use the NCEP ATP-III as recently modified by lowering the fasting glucose level of 100 mg/dL (5.6 mmolar) (5).

CENTRAL ADIPOSITY AND VISCERAL FAT

Visceral fat is a central component of the metabolic syndrome and it is a required component of the definition proposed by the International Diabetes Federation and one of the five components for the ATP-III and ATP-III-revised systems. There are a number of techniques for reducing visceral fat, including decreasing body fat, exercise, and hormones. All of these, of course, work on a genetic background (6). There is also considerable evidence showing that genetic factors are important in the development of the metabolic syndrome, and no doubt in its response to therapy.

Effects of Weight Loss on Central Adiposity

Weight loss is associated with a decrease in visceral fat (7) and will improve most of the features of the metabolic syndrome (8). Convincing evidence for this proposition is found in the Diabetes Prevention Program (8). A total of 1,711 of the 3,234 participants (53%) had the metabolic syndrome at randomization (Table 4.1). This is comparable to the data for this age group provided by the National Center for Health Statistics (9). The prevalence did not vary by gender or age groups (<45; 45–60; >60). However, ethnicity did affect the prevalence, which was lowest in Asians (41%) and highest in whites (57%).

Components of the metabolic syndrome (MS) varied by ethnic groups. Among African Americans, triglycerides were elevated in only 20.6%, compared with 47 to 53% for the Caucasian, Hispanic, Asian, and Native Americans. Among Native Americans, the prevalence of hypertension and impaired fasting glucose was lower than in

Table 4.1
Prevalence (*n* (%)) of the Metabolic Syndrome (NCEP ATP-III Criteria) and its Components by Age
and Gender in the Diabetes Prevention Program

	Total	Age (yrs)			Gender	
		<45	45–59	60+	Men	Women
Number participants	**3234**	**1000**	**1586**	**648**	**1043**	**2191**
Metabolic syndrome	1711 (53%)	521 (52%)	868 (55%)	322 (50%)	550 (53%)	1161 (53%)
Waist circumference*[†]	2532 (78%)	818 (82%)	1240 (78%)	474 (73%)	656 (63%)	1876 (86%)
Low HDLc*[†]	1838 (57%)	698 (70%)	883 (56%)	257 (40%)	529 (51%)	1309 (60%)
High triglycerides or Rx[†]	1472 (46%)	423 (42%)	764 (48%)	285 (44%)	522 (50%)	950 (43%)
High FPG*[†]	1060 (33%)	307 (31%)	526 (33%)	227 (35%)	435 (42%)	625 (28%)
High blood pressure*	1460 (45%)	310 (31%)	740 (47%)	410 (63%)	569 (55%)	891 (41%)

*$p < 0.05$ comparing across all age groups.
[†]p across all gender groups.

the other groups. Approximately half of IGT subjects have the MS with little difference by age, but differences by component. Lifestyle and metformin both reduced the incidence of metabolic syndrome, but lifestyle was more effective than metformin in this regard.

The effects of weight loss on visceral fat are proportionately greater than on total fat (7). This is again shown in the Diabetes Prevention Program, a multicenter study of weight loss on the development of diabetes in individuals with impaired glucose tolerance (10). In this study, 745 participants had an abdominal CT at baseline and 1 year. Weight loss for men in the lifestyle intervention group was −8.3 ± 7.1 (m ± SD), and for the women it was −7.0 ± 7.1 (m ± SD). The visceral adipose tissue (VAT) at the L4-5 cross-sectional area decreased by 48 cm, or 26%, after a weight loss of 7% of body weight. Subcutaneous adipose decreased by 58 cm or 17%, which was significantly less than the percent decrease in VAT. Thus relatively, the VAT was more responsive to weight loss than the subcutaneous fat.

Weight loss in the Diabetes Prevention Program was associated with reversal of the metabolic syndrome (Table 4.2). This table shows the overall prevalence at baseline and the increase over the 3.2 years of follow-up. It also shows that there was a significant reversal of the metabolic syndrome that was lowest in the placebo group (18%) and rose to 38% reduction in the lifestyle group that initially lost 7% of their body weight and maintained an average loss of 5.5%.

Exercise and Loss of Body Weight and Visceral Fat

Exercise also decreases VAT and there is a genetic component to this response. A group of 12 overweight identical male twins were recruited to lose body weight and fat by exercise. Five pairs discontinued the study, but there was a correlation of $r = 0.84$ in the decrease in visceral fat between the two sets of twins. The decrease in visceral fat, body fat, and body weight was significantly greater within pairs of twins than

Table 4.2
Development and Reversal of the Metabolic Syndrome in the DPP

Overall prevalence at 3.2 years:		
Placebo	61%	+6% from baseline
Metformin	55%	+2% from baseline
Lifestyle	42%	−9% from baseline
Reversal at 3.2 years:		
Placebo	18%	
Metformin	23%	
Lifestyle	38%	

Source: Adapted from Orchard DPP, *Ann Int Med* 2005.

between them, indicating that exercise will decrease visceral fat, and that there is a significant genetic component to this effect (11).

The effect of exercise and diet is shown further in a year-long study by Wood et al. (Table 4.3) (12). They reported a decrease of −7.2 kg in body weight in the group receiving the dietary prescription and a decrease of −4.0 kg in body weight in the group participating in the exercise intervention.

As with the other components of the metabolic syndrome, the dyslipidemias are responsive to both diet and exercise. The effect of diet can be seen in the responses from the lifestyle arm of the Diabetes Prevention Program. This group lost an average of 7% of their body weight during the first 6 months of the trial and maintained it for the next 6 months. Triglyceride levels fell significantly more in the Intensive Lifestyle group than in the other groups as anticipated from the greater weight loss (−25.4 mg/dl vs. −7.4 mg/dl in the lifestyle and placebo groups, respectively; $p = 0.001$). The Intensive Lifestyle group also demonstrated a greater increase in HDL cholesterol than the placebo group, respectively (+1.0 mg/dl vs. −0.1 mg/dl; $p = 0.002$). Furthermore, Intensive Lifestyle favorably altered LDL phenotype, with a reduction in the incidence of phenotype B representing a smaller, denser more atherogenic LDL particle.

With both diet and exercise, there was a decrease in LDL-cholesterol and triglycerides and an increase in HDL-cholesterol. These effects occurred in both men and women. In a meta-analysis of changes in lipids with diet and exercise, Dattillo et al.

Table 4.3
Effect of Diet and Exercise on Plasma Lipids During One Year of Adherence to a Diet or Exercise Program

Change from Baseline	Control	Diet	Exercise
Weight (kg)	+0.6	−9.3	−4.1
Triglyceride	+0.08	−0.27	−0.17
LDL-cholesterol	−0.21	−0.31	−0.25
HDL-cholesterol	−0.03	+0.24	+0.21

Source: Adapted from Wood et al., *NEJM* 1989.

(13) found that for each decrease of 1 kg in body weight there was a decrease of −0.75 mg/dL in total cholesterol, a decrease of 0.6 mg/dL in triglycerides, and a change in HDL-cholesterol that depended on whether body weight was stable or body weight was still declining. If it was stable, HDL-cholesterol increased +0.35 mg/dL, but if weight loss was still occurring, HDL-cholesterol was −0.25 mg/dL lower.

Diet and exercise are also effective in lowering blood pressure. Even without weight loss, a diet rich in fruits and vegetables produced a significant reduction in blood pressure. When this dietary pattern was modified by adding low-fat dairy products (the DASH diet), the reduction in blood pressure was even more substantial. The DASH diet also lowered blood pressure at normal and elevated levels of dietary sodium intake (14–16). Because of these important effects on blood pressure, the DASH (Dietary Approaches to Stop Hypertension) diet has been included in the 2005 Dietary Guidelines.

In the Trials of Hypertension Prevention II (TOPH II), Stevens et al. reported a graded reduction in both systolic and diastolic blood pressure with increasing weight loss. For a weight loss of >9.5 kg, the change in SBP/DBP was −9.4/−8.4 mmHg. With a weight loss between 4.5 and 9.5 kg, the blood pressure declined −6.4/−6.4, whereas a loss of 1.0 to 2.0 kg was associated with only a small change in blood pressure of −4.4/−2.5 mmHg after 18 months of treatment with a behavioral weight loss program. In a further follow-up, they reported that the participants in the weight loss program who maintained their weight loss maintained a significantly lower blood pressure as compared to individuals who regained their body weight (17). In the Swedish Obese Subjects study, Sjostrom et al. reported a nearly linear change in both systolic and diastolic blood pressure with change in body weight.

Medications

Weight loss can be produced by treatment with a variety of medications. In this chapter, I will consider rimonabant, orlistat and sibutramine.

RIMONABANT

There are two cannabinoid receptors, CB-1 (470 amino acids in length) and CB-2 (360 amino acids in length). The CB-1 receptor has almost all the amino acids that comprise the CB-2 receptor and additional amino acids at both ends. CB-1 receptors are distributed throughout the brain in the areas related to feeding, on fat cells, and in the gastrointestinal tract. CB-2 receptors are found primarily on immune cells. Marijuana and tetrahydrocannabinol, which stimulate the CB-1 receptor, also increase the intake of high-fat and high-sweet foods. Fasting increases the levels of endocannabinoids. The rewarding properties of cannabinoid agonists are mediated through the meso-limbic dopaminergic system. Rimonabant is a specific antagonist of the CB-1 receptor that inhibits sweet-food intake in marmosets as well as high-fat food intake in rats, but it does not inhibit food intake in rats eating standard chow. Rimonabant is thus specific in inhibiting the intake of highly palatable food intake. Pair-feeding experiments in diet-induced obese rats suggest, at least in rodents, that rimonabant increases energy expenditure in addition to reducing food intake. Rimonabant-treated animals lost 21% of their body weight compared to 14% in the pair-fed controls. CB-1 knockout mice are lean and resistant to diet-induced weight gain. CB-1 receptors are upregulated on adipocytes in diet-induced obese mice, and rimonabant increases adiponectin, a fat cell hormone associated with insulin sensitivity (18–21), suggesting peripheral as well as central effects of this drug.

Rimonabant Weight Loss and Reversal of the Metabolic Syndrome. The results of four phase-III trials of rimonabant for the treatment of overweight have been presented and published. The first trial, called the Rimonabant in Obesity (RIO)-Europe trial, was reported in 2005 (22) and typifies the results. A total of 1,057 patients with a BMI > 30 kg/m2 without co-morbidities or >27 kg/m^2 with hypertension or dyslipidemia were stratified on whether they lost more or less than 2 kg during run-in and then randomized in a ratio of 1 : 2 : 2 to receive placebo, rimonabant 5 mg/d, or rimonabant 20 mg/d. The energy content of the diet was calculated by subtracting 600 kcal/d from the energy requirements calculated from the Harris-Benedict equation. The trial consisted of a 4-week run-in period followed by 52 weeks of treatment. Of those who started, 61% (920) completed the first year. Weight loss was 2% in the placebo group and 8.5% in the 20 mg rimonabant group. Baseline weight was between 98.5 kg (placebo group) and 102.0 kg (for the rimonabant 20 mg dose). During run-in there was a mean −1.9 kg weight loss. From baseline at the end of run-in, only among those in each group who completed the trial, those on placebos lost an additional −2.3 kg; the low-dose rimonabant group lost −3.6 kg; and the high-dose group lost −8.6 kg. On an intent-to-treat (ITT-LOCF) basis, these numbers were a weight loss of −1.8 kg for the placebo group, −3.4 kg for the 5 mg/d, and -6.6 kg for the 20 mg/d group. Expressing the data as a responder analysis, the authors reported that 30.5% of the placebo group lost 5% or more, compared to 44.2% for the 5 mg/d and 67.4% for the 20 mg/d dose of rimonabant. A weight loss of 10% or more was achieved in 12.4% of the placebo group, 15.3% of the 5 mg/d group, and 39% of the 20 mg/d dose of rimonabant. Waist circumference was also reduced by treatment. Using the ITT analysis, waist declined 2.4 cm in the placebo group, 3.9 cm in the 5 mg/d group, and 6.5 cm with the 20 mg/d dose. Triglycerides were reduced by 6.8% in the 20 mg/d group compared to a rise of 8.3% in the placebo group. HDL cholesterol increased by 22.3% in the 20 mg/d group compared to 13.4% in the placebo group. These changes in metabolic parameters were reflected in a change in the prevalence of the metabolic syndrome. Among the completers there was a 33.9% reduction in the prevalence of the metabolic syndrome, compared to 34.8% in the 5 mg/d dose group and 64.8% in the 20 mg/d rimonabant dose group. In the 20 mg/d group, the LDL particle size increased, adiponectin increased, glucose decreased, insulin decreased, C-reactive protein decreased, and the metabolic syndrome prevalence was cut in half. There was no significant change in blood pressure or pulse between groups.

The metabolic syndrome also improved during treatment of rimonanbant. The prevalence of the metabolic syndrome was about 50% in the clinical trials with this drug. In the placebo groups after one year of treatment, the metabolic syndrome was still present in 53% of the subjects in the RIO-Europe study (22), 51% of those in the RIO lipids study (23), and 38% of those in the RIO–North America study (24). Substantial decreases occurred in the rimonabant treatment groups. For the RIO-Europe and RIO-lipids group, only 21% still had the metabolic syndrome, a 60% decrease. For the RIO–North America group it was 7.9%, a decrease of almost 60% (22–24).

ORLISTAT

Orlistat is a drug that blocks pancreatic lipase in the intestine and thus reduces the digestion of triglycerides. In people eating a 30% fat diet, orlistat reduced the digestion of fat by about 30% at the currently recommended dose.

Orlistat, Weight Loss, and Reversal of the Metabolic Syndrome. A number of 1- to 2-year long-term clinical trials with orlistat have been published. The study reported by Sjostrom et al. (25) consisted of two parts. In the first year, patients received a hypocaloric diet calculated to be 500 kcal per day less than the patient's requirements. During the second year, the diet was calculated to maintain body weight. By the end of year 1, the placebo-treated patients lost −6.1% of their initial body weight and the drug-treated patients lost −10.2%. The patients were randomized again at the end of year 1. Those switched from orlistat to placebo gained weight from −10% to −6% below baseline. Those switched from placebo to orlistat lost weight from −6% to −8.1% below baseline, which was essentially identical to the −7.9% loss in the patients treated with orlistat for the full 2 years.

Orlistat and the Metabolic Syndrome. Orlistat also improved features of the metabolic syndrome. For this analysis, patients who had participated in previously reported studies were divided into the highest and lowest quintiles for triglyceride and HDL cholesterol levels (26). Those with high triglyceride and low HDL cholesterol levels were labeled "syndrome X," and those with the lowest triglyceride levels and highest HDL cholesterol levels were the "nonsyndrome X" controls. In this classification, there were almost no men in the nonsyndrome X group, compared with an equal sex breakdown in the syndrome X group. In addition, the syndrome X group had slightly higher systolic and diastolic blood pressure levels and a nearly twofold higher level of fasting insulin. The subgroup with syndrome X showed a significantly greater decrease in triglyceride and insulin levels than those without syndrome X. Levels of HDL cholesterol increased more in the syndrome X group, but LDL cholesterol levels showed a smaller decrease than in the nonsyndrome X group.

All of the clinical studies with orlistat have shown significant decreases in serum cholesterol and LDL cholesterol levels that usually are greater than can be accounted for by weight loss alone (27). One study showed that orlistat reduces the absorption of cholesterol from the GI tract, thus providing a mechanism for the clinical observations (28).

Orlistat in Diabetics. Diabetes is a cardiovascular risk factor in its own right, and there is debate about whether to include it in the concept of a metabolic syndrome. However, orlistat, like other weight-loss medications, can improve diabetes as well as the metabolic syndrome. Patients with diabetes treated with orlistat, 120 mg three times daily for 1 year, lost more weight than the placebo-treated group (29–31). The subjects with diabetes also showed a significantly greater decrease in hemoglobin A1c levels. In another study of orlistat and weight loss, investigators pooled data on 675 subjects from three of the 2-year studies described previously in which glucose tolerance tests were available (32). During treatment, 6.6% of the patients taking orlistat converted from a normal to an impaired glucose tolerance test, compared with 10.8% in the

Table 4.4
Effect of Sibutramine and Orlistat on Lipids and Blood Pressure

Variable	Sibutramine	Orlistat
Cholesterol (nmol/L)	0.01 (−0.15 to 0.18)	−0.34 (−0.41 to −0.27)
LDL-cholesterol (nmol/L)	−0.08 (−0.23 to 0.07)	−0.29 (0.34 to −0.24)
HDL-cholesterol (nmol/L)	**0.10 (0.04 to 0.15)**	**−0.03 (−0.05 to −0.01)**
Triglycerides (nmol/L)	**−0.16 (−0.26 to −0.05)**	0.03 (−0.04 to 0.10)
Systolic blood pressure	1.16 (−0.60 to 2.93)	**−2.02 (−2.87 to −1.17)**
Diastolic blood pressure	**2.04 (0.89 to 3.20)**	**−1.64 (−2.20 to −1.09)**

Effect size from a meta-analysis (adapted from Avenell, ref. 35). Significant differences are highlighted in bold.

placebo-treated group. None of the orlistat-treated patients who originally had normal glucose tolerance developed diabetes, compared with 1.2% in the placebo-treated group. Of those who initially had normal glucose tolerance, 7.6% in the placebo group but only 3% in the orlistat-treated group developed diabetes. The effect of orlistat in preventing diabetes has been assessed in a four-year study (33). In this trial, body weight was reduced by 2.8 kg (95% CI 1.1 to 4.5 kg) compared to placebo, and the conversion rate of diabetes was reduced from 9% to 6% for a relative risk reduction of 0.63 (95% CI 0.46 to 0.86) (34).

Orlistat and Lipids and Blood Pressure. A comparison of the effects of orlistat and sibutramine on lipids and blood pressure is shown in Table 4.4. These data are from a meta-analysis by Avenell et al. (35). The significant changes have been bolded. It can be seen that orlistat slightly lowered HDL-cholesterol, but had significant positive effects on blood pressure with a −2.02/−1.64 mmHg change during 1 year of treatment. In contrast, sibutramine (discussed below) produced a significant reduction in triglycerides and a significant increase in HDL-cholesterol but also increased blood pressure by 1.16/2.04 mmHg on average. Thus a reduction in the metabolic syndrome with sibutramine would depend on a decrease in waist circumference and improved atherogenic lipid profile.

SIBUTRAMINE

Sibutramine is a serotonin-norepinephrine reuptake inhibitor that reduces food intake in experimental animals and human beings.

Weight Loss. Sibutramine has been evaluated extensively in several multicenter trials lasting 6–24 months. In a 6-month dose-ranging study of 1,047 patients, 67% treated with sibutramine achieved a 5% weight loss from baseline, and 35% lost 10% or more. There was a clear dose-response effect in this 24-week trial, and patients regained weight when the drug was stopped, indicating that the drug remained effective when used (36). Although sibutramine improves lipid profiles and reduces waist circumference, and thus central adiposity, it does not lower blood pressure, and in most studies increases blood pressure, particularly diastolic blood pressure, as well as pulse rate.

In a 1-year trial of 456 patients who received sibutramine (10 mg or 15 mg per day) or placebo, 56% of those who stayed in the trial for 12 months lost at least 5% of their initial body weight, and 30% of the patients lost 10% of their initial body weight while taking the 10-mg dose (37).

Maintenance of Weight Loss. Three trials have assessed the value of using sibutramine to prevent regain of body weight. In the first multicenter trial, participants were initially given a very-low-calorie diet (VLCD) for 6 weeks to induce weight loss (38). Of the initial 181 subjects enrolled, 142 were randomized to either 10 mg/d of sibutramine or placebo after losing −6 kg or more on the VLCD. After another 12 months, those receiving the drug had lost an additional −6.4 kg compared to a small weight gain of +0.2 kg for those receiving placebo. The authors concluded that sibutramine had effectively enhanced the initial weight loss and maintained it for an additional 12 months.

The second weight maintenance trial was the Sibutramine Trial of Obesity Reduction and Maintenance (STORM) (39). Patients were initially enrolled in an open-label phase and treated with 10 mg per day of sibutramine for 6 months. Of the patients who lost more than −8 kg, two-thirds were then randomized to sibutramine and one-third to placebo. During the 18-month double-blind phase of this trial, the placebo-treated patients steadily regained weight, maintaining only 20% of their weight loss at the end of the trial. In contrast, the subjects treated with sibutramine maintained their weight for 12 months and then regained an average of only 2 kg, thus maintaining 80% of their initial weight loss after 2 years (39). Despite the higher weight loss with sibutramine at the end of the 18 months of controlled observation, the blood pressure levels of the sibutramine-treated patients were still higher than in the patients treated with placebo. Again, waist circumference and lipids improved, but blood pressure did not.

In the final multicenter trial for weight maintenance, patients were initially treated in a hospital outpatient setting before referral to their primary care physicians. A total of 221 patients began the very-low-calorie diet (VLCD) phase. Of these patients, 189 lost the required −10 kg or more during 3 months and were randomized to sibutramine 10 mg/d or placebo for the remaining 15 months. Mean weight loss during the VLCD period for the successful subjects was 14.5% from baseline. Following 2 additional months of treatment in the hospital clinic, the final 13 months were conducted in the GP's offices. At 18 months, the odds ratio was 1.76 (95% CI 1.06, 2.93) favoring weight loss with sibutramine ($p = 0.03$). Using the intent-to-treat analysis, >80% of the weight loss at the end of the VLCD was maintained by 70%, 51%, and 30% of those on sibutramine at 6, 12, and 18 months compared to 48%, 31%, and 20% for those receiving placebo and these differences were significant at all time points ($p \leq 0.03$) (40).

Sibutramine in Diabetic Patients. A number of studies have examined the effect of sibutramine in diabetic patients. In a 3-month (12-week) trial, diabetic patients who were treated with 15 mg/d of sibutramine lost −2.4 kg (2.8%), compared with −0.1 kg (0.12%) in the placebo group (41). In this study, hemoglobin A1c levels decreased 0.3% in the drug-treated group and remained stable in the placebo group. Fasting glucose values decreased 0.3 mg/dL in the drug-treated patients and increased 1.4 mg/dL in the placebo-treated group. In a 24-week trial, the dose of sibutramine was increased from 5 mg to 20 mg per day over 6 weeks (42). Among those who completed the treatment, weight loss was −4.3 kg (4.3%) in the sibutramine-treated patients, compared with

−0.3 kg (0.3%) in placebo-treated patients. Hemoglobin A1C levels decreased 1.67% in the drug-treated group, compared with 0.53% in the placebo-treated group. These changes in glucose and hemoglobin A1C levels were expected from the amount of weight loss associated with drug treatment. In a 12-month multicenter, randomized placebo-controlled study (43), 194 diabetics receiving metformin were assigned to placebo ($N = 64$), sibutramine 15 mg/d ($N = 68$), or sibutramine 20 mg/d ($N = 62$). At 12 months, weight loss in the 15 mg/d group was $−5.5 \pm 0.6$ kg, and in the 20 mg/d group it was $−8.0 \pm 0.9$ kg compared to 0.2 ± 0.5 kg in the placebo group. Glycemic control improved in parallel with weight loss. Sibutramine raised sitting diastolic blood pressure by more than 5 mmHg in 43% of those receiving 15 mg/d of sibutramine compared to 25% for the placebo group ($P < 0.05$). Pulse rate increased more than 10 beats/minute in 42% of those on sibutramine, compared to 17% for those on placebo.

The final trial in diabetics that I will discuss here lasted 2 years (44). It was a double-blind, randomized placebo-controlled trial that had a crossover for the control group after the first year. The treatment group received sibutramine 10 mg/d for the entire 2 years. In addition, they had a portion-controlled diet used for 7 days at the end of each 2 months. There was a significantly greater weight loss in the drug-treated group that reached −9.7 kg at 12 months, compared to −1.6 kg in the placebo-treated group. During the second year, those receiving sibutramine continuously regained weight slowly rising to a maximal loss of −6.3 kg at 24 months. In contrast, the group that got sibutramine during the second year weighed less at 24 months than those receiving sibutramine continuously (−6.3 kg in continuous treatment vs. −9.7 kg for the crossover group). There was an improvement in diabetic control associated with the weight loss.

A meta-analysis of eight studies in diabetic patients receiving sibutramine (45) that examined changes in body weight, waist circumference, glucose, hemoglobin A1c, tri-glycerides, and HDL-cholesterol favored sibutramine. The mean weight loss was $−5.53 \pm 2.2$ for those treated with sibutramine and $−0.90 \pm 0.17$ for the placebo-treated patients. There was no significant change in systolic blood pressure, but diastolic blood pressure was significantly higher in the sibutramine-treated patients (45). In the meta-analysis by Norris et al. (46), the net weight loss over 12–26 weeks in 4 trials including 391 diabetics was −4.5 kg (95% CI −7.2 to −1.8 kg).

Surgery

Surgical intervention is the most drastic method of producing weight loss, but one of the most effective. In the following sections I will examine the effects of this surgery on components of the metabolic syndrome and will discuss two types of surgery for weight loss, one of which improves the features of the metabolic syndrome and another that does not.

LAPAROSCOPIC PLACEMENT OF A GASTRIC BAND

One randomized clinical trial compared intensive medical management versus lapa-roscopic insertion of an adjustable gastric band (LAP-BAND system). Included in the trial were individuals who had a BMI between 30 and 35 kg/m^2, who also had co-morbid conditions such as hypertension, dyslipidemia, diabetes, obstructive sleep apnea, or gastroesophageal reflux disease, severe physical limitations, or clinically significant psychosocial problems. The intensive medical program consisted of a very-low-calorie (energy) diet and behavior modification for 12 weeks, followed by a transition phase over 4 weeks combining some VLCD meals with 120 mg of orlistat and then orlistat 120 mg before all meals. Surgery was performed by two surgeons. Of the 40 patients in each group, one withdrew before surgery, leaving 39 at the end of 2 years. Seven dropped out of the intensive intervention, leaving 33 patients who completed treatment. Both groups had an identical 13.8% weight loss at 6 months. The surgical group continued to lose weight and were 21.6% below baseline at 2 years. The nonsurgical group regained weight from 6 to 24 months, at which time they were on average 5.5% below baseline weight. At 2 years, the surgically treated group had significantly greater improvements in diastolic blood pressure, fasting plasma glucose level, insulin sensitivity index, and HD-cholesterol level. Quality of life improved more in the surgical group. Physical function, vitality, and mental health domains of the SF-36 were improved in the surgical group. Thus laparoscopic insertion of an adjustable gastric band may be beneficial to patients at high risk for diabetes or sleep apnea with body mass index in the range of 30 to 35 kg/m^2, which is below those usually recommended for this procedure (47).

The Swedish Obese Subjects Trial

The Swedish Obese Subjects (SOS) Trial is a second controlled, but nonrandomized, trial directly comparing surgical and nonsurgical treatment for obesity, and is the largest trial comparing surgical versus medical treatment of excessive weight (48–51). A total of 6,328 obese (BMI > 34 for men and >38 kg/m^2 for women) subjects were recruited, of whom 2,010 underwent surgery for obesity (gastric banding, gastroplasty, or gastric bypass) while 2,037 chose conventional treatment. Operated participants were matched on a number of criteria to a group of 6,322 overweight men and women in the SOS registry who were not operated on. The SOS study began in 1987. Prior to surgery there were an average of 7.6 weight-loss attempts for the men and 18.2 for the women. The mean for the largest weight loss prior to surgery was 17.7 kg for the men and 18.2 kg for the women, but they were able to maintain this for only 7 to 10 months.

The incidence of other medical complications was also reduced. There was a linear reduction in the systolic and diastolic blood pressure with the degree of weight loss (52) and the odds ratio (OR) for incident hypertension was 0.38. Triglyceride and insulin levels also showed a linear decrease with weight loss (OR 0.28 for hypertriglyceridemia), and there was a marked reduction in the incidence of new cases of diabetes in the surgically treated groups. The concentration of HDL-cholesterol increased linearly with weight loss (OR 0.28), but cholesterol did not decline significantly until weight loss had exceeded 25 kg (OR 1.24) (53).

Liposuction and Omentectomy

Liposuction and the Metabolic Syndrome. Liposuction, which is also known as *lipoplasty* or *suction-assisted lipectomy*, is the most common esthetic procedure performed in the United States, with over 400,000 cases performed annually (54). Although liposuction is not generally considered to be a bariatric procedure, removal of fat by aspiration after injection of physiologic saline has been used to diminish and contour subcutaneous fat. As the techniques have improved it is now possible to remove significant amounts of subcutaneous adipose tissue without affecting the amount of visceral fat. In a study to examine the effects of this procedure, Klein et al. (54) studied 7 overweight diabetic women and 8 overweight women with normal glucose tolerance before and after liposuction. One week after assessing insulin sensitivity, the subjects underwent large-volume tumescent liposuction, which consists of removing more than 4 liters of aspirate injected into the fat beneath the skin. There was a significant loss of subcutaneous fat, as expected, but no change in the visceral fat. Subjects were reassessed 10–12 weeks after the surgery, when the nondiabetic women had lost −6.3 kg of body weight and −9.1 kg of body fat, which reduced body fat by −6.3%. The diabetic women had a similar response, with a weight loss of −7.9 kg, a reduction in body fat of −10.5 kg, and reduction in percent fat of −6.7%. Waist circumference was also significantly reduced. In spite of these significant reductions in body fat and waist circumference, there were no improvements in blood pressure, lipids, or cytokines (tumor necrosis factor-a, interleukin-6) or C-reactive protein. There was also no improvement in insulin sensitivity, suggesting that removal of subcutaneous adipose tissue without reducing visceral fat has little influence on the risk factors related to being overweight.

Omentectomy and the Metabolic Syndrome. Omentectomy is the direct removal of the intraabdominal fat by surgical means. One randomized controlled trial in 50 overweight subjects compared the effect of an adjustable lap-band alone with a lap-band plus removal of the omentum (55). Of the original 50 operated patients, 37 were reevaluated at the end of 2 years after the surgery. The reduction in body weight was 27 kg in the lap-band group and 36 kg in the lap-band + omentectomy group ($p = 0.07$). Both glucose and insulin improved more in the subjects with omentectomy than in those without it, which may be in part due to the greater weight loss. This study complements the one by Klein described earlier by showing that removal of extra visceral fat can have a small but significant effect, while decreasing subcutaneous fat alone without dietary restriction or other procedures to reduce visceral fat has little impact.

HORMONAL INFLUENCES ON CENTRAL ADIPOSITY

Several hormones directly affect visceral fat. They include growth hormone (GH), testosterone, dehydroepiandrosterone (DHEA), and cortisol.

Growth Hormone

Chronic treatment with growth hormone reduces the visceral fat compartment more than the subcutaneous one (56–58). In a one-year study, body weight decreased 1.2 kg in the GH-treated group compared to 0.9 kg in the placebo-treated group (56). This was accompanied by a decrease of 1.5 kg of body fat in the GH-treated subjects compared to 1.0 kg in the placebo group. Subcutaneous adipose tissue increased 1.8 cm^2 and VAT decreased −6.6 cm^2 in the GH-treated group compared with a decrease of −0.4 cm2 in SAT and an increase of 11 cm^2 in the VAT compartment in the placebo-group. This differential effect on VAT and SAT suggests that these two compartments have different hormonal controls for maintaining their mass.

Testosterone and Anabolic Steroids

Testosterone and anabolic steroids affect visceral fat more than subcutaneous fat. Plasma testosterone declines with age (59,60). It also decreases with obesity and with the number of features of the metabolic syndrome that are present (61). In a study of older men with low levels of testosterone, Marin et al. (62) applied testosterone, dihydrotestosterone, or placebo cream to the arms of overweight men for 9 months and measured their visceral fat by computed tomography before and after treatment. The placebo- and dihydrotestosterone-treated groups showed no change in body weight and a small increase in visceral and subcutaneous fat. In contrast, among the testosterone-treated group whose weight also did not change much, visceral fat was significantly reduced by −9.3 % and subcutaneous fat by −6.1 %. The men treated with testosterone also showed an improvement in insulin sensitivity using the glucose-clamp technique (62).

A second weight-loss study using anabolic steroids reached similar conclusions (63).

Dehydroepiandrosterone

A study with dehydroepiandrosterone (DHEA) was also conducted in older men and women. Fifty-six elderly men and women aged 65–78 years were randomly assigned to either placebo or 50 mg/d of DHEA for 6 months. Compliance with the intervention was 97%. After 6 months of treatment, body weight declined by −0.9 kg in the DHEA-treated group compared with a small gain of +0.6 kg in the placebo-treated group. Visceral fat decreased by −13 cm^2 in the DHEA-treated group corresponding to 10.2% reduction for women and 7.4% for men, compared with a small gain of +0.3 cm^2 ($p < 0.001$) in the placebo-treated group. There were similar changes in subcutaneous fat (−13 cm^2 in the DHEA group and +2 cm^2 in the placebo group, $p < 0.003$). The insulin response after an oral-glucose tolerance test was improved in the DHEA group and glucose response was unchanged, indicating improved insulin sensitivity after treatment with DHEA (64). Thus DHEA can have significant effects on visceral fat.

Cortisol

Cortisol also affects visceral fat. Following treatment of Cushing's Disease, a disease that results from excess secretion of cortisol from the adrenal gland, visceral adipose tissue decreased by 37% and subcutaneous adipose tissue by 33% (65). In experimental animals, manipulation of the genes that metabolize cortisol has significant effects on the visceral adipose tissue.

Evidence from experimental animals even suggests that increasing visceral fat may reflect altered metabolism of cortisol by visceral fat cells. When cortisol dehydrogenase type 1 is overexpressed in fat of mice, the rate of conversion from the inactive steroid cortisone to the active cortisol form is increased (66) and this is accompanied by an increase in visceral adipose tissue in these animals. Overactivity of this enzyme that produces cortisol has been suggested as a cause of centrally deposited fat in human beings.

CONCLUSION

The discussion in this chapter has shown that weight loss using many strategies can decrease visceral fat (central adiposity) and other components of the metabolic syndrome. It has also shown that a variety of strategies, mainly hormonal, can change visceral fat differentially from subcutaneous fat. The clear demonstration from the liposuction, which removes only subcutaneous fat and did not improve the metabolic risk factors in either obese or obese-diabetic women, indicates the importance of strategies that will reduce visceral fat as a requirement for improvements in the metabolic components of the metabolic syndrome.

REFERENCES

 1. Stamler J, Wentworth D, Neaton JD. Is relationship between serum cholesterol and risk of premature death from coronary heart disease continuous and graded? Findings in 356,222 primary screenees of the Multiple Risk Factor Intervention Trial (MRFIT). *JAMA* 1986; 256:2823–2828.
 2. Wilson PW, Castelli WP, Kannel WB. Coronary risk prediction in adults (the Framingham Heart Study). *Am J Cardiol* 1987; 59:91G–94G.
 3. Yusuf S, Hawken S, Ounpuu S, Bautista L, Franzosi MG, Commerford P et al. Obesity and the risk of myocardial infarction in 27,000 participants from 52 countries: A case-control study. *Lancet* 2005; 366:1640–1649.
 4. Kahn R, Buse J, Ferrannini E, Stern M. The metabolic syndrome—time for a critical appraisal: Joint statement from the American Diabetes Association and the European Association for the Study of Diabetes. *Diabetes Care* 2005; 28:2289–2304.
 5. Executive summary of the third report of the National Cholesterol Education Program (NCEP) Expert Panel on Detection, Evaluation, and Treatment of High Blood Cholesterol in Adults (Adult Treatment Panel III). *JAMA* 2001; 285:2486–2497.
 6. Bouchard C, Despres JP, Mauriege P. Genetic and nongenetic determinants of regional fat distribution. *Endocr Rev* 1993; 14:72–93.
 7. Smith SR, Zachwieja JJ. Visceral adipose tissue: A critical review of intervention strategies. *Int J Obes Relat Metab Disord* 1999; 23:329–335.
 8. Orchard TJ, Temprosa M, Goldberg R, Haffner S, Ratner R, Marcovina S et al. The effect of metformin and intensive lifestyle intervention on the metabolic syndrome: The Diabetes Prevention Program randomized trial. *Ann Intern Med* 2005; 142:611–619.
 9. Ford ES, Giles WH. A comparison of the prevalence of the metabolic syndrome using two proposed definitions. *Diabetes Care* 2003; 26:575–581.
10. Fujimoto WY. Background and recruitment data for the U.S. Diabetes Prevention Program. *Diabetes Care* 2000; 23(suppl 2):B11–13.
11. Bouchard C, Tremblay A, Despres JP, Theriault G, Nadeau A, Lupien PJ et al. The response to exercise with constant energy intake in identical twins. *Obes Res* 1994; 2:400–410.
12. Wood PD, Stefanick ML, Dreon DM, Frey-Hewitt B, Garay SC, Williams PT et al. Changes in plasma lipids and lipoproteins in overweight men during weight loss through dieting as compared with exercise. *N Engl J Med* 1988; 319:1173–1179.
13. Dattilo AM, Kris-Etherton PM. Effects of weight reduction on blood lipids and lipoproteins: A meta-analysis. *Am J Clin Nutr* 1992; 56:320–328.
14. Appel LJ, Moore TJ, Obarzanek E, Vollmer WM, Svetkey LP, Sacks FM et al. A clinical trial of the effects of dietary patterns on blood pressure: DASH Collaborative Research Group. *N Engl J Med* 1997; 336:1117–1124.
15. Sacks FM, Svetkey LP, Vollmer WM, Appel LJ, Bray GA, Harsha D et al. Effects on blood pressure of reduced dietary sodium and the Dietary Approaches to Stop Hypertension (DASH) diet: DASH-Sodium Collaborative Research Group. *N Engl J Med* 2001; 344:3–10.
16. Bray GA, Vollmer WM, Sacks FM, Obarzanek E, Svetkey LP, Appel LJ. A further subgroup analysis of the effects of the DASH diet and three dietary sodium levels on blood pressure: Results of the DASH-Sodium Trial. *Am J Cardiol* 2004; 94:222–227.
17. Stevens VJ, Obarzanek E, Cook NR, Lee IM, Appel LJ, Smith West D et al. Long-term weight loss and changes in blood pressure: Results of the Trials of Hypertension Prevention, phase II. *Ann Intern Med*. 2001; 134:1–11.
18. Bensaid M, Gary-Bobo M, Esclangon A, Maffrand JP, Le Fur G, Oury-Donat F et al. The cannabinoid CB1 receptor antagonist SR141716 increases Acrp30 mRNA expression in adipose tissue of obese fa/fa rats and in cultured adipocyte cells. *Mol Pharmacol* 2003; 63:908–914.
19. Pagotto U, Marsicano G, Cota D, Lutz B, Pasquali R. The emerging role of the endocannabinoid system in endocrine regulation and energy balance. *Endocr Rev* 2006; 27:73–100.
20. Kirkham TC. Endocannabinoids in the regulation of appetite and body weight. *Behav Pharmacol* 2005; 16:297–313.

21. Juan-Pico P, Fuentes E, Javier Bermudez-Silva F, Javier Diaz-Molina F, Ripoll C, Rodriguez de Fonseca F et al. Cannabinoid receptors regulate Ca(2+) signals and insulin secretion in pancreatic beta-cell. *Cell Calcium* 2006; 39:155–162.
22. Van Gaal LF, Rissanen AM, Scheen AJ, Ziegler O, Rossner S. Effects of the cannabinoid-1 receptor blocker rimonabant on weight reduction and cardiovascular risk factors in overweight patients: One-year experience from the RIO-Europe study. *Lancet* 2005; 365:1389–1397.
23. Despres JP, Golay A, Sjostrom L. Effects of rimonabant on metabolic risk factors in overweight patients with dyslipidemia. *N Engl J Med* 2005; 353:2121–2134.
24. Pi-Sunyer FX, Aronne LJ, Heshmati HM, Devin J, Rosenstock J. Effect of rimonabant, a cannabinoid-1 receptor blocker, on weight and cardiometabolic risk factors in overweight or obese patients: RIO–North America—a randomized controlled trial. *JAMA* 2006; 295:761–775.
25. Sjostrom L, Rissanen A, Andersen T, Boldrin M, Golay A, Koppeschaar HP et al. Randomised placebo-controlled trial of orlistat for weight loss and prevention of weight regain in obese patients: European Multicentre Orlistat Study Group. *Lancet* 1998; 352:167–172.
26. Reaven G, Segal K, Hauptman J, Boldrin M, Lucas C. Effect of orlistat-assisted weight loss in decreasing coronary heart disease risk in patients with syndrome X. *Am J Cardiol* 2001; 87:827–831.
27. Bray GA, Greenway FL. Current and potential drugs for treatment of obesity. *Endocr Rev* 1999; 20:805–875.
28. Mittendorfer B, Ostlund RE Jr., Patterson BW, Klein S. Orlistat inhibits dietary cholesterol absorption. *Obes Res* 2001; 9:599–604.
29. Hollander PA, Elbein SC, Hirsch IB, Kelley D, McGill J, Taylor T et al. Role of orlistat in the treatment of obese patients with type 2 diabetes: A 1-year randomized double-blind study. *Diabetes Care* 1998; 21:1288–1294.
30. Kelley DE, Bray GA, Pi-Sunyer FX, Klein S, Hill J, Miles J et al. Clinical efficacy of orlistat therapy in overweight and obese patients with insulin-treated type 2 diabetes: A 1-year randomized controlled trial. *Diabetes Care* 2002; 25:1033–1041.
31. Miles JM, Leiter L, Hollander P, Wadden T, Anderson JW, Doyle M et al. Effect of orlistat in overweight and obese patients with type 2 diabetes treated with metformin. *Diabetes Care* 2002; 25:1123–1128.
32. Heymsfield SB, Segal KR, Hauptman J, Lucas CP, Boldrin MN, Rissanen A et al. Effects of weight loss with orlistat on glucose tolerance and progression to type 2 diabetes in obese adults. *Arch Intern Med* 2000; 160:1321–1326.
33. Torgerson JS, Hauptman J, Boldrin MN, Sjostrom L. XENical in the prevention of diabetes in obese subjects (XENDOS) study: A randomized study of orlistat as an adjunct to lifestyle changes for the prevention of type 2 diabetes in obese patients. *Diabetes Care* 2004; 27:155–161.
34. Padwal R, Majumdar SR, Johnson JA, Varney J, McAlister FA. A systematic review of drug therapy to delay or prevent type 2 diabetes. *Diabetes Care* 2005; 28:736–744.
35. Avenell A, Broom J, Brown TJ, Poobalan A, Aucott L, Stearns SC et al. Systematic review of the long-term effects and economic consequences of treatments for obesity and implications for health improvement. *Health Technol Assess* 2004; 8:iii–iv, 1–182.
36. Bray GA, Blackburn GL, Ferguson JM, Greenway FL, Jain AK, Mendel CM et al. Sibutramine produces dose-related weight loss. *Obes Res* 1999; 7:189–198.
37. Smith IG, Goulder MA. Randomized placebo-controlled trial of long-term treatment with sibutramine in mild to moderate obesity. *J Fam Pract* 2001; 50:505–512.
38. Apfelbaum M, Vague P, Ziegler O, Hanotin C, Thomas F, Leutenegger E. Long-term maintenance of weight loss after a very-low-calorie diet: A randomized blinded trial of the efficacy and tolerability of sibutramine. *Am J Med* 1999; 106:179–184.
39. James WP, Astrup A, Finer N, Hilsted J, Kopelman P, Rossner S et al. Effect of sibutramine on weight maintenance after weight loss: A randomised trial. STORM Study Group: Sibutramine trial of obesity reduction and maintenance. *Lancet* 2000; 356:2119–2125.
40. Mathus-Vliegen EM. Long-term maintenance of weight loss with sibutramine in a GP setting following a specialist guided very-low-calorie diet: A double-blind, placebo-controlled, parallel group study. *Eur J Clin Nutr* 2005; 59(suppl 1):S31–38; discussion S9.
41. Finer N, Bloom SR, Frost GS, Banks LM, Griffiths J. Sibutramine is effective for weight loss and diabetic control in obesity with type 2 diabetes: A randomised, double-blind, placebo-controlled study. *Diabetes Obes Metab* 2000; 2:105–112.

42. Fujioka K, Seaton TB, Rowe E, Jelinek CA, Raskin P, Lebovitz HE et al. Weight loss with sibutramine improves glycaemic control and other metabolic parameters in obese patients with type 2 diabetes mellitus. *Diabetes Obes Metab* 2000; 2:175–187.
43. McNulty SJ, Ur E, Williams G. A randomized trial of sibutramine in the management of obese type 2 diabetic patients treated with metformin. *Diabetes Care* 2003; 26:125–131.
44. Redmon JB, Reck KP, Raatz SK, Swanson JE, Kwong CA, Ji H et al. Two-year outcome of a combination of weight loss therapies for type 2 diabetes. *Diabetes Care* 2005; 28:1311–1315.
45. Vettor R, Serra R, Fabris R, Pagano C, Federspil G. Effect of sibutramine on weight management and metabolic control in type 2 diabetes: A meta-analysis of clinical studies. *Diabetes Care* 2005; 28:942–949.
46. Norris SL, Zhang X, Avenell A, Gregg E, Schmid CH, Kim C et al. Efficacy of pharmacotherapy for weight loss in adults with type 2 diabetes mellitus: A meta-analysis. *Arch Intern Med* 2004; 164:1395–1404.
47. O'Brien PE, Dixon JB, Laurie C, Skinner S, Proietto J, McNeil J et al. Treatment of mild to moderate obesity with laparoscopic adjustable gastric banding or an intensive medical program: A randomized trial. *Ann Intern Med* 2006; 144:625–633.
48. Sjostrom L, Lindroos AK, Peltonen M, Torgerson J, Bouchard C, Carlsson B et al. Lifestyle, diabetes, and cardiovascular risk factors 10 years after bariatric surgery. *N Engl J Med* 2004; 351:2683–2693.
49. Karlsson J, Sjostrom L, Sullivan M. Swedish obese subjects (SOS)—an intervention study of obesity: Two-year follow-up of health-related quality of life (HRQL) and eating behavior after gastric surgery for severe obesity. *Int J Obes Relat Metab Disord* 1998; 22:113–126.
50. Torgerson JS, Sjostrom L. The Swedish Obese Subjects (SOS) study: Rationale and results. *Int J Obes Relat Metab Disord* 2001; 25(suppl 1):S2–4.
51. Sjostrom L, Larsson B, Backman L, Bengtsson C, Bouchard C, Dahlgren S et al. Swedish obese subjects (SOS): Recruitment for an intervention study and a selected description of the obese state. *Int J Obes Relat Metab Disord* 1992; 16:465–479.
52. Sjostrom CD, Lissner L, Sjostrom L. Relationships between changes in body composition and changes in cardiovascular risk factors: The SOS Intervention Study (Swedish Obese Subjects). *Obes Res* 1997; 5:519–530.
53. Sjostrom CD, Lissner L, Wedel H, Sjostrom L. Reduction in incidence of diabetes, hypertension and lipid disturbances after intentional weight loss induced by bariatric surgery: The SOS Intervention Study. *Obes Res* 1999; 7:477–484.
54. Klein S, Fontana L, Young VL, Coggan AR, Kilo C, Patterson BW et al. Absence of an effect of liposuction on insulin action and risk factors for coronary heart disease. *N Engl J Med* 2004; 350:2549–2557.
55. Thorne A, Lonnqvist F, Apelman J, Hellers G, Arner P. A pilot study of long-term effects of a novel obesity treatment: Omentectomy in connection with adjustable gastric banding. *Int J Obes Relat Metab Disord* 2002; 26:193–199.
56. Franco C, Brandberg J, Lonn L, Andersson B, Bengtsson BA, Johannsson G. Growth hormone treatment reduces abdominal visceral fat in postmenopausal women with abdominal obesity: A 12-month placebo-controlled trial. *J Clin Endocrinol Metab* 2005; 90:1466–1474.
57. Hoffman AR, Kuntze JE, Baptista J, Baum HB, Baumann GP, Biller BM et al. Growth hormone (GH) replacement therapy in adult-onset gh deficiency: Effects on body composition in men and women in a double-blind, randomized, placebo-controlled trial. *J Clin Endocrinol Metab* 2004; 89:2048–2056.
58. Nam SY, Kim KR, Cha BS, Song YD, Lim SK, Lee HC et al. Low-dose growth hormone treatment combined with diet restriction decreases insulin resistance by reducing visceral fat and increasing muscle mass in obese type 2 diabetic patients. *Int J Obes Relat Metab Disord* 2001; 25:1101–1107.
59. Harman SM, Metter EJ, Tobin JD, Pearson J, Blackman MR. Longitudinal effects of aging on serum total and free testosterone levels in healthy men: Baltimore Longitudinal Study of Aging. *J Clin Endocrinol Metab* 2001; 86:724–731.
60. Feldman HA, Longcope C, Derby CA, Johannes CB, Araujo AB, Coviello AD et al. Age trends in the level of serum testosterone and other hormones in middle-aged men: Longitudinal results from the Massachusetts male aging study. *J Clin Endocrinol Metab* 2002; 87:589–598.
61. Meehan AG, Shah AK, Heymsfield SB. Obesity and the metabolic syndrome are associated with lower serum testosterone levels in aging men: What are the implications of this for the relatively high incidence of erectile dysfunction seen in these patients? *Obesity Reviews* 2006; 7(suppl 2):Abs.

62. Marin P, Holmang S, Gustafsson C, Jonsson L, Kvist H, Elander A et al. Androgen treatment of abdominally obese men. *Obes Res.* 1993; 1:245–251.
63. Lovejoy JC, Bray GA, Greeson CS, Klemperer M, Morris J, Partington C et al. Oral anabolic steroid treatment, but not parenteral androgen treatment, decreases abdominal fat in obese, older men. *Int J Obes Relat Metab Disord* 1995; 19:614–624.
64. Villareal DT, Holloszy JO. Effect of DHEA on abdominal fat and insulin action in elderly women and men: A randomized controlled trial. *JAMA* 2004; 292:2243–2248.
65. Lonn L, Kvist H, Ernest I, Sjostrom L. Changes in body composition and adipose tissue distribution after treatment of women with Cushing's syndrome. *Metabolism* 1994; 43:1517–1522.
66. Masuzaki H, Paterson J, Shinyama H, Morton NM, Mullins JJ, Seckl JR et al. A transgenic model of visceral obesity and the metabolic syndrome. *Science* 2001; 294:2166–2170.

5 Insulin Resistance, Metabolic Syndrome, and Cardiovascular Disease
An Epidemiological Perspective

Earl S. Ford and Simin Liu

CONTENTS

Insulin resistance has been defined as a state (of a cell, tissue, system, or body) in which greater-than-normal amounts of insulin are required to elicit a quantitatively normal response (1). The list of adverse events to which insulin resistance potentially contributes has grown as researchers have examined the critical links underlying these relationships. One of the most important of these is the increased risk from cardiovascular disease. The link between concentrations of insulin and coronary heart disease was first made in the late 1960s (2). Since then, a solid body of evidence that supports insulin resistance syndrome as a risk factor for cardiovascular disease has accumulated. In this chapter, the epidemiologic evidence linking insulin resistance to cardiovascular disease will be reviewed. The focus will be on prospective studies of mostly population samples.

INSULIN RESISTANCE AND SURROGATE MEASURES FOR INSULIN RESISTANCE

There are several "gold-standard" methods for measuring insulin resistance, including the hyperinsulinemic-euglycemic clamp technique, the frequently sampled intravenous glucose tolerance test, and the insulin infusion sensitivity test (3,4). Because of the technical and logistic requirements of performing these techniques, they have been

From: *Contemporary Endocrinology: The Metabolic Syndrome: Epidemiology, Clinical Treatment, and Underlying Mechanisms*
Edited by: B.C. Hansen and G.A. Bray © Humana Press, Totowa, NJ

One of the largest analyses of the association between insulin resistance and cardio-vascular disease was done in the context of the Diabetes Epidemiology: Collaborative Analysis of Diagnostic Criteria in Europe (DECODE) study (42). In 11 cohorts that included 6,156 men and 5,351 women aged 30–89 years who were followed for 8.8 years, the risk of dying from cardiovascular disease was higher among participants whose fasting plasma concentration of insulin was in the highest quartile compared with those whose concentration of insulin was in the lowest quartile (men: hazard ratio (HR) 1.54, 95% confidence interval (CI) = 1.16–2.03; women: HR = 2.66, 95% CI = 1.45–4.90). Results based on the use of HOMA were similar (men: HR = 1.58, 95% CI = 1.20–2.09; women: HR = 2.35, 95% CI = 1.27–4.37). However, concentrations of 2-hour insulin were not significantly associated with death from cardiovascular disease.

In addition, surrogate measures of insulin resistance have been linked prospectively to cardiovascular disease among people with type 1 diabetes (43), patients with type 2 diabetes (44,45), patients with end-stage renal disease (46), and patients with coronary artery disease (47).

THE METABOLIC SYNDROME AND CARDIOVASCULAR DISEASE

Interest in the metabolic syndrome, as judged by the number of publications listing the insulin resistance syndrome or the metabolic syndrome in their title, has increased tremendously since the late 1990s. The *metabolic syndrome*, which increasingly has become the preferred term among a dozen or so synonyms, constitutes a constellation of anthropometric, blood pressure, lipid, and glycemic abnormalities that occur more frequently than expected by chance. Based on these and other abnormalities, defining the metabolic syndrome has been a major challenge. Numerous attempts using factor analysis or related methods have been used to delineate an underlying structure among these variables (48,49). Such studies have in general identified 2 to 4 factors, with a factor that includes measures of central adiposity, dysglycemia, insulin resistance, hypertriglyceridemia, and low concentrations of high-density lipoprotein cholesterol accounting for the largest proportion of the variance (50). However, the use of factor analysis has been controversial (51).

Several major organizations have endorsed different definitions of the syndrome (52–56). Of relevance to this chapter is that insulin resistance is proposed by many as an important pathogenetic mechanism of the syndrome (57). However, insulin resistance measured by reference methods (hyperinsulinemic euglycemic clamp, frequently sampled intravenous glucose tolerance test, or insulin suppression test) has been shown to be present in only about 32% to 76% of people with the metabolic syndrome (58–61). However, the sensitivities range from 20% to 66%.

The major components (obesity, hypertriglyceridemia, low concentrations of high-density lipoprotein cholesterol, elevated blood pressure, dysglycemia, microalbumin-uria, insulin resistance) used in the definitions of the metabolic syndrome have all been associated with an increased risk for cardiovascular disease (57,62–69). This certainly suggested that people with the metabolic syndrome would be expected to be at increased risk for developing cardiovascular disease.

Over a dozen prospective studies have examined whether the metabolic syndrome is an independent risk factor for cardiovascular disease (70–74). In a meta-analysis of prospective studies, the presence of the metabolic syndrome conferred an increased risk of developing or dying from cardiovascular disease (National Cholesterol Education Program (NCEP) definition: summary RR = 1.65, 95% CI = 1.38–1.99; World Health Organization (WHO) definition: summary RR = 1.89, 95% CI = 1.50–2.37) (70). A more recent study conducted among 557 postmenopausal women followed for an average of 8.5 years of whom 36 died of cardiovascular disease reported that the presence of the metabolic syndrome increased the risk of dying from cardiovascular disease (HR = 3.2, 95% CI = 1.5–6.5) (71). However, in a study of Finnish men aged 70–89 years who were followed for 8 years, the percentage dying from cardiovascular disease did not differ significantly by status of metabolic syndrome (72). Over the course of about 11 years, the risk of fatal or nonfatal CVD was elevated among men, but not women, with the metabolic syndrome compared with those without the syndrome in the Hoorn Study (men: HR = 1.88, 95% CI = 1.28–2.86; women: 1.44, 95% CI = 0.95–2.19) (73). Finally, the metabolic syndrome was associated with an increased risk of incident coronary heart disease or stroke among 2,175 participants aged about 65 years of the Cardiovascular Health Study (median follow-up time of 4.1 years) (NCEP: HR = 2.04, 95% CI = 1.69–2.46; WHO: HR = 1.63, 95% CI = 1.33–2.01) (74). In addition, studies conducted among people with diabetes (75–78) or cardiovascular disease (78–80) have also reported increased adverse events among participants who had the metabolic syndrome compared with those who did not have this syndrome.

The impact of the metabolic syndrome on other cardiovascular disease parameters has been investigated. In a 3-year follow-up of 316 Swedish men aged 58 years, men with the metabolic syndrome experienced larger increases in carotid artery intima-media thickness than those without the syndrome (81). In a study of 901 Dutch patients who had a percutaneous coronary intervention, patients with the metabolic syndrome had a nonsignificantly elevated risk of dying from any cause or from cardiac-related causes during a median of 9.6 months of follow-up (82).

MECHANISMS

Insulin resistance has been linked to numerous risk factors for cardiovascular disease (83,84). Also, insulin resistance may reflect the combined influences of obesity, especially abdominal obesity, dietary patterns, and sedentary lifestyle. Numerous studies have linked hyperinsulinemia or insulin resistance to hypertension (85). Furthermore, insulin resistance results in dysglycemia, dyslipidemia, inflammation, and a prothrombotic environment.

In recent years, more is being learned about the relationships between insulin resistance, inflammation, and endothelial dysfunction (86–88). A growing body of research has linked insulin resistance to inflammation (89–91) that in turn contributes to the endothelial dysfunction seen in prediabetic states, diabetes, and cardiovascular disease (87). Under normal circumstances, insulin stimulates the production of nitric oxide by endothelial cells (92). However, the presence of insulin resistance and compensatory hyperinsulinemia promotes the interaction between endothelial cells with circulating leukocytes. Furthermore, the homeostatic effect of insulin on vascular smooth muscle cells is lost in insulin resistance. Finally, hyperinsulinemia in the presence of insulin resistance leads to increased activity of the farnesyltransferase and geranylgeranyltransferase.

SUMMARY

In summary, few studies prospectively relate insulin resistance measured with reference methods to cardiovascular events. The complexity of measuring insulin resistance using gold-standard methods in large numbers of people makes it unlikely that many such studies will be done. One such effort is currently being conducted by the European Group for the Study of Insulin Resistance (93). In contrast, quite a few studies have examined the associations between surrogate markers of insulin resistance and the incidence or mortality from cardiovascular disease. The majority of these studies reported significant associations between these markers and cardiovascular events, thus lending support to the notion that insulin resistance may be an independent risk factor for cardiovascular disease. Because the validity of these measures compared with gold-standard methods remains a matter of debate and because of the paucity of prospective studies measuring insulin resistance by reference methods, more research clarifying various aspects of the association between insulin resistance and cardiovascular disease is needed.

REFERENCES

1. Yalow RS, Berson SA. Dynamics of insulin secretion in early diabetes in humans. *Adv Metab Disord* 1970; 1(suppl 1):95ff.
2. Stout RW, Vallance-Owen J. Insulin and atheroma. *Lancet* 1969 May 31; 1(7605):1078–1080.
3. Wallace TM, Matthews DR. The assessment of insulin resistance in man. *Diabet Med* 2002; 19:527–534.
4. Monzillo LU, Hamdy O. Evaluation of insulin sensitivity in clinical practice and in research settings. *Nutr Rev* 2003; 61:397–412.
5. Yip J, Facchini FS, Reaven GM. Resistance to insulin-mediated glucose disposal as a predictor of cardiovascular disease. *J Clin Endocrinol Metab* 1998; 83:2773–2776.
6. Facchini FS, Hua N, Abbasi F, Reaven GM. Insulin resistance as a predictor of age-related diseases. *J Clin Endocrinol Metab* 2001; 86:3574–3578.
7. Nosadini R, Manzato E, Solini A, Fioretto P, Brocco E, Zambon S, Morocutti A, Sambataro M, Velussi M, Cipollina MR et al. Peripheral, rather than hepatic, insulin resistance and atherogenic lipoprotein phenotype predict cardiovascular complications in NIDDM. *Eur J Clin Invest* 1994; 24:258–266.
8. Shen SW, Reaven GM, Farquhar JW. Comparison of impedance to insulin-mediated glucose uptake in normal subjects and in subjects with latent diabetes. *J Clin Invest* 1970; 49:2151–2160.
9. Sherwin RS, Kramer KJ, Tobin JD, Insel PA, Liljenquist JE, Berman M, Andres R. A model of the kinetics of insulin in man. *J Clin Invest* 1974; 53:1481–1492.
10. DeFronzo RA, Tobin JD, Andres R. Glucose clamp technique: A method for quantifying insulin secretion and resistance. *Am J Physiol* 1979; 237:E214–223.
11. Bergman RN, Phillips LS, Cobelli C. Physiologic evaluation of factors controlling glucose tolerance in man: measurement of insulin sensitivity and beta-cell glucose sensitivity from the response to intravenous glucose. *J Clin Invest* 1981; 68:1456–1467.
12. Sluiter WJ, Erkelens DW, Terpstra P, Reitsma WD, Doorenbos H. Glucose tolerance and insulin release, a mathematical approach. II: Approximation of the peripheral insulin resistance after oral glucose loading. *Diabetes* 1976; 25:245–249.
13. Matthews DR, Hosker JP, Rudenski AS, Naylor BA, Treacher DF, Turner RC. Homeostasis model assessment: Insulin resistance and beta-cell function from fasting plasma glucose and insulin concentrations in man. *Diabetologia* 1985; 28:412–419.
14. Hosker JP, Matthews DR, Rudenski AS, Burnett MA, Darling P, Bown EG, Turner RC. Continuous infusion of glucose with model assessment: Measurement of insulin resistance and beta-cell function in man. *Diabetologia* 1985; 28:401–411.
15. Belfiore F, Iannello S, Camuto M, Fagone S, Cavaleri A. Insulin sensitivity of blood glucose versus insulin sensitivity of blood free fatty acids in normal, obese, and obese-diabetic subjects. *Metabolism* 2001; 50:573–582.

16. Laakso M. How good a marker is insulin level for insulin resistance? *Am J Epidemiol* 1993; 137:959–965.
17. Duncan MH, Singh BM, Wise PH, Carter G, Alaghband-Zadeh J. A simple measure of insulin resistance. *Lancet* 1995; 346:120–121.
18. Raynaud E, Perez-Martin A, Brun JF, Benhaddad AA, Mercier J. Revised concept for the estimation of insulin sensitivity from a single sample. *Diabetes Care* 1999; 22:1003–1004.
19. Katz A, Nambi SS, Mather K, Baron AD, Follmann DA, Sullivan G, Quon MJ. Quantitative insulin sensitivity check index: A simple, accurate method for assessing insulin sensitivity in humans. *J Clin Endocrinol Metab* 2000; 85:2402–2410.
20. Hanson RL, Pratley RE, Bogardus C, Narayan KM, Roumain JM, Imperatore G, Fagot-Campagna A, Pettitt DJ, Bennett PH, Knowler WC. Evaluation of simple indices of insulin sensitivity and insulin secretion for use in epidemiologic studies. *Am J Epidemiol* 2000; 151:190–198.
21. McAuley KA, Williams SM, Mann JI, Walker RJ, Lewis-Barned NJ, Temple LA, Duncan AW. Diagnosing insulin resistance in the general population. *Diabetes Care* 2001; 24:460–464.
22. Levine R, Haft DE. Carbohydrate homeostasis. *N Engl J Med* 1970 July 30; 283(5):237–246.
23. Cederholm J, Wibell L. Insulin release and peripheral sensitivity at the oral glucose tolerance test. *Diabetes Res Clin Pract* 1990; 10:167–175.
24. Avignon A, Boegner C, Mariano-Goulart D, Colette C, Monnier L. Assessment of insulin sensitivity from plasma insulin and glucose in the fasting or post oral glucose-load state. *Int J Obes Relat Metab Disord* 1999; 23:512–517.
25. Matsuda M, DeFronzo RA. Insulin sensitivity indices obtained from oral glucose tolerance testing: comparison with the euglycemic insulin clamp. *Diabetes Care* 1999; 22:1462–1470.
26. Gutt M, Davis CL, Spitzer SB, Llabre MM, Kumar M, Czarnecki EM, Schneiderman N, Skyler JS, Marks JB. Validation of the insulin sensitivity index (ISI(0,120)): Comparison with other measures. *Diabetes Res Clin Pract* 2000; 47:177–184.
27. Stumvoll M, Mitrakou A, Pimenta W, Jenssen T, Yki-Jarvinen H, Van Haeften T, Renn W, Gerich J. Use of the oral glucose tolerance test to assess insulin release and insulin sensitivity. *Diabetes Care* 2000; 23:295–301.
28. Mari A, Pacini G, Murphy E, Ludvik B, Nolan JJ. A model-based method for assessing insulin sensitivity from the oral glucose tolerance test. *Diabetes Care* 2001; 24:539–548.
29. Soonthornpun S, Setasuban W, Thamprasit A, Chayanunnukul W, Rattarasarn C, Geater A. Novel insulin sensitivity index derived from oral glucose tolerance test. *J Clin Endocrinol Metab* 2003; 88:1019–1023.
30. Ruige JB, Assendelft WJ, Dekker JM, Kostense PJ, Heine RJ, Bouter LM. Insulin and risk of cardiovascular disease: a meta-analysis. *Circulation* 1998; 97:996–1001.
31. Smiley T, Oh P, Shane LG. The relationship of insulin resistance measured by reliable indexes to coronary artery disease risk factors and outcomes–a systematic review. *Can J Cardiol* 2001; 17:797–805.
32. Folsom AR, Szklo M, Stevens J, Liao F, Smith R, Eckfeldt JH. A prospective study of coronary heart disease in relation to fasting insulin, glucose, and diabetes: The Atherosclerosis Risk in Communities (ARIC) Study. *Diabetes Care.* 1997; 20:935–942.
33. Folsom AR, Rasmussen ML, Chambless LE, Howard G, Cooper LS, Schmidt MI, Heiss G. Prospective associations of fasting insulin, body fat distribution, and diabetes with risk of ischemic stroke: The Atherosclerosis Risk in Communities (ARIC) Study Investigators. *Diabetes Care* 1999; 22:1077–1083.
34. Pyorala M, Miettinen H, Laakso M, Pyorala K. Hyperinsulinemia predicts coronary heart disease risk in healthy middle-aged men: The 22-year follow-up results of the Helsinki Policemen Study. *Circulation* 1998; 98:398–404.
35. Pyorala M, Miettinen H, Laakso M, Pyorala K. Hyperinsulinemia and the risk of stroke in healthy middle-aged men: The 22-year follow-up results of the Helsinki Policemen Study. *Stroke* 1998; 29:1860–1866.
36. Yarnell JW, Patterson CC, Bainton D, Sweetnam PM. Is metabolic syndrome a discrete entity in the general population? Evidence from the Caerphilly and Speedwell population studies. *Heart* 1998; 79:248–252.
37. Wannamethee SG, Perry IJ, Shaper AG. Nonfasting serum glucose and insulin concentrations and the risk of stroke. *Stroke* 1999; 30:1780–1786.

38. Hanley AJ, Williams K, Stern MP, Haffner SM. Homeostasis model assessment of insulin resistance in relation to the incidence of cardiovascular disease: The San Antonio Heart Study. *Diabetes Care* 2002; 25:1177–1184.
39. Resnick HE, Jones K, Ruotolo G, Jain AK, Henderson J, Lu W, Howard BV, Strong Heart Study. Insulin resistance, the metabolic syndrome, and risk of incident cardiovascular disease in nondiabetic American Indians: The Strong Heart Study. *Diabetes Care* 2003; 26:861–867.
40. Welin L, Bresater LE, Eriksson H, Hansson PO, Welin C, Rosengren A. Insulin resistance and other risk factors for coronary heart disease in elderly men: The Study of Men Born in 1913 and 1923. *Eur J Cardiovasc Prev Rehabil* 2003; 10:283–288.
41. Bataille V, Perret B, Troughton J, Amouyel P, Arveiler D, Woodside J, Dallongeville J, Haas B, Bingham A, Ducimetiere P, Ferrieres J. Fasting insulin concentrations and coronary heart disease incidence in France and Northern Ireland: The PRIME study. *Int J Cardiol* 2006; 108:189–196.
42. Hu G, Qiao Q, Tuomilehto J, Eliasson M, Feskens EJ, Pyorala K, DECODE Insulin Study Group. Plasma insulin and cardiovascular mortality in non-diabetic European men and women: A meta-analysis of data from eleven prospective studies. *Diabetologia* 2004; 47:1245–1256.
43. Orchard TJ, Olson JC, Erbey JR, Williams K, Forrest KY, Smithline Kinder L, Ellis D, Becker DJ. Insulin resistance–related factors, but not glycemia, predict coronary artery disease in type 1 diabetes: Ten-year follow-up data from the Pittsburgh Epidemiology of Diabetes Complications Study. *Diabetes Care* 2003; 26:1374–1379.
44. Wasada T, Katsumori K, Kuroki H, Iwamoto Y. Insulin resistance facilitates the development of coronary artery disease in Japanese type II diabetic patients: A single hospital-based follow-up study. *Diabetologia* 1999; 42:1264–1265.
45. Bonora E, Formentini G, Calcaterra F, Lombardi S, Marini F, Zenari L, Saggiani F, Poli M, Perbellini S, Raffaelli A, Cacciatori V, Santi L, Targher G, Bonadonna R, Muggeo M. HOMA-estimated insulin resistance is an independent predictor of cardiovascular disease in type 2 diabetic subjects: Prospective data from the Verona Diabetes Complications Study. *Diabetes Care* 2002; 25:1135–1141.
46. Shinohara K, Shoji T, Emoto M, Tahara H, Koyama H, Ishimura E, Miki T, Tabata T, Nishizawa Y. Insulin resistance as an independent predictor of cardiovascular mortality in patients with end-stage renal disease. *J Am Soc Nephrol* 2002; 13:1894–1900.
47. Yanase M, Takatsu F, Tagawa T, Kato T, Arai K, Koyasu M, Horibe H, Nomoto S, Takemoto K, Shimizu S, Watarai M. Insulin resistance and fasting hyperinsulinemia are risk factors for new cardiovascular events in patients with prior coronary artery disease and normal glucose tolerance. *Circ J* 2004; 68:47–52.
48. Edwards KL, Austin MA, Newman B, Mayer E, Krauss RM, Selby JV. Multivariate analysis of the insulin resistance syndrome in women. *Arterioscler Thromb* 1994; 14:1940–1945.
49. Meigs JB, D'Agostino RB Sr, Wilson PW, Cupples LA, Nathan DM, Singer DE. Risk variable clustering in the insulin resistance syndrome: The Framingham Offspring Study. *Diabetes* 1997; 46:1594–1600.
50. Ford ES. Factor analysis and defining the metabolic syndrome. *Ethn Dis* 2003; 13:429–437.
51. Lawlor DA, Ebrahim S, May M, Davey Smith G. (Mis)use of factor analysis in the study of insulin resistance syndrome. *Am J Epidemiol* 2004; 159:1013–1018.
52. Alberti KG, Zimmet PZ. Definition, diagnosis and classification of diabetes mellitus and its complications. Part 1: Diagnosis and classification of diabetes mellitus provisional report of a WHO consultation. *Diabet Med* 1998; 15:539–553.
53. World Health Organization. Definition, diagnosis and classification of diabetes mellitus and its complications: Report of a WHO consultation. Geneva, 1999; WHO/NCD/NCS 99.2.
54. National Institutes of Health. Third report of the National Cholesterol Education Program Expert Panel on Detection, Evaluation, and Treatment of High Blood Cholesterol in Adults (Adult Treatment Panel III): Executive summary. NIH Publication no. 01–3670, 2001.
55. Balkau B, Charles MA. Comment on the provisional report from the WHO consultation: European Group for the Study of Insulin Resistance (EGIR). *Diabet Med* 1999; 16:442–443.
56. Grundy SM, Brewer HB Jr, Cleeman JI, Smith SC Jr, Lenfant C; American Heart Association; National Heart, Lung, and Blood Institute. Definition of metabolic syndrome: Report of the National Heart, Lung, and Blood Institute/American Heart Association conference on scientific issues related to definition. *Circulation* 2004; 109:433–438.

57. Reaven GM. Banting lecture 1988: Role of insulin resistance in human disease. *Diabetes* 1988; 37:1595–1607.
58. Hanley AJ, Wagenknecht LE, D'Agostino RB Jr, Zinman B, Haffner SM. Identification of subjects with insulin resistance and beta-cell dysfunction using alternative definitions of the metabolic syndrome. *Diabetes* 2003; 52:2740–2747.
59. Ascaso JF, Pardo S, Real JT, Lorente RI, Priego A, Carmena R. Diagnosing insulin resistance by simple quantitative methods in subjects with normal glucose metabolism. *Diabetes Care*. 2003; 26:3320–3325.
60. Liao Y, Kwon S, Shaughnessy S, Wallace P, Hutto A, Jenkins AJ, Klein RL, Garvey WT. Critical evaluation of adult treatment panel III criteria in identifying insulin resistance with dyslipidemia. *Diabetes Care* 2004; 27:978–983.
61. Cheal KL, Abbasi F, Lamendola C, McLaughlin T, Reaven GM, Ford ES. Relationship to insulin resistance of the adult treatment panel III diagnostic criteria for identification of the metabolic syndrome. *Diabetes* 2004; 53:1195–1200.
62. Austin MA, Hokanson JE, Edwards KL. Hypertriglyceridemia as a cardiovascular risk factor. *Am J Cardiol* 1998; 81:7B–12B.
63. Patel A, Barzi F, Jamrozik K, Lam TH, Ueshima H, Whitlock G, Woodward M, Asia Pacific Cohort Studies Collaboration. Serum triglycerides as a risk factor for cardiovascular diseases in the Asia-Pacific region. *Circulation* 2004; 110:2678–2686.
64. Gordon DJ, Probstfield JL, Garrison RJ, Neaton JD, Castelli WP, Knoke JD, Jacobs DR Jr, Bangdiwala S, Tyroler HA. High-density lipoprotein cholesterol and cardiovascular disease: Four prospective American studies. *Circulation* 1989; 79:8–15.
65. Robins SJ, Collins D, Wittes JT, Papademetriou V, Deedwania PC, Schaefer EJ, McNamara JR, Kashyap ML, Hershman JM, Wexler LF, Rubins HB, VA-HIT Study Group. Veterans Affairs High-Density Lipoprotein Intervention Trial. Relation of gemfibrozil treatment and lipid levels with major coronary events: VA-HIT—a randomized controlled trial. *JAMA* 2001; 285:1585–1591.
66. Rashid P, Leonardi-Bee J, Bath P. Blood pressure reduction and secondary prevention of stroke and other vascular events: A systematic review. *Stroke* 2003; 34:2741–2748.
67. Levitan EB, Song Y, Ford ES, Liu S. Is nondiabetic hyperglycemia a risk factor for cardiovascular disease? A meta-analysis of prospective studies. *Arch Intern Med* 2004; 164:2147–2155.
68. McGee DL, Diverse Populations Collaboration. Body mass index and mortality: A meta-analysis based on person-level data from 26 observational studies. *Ann Epidemiol* 2005; 15:87–97.
69. Arnlov J, Evans JC, Meigs JB, Wang TJ, Fox CS, Levy D, Benjamin EJ, D'Agostino RB, Vasan RS. Low-grade albuminuria and incidence of cardiovascular disease events in nonhypertensive and non-diabetic individuals: The Framingham Heart Study. *Circulation* 2005; 112:969–975.
70. Ford ES. Risks for all-cause mortality, cardiovascular disease, and diabetes associated with the metabolic syndrome: A summary of the evidence. *Diabetes Care* 2005; 28:1769–1778.
71. Tanko LB, Bagger YZ, Qin G, Alexandersen P, Larsen PJ, Christiansen C. Enlarged waist combined with elevated triglycerides is a strong predictor of accelerated atherogenesis and related cardiovascular mortality in postmenopausal women. *Circulation* 2005; 111:1883–1890.
72. Kalme T, Seppala M, Qiao Q, Koistinen R, Nissinen A, Harrela M, Loukovaara M, Leinonen P, Tuomilehto J. Sex hormone–binding globulin and insulin-like growth factor–binding protein-1 as indicators of metabolic syndrome, cardiovascular risk, and mortality in elderly men. *J Clin Endocrinol Metab* 2005; 90:1550–1556.
73. Dekker JM, Girman C, Rhodes T, Nijpels G, Stehouwer CD, Bouter LM, Heine RJ. Metabolic syndrome and 10-year cardiovascular disease risk in the Hoorn Study. *Circulation* 2005; 112:666–673.
74. Scuteri A, Najjar SS, Morrell CH, Lakatta EG, Cardiovascular Health Study. The metabolic syndrome in older individuals—prevalence and prediction of cardiovascular events: The Cardiovascular Health Study. *Diabetes Care* 2005; 28:882–887.
75. Bonora E, Targher G, Formentini G, Calcaterra F, Lombardi S, Marini F, Zenari L, Saggiani F, Poli M, Perbellini S, Raffaelli A, Gemma L, Santi L, Bonadonna RC, Muggeo M. The Metabolic Syndrome is an independent predictor of cardiovascular disease in Type 2 diabetic subjects: Prospective data from the Verona Diabetes Complications Study. *Diabet Med* 2004; 21:52–58.
76. Bruno G, Merletti F, Biggeri A, Bargero G, Ferrero S, Runzo C, Prina Cerai S, Pagano G, Cavallo-Perin P, Casale Monferrato Study. Metabolic syndrome as a predictor of all-cause and cardiovascular mortality in type 2 diabetes: The Casale Monferrato Study. *Diabetes Care* 2004; 27:2689–2694.

77. Sone H, Mizuno S, Fujii H, Yoshimura Y, Yamasaki Y, Ishibashi S, Katayama S, Saito Y, Ito H, Ohashi Y, Akanuma Y, Yamada N. Is the diagnosis of metabolic syndrome useful for predicting cardiovascular disease in Asian diabetic patients? Analysis from the Japan Diabetes Complications Study. *Diabetes Care* 2005; 28:1463–1471.
78. Saely CH, Aczel S, Marte T, Langer P, Hoefle G, Drexel H. The metabolic syndrome, insulin resistance, and cardiovascular risk in diabetic and nondiabetic patients. *J Clin Endocrinol Metab* 2005 Aug 9.
79. Marroquin OC, Kip KE, Kelley DE, Johnson BD, Shaw LJ, Bairey Merz CN, Sharaf BL, Pepine CJ, Sopko G, Reis SE, Women's Ischemia Syndrome Evaluation Investigators. Metabolic syndrome modifies the cardiovascular risk associated with angiographic coronary artery disease in women: A report from the Women's Ischemia Syndrome Evaluation. *Circulation* 2004; 109:714–721.
80. Levantesi G, Macchia A, Marfisi R, Franzosi MG, Maggioni AP, Nicolosi GL, Schweiger C, Tavazzi L, Tognoni G, Valagussa F, Marchioli R, GISSI-Prevenzione Investigators. Metabolic syndrome and risk of cardiovascular events after myocardial infarction. *J Am Coll Cardiol* 2005; 46:277–283.
81. Wallenfeldt K, Hulthe J, Fagerberg B. The metabolic syndrome in middle-aged men according to different definitions and related changes in carotid artery intima-media thickness (IMT) during 3 years of follow-up. *J Intern Med* 2005; 258:28–37.
82. Rana JS, Monraats PS, Zwinderman AH, de Maat MP, Kastelein JJ, Doevendans PA, de Winter RJ, Tio RA, Frants RR, van der Laarse A, van der Wall EE, Jukema JW, GENDER study. Metabolic syndrome and risk of restenosis in patients undergoing percutaneous coronary intervention. *Diabetes Care* 2005; 28:873–877.
83. Lind L, Lithell H, Pollare T. Is it hyperinsulinemia or insulin resistance that is related to hypertension and other metabolic cardiovascular risk factors? *J Hypertens Suppl* 1993; 11:S11–16.
84. Lindahl B, Asplund K, Hallmans G. High serum insulin, insulin resistance and their associations with cardiovascular risk factors: The Northern Sweden MONICA Population Study. *J Intern Med* 1993; 234:263–270.
85. Denker PS, Pollock VE. Fasting serum insulin levels in essential hypertension: A meta-analysis. *Arch Intern Med* 1992; 152:1649–1651.
86. Hsueh WA, Lyon CJ, Quinones MJ. Insulin resistance and the endothelium. *Am J Med.* 2004; 117:109–117.
87. Caballero AE. Endothelial dysfunction, inflammation, and insulin resistance: A focus on subjects at risk for type 2 diabetes. *Curr Diab Rep.* 2004; 4:237–246.
88. Wang CC, Goalstone ML, Draznin B. Molecular mechanisms of insulin resistance that impact cardiovascular biology. *Diabetes* 2004; 53:2735–2740.
89. Yudkin JS, Stehouwer CD, Emeis JJ, Coppack SW. C-reactive protein in healthy subjects—associations with obesity, insulin resistance, and endothelial dysfunction: A potential role for cytokines originating from adipose tissue? *Arterioscler Thromb Vasc Biol* 1999; 19:972–978.
90. Ford ES. Body mass index, diabetes, and C-reactive protein among U.S. adults. *Diabetes Care* 1999; 22:1971–1977.
91. McLaughlin T, Abbasi F, Lamendola C, Liang L, Reaven G, Schaaf P, Reaven P. Differentiation between obesity and insulin resistance in the association with C-reactive protein. *Circulation* 2002; 106:2908–2912.
92. Westerbacka J, Bergholm R, Tiikkainen M, Yki-Jarvinen H. Glargine and regular human insulin similarly acutely enhance endothelium-dependent vasodilatation in normal subjects. *Arterioscler Thromb Vasc Biol* 2004; 24:320–324.
93. Hills SA, Balkau B, Coppack SW, Dekker JM, Mari A, Natali A, Walker M, Ferrannini E, EGIR-RISC Study Group. The EGIR-RISC Study (The European group for the study of insulin resistance: Relationship between insulin sensitivity and cardiovascular disease risk): I. Methodology and objectives. *Diabetologia* 2004; 47:566–570.

6 The Sympatho-Adrenal System in the Metabolic Syndrome

Lewis Landsberg

CONTENTS

The sympathetic nervous system (SNS) and the adrenal medulla are intimately involved in the pathogenesis and clinical expression of the metabolic syndrome. This chapter will address that involvement. Obesity and insulin resistance are the primary components of the syndrome (1–3); the sympatho-adrenal contributions may be viewed as physiologic responses to these primary components and as significant causal factors in the pathogenesis of the major clinical manifestations (4,5).

A strong case can be made, for example, that increased activity of the SNS is involved in the pathogenesis of the hypertension commonly noted in patients with the metabolic syndrome, and that diminished secretion of epinephrine from the adrenal medulla contributes to the characteristic dyslipidemia. Insulin resistance and consequent hyperinsulinemia stimulate central sympathetic activity and promote triglyceride synthesis in liver. The increased sympathetic activity may also worsen insulin resistance

From: *Contemporary Endocrinology: The Metabolic Syndrome: Epidemiology, Clinical Treatment, and Underlying Mechanisms*
Edited by: B.C. Hansen and G.A. Bray © Humana Press, Totowa, NJ

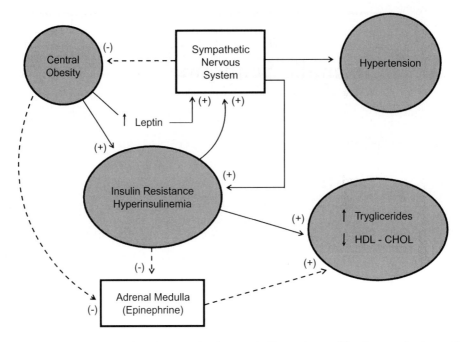

Figure 6.1. The sympatho-adrenal system in the metabolic syndrome. The four cardinal manifestations of the metabolic syndrome are shown in shaded circles and ovals, and the sympatho-adrenal system in open rectangles. Positive or stimulatory influences are shown by the solid lines, and negative or inhibitory by the broken lines.

and increase hyperinsulinemia by antagonizing insulin mediated glucose uptake in skeletal muscle. Central obesity, the other major manifestation of the syndrome, is a prominent cause of the insulin resistance and hyperinsulinemia. The relationships between these cardinal manifestations of the metabolic syndrome are shown schematically in Figure 6.1, where the shaded circles and ovals represent the defining abnormalities and the open rectangles the sympatho-adrenal responses.

SYMPATHETIC NERVOUS SYSTEM (SNS) ACTIVITY IS INCREASED IN THE METABOLIC SYNDROME

Two recent studies (6,7) measuring impulses from implanted electrodes in the peroneal nerve (microneurography) report muscle sympathetic nerve activity (MSNA) in subjects with and without the metabolic syndrome, as defined by the National Cholesterol Education Program (NCEP) Adult Treatment Panel III (ATP III). The findings were remarkably similar in both studies: increased MSNA in metabolic syndrome patients as compared with controls and a further increase in MSNA in those patients with the syndrome who were hypertensive. The demonstration that higher MSNA was associated with higher blood pressures in these subjects is consistent with a role for the SNS in the pathogenesis of the hypertension. Although the numbers of subjects with the metabolic syndrome in these studies were relatively small (18 in one; 48 in the other), the validity of the observations is strongly supported by the well-documented increase in SNS activity that occurs with obesity (8–11), and the well-established effect of insulin to stimulate the SNS (12,13).

Increased SNS Activity in Obesity

Since several genetic rodent models of obesity have decreased sympathetic activity (14), and since catecholamines increase energy output (15), it had long been supposed that human obesity was associated with a decrease in SNS activity. Measurements of urinary norepinephrine excretion in a population-based study, however, showed a direct correlation with body mass index and waist/hip ratio, demonstrating that sympathetic activity was stimulated, not suppressed, with increasing central obesity (Fig. 6.2) (8,16). Subsequent application of microneurography by several groups clearly demonstrated increased MSNA in obese as compared with lean subjects (10,11) and a direct correlation of MSNA with body mass index (9). It is, therefore, conclusively established that human obesity is associated with increased SNS activity. Further, it is a reasonable inference that the central obesity in the metabolic syndrome is the cause of the increased SNS activity in this syndrome. In fact, it has been demonstrated that MSNA is greater in subjects with central obesity as compared with the peripheral form (17); and in the study of Grassi et al. described earlier, MSNA was directly correlated with body mass index and waist circumference (7).

Insulin Stimulates the SNS

It has been known for 25 years that insulin stimulates sympathetic activity (12). Measurements of plasma norepinephrine and the application of microneurography during euglycemic, hyperinsulinemic clamps (13) in which insulin is infused along with sufficient glucose to keep the blood glucose constant ("clamped") have established definitively the stimulatory effects of insulin on the SNS. This stimulation, moreover, occurs at physiological insulin concentrations (13). Since insulin both stimulates the

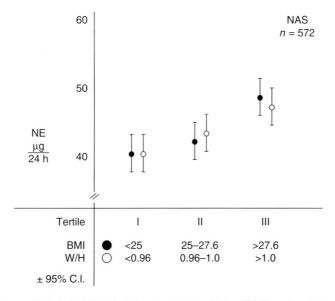

Figure 6.2. Urinary NE excretion in relation to body mass index (BMI) and waist-to-hip ratio (W/H). With increasing weight (BMI) and central body fat distribution (W/H) 24 hour NE excretion (a measure of SNS activity) increases. Brackets indicate 95% confidence intervals (CI). Data are from 572 men enrolled in the Normative Aging Study (NAS). (From ref. 16, with permission.)

SNS and links obesity with sympathetic stimulation, it is reasonable to infer that the insulin resistance and hyperinsulinemia of the metabolic syndrome underlie the increase in SNS activity that characterizes this syndrome. This interpretation is supported by the direct correlation between insulin and MSNA in the studies of Huggett et al. and Grassi et al. described earlier (6,7).

Insulin Is Associated with Hypertension

A link between hypertension and insulin has been clearly established in numerous clinical and epidemiologic studies (18–22). The relationship is noted in obese and non-obese individuals. In fact, the parallel tracking of insulin resistance and elevated blood pressures in the centrally obese was of historical importance in unraveling the pathogenesis of obesity-related hypertension (23). Controversy, however, has surrounded the relationship between insulin and hypertension, the literature referred to earlier notwithstanding. The confusion results from the complexity of the relationship between insulin and blood pressure. Insulin is a direct vasodilator and in some species, such as the dog, chronic insulin administration does not elevate blood pressure (24). In rats, however, insulin does increase blood pressure (25) and obese humans have been shown to be resistant to the vasodilatory effects of insulin (26). Different interventions that lower insulin levels and improve insulin sensitivity, moreover, such as weight loss (27) and treatment with thiazolidenediones (28), also decrease blood pressure and it is now generally accepted that insulin is linked to hypertension.

Thus, obesity and insulin resistance are likely explanations for hypertension in the metabolic syndrome. Two mechanisms have been identified that might contribute to the pro-hypertensive actions of insulin: augmentation of renal sodium reabsorption, and stimulation of the SNS described above.

INSULIN ENHANCES RENAL SODIUM REABSORPTION

Insulin stimulates sodium reabsorption via direct effects on the renal tubules (29–31). Factors that promote renal sodium retention alter the pressure natriuresis relationship (32,33) so that higher renal perfusion pressures are required to balance sodium excretion with sodium intake. The pro-hypertensive diathesis thus established would display itself in the face of high salt intakes. The hypertension that occurs in the obese is, in fact, salt sensitive (34).

LEPTIN STIMULATES SNS ACTIVITY

The protein product of the ob/ob gene, leptin, suppresses appetite and stimulates the SNS. Synthesized in and released from adipose tissue, leptin levels are directly correlated with body fat mass (35). In experimental animals, infusions of leptin increase SNS activity (36) by central nervous system mechanisms that have not yet been well characterized. Leptin's actions on appetite and the SNS serve, therefore, to limit fat accumulation. Infusions of leptin also increase blood pressure (37), and elevated leptin levels have been reported in patients with essential hypertension and correlated with blood pressure (38).

Both insulin and leptin, therefore, provide a link between obesity and the SNS, and both, therefore, are potential mediators of obesity-related hypertension and the blood pressure elevation that occurs in the metabolic syndrome. Sympathetic stimulation of the heart (increased cardiac output), the blood vessels (vasoconstriction), and the kidneys (renal sodium reabsorption, renin secretion) would all contribute a pro-hypertensive effect. This effect is pro-hypertensive since not all patients with obesity or the metabolic syndrome have hypertension.

HOW AND WHY INSULIN STIMULATES THE SNS

Since teleology is the handmaiden of integrative physiology, it is reasonable to ask why insulin, the major anabolic hormone of the fed state, might stimulate the SNS. The answer, rooted in the relationship between dietary intake and sympathetic activity, illuminates the important interface between metabolism and the cardiovascular system.

Insulin Mediates Dietary Changes in SNS Activity

It has been known since the late 1970s that dietary intake exerts important effects on the SNS: Fasting suppresses while overfeeding stimulates sympathetic activity (39–42). These observations implied a mechanism for linking diet with central sympathetic outflow. Studies in laboratory rodents demonstrated that insulin-mediated glucose uptake in neurons of the ventromedial hypothalamus was importantly involved in this link between diet and the SNS (43–46). A schematic model based on these experiments is presented in Figure 6.3 (47). During fasting, a small fall in glucose level and a larger fall in insulin decreases glucose metabolism in a group of hypothalamic regulatory neurons; this decrease in glucose utilization stimulates an inhibitory pathway from the hypothalamus to tonically active brainstem sympathetic centers, thereby resulting in a suppression of sympathetic outflow. This is an example of neural regulation by descending inhibition. Conversely, during carbohydrate intake, or in the presence of insulin resistance, a small increase in glucose and a larger increase in insulin enhances glucose metabolism in these regulatory neurons thereby diminishing the inhibitory output from

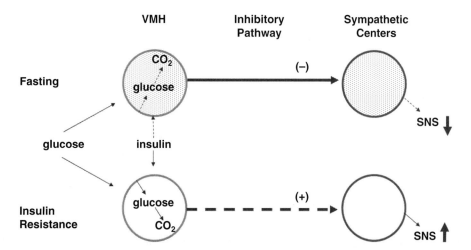

Figure 6.3. Model of the effect of insulin and glucose on central regulation of SNS outflow. See text for details. In the presence of insulin resistance insulin-mediated glucose metabolism depresses an inhibitory pathway between the hypothalamus and the brainstem leading to disinhibition of tonically active SNS centers and thus an increase in SNS activity. (From ref. 47, with permission.)

the hypothalamus, releasing the restraint on the lower sympathetic centers, and increasing central sympathetic outflow. Central mechanisms, therefore, have been identified that link insulin resistance and hyperinsulinemia with sympathetic activity in obesity and in the metabolic syndrome.

Insulin-Mediated Sympathetic Stimulation Underlies Dietary Thermogenesis

The function subserved by dietary changes in SNS activity relates to energy production (15). These sympathetically mediated changes in metabolic rate are a component of overall energy production known as *adaptive thermogenesis*, the latter occurring principally in response to cold exposure or diet. During fasting or decreased caloric intake, suppression of sympathetically mediated energy output occurs with a fall in metabolic rate of up to 10%. The survival value of decreasing energy production at a time of diminished nutrient availability is obvious as it would prolong survival during periods of low energy intake such as those imposed by famine.

Conversely, during overfeeding, sympathetic stimulation increases energy output by as much as 10%. Less obvious is the survival value of increasing metabolic rate with overfeeding, the well-established phenomenon known as *dietary thermogenesis*. The latter may have evolved in the context of diets deficient in one or more essential nutrients; by overeating such a subsistence diet, an organism might achieve adequate intake of the required nutrient while dissipating the excess calories as heat, thereby avoiding excessive fuel storage as fat. Since access to adequate amounts of protein for growth and development appears to have been a high priority over the course of mammalian evolution, dietary thermogenesis may have its origins in the response to diets low in protein. The capacity for dietary thermogenesis would permit an animal to achieve adequate nitrogen intake by overfeeding without becoming obese. This hypothesis is supported by experiments that demonstrate a striking stimulatory effect of low-protein diets on sympathetic activity (48), and by the fact that protein does not stimulate the SNS (49) while carbohydrate and fat are highly stimulatory (50,51). Whatever the evolutionary origins, however, it should be clear that dietary thermogenesis conveys the possibility for resisting excessive fat storage by increasing the range of energy intakes over which energy balance can be maintained. It is of interest and importance that individuals differ in their capacity for dietary thermogenesis; those with lower capacity have been endowed with greater metabolic efficiency (a "thrifty" trait) (52).

THE ADAPTIVE SIGNIFICANCE OF INSULIN RESISTANCE

Since skeletal muscle is the major site of glucose uptake, it is no surprise that the defining abnormality in insulin resistance is an impediment to insulin-mediated glucose uptake in muscle. Insulin resistance during fasting conveys a survival advantage by directing glucose from skeletal muscle, which can utilize other substrates such as free fatty acids, to the central nervous system, an obligate glucose utilizer that does not depend on insulin for glucose uptake and metabolism. This shift in substrate utilization induced by insulin resistance lessens the need for gluconeogenesis, thereby preserving muscle protein and lengthening survival during fasting. Sensitivity (and conversely resistance) to insulin action is known to vary widely in different individuals.

THRIFTY METABOLIC TRAITS INVOLVE THERMOGENESIS AND INSULIN RESISTANCE

Since individuals differ in both the capacity for dietary thermogenesis and sensitivity to insulin, it follows that individuals differ in their propensity to become obese and develop type 2 diabetes (52,53). These thrifty traits, evolved in the setting of intermittent famine, would prolong survival in times of inadequate food supply; in the presence of abundant food and dietary excess, however, these same traits would predispose to obesity and type 2 diabetes. The current worldwide epidemic of obesity, and its offspring, the metabolic syndrome, may thus have its origin in metabolic traits suited to ensure survival in an environment characterized by wide swings in nutrient availability. The Pima Indians of the southwestern United States, and other indigenous populations, once lean but now suffering the ravages of obesity and its complications, may be living examples of the maladaptive potential of thrifty metabolic traits when combined with dietary excess.

INSULIN RESISTANCE AND THE METABOLIC ECONOMY OF THE OBESE STATE

Resistance to the effect of insulin on muscle glucose uptake begets hyperinsulinemia, the latter stimulated by the rise in glucose that reflects diminished insulin action. When pancreatic beta-cell reserve is insufficient to meet the demands imposed by the insulin-resistant state, type 2 diabetes mellitus develops. Obesity is the major environmental cause of insulin resistance, although as noted above, individuals differ in their innate sensitivity to insulin, accounting for, along with inherited differences in beta-cell reserve, the genetic propensity to develop type 2 diabetes.

Insulin Resistance as a Compensatory Mechanism

On a cellular level it seems obvious that, in the face of hyperinsulinemia, resistance to the effects of insulin on fuel synthesis and storage would have to develop to prevent disruption of adipocytes and muscle cells from triglyceride or glycogen engorgement respectively. That engorgement may, parenthetically, contribute to insulin resistance by alteration of cell membrane structural components that contain portions of the insulin response elements.

At the level of the whole organism, hyperinsulinemia, by driving sympathetically mediated thermogenic mechanisms (dietary thermogenesis) and increasing energy output, would tend to restore energy balance and limit further fuel storage (Fig. 6.4) (54). The sympathetic stimulation that occurs in obesity, according to this formulation, is a compensatory mechanism engendered by insulin resistance to restrain further weight gain. Like all compensatory mechanisms, however, there is a price to pay, in this case hyperinsulinemia and sympathetic stimulation. The latter, by effects on the kidneys, the heart, and the vessels, exerts a pro-hypertensive effect that elevates the blood pressure in predisposed individuals. The effect is pro-hypertensive since not all obese, despite sympathetic stimulation, have hypertension. The schema presented in Figure 6.4 has been tested in clinical and population-based studies (4).

SELECTIVE INSULIN RESISTANCE

The formulation in Figure 6.4 depends on the selectivity of insulin resistance in different tissues, with the obese retaining sensitivity to the effects of insulin on the SNS, despite resistance in skeletal muscle and adipose tissue. This in fact has been demonstrated to be the case. The obese are not resistant to the effects of insulin on the SNS (55) despite marked resistance to the effect on muscle glucose uptake.

INCREASED SYMPATHETIC ACTIVITY IN OBESITY DEPENDS ON INSULIN AND IS LINKED TO BLOOD PRESSURE

Increased SNS activity in the obese is central to the schema in Figure 6.4. As noted in detail earlier, enhanced SNS activity in the obese is firmly established. The schema, moreover, depends on a causal relationship between increased insulin levels and stimulation of the SNS. Such a relationship has been convincingly demonstrated in clinical studies (17) that correlate measures of insulin resistance with MSNA. A link to hyper-

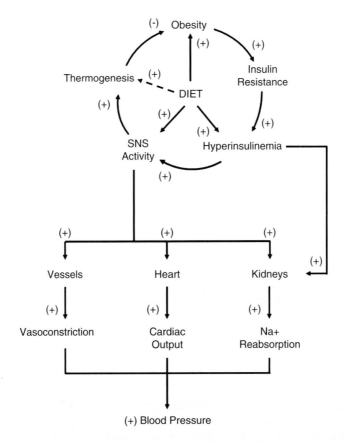

Figure 6.4. Hypothetical relationship between obesity and hypertension. Insulin resistance is associated with central obesity. According to this formulation, the resultant hyperinsulinemia drives sympathetically mediated thermogenic mechanisms in order to restore energy balance. The sympathetic stimulation of the heart, kidneys, and blood vessels exerts a pro-hypertensive effect. Viewed in this light, the hypertension of obesity is a byproduct of mechanisms recruited in the obese to limit further weight gain. (From ref. 54, with permission.)

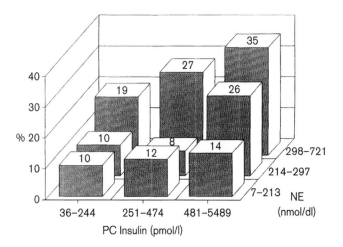

Figure 6.5. Relationship of hypertension to insulin levels and SNS activity in men from the Normative Aging Study (NAS). Data from 572 population-based subjects were analyzed. Percentage (%) of the population with hypertension (>160/90 BP, or treatment) is shown for tertiles of postprandial (PC) insulin level and urinary NE excretion. The incidence of hypertension increases 3.5-fold from those in the lowest tertiles of insulin and NE to those in the highest tertile of each. (From ref. 56, with permission.)

tension is established by correlations between MSNA and diastolic pressure (7) and in a population-based study (Fig. 6.5) (56). Highly significant in this regard as well is the marked fall in MSNA activity and blood pressure when insulin sensitivity increases following weight loss (27). Additional support for the linkage between insulin and blood pressure comes from the effect of thiazolidinediones, insulin sensitizers that also lower blood pressure (28,57).

Taken together, therefore, the evidence is compatible with an important role for insulin-mediated sympathetic stimulation in the pathogenesis of obesity-related hypertension, and thus, the hypertension of the metabolic syndrome. It suggests, further, that insulin resistance and sympathetic stimulation are compensatory mechanisms recruited in the obese to restore energy balance. This does not, of course, preclude a role for other mechanisms, as redundancy is the hallmark of important physiological responses. It seems likely, for example, that leptin is also an important mediator of sympathetic stimulation in the obese (58).

CAN INCREASED SNS ACTIVITY BE THE PRIMARY ABNORMALITY IN THE METABOLIC SYNDROME?

The earlier discussion relates activation of the SNS to obesity and insulin resistance as a homeostatic mechanism integrated into the physiology of the obese state to limit further weight gain. SNS involvement, as portrayed, is secondary to the insulin resistance and obesity. It provides an explanation for the close but hitherto elusive association between obesity and hypertension first noted when blood pressure was measured in populations at the turn of the last century. It is reasonable to ask, however, as some investigators have, whether the phenomena described earlier may be explained differently. An alternative hypothesis has been advanced postulating the primacy of sympathetic stimulation in the underlying pathogenesis of the entire syndrome including obesity (59,60). This formulation, however, cannot be convincingly supported by the evidence, as detailed below.

The "Chicken-and-Egg" Question

The argument in favor of a primary role for the SNS is based on the following observations: (1) SNS stimulation causes insulin resistance by a combination of vascular (vasoconstriction) and cellular processes (61); (2) enhanced SNS activity is a well-recognized factor in the pathogenesis of hypertension; and (3) there is evidence from the Framingham study (62) showing that hypertension predicts the subsequent development of obesity, as well as the other way around. This hypothesis postulates downregulation of adrenergic beta receptors in the face of a primary increase in SNS activity, which in turn diminishes sympathetically mediated energy expenditure, thereby predisposing to obesity (60). Although superficially plausible, this formulation runs afoul of a well-established body of evidence dealing with the SNS and energy production, and is not compatible with the well-established observation that weight loss decreases SNS activity.

Evidence Against a Primary Role for the SNS

A major problem with the contention that SNS activation is a primary abnormality is the lack of a predicate for desensitization of sympathetically mediated energy expenditure. Although cardiovascular beta receptor–mediated responses show downregulation, a large body of evidence developed around cold exposure and cold acclimation indicates enhancement, not attenuation, of sympathetically mediated thermogenesis in the setting of chronic sympathetic stimulation (15,63). This enhancement in fact defines the cold-acclimated state. Cold-induced thermogenesis and diet-induced thermogenesis, moreover, are known to have a similar physiological basis (15). A recent study purporting to show such desensitization of energy expenditure in hypertensive subjects is not convincing in this regard (64,65). To the contrary, obese hypertensives have been shown to have a greater fall in metabolic rate after beta blockade than nonobese hypertensives, consistent with enhanced (not diminished) sympathetically mediated thermogenesis in obese hypertensives (66). In population-based studies, furthermore, MSNA correlates directly with energy expenditure, not inversely as predicted by the hypothesis of desensitization (67), and similarly a direct correlation between metabolic rate and blood pressure (68) has been reported. Finally, weight loss results in a marked fall in SNS activity (27), an observation seemingly incompatible with SNS activity as the cause of the weight gain in the first place. For all these reasons, it seems unlikely that a primary increase in SNS activity causes the full-blown metabolic syndrome; the data appear more consistent with a primary role for insulin and obesity.

This does not preclude the possibility that sympathetic stimulation worsens insulin resistance (Fig. 6.1) by antagonizing insulin-mediated glucose uptake in muscle. If such an antagonism was sustained it would create a vicious cycle and exacerbate the whole cycle shown in Figure 6.4.

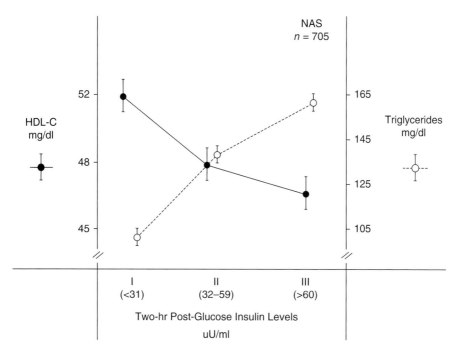

Figure 6.6. Relationship between insulin levels and plasma HDL-cholesterol and triglyceride levels. Data are from 705 subjects from the NAS. Higher post-glucose insulin levels are associated with higher triglycerides and lower HDL-C levels. Similar patterns have been noted in many studies. (From ref. 70, with permission.)

DECREASED EPINEPHRINE SECRETION CONTRIBUTES TO THE DYSLIPIDEMIA OF THE METABOLIC SYNDROME

Insulin is well known to influence plasma lipid concentrations. Elevated levels of insulin are directly correlated with high levels of triglycerides and low levels of HDL-cholesterol (Fig. 6.6) (69,70). A population-based study has also demonstrated a role for epinephrine, the circulating hormone of the adrenal medulla, in the characteristic dyslipidemia of the metabolic syndrome (71).

Adrenal Medullary Activity Is Diminished in Obesity

The level of activity of the SNS and the secretion of adrenal medullary epinephrine is always coordinated but not always congruent. Hypoglycemia, for example, stimulates the adrenal medulla and suppresses the SNS, while cold exposure and exercise stimulate both. Obesity provides another example of dissociated responses. Adrenal medullary activity is diminished in the obese (Fig. 6.7) (8,72–74) while, as noted above, the SNS is activated (Fig. 6.2).

Low Levels of Epinephrine Are Related to High Triglyceride and Low HDL-Cholesterol Levels

In addition to elevated insulin levels (Fig. 6.6), the decreased excretion of epinephrine appears to play a role in the pathogenesis of the circulating lipid abnormalities that accompany obesity (Fig. 6.8) (70,71); as epinephrine excretion diminishes, triglycerides

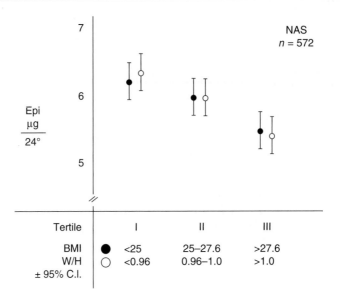

Figure 6.7. Urinary epinephrine excretion in relation to BMI and W/H. In contrast to NE excretion (Fig. 6.2), epinephrine excretion diminishes with increasing BMI and W/H ratio. While SNS activity is increased in the obese, adrenal medullary activity is diminished. Data are from the same subjects as shown in Figure 6.2. (From ref. 74, with permission.)

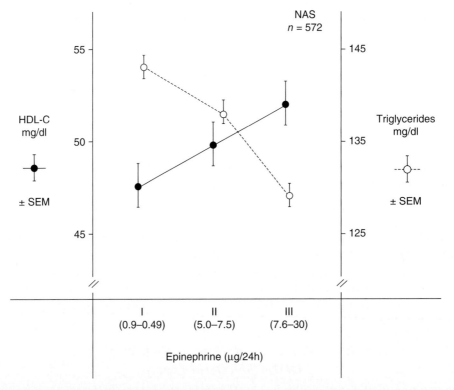

Figure 6.8. Relationship between epinephrine excretion and plasma HDL-C and triglyceride levels. Data are from the same subjects shown in Figure 6.6. Note that as epinephrine excretion goes up, triglycerides fall and HDL-C levels rise. (From ref. 70, with permission.)

rise and HDL-cholesterol falls. Interestingly, these lipid changes are reminiscent of those seen in patients receiving beta receptor blocking agents, implying that the effect of beta blockers on plasma lipids may be mediated, at least in part, by antagonizing the actions of circulating epinephrine on lipid metabolism.

TWO NEWLY RECOGNIZED FACTORS THAT INVOLVE THE SNS AND THAT MAY INFLUENCE THE DEVELOPMENT OF THE METABOLIC SYNDROME

Sleep Disorders

An interesting body of evolving research has highlighted an association between altered sleep patterns and the development of physiological changes characteristic of the metabolic syndrome, including SNS stimulation. These observations have long-term public health implications (75) and may illuminate some potential factors in the pathogenesis of the metabolic syndrome.

OBSTRUCTIVE SLEEP APNEA

Obstructive sleep apnea is a well-known complication of obesity. It is also well recognized that sleep apnea is associated with prolonged increases in sympathetic activity (76) that persist beyond the apneic and hypoxic periods of disturbed sleep and that increased SNS activity can be demonstrated during daytime wakefulness. It is a reasonable inference that the hypertension that accompanies sleep apnea is caused, at least in part, by sympathetic stimulation since effective treatment lowers both MSNA and blood pressure (77). The physiological abnormalities that occur in obstructive sleep apnea may be relevant to other disorders associated with disturbed sleep, especially since it has been suggested that there is enhanced SNS activity with sleep deprivation.

SLEEP DEBT IS ASSOCIATED WITH INCREASED CORTISOL LEVELS AND INSULIN RESISTANCE

Cushing's syndrome, the prototype of central obesity, has long suggested a role for glucocorticoid excess in the body fat distribution that accompanies obesity-related hypertension and the metabolic syndrome. A plausible connection between body fat distribution and glucocorticoid action has been suggested by studies demonstrating that omental fat has higher levels of 11 beta-hydroxysteroid dehydrogenase-1 than subcutaneous fat (78,79). The higher levels of enzyme activity in intraabdominal fat depots might generate formation of the active glucocorticoid, *cortisol*, from the inactive metabolite, *cortisone*. It has been postulated that cortisol, acting locally in fat cells in these sites, might stimulate expansion of the intraabdominal fat mass, contributing to the central form of obesity.

It is also possible that subtle increases in cortisol secretion might induce the central body fat distribution pattern. Particularly interesting in this regard is evidence of an increase in cortisol levels in sleep-deprived subjects (80,81). Six days of imposed sleep debt (4 hours sleep per night for 6 nights) was shown to cause reversible increases in PM cortisol levels. Insulin resistance was also noted in these sleep-deprived subjects, perhaps a consequence of the increase in cortisol and/or enhanced SNS activity. These data have raised the possibility that disordered sleep might play a role in the pathogenesis of the metabolic syndrome, given the underlying importance of central obesity and insulin resistance in the latter.

LOW BIRTH WEIGHT

Epidemiological evidence has suggested an association between low birth weight and the subsequent development during adulthood of type 2 diabetes (82–84), central obesity (85), cardiovascular disease (82), and hypertension (86). Fetal and neonatal environment have been shown to influence the development of the SNS (87), and increased MSNA during young adulthood (88) has been demonstrated in low-birth-weight individuals, suggesting a possible mechanism for the development of high blood pressure in this cohort. These data raise the interesting possibility that low birth weight predisposes to the development of the metabolic syndrome. The startling incidence of obesity and impaired glucose tolerance in the infants of diabetic mothers (89) underlines the potential importance of prenatal factors as antecedents of adult hypertension and obesity. Further studies of the pre- and neonatal antecedents of adult disease will undoubtedly be of interest and may shed further light on the pathogenesis of the metabolic syndrome (90).

IMPLICATIONS FOR TREATMENT

Since the risk of cardiovascular events is high in patients with the metabolic syndrome, aggressive treatment of hypertension, obesity, and the lipid abnormalities is warranted. In the absence of controlled studies, but cognizant of the overriding importance of blood pressure control in patients with diabetes (91), as well as in other high-risk groups, many authorities recommend low blood pressure thresholds (140/90 mmHg) for the initiation of treatment and aggressive blood pressure targets (130–120/80) in this group.

Lifestyle Modifications

The cornerstone of treatment for subjects with the metabolic syndrome involves changes in diet, weight loss, exercise, and moderation of alcohol intake (92). All of these recommendations affect insulin sensitivity and/or the SNS, thereby addressing the underlying pathophysiology of the syndrome. The effectiveness and feasibility of lifestyle changes as a long-term strategy has been amply shown by many studies (93), including the Treatment of Mild Hypertension Study (TOMHS), which demonstrated falls in systolic and diastolic blood pressure of 8–10 mmHg that were sustained over a four-year period (94).

DIETARY RECOMMENDATIONS

Since obesity plays a critical role in the pathogenesis of the metabolic syndrome, and since obesity-related hypertension is salt sensitive, it is no surprise that restriction of salt and calories are central recommendations (93,94). Moderate salt restriction (2 g Na/day) and modest weight loss frequently produce meaningful results. Exercise aids weight loss while increasing insulin sensitivity and decreasing sympathetic activation as well as lowering blood pressure. Excessive alcohol intake is associated with hypertension and has been reported to affect body fat distribution (95). Alcohol restriction to two drinks per day is generally recommended (96). In addition to these changes, specific alterations in macronutrient intake have been shown to lower blood pressure on a constant intake of calories or salt, the so-called *DASH diet* (97).

The DASH Diet. The Dietary Approaches to Stop Hypertension (DASH) trial has demonstrated convincingly that eight weeks of a diet rich in fruits and vegetables, high in fiber, high in protein and low-fat dairy products but low in saturated fat (97) produces a meaningful decrease in blood pressure. Blood pressure reduction is greater in hypertensive than normotensive subjects. Although not dependent on sodium restriction, when sodium is lowered the effect on blood pressure is accentuated. The DASH diet is high in potassium, calcium, and magnesium and it seems likely that these minerals play a role in the response. The diet also has been reported to increase insulin sensitivity (98).

Pharmacological Treatment

If blood pressure and plasma lipids are not normalized by the lifestyle changes outlined earlier, appropriate pharmacological agents should be added to the regimen. The lifestyle changes should of course be maintained for their impact on cardiovascular risk factors and because they are synergistic with, and improve the response to, the pharmacological agents.

HYPERTENSION

Although lowering the blood pressure is the overarching concern, not all agents are equally beneficial in the context of the metabolic syndrome. Thiazide diuretics and beta blockers worsen insulin resistance (99) and increase the risk of developing type 2 diabetes while ACE inhibitors and A II receptor blockers improve insulin resistance and lessen the likelihood of developing diabetes (100–103). Diuretics will frequently be required to control the blood pressure, so prudence dictates using as low a dose of a thiazide as possible or trying another class of agent. Beta blockers should be reserved for those patients with ischemic heart disease.

THIAZOLIDINEDIONES

The thiazolidinedione class of insulin-sensitizing agents has been of use in the treatment of type 2 diabetes (104). These agents enhance insulin action by binding with PPAR-gamma, an intranuclear transcription factor that regulates insulin action, adipocyte differentiation, and adipogenesis. Troglitozone, the prototype of the class, has been withdrawn from the market because of hepatotoxicity; currently rosiglitazone and pioglitazone are being studied for use in the metabolic syndrome and type 2 diabetes. These agents appear to be safe and may have value in the treatment of the metabolic syndrome since they increase insulin sensitivity and lower blood pressure, without a clear-cut impact on the dyslipidemia (28,57,105). As with lifestyle changes (106), they may also prevent or forestall the development of type 2 diabetes in those at high risk for the disease (107). Weight gain and increase in body fat, particularly in the subcutaneous regions, have been regularly noted and have been a cause of concern.

CONCLUSIONS: FEAST OR FAMINE—THE LEGACY OF THRIFTY METABOLIC TRAITS IN THE FACE OF AN ABUNDANT FOOD SUPPLY

The sympatho-adrenal system is involved in the pathogenesis of the hypertension (increased SNS activity) and the dyslipidemia (diminished adrenal medullary activity) that occur in the metabolic syndrome. These effects appear to be secondary to obesity and insulin resistance, the primary abnormalities of the syndrome. Enhanced sympathetic activity may be a compensatory mechanism, recruited in the obese to restore energy balance. An inherited tendency to insulin resistance and a diminished capacity for sympathetically mediated dietary thermogenesis may be examples of thrifty metabolic traits that serve well in periods of scarcity (famine) but not during periods of abundance where dietary excess (feast) leads to obesity and the metabolic syndrome.

Treatment should be aggressive and directed at the major manifestations of the metabolic syndrome: obesity, insulin resistance, hypertension, and lipid abnormalities. Lifestyle modifications that enhance insulin sensitivity play a central role, but pharmacological agents that address the specific manifestations, without worsening insulin resistance, frequently will be required.

REFERENCES

1. Natali A, Ferrannini E. Hypertension, insulin resistance, and the metabolic syndrome. *Endocrinol Metab Clin N Am* 2004; 33:417–429.
2. Reaven GM. Insulin resistance/compensatory hyperinsulinemia, essential hypertension, and cardiovascular disease. *J Clin Endocrinol Metab* 2003; 88:2399–2403.
3. Reaven GM, Lithell H, Landsberg L. Hypertension and associated metabolic abnormalities: The role of insulin resistance and the sympathoadrenal system. *NEJM* 1996; 343:374–381.
4. Landsberg L. Insulin-mediated sympathetic stimulation: Role in the pathogenesis of obesity-related hypertension (or, How insulin affects blood pressure and why). *J Hypertens* 2001; 19:523–528.
5. Landsberg L. Insulin resistance and the metabolic syndrome. *Diabetologia* 2005; 48:1244–1246.
6. Huggett RJ, Burns J, Mackintosh AF, Mary DA. Sympathetic neural activation in nondiabetic metabolic syndrome and its further augmentation by hypertension. *Hypertension* 2004; 44:847–852.
7. Grassi G, Dell'Oro R, Quarti-Trevano F, Scopelliti F, Seravalle G, Paleari F, Gamba PL, Mancia G. Neuroadrenergic and reflex abnormalities in patients with metabolic syndrome. *Diabetologia* 2005; 48:1359–1365.
8. Troisi RJ, Weiss ST, Parker DR, Sparrow D, Young JB, Landsberg L. Relation of obesity and diet to sympathetic nervous system activity. *Hypertension* 1991; 17:669–677.
9. Scherrer U, Randin D, Tappy L, Vollenweider P, Jéquier E, Nicod P. Body fat and sympathetic nerve activity in healthy subjects. *Circulation* 1994; 89:2634–2640.
10. Vollenweider P, Randin D, Tappy L, Jéquier E, Nicod P. Scherrer U. Impaired insulin-induced sympathetic neural activation and vasodilation in skeletal muscle in obese humans. *J Clin Invest* 1994; 93:2365–2371.
11. Grassi G, Seravalle G, Cattaneo BM, Bolla GB, Lanfranchi A, Colombo M, Giannattasio C, Brunani A, Cavagnini F, Mancia G. Sympathetic activation in obese normotensive subjects. *Hypertension* 1995; 25:560–563.
12. Rowe JW, Young JB, Minaker KL, Stevens AL, Pallotta J, Landsberg L. Effect of insulin and glucose infusions on sympathetic nervous system activity in normal man. *Diabetes* 1981; 30:219–225.
13. Hausberg M, Mark AL, Hoffman RP, Sinkey CA, Anderson EA. Dissociation of sympathoexcitatory and vasodilator actions of modestly elevated plasma insulin levels. *J Hypertens* 1995; 13:1015–1021.
14. Young JB, Landsberg L. Diminished sympathetic nervous system activity in the genetically obese mouse. *Am J Physiol* 1983; 245:E148–E154.
15. Landsberg L, Saville ME, Young JB. The sympathoadrenal system and regulation of thermogenesis. Am J Physiol 1984; 247:E181–E189.
16. Landsberg L, Young JB. Sympathoadrenal activity and obesity: Physiological rationale for the use of adrenergic thermogenic drugs. *Int J Obesity* 1993; 17:S29–S34.
17. Grassi G, Dell'Oro R, Facchini A, Trevano FQ, Bolla GB, Mancia G. Effect of central and peripheral body fat distribution on sympathetic and baroreflex function in obese normotensives. *J Hypertens* 2004; 22:2363–2369.

18. Modan M, Halkin H, Almog S et al. Hyperinsulinemia: A link between hypertension obesity and glucose intolerance. *J Clin Invest* 1985; 75:809–817.
19. Manicardi V, Camellini L, Bellodi G, Coscelli C, Ferrannini E. Evidence for an association of high blood pressure and hyperinsulinemia in obese man. *J Clin Endocrinol Metab* 1986; 62:1302–1304.
20. Ferrannini E, Buzzigoli G, Bonadonna R et al. Insulin resistance in essential hypertension. *N Engl J Med* 1987; 317:350–357.
21. Nilsson PM, Lind L, Andersson PE, Hanni A, Berne C, Baron J, Lithell HO. On the use of ambulatory blood pressure recordings and insulin sensitivity measurements in support of the insulin-hypertension hypothesis. *J Hypertens* 1994; 12:965–969.
22. Zavaroni I, Mazza S, Dall'Aglio E, Gasparini P, Passeri M, Reaven GM. Prevalence of hyperinsulinaemia in patients with high blood pressure. J Intern Med 1992; 231:235–240.
23. Kissebah AH, Vydelingum N, Murray R, Evans DJ, Hartz AJ, Kalkhoff RK, Adams PW. Relation of body fat distribution to metabolic complications of obesity. *J Clin Endocrinol Metab* 1982; 54:254–260.
24. Hall JE, Brands MW, Mizelle HL, Gaillard CA, Hildebrandt DA. Chronic intrarenal hyperinsulinemia does not cause hypertension. *Am J Physiol* 1991; 260:F663–F669.
25. Brands MW, Lee WF, Keen HL, Alonso-Galicia M, Zappe DH, Hall JE. Cardiac output and renal function during insulin hypertension in Sprague-Dawley rats. *Am J Physiol* 1996; 271:R276–R281.
26. Baron AD, Brechtel-Hook G, Johnson A, Hardin D. Skeletal muscle blood flow: A possible link between insulin resistance and blood pressure. *Hypertension* 1993; 21:129–135.
27. Grassi G, Seravalle G, Colombo M, Bolla GB, Cattaneo BM, Cavagnini F, Mancia G. Body weight reduction, sympathetic nerve traffic, and arterial baroreflex in obese normotensive humans. *Circulation* 1998; 97:2037–2042.
28. Yosefy C, Magen E, Kiselevich A, Priluk R, London D, Volchek L, Viskoper RJ Jr. Rosiglitazone improves, while Glibenclamide worsens blood pressure control in hypertensive diabetic and dyslipidemic subjects via modulation of insulin resistance and sympathetic activity. *J Cardiovasc Pharmacol* 2004; 44:215–222.
29. Herrera FC. Effect of insulin on short-circuit current and sodium transport across toad urinary bladder. *Am J Physiol* 1965; 209:819–824.
30. Saudek CD, Boulter PR, Knopp RH, Arky RA. Sodium retention accompanying insulin treatment of diabetes mellitus. *Diabetes* 1974; 23:240–246.
31. DeFronzo RA. Insulin and renal sodium handling: Clinical implications. *Int J Obes* 1981; 5(suppl.):93–104.
32. Guyton AC, Coleman TG, Cowley AW Jr, Scheel KW, Manning RD Jr, Norman RA Jr. Arterial pressure regulation: Overriding dominance of the kidneys in long-term regulation and in hypertension. *Am J Med* 1972; 52:584–594.
33. Hall JR, Guyton AC, Coleman TG, Mizelle HL, Woods LL. Regulation of arterial pressure: Role of pressure natriuresis and diuresis. *Fed Proc* 1986; 45:2897–2903.
34. Rocchini AP, Key J, Bondie D et al. The effect of weight loss on the sensitivity of blood pressure to sodium in obese adolescents. *NEJM* 1989; 321:580–585.
35. Kennedy A, Gettys TW, Watson P, Wallace P, Ganaway E, Pan Q, Garvey WT. The metabolic significance of leptin in humans: Gender-based differences in relationship to adiposity, insulin sensitivity, and energy expenditure. *J Clin Endocrinol Metab* 1997; 82:1293–1300.
36. Haynes WG, Morgan DA, Walsh SA, Mark AL, Sivitz WI. Receptor-mediated regional sympathetic nerve activation by leptin. *J Clin Invest* 1997; 100:270–278.
37. Shek EW, Brands MW, Hall JE. Chronic leptin infusion increases arterial pressure. *Hypertension* 1998; 31(part 2):409–414.
38. Agata J, Masuda A, Takada M, Higashiura K, Murakami H, Miyazaki Y, Shimamoto K. High plasma immunoreactive leptin level in essential hypertension. *Am J Hypertens* 1997; 10:1171–1174.
39. Young JB, Landsberg L. Suppression of sympathetic nervous system during fasting. *Science* 1977; 196:1473–1475.
40. Young JB, Landsberg L. Stimulation of the sympathetic nervous system during sucrose feeding. *Nature* 1977; 269:615–617.
41. Young JB, Saville E, Rothwell NJ, Stock MJ, Landsberg L. Effect of diet and cold exposure on norepinephrine turnover in brown adipose tissue in the rat. *J Clin Invest* 1982; 69:1061–1071.
42. O'Dea K, Esler M, Leondard P, Stockigt JR, Nestel P. Noradrenaline turnover during under- and overeating in normal weight subjects. *Metabolism* 1982; 31:896–899.

43. Young JB, Landsberg L. Sympathoadrenal activity in fasting pregnant rats: Dissociation of adrenal medullary and sympathetic nervous system responses. *J Clin Invest* 1979; 64:109–116.

44. Landsberg L, Greff L, Gunn S, Young JB. Adrenergic mechanisms in the metabolic adaptation to fasting and feeding: Effects of phlorizin on diet-induced changes in sympathoadrenal activity in the rat. *Metabolism* 1980; 29:1128–1137.

45. Rappaport EB, Young JB, Landsberg L. Effects of 2-deoxy-glucose on the cardiac sympathetic nerves and the adrenal medulla in the rat: Further evidence for a dissociation of sympathetic nervous system and adrenal medullary responses. *Endocrinology* 1982; 110:650–656.

46. Young JB, Landsberg L. Impaired suppression of sympathetic activity during fasting in the gold thioglucose-treated mouse. *J Clin Invest* 1980; 65:1086–1094.

47. Landsberg L, Young JB. Diet and the sympathetic nervous system: Relationship to hypertension. *Int J Obesity* 1981; 5(suppl 1):79–91.

48. Young JB, Kaufman LN, Saville ME, Landsberg L. Increased sympathetic nervous system activity in rats fed a low protein diet: Evidence against a role for dietary tyrosine. *Am J Physiol* 1985; 248: R627–R637.

49. Kaufman LN, Young JB, Landsberg L. Effect of protein on sympathetic nervous system activity in the rat: Evidence for nutrient-specific responses. *J Clin Invest* 1986; 77:551–558.

50. Schwartz JH, Young JB, Landsberg L. Effect of dietary fat on sympathetic nervous system activity in the rat. *J Clin Invest* 1983; 72:361–370.

51. Walgren MC, Young JB, Kaufman LN, Landsberg L. The effects of various carbohydrates on sympathetic activity in heart and interscapular brown adipose tissue (IBAT) of the rat. *Metabolism* 1987; 6(6):585–594.

52. Neel JV. Diabetes mellitus: A "thrifty" genotype rendered detrimental by "progress"? *Am J Hum Genetics* 1962; 14:353–362.

53. Reaven GM. Insulin resistance: A chicken that has come to roost. In: *The Metabolic Syndrome X*, Hansen BC, Saye J, Wennogle LP (eds.), *Annals NY Acad Sci*, 1999; 892:45–57.

54. Landsberg L. Diet, obesity and hypertension: An hypothesis involving insulin, the sympathetic nervous system, and adaptive thermogenesis. *QJ Med* 1986; 236:1081–1090.

55. O'Hare JA, Minaker KL, Meneilly GS, Rowe JW, Pallotta JA, Young JB. Effect of insulin on plasma norepinephrine and 3,4-dihydroxyphenylalanine in obese men. *Metabolism*. 1989; 38:322–329.

56. Ward KD, Sparrow D, Landsberg L, Young JB, Vokonas PS, Weiss ST. Influence of obesity, insulin, and sympathetic nervous system activity on blood pressure: The Normative Aging Study. *J of Hypertension* 1996; 14:301–308.

57. Sarafidis PA, Lasaridis AN, Nilsson PM, Pagkalos EM, Hitoglou-Makedou AD, Pliakos CI, Kazakos KA, Yovos JG, Zebekakis PE, Tziolas IM, Tourkantonis AN. Ambulatory blood pressure reduction after rosiglitazone treatment in patients with type 2 diabetes and hypertension correlates with insulin sensitivity increase. *J Hypertens* 2004; 22:1769–1777.

58. Mark AL, Correia MLG, Rahmouni K, Haynes WG. Selective leptin resistance: A new concept in leptin physiology with cardiovascular implications. *J Hypertens* 2002; 20:1245–1250.

59. Julius S, Jamerson K. Sympathetics, insulin resistance and coronary risk in hypertension: The "chicken and egg" question. *J Hypertens* 1994; 12:495–502.

60. Julius S, Valentini M, Palatini P. Overweight and hypertension a 2-way street? *Hypertension* 2000; 35:807–813.

61. Jamerson KA, Julius S, Gudbrandsson T, Andersson O, Brant DO. Reflex sympathetic activation induces acute insulin resistance in the human forearm. *Hypertension* 1993; 21:618–623.

62. Kannel WB, Brand N, Skinner JJ Jr, Dawber TR, McNamara PM. The relation of adiposity to blood pressure and development of hypertension. *Ann Intern Med* 1967; 67(1):48–59.

63. Hsieh ACL, Carlson LD, Gray G. Role of the sympathetic nervous system in the control of chemical regulation of heat production. *Am J Physiol* 1957; 190:247–251.

64. Valentini M, Julius S, Palatini P, Brook RD, Bard RL, Bisognano JD, Kaciroti N. Attenuation of haemodynamic, metabolic and energy expenditure responses to isoproterenol in patients with hypertension. *J Hypertens* 2004; 22:1999–2006.

65. Calhoun DA, Grassi G. Weight gain and hypertension: The chicken-egg question revisited. *J Hypertens* 2004; 22:1869–1871.

66. Kunz I, Schorr U, Klaus S, Sharma AM. Resting metabolic rate and substrate use in obesity hypertension. *Hypertension* 2000; 36:26–32.

67. Spraul M, Ravussin E, Fontvieille AM, Rising R, Larson DE, Anderson EA. Reduced sympathetic nervous activity (a potential mechanism predisposing to body weight gain). *J Clin Inv* 1993; 92:1730–1735.
68. Saad MF, Lillioja S, Nyomba BL, Castillo C, Ferraro R, De Gregorio M, Ravussin E, Knowler WC, Bennett PH, Howard BV et al. Racial differences in the relation between blood pressure and insulin resistance. *NEJM* 1991; 324:733–739.
69. Ward KD, Sparrow D, Vokonas PS, Willett W, Landsberg L, Weiss ST. The relationships of abdominal obesity, hyperinsulinemia and saturated fat intake to serum lipid levels: The Normative Aging Study. *Intl J Obes* 1994; 18:137–144.
70. Landsberg L. Pathophysiology of obesity-related hypertension: Role of insulin and the sympathetic nervous system. *J Cardiovasc Pharmacol* 1994; 23(suppl 1):S1–S8.
71. Ward KD, Sparrow D, Landsberg L, Young JB, Vokonas PS, Weiss ST. The relationship of epinephrine excretion to serum lipid levels: The Normative Aging Study. *Metabolism* 1994; 43:509–513.
72. Young JB, Macdonald IA. Sympathoadrenal activity in human obesity: Heterogeneity of findings since 1980. *Int J Obesity* 1992; 16:959–967.
73. Del Rio G. Adrenomedullary function and its regulation in obesity. *Int J Obesity* 2000; 24(suppl 2)S89–S91.
74. Landsberg L, Young JB. Sympathoadrenal activity and obesity: Physiological rationale for the use of adrenergic thermogenic drugs. *Int J Obes* 1993; 17(suppl 1) S29–S34.
75. Van Cauter E, Spiegel K. Sleep as a mediator of the relationship between socioeconomic status and health: A hypothesis. *Annals NY Acad Sci* 1999; 896:254–261.
76. Narkiewicz K, Somers VK. Sympathetic nerve activity in obstructive sleep apnoea. *Acta Physiol Scand* 2003; 177:385–390.
77. Wolk R, Shamsuzzaman ASM, Somers VK. Obesity, sleep apnea, and hypertension. *Hypertension* 2003; 42:1067–1074.
78. Bujalska IJ, Kumar S, Stewart PM. Does central obesity reflect "Cushing's disease of the omentum?" *Lancet* 1997; 349:1210–1213.
79. Stewart PM. Tissue-specific Cushing's syndrome: 11β-hydroxysteroid dehydrogenases and the redefinition of corticosteroid hormone action. *Eur J Endocrinol* 2003; 149:163–168.
80. Spiegel K, Leproult R, Van Cauter E. Impact of sleep debt on metabolic and endocrine function. *Lancet* 1999; 354:1435–1439.
81. Spiegel K, Leproult R, L'Hermite-Balériaux, Copinschi G, Penev PD, Van Cauter E. Leptin levels are dependent on sleep duration: Relationships with sympathovagal balance, carbohydrate regulation, cortisol, and thyrotropin. *J Clin Endocrinol Metab* 2004; 89:5762–5771.
82. Barker DJP. Fetal programming of coronary heart disease. *Trends in Endocrinol Metab* 2002; 13:364–368.
83. Lithell HO, McKeigue PM, Berglund L, Mohsen R, Lithell UB, Leon DA. Relation of size at birth to non-insulin dependent diabetes and insulin concentrations in men aged 50–60 years. *BMJ* 1996; 312:406–410.
84. Forsén T, Eriksson J, Tuomilehto J, Reunanen A, Osmond C, Barker D. The fetal and childhood growth of persons who develop type 2 diabetes. *Ann Intern Med* 2000; 133:176–182.
85. Oken E, Gillman MW. Fetal origins of obesity. *Obes Res* 2003; 11:496–506.
86. Law CM, Shiell AW. Is blood pressure inversely related to birth weight? The strength of evidence from a systematic review of the literature. *J Hypertens* 1996; 14:935–941.
87. Young JB, Morrison SF. Effects of fetal and neonatal environment on sympathetic nervous system development. *Diabetes Care* 1998; 21(suppl 2):B156–B160.
88. Boguszewski MCS, Johannsson G, Fortes LC, Sverrisdóttir YB. Low birth size and final height predict high sympathetic nerve activity in adulthood. *J Hypertens* 2004; 22:1157–1163.
89. Silverman BL, Landsberg L, Metzger BE. Fetal hyperinsulinism in offspring of diabetic mothers: Association with the subsequent development of childhood. *Annals NY Acad Sci* 1993; 699:36–45.
90. Hausberg M, Barenbrock M, Kosch M. Elevated sympathetic nerve activity: The link between low birth size and adult-onset metabolic syndrome? *J Hypertens* 2004; 22:1087–1089.
91. Landsberg L, Molitch M. Diabetes and hypertension: Pathogenesis, prevention and treatment. *Clin and Exp Hypertens* 2004; 26(7&8):621–628.
92. Daskalopoulou SS, Mikhailidis DP, Elisaf M. Prevention and treatment of the metabolic syndrome. *Angiology* 2004; 55:589–612.

93. Beilin LJ. Non-pharmacological management of hypertension: Science, consensus and controversies. In: *Handbook of Hypertension,* Birkenhäger WH, Robertson JIS, Zanchetti A (eds.), *Hypertension in the Twentieth Century* 2004; 22:417–456.

94. Elmer PJ, Grimm R Jr., Laing B, Grandits G, Svendsen K, Van Heel N, Betz E, Raines J, Link M, Stamler J, Neaton J. Lifestyle intervention: Results of the treatment of mild hypertension study (TOMHS). *Preventive Med* 1995; 24:378–388.

95. Troisi RJ, Weiss ST, Segal MR, Cassano PA, Vokonas PS, Landsberg L. The relationship of body fat distribution to blood pressure in normotensive men: The Normative Aging Study. *Int J Obesity* 1990; 14:515–525.

96. Beilin LJ. Non-pharmacological management of hypertension: Optimal strategies for reducing cardiovascular risk. *J Hypertens* 1994; 12(suppl 10):S71–S81.

97. Appel LJ, Moore TJ, Obarzanek E, Vollmer WM, Svetkey LP, Sacks FM, Bray GA, Vogt TM, Cutler JA, Windhauser MM, Lin PH, Karanja N. A clinical trial of the effects of dietary patterns on blood pressure. *NEJM* 1997; 336:1117–1124.

98. Ard JD, Slentz CA, Grambow SC, Kraus WE, Liu D, Svetkey LP. The effect of the premier interventions on insulin sensitivity. *Diabetes Care* 2004; 27:340–347.

99. Reaven G, Lithell H, Landsberg L. Hypertension and associated metabolic abnormalities: The role of insulin resistance and the sympathoadrenal system. *NEJM* 1996; 334(6):374–381.

100. Yusuf S, Gerstein H, Hoogwerf B, Pogue J, Bosch J, Wolffenbuttel BHR, Zinman B. Ramipril and the development of diabetes. *JAMA* 2001; 286:1882–1885.

101. Dahlöf B, Devereux RB, Kjeldsen SE, Julius S, Beevers G, de Faire U, Fyhrquist F, Ibsen H, Kristiansson K, Lederballe-Pedersen O, Lindholm LH, Nieminen MS, Omvik P, Oparil S, Wedel H. Cardiovascular morbidity and mortality in the Losartan Intervention for Endpoint Reduction in Hypertension Study (LIFE): A randomised trial against atenolol. *Lancet* 2002; 359:995–1003.

102. Lindholm LH, Ibsen H, Borch-Johnsen K, Olsen MH; Wachtell K, Dahlöf B, Devereux RB, Beevers G, de Faire U, Fyhrquist F, Julius S, Kjeldsen SE, Kristianson K, Lederballe-Pedersen O, Nieminen MS, Omvik P, Oparil S, Wedel H, Aurup P, Edelman JM, Snapinn S, LIFE Study Group. Risk of new-onset diabetes in the Losartan Intervention for Endpoint Reduction in Hypertension Study. *J Hypertens* 2002; 20:1879–1886.

103. Grassi G, Seravalle G, Dell'Oro R, Trevano FQ, Bombelli M, Scopelliti F, Facchini A, Mancia G. Comparative effects of candesartan and hydrochlorothiazide on blood pressure, insulin sensitivity, and sympathetic drive in obese hypertensive individuals: Results of the CROSS study. *J Hypertens* 2003; 21:1761–1769.

104. Lebovitz HE. Rationale for and role of thiazolidinediones in type 2 diabetes mellitus. *Am J Cardiol* 2002; 90(suppl):34G–41G.

105. Rajagopalan R, Iyer S, Khan M. Effect of pioglitazone on metabolic syndrome risk factors: Results of double-blind, multicenter, randomized clinical trials. *Curr Med Res Opin* 2005; 21:163–172.

106. Tuomilehto J, Lindström J, Eriksson JG, Valle TT, Hämäläinen H, Ilanne-Parikka P, Keinänen-Kiukaanniemi S, Laakso M, Louheranta A, Rastas M, Salminen V. Prevention of type 2 diabetes mellitus by changes in lifestyle among subjects with impaired glucose tolerance. *NEJM* 2001; 344:1343–1350.

107. Buchanan TA, Xiang AH, Peters RK, Kjos SL, Marroquin A, Goico J, Ochoa C, Tan S, Berkowitz K, Hodis HN, and Azen SP. Preservation of pancreatic β-cell function and prevention of type 2 diabetes by pharmacological treatment of insulin resistance in high-risk Hispanic women. *Diabetes* 2002; 51:2796–2803.

II

ENDOTHELIAL FUNCTION, INFLAMMATION, AND DYSLIPIDEMIA

7

Insulin Action and Endothelial Function

Kieren J. Mather, Alain Baron, and Michael J. Quon

CONTENTS

INTRODUCTION
MOLECULAR MECHANISMS OF INSULIN SIGNALING IN
THE VASCULATURE
PHYSIOLOGICAL MECHANISMS OF INSULIN ACTION IN
THE VASCULATURE
CONCURRENT METABOLIC AND VASCULAR INSULIN RESISTANCE
GENERALIZED VASCULAR DYSFUNCTION IN
INSULIN RESISTANCE
EXOGENOUS INSULIN RESISTANCE INDUCES
VASCULAR DYSFUNCTION
CLINICAL IMPLICATIONS
FUTURE DIRECTIONS
ACKNOWLEDGMENTS

INTRODUCTION

The endothelium is a diaphanous cellular monolayer lining the lumen of the vasculature throughout the body and weighs approximately 1.8 kg in a 70 kg man. In addition to its well-recognized passive barrier and transport functions, the endothelium actively participates in processes related to local vascular and tissue health. These include active control of vascular tone (1,2), regulation of blood fluidity (3), and modulation of monocyte adhesion (4,5), inflammation (6,7), and lipid peroxidation (8–10), to name but a few processes. More recently, the endothelium has been recognized as an endocrine organ. Indeed, the endothelium produces a variety of hormones acting in a paracrine fashion to regulate vascular tone as well as growth and remodeling of the vascular wall (11–14). The endothelium also possesses receptors for humoral ligands. These receptors, whose predominant role was initially thought to be transendothelial transfer of

From: *Contemporary Endocrinology: The Metabolic Syndrome: Epidemiology, Clinical Treatment, and Underlying Mechanisms*
Edited by: B.C. Hansen and G.A. Bray © Humana Press, Totowa, NJ

hormones, are now known to directly activate signaling cascades and physiological responses.

This chapter discusses the evidence and functional implications of the endothelium as a target tissue for insulin action and the pathophysiological consequences of insulin resistance. We present evidence from *in vitro* and *in vivo* studies demonstrating that the vascular endothelium responds to insulin by increasing the release of nitric oxide (the dominant endothelium-derived vasodilator and anti-atherosclerotic factor), and that this action is impaired in states of insulin resistance. More recent data implicating insulin and other metabolic factors in the regulation of endothelin (the primary endothelium-derived vasoconstrictor and pro-atherosclerotic agent) are also reviewed. Pathophysiological implications relevant to cardiovascular disease in insulin resistance and the opportunities for novel treatment approaches are discussed.

MOLECULAR MECHANISMS OF INSULIN SIGNALING IN THE VASCULATURE

Insulin Signaling Pathways Regulating Production of NO

One important biological action of insulin in vascular endothelium is to directly stimulate production of nitric oxide (NO), a potent vasodilator (15,16). Classical vasodilators such as acetylcholine bind and activate specific G-protein-coupled receptors on the surface of endothelial cells, leading to generation of inositol trisphosphate (IP3) and subsequent increases in intracellular Ca2+ levels.

Ca2+/calmodulin complexes bind to a specific region on eNOS that promotes dissociation of eNOS from caveolin-1 and enhances activation of eNOS (Fig. 7.1) (17,18). Signaling pathways leading from the insulin receptor to activation of eNOS are distinct and separable from the classical signaling pathways linking G-protein-coupled receptors to eNOS (19). Studies of endothelial cells in primary culture have elucidated a complete biochemical signaling pathway leading from the insulin receptor to activation of eNOS (19–22). This pathway requires activation of the insulin receptor tyrosine kinase, subsequent phosphorylation of IRS-1, binding and activation of PI 3-kinase, and activation of the serine kinase PDK-1 that in turn phosphorylates and activates Akt, which then directly phosphorylates and activates eNOS, leading to increased production of NO within a matter of minutes (Fig. 7.1).

INSULIN RECEPTOR TYROSINE KINASE

In endothelial cells, insulin receptors are expressed on the cell surface. However, they are approximately tenfold less abundant than the related IGF-1 receptor (~40,000 insulin and ~400,000 IGF-1 receptors per human endothelial cell) (20). The first study directly demonstrating that insulin can stimulate production of NO from endothelial cells used an NO-selective electrode to show that levels of NO produced in human umbilical vein endothelial cells (HUVEC) in response to a maximally stimulating concentration of insulin are approximately twice those that can be elicited by IGF-1 stimulation. This process is dependent on insulin receptor autophosphorylation (20). Moreover, transfection of wild-type insulin receptors into HUVEC results in a threefold increase in insulin-stimulated NO production (not seen with mutant kinase-deficient insulin receptors) (21). These data suggest an essential role for insulin receptor tyrosine kinase activity in activation of eNOS in response to insulin.

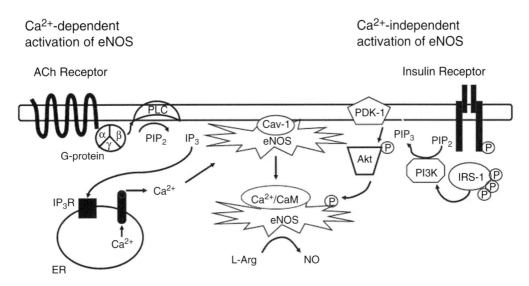

Figure 7.1. Insulin signaling pathways regulating production of NO in vascular endothelium. Phosphorylation-dependent pathway used by insulin to activate eNOS is completely independent and separable from the classical calcium-dependent pathway used by acetylcholine (19).

INSULIN RECEPTOR SUBSTRATES

After autophosphorylation of the insulin receptor and activation of its tyrosine kinase activity, the next step in insulin signaling is the tyrosine phosphorylation of various intracellular substrates by the insulin receptor. Substrates of the insulin receptor include insulin receptor substrate (IRS) family members IRS-1, -2, -3, -4 (23). Overexpression of wild-type IRS-1 in bovine aortic endothelial cells (BAEC) results in a threefold increase in NO production in response to a maximally stimulating concentration of insulin (as determined using the NO-specific fluorescent dye DAF-2) (22). These results suggest that IRS-1 is capable of mediating insulin-stimulated activation of eNOS. All IRS family members contain multiple YXXM motifs whose tyrosine residues can be phosphorylated by the insulin receptor. These phosphorylated motifs are predicted to bind to SH2 domains in the p85 regulatory subunit of phosphatidylinositol (PI) 3-kinase, resulting in activation of the preassociated p110 catalytic subunit. Expression of a mutant IRS-1 (IRS1-F6), where 6 YXXM motifs have substitutions of Phe for Tyr at positions 465, 612, 632, 662, 989, and 941, inhibits both insulin-stimulated PI3-kinase activity and NO production in endothelial cells (22). It is important to note that introduction of an IRS-1 ribozyme into endothelial cells substantially reduces insulin-stimulated production of NO (24).

Taken together, these results suggest that IRS-1 is a necessary component (and predominant insulin receptor substrate) of the insulin signaling pathway leading to activation of PI 3-kinase that then enhances activation of eNOS.

PHOSPHATIDYLINOSITOL 3-KINASE

Signaling downstream from IRS-1 involves the binding of SH2-domain containing signaling molecules to tyrosine phosphorylated motifs in IRS-1. Support for the essential role of PI 3-kinase includes studies demonstrating that preincubation of

HUVEC with wortmannin (PI 3-kinase inhibitor) partially blocks NO production in response to insulin (20).

More important, overexpression of a dominant inhibitory mutant of the p85 regulatory subunit of PI 3-kinase significantly and substantially inhibits insulin-mediated production of NO in transfected HUVEC (21).

Phosphoinositide-Dependent Kinase 1 (PDK-1)

Downstream from PI 3-kinase, PDK-1 is autophosphorylated and activated upon binding of the PI 3-kinase product PI(3,4,5)P3 to the PH domain of PDK-1. PDK-1 then goes on to phosphorylate and activate a host of intracellular kinases including Akt, PKC-zeta, SGK, and p70 S6 kinase. Overexpression of wild-type PDK-1 in BAEC results in a twofold increase in insulin responsiveness with respect to production of NO (22). Furthermore, expression of a kinase-deficient PDK-1 mutant significantly blocks insulin-mediated production of NO.

Taken together, these data strongly suggest that PDK-1 is an essential component of the insulin-signaling pathway leading to production of NO in vascular endothelial cells.

Role of Akt/PKB

Akt (also known as PKB) is a serine/threonine kinase that is directly phosphorylated and activated by PDK-1. Overexpression of mutant Akt proteins (Ala substituted for Lys179 at the ATP binding site or Akt-AAA with Ala substitutions for Ser at position 179, and at regulatory PDK-1 and -2 phosphorylation sites at 308 and 473) in HUVEC nearly completely inhibits production of NO in response to insulin (19,21). Interestingly, although Akt is a necessary signaling molecule for insulin-stimulated activation of eNOS, activation of Akt per se is not sufficient for activation of eNOS (19). For example, insulin or PDGF treatment of endothelial cells results in comparable phosphorylation and activation of endogenous Akt (19,20). However, only insulin treatment, but not PDGF treatment, results in phosphorylation and activation of eNOS with resultant production of NO. Thus, Akt activation is necessary, but not sufficient, for activation of eNOS in response to insulin.

Characteristic Features of eNOS Activation in Response to Insulin

Akt directly phosphorylates human eNOS at Ser1177 (equivalent to Ser1179 in bovine eNOS), resulting in enhanced eNOS activity (25). With respect to insulin signaling, the Akt phosphorylation site on eNOS is absolutely essential for activation of eNOS, since cells expressing a mutant eNOS with a disrupted Akt phosphorylation site (Ala substituted for Ser1179) are unable to produce NO in response to insulin. Moreover, pretreatment of cells with the Ca2+ chelator BAPTA does not inhibit the ability of insulin to either stimulate phosphorylation of eNOS at Ser1179 or enhance eNOS activity. This suggests that insulin-stimulated production of NO is Ca2+-independent (19). The NO response to ligands such as lysophosphatidic acid (LPA) that depend on increased intracellular calcium levels is completely blocked by BAPTA. In addition, the S1179A eNOS mutant can produce NO in a normal fashion in response to LPA but not in response to insulin (19).

Taken together, these data suggest that the phosphorylation-dependent mechanism used by insulin to stimulate activation of eNOS is distinct and separable from the classical calcium-dependent pathway for activation of eNOS. Furthermore, Akt represents a final direct link to eNOS in a complete biochemical pathway involving the

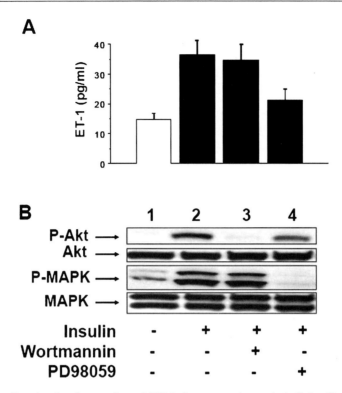

Figure 7.2. Insulin-stimulated secretion of ET-1 from vascular endothelial cells is mediated by MAP-kinase-dependent pathways but not PI 3-kinase-dependent pathways. Panel A, ET-1 levels in cultured medium. Panel B, Western blots demonstrating MAPK-specific signaling of insulin to ET-1 production.

insulin receptor, IRS-1, PI 3-kinase, PDK-1, Akt, and eNOS that regulates activation of eNOS in endothelium in response to insulin (Fig. 7.1).

Insulin-Stimulated Secretion of ET-1

Much less is known about endothelial insulin signaling pathways regulating secretion of the vasoconstrictor endothelin (ET)-1. Recent work from our lab using bovine aortic endothelial cells (BAEC) demonstrates that MAP-kinase signaling is required for this process while PI 3-kinase signaling is not (26).

Levels of ET-1 in conditioned media from BAEC were measured under basal conditions, and after acute insulin stimulation (100 nM, 5 min) without or with pretreatment with wortmannin (PI 3-kinase inhibitor) or PD-98059 (MEK inhibitor) (Fig. 7.2). Insulin treatment induced a twofold increase in ET-1 levels in conditioned media. Pretreatment with wortmannin did not significantly affect insulin-stimulated ET-1 secretion. By contrast, pretreatment with PD-98059 completely blocked this effect of insulin. Cell lysates from these experiments were immunoblotted with phospho-specific antibodies to monitor PI 3-kinase- and MAP-kinase-dependent insulin signaling (Fig. 7.2). As expected, insulin-stimulated phosphorylation of Akt was completely blocked by wortmannin treatment while MAP-kinase phosphorylation was unaffected. Moreover, insulin-stimulated phosphorylation of MAP-kinase was completely blocked by PD-98059 pretreatment while Akt phosphorylation was unaffected.

Taken together, these results directly demonstrate that insulin-stimulated secretion of ET-1 in endothelial cells is mediated by MAPK-dependent signaling pathways independent of PI 3-kinase-dependent signaling.

Insulin-Stimulated Expression of Adhesion Molecules

Another insulin action that regulates vascular function is stimulation of expression of vascular cellular adhesion molecule-1 (VCAM-1) and E-selectin on the endothelium. MAP-kinase-dependent signaling pathways (but not PI3-kinase pathways) regulate these functions of insulin (22). Some human data support the notion that hyperinsulinemia/insulin resistance may be associated with detrimental activation of endothelium (27–29). Nevertheless, in healthy subjects without insulin resistance, the response to exogenous insulin does not include abnormal production of adhesion molecules (30).

Other Hormones that Mimic Insulin Signaling in Endothelium

In addition to insulin, there is a growing list of hormones involved in regulation of vascular and metabolic physiology that acutely activate eNOS in vascular endothelium by PI 3-kinase-dependent signaling mechanisms, leading to phosphorylation of eNOS. This list includes leptin (31), adiponectin (32), HDL (33), estrogen (34), glucocorticoids (35), and dehydroepiandrosterone (DHEA) (36). Moreover, DHEA has acute nongenomic vascular actions to stimulate secretion of ET-1 from endothelium by a MAP-kinase-dependent mechanism similar to that used by insulin (36).

PHYSIOLOGICAL MECHANISMS OF INSULIN ACTION IN THE VASCULATURE

Insulin and Nitric Oxide–Dependent Vasodilation

Insulin has a dose-dependent effect to vasodilate skeletal muscle vasculature (37). This vasodilation occurs at physiological insulin concentrations with an EC50 (concentration to reach half-maximal effect) of 44 µU/mL and with a t1/2 (time to reach half maximal vasodilation) of approximately 35 min (38). Figure 7.3 illustrates the effect of

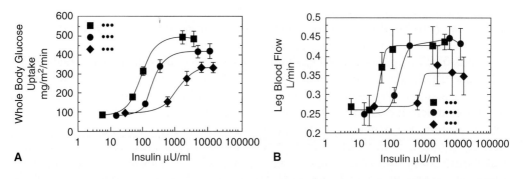

Figure 7.3. Rates of whole-body glucose uptake (left-hand graph) and leg blood flow (right-hand graph), measured by thermodilution, as a function of prevailing serum insulin level during euglycemic clamp studies in lean subjects (closed squares), obese nondiabetic subjects (closed circles), and subjects with type 2 diabetes (closed diamonds). Note the log scale on the abscissa. (Reprinted with permission from ref. 38.)

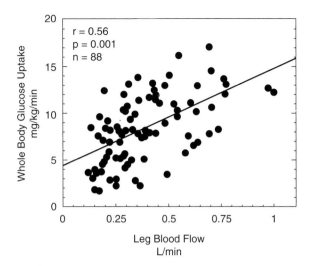

Figure 7.4. Correlation between rates of whole-body glucose uptake and rates of leg blood flow in lean and obese nondiabetic subjects measured during euglycemic hyperinsulinemic clamp studies over a wide range of steady-state serum insulin concentrations. (Reprinted with permission from ref. 39.)

physiological concentrations of insulin, administered under constant euglycemic conditions, to cause an approximately twofold increase in leg blood flow above baseline in lean insulin-sensitive individuals. The robust correlation between the rate of insulin-stimulated glucose uptake and the extent of insulin-mediated vasodilation in Figure 7.4 (39) indicates that the metabolic and vasodilator responses to insulin are highly correlated in vivo in humans. Systemic administration of insulin induces changes in both systemic and leg vascular resistance, but the fall in systemic vascular resistance is modest (~15%) compared to the reduction in leg vascular resistance (~40%), suggesting a differential and specific effect of insulin to dilate skeletal muscle vasculature (40).

Nitric oxide (NO) is a gas that is continuously released from the endothelium, where it is synthesized from the precursor L-arginine in a reaction catalyzed by nitric oxide synthase (eNOS isoform in endothelium). In intact tissues, NO released from the endothelium diffuses across the subendothelial space to the underlying smooth muscle, where it binds to the heme group of guanylate cyclase and stimulates the generation of cyclical GMP, which then mediates smooth muscle relaxation and results in vasodilation. Insulin-mediated vasodilation is dependent on the release of endothelium-derived NO.

As illustrated in Figure 7.5, following the establishment of steady-state hyperinsulinemia under euglycemic clamp conditions, the infusion of L-NMMA (a competitive antagonist of eNOS) completely abrogated the insulin-induced vasodilation, suggesting that insulin-mediated vasodilation is entirely NO dependent. (41). This has also been seen in the forearm (42).

It is possible that this effect of insulin is exerted by enhancing nitrate-induced vasodilation, rather than directly stimulating NO production. In our laboratory we have taken two approaches to evaluating this possibility. One approach examines effects of subvasodilatory insulin doses (~25 µU/mL) to enhance the vasodilatory response to a

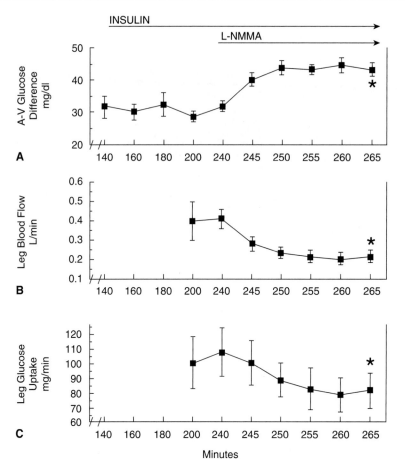

Figure 7.5. Effect of intrafemoral artery infusion of the nitric oxide synthase inhibitor N-G-monomethyl-L-arginine (L-NMMA; 16 mg/min) on leg blood flow during hyperinsulinemic (120 mU/m2/min) euglycemic clamp studies. *$p < 0.05$, **$p < 0.01$. Panel A, leg glucose extraction; Panel B, leg blood flow; Panel C, leg glucose uptake. (Adapted with permission from ref. 41.)

classical endothelium-dependent vasodilator (e.g., methacholine chloride). Studies performed in the leg and forearm by us and others demonstrate that endothelium-dependent vasodilation is enhanced in the presence of insulin (27,43). By contrast, the response to the NO donor sodium nitroprusside is unaltered by co-infusion of insulin, suggesting that insulin is specifically enhancing the endothelial response to the endothelium-dependent vasodilator methacholine chloride (27,44). Using a complementary approach, we measured femoral venous efflux of the stable oxidative end products of nitric oxide, nitrate (NO3), and nitrite (NO2) (together commonly referred to as NOx).

NOx concentrations were measured by a chemiluminescence technique. Femoral venous NOx fluxes (NOx multiplied by leg blood flow) were measured under basal conditions and after a period of euglycemic hyperinsulinemia designed to stimulate NO production. Insulin caused a net increase in NOx release from the leg, and this effect of insulin was reversed by the application of L-NMMA (45).

Together, these data suggest that insulin vasodilates skeletal muscle vasculature by stimulating the net release of endothelium-derived NO. While it is possible that insulin is causing production of NO via the stimulation of NOS isoforms residing in cells other than the endothelium (45,46), this seems unlikely as vasodilation in response to intra-arterial methacholine chloride (an endothelium-dependent vasodilator) was specifically enhanced by insulin (41). Together these data are consistent with a direct in vivo effect of insulin to stimulate NO release from the endothelium.

Insulin Action Couples Hemodynamic and Glucose Homeostasis

Vasodilator actions of insulin may play a central physiological role in coupling hemodynamic and metabolic homeostasis under healthy conditions (Fig. 7.6). Evidence supporting this hypothesis has emerged from investigations of insulin signaling pathways in skeletal muscle, adipose tissue, and vascular endothelium, as well as from physiological studies manipulating blood flow and glucose metabolism (47).

PARALLEL INSULIN SIGNALING PATHWAYS IN METABOLIC AND VASCULAR TISSUES

Insulin-stimulated glucose uptake in skeletal muscle and adipose tissue is mediated by translocation of the insulin-responsive glucose transporter GLUT4 to the cell surface (23). This requires PI 3-kinase-dependent signaling pathways that involve the insulin receptor, IRS-1, PI 3-kinase, PDK-1, and Akt. Ras/MAP kinase pathways do not contribute significantly to insulin-stimulated translocation of GLUT4. While activation of PI 3-kinase and Akt is necessary, it is not sufficient for GLUT4 translocation since PDGF stimulates activation of PI 3-kinase and Akt without causing translocation of

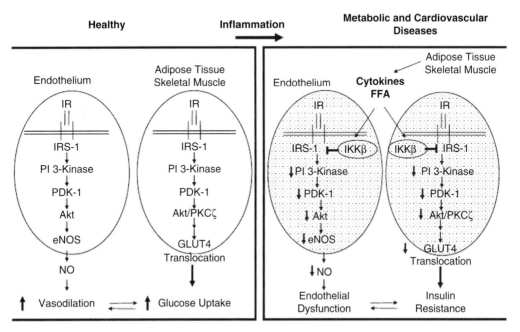

Figure 7.6. (Left) Parallel PI 3-kinase-dependent insulin signaling pathways in metabolic and vascular tissues synergistically couples metabolic and vascular physiology under healthy conditions. (Right) Parallel impairment in insulin signaling pathways under pathological conditions contributes to synergistic coupling of insulin resistance and endothelial dysfunction.

The concept of pathway-specific insulin resistance may help to explain these observations. Metabolic insulin resistance due to molecular defects in the IR/IRS- 1/PI 3-kinase/PDK-1Akt/GLUT4 pathways (discussed in detail above) results in compensatory hyperinsulinemia. In the vasculature and elsewhere, hyperinsulinemia will overdrive unaffected MAP-kinase-dependent pathways leading to an imbalance between PI 3-kinase- and MAP-kinase-dependent functions of insulin. Pro-hypertensive effects of insulin to promote secretion of ET-1, activate cation pumps, and increase expression of VCAM-1 and other adhesion molecules are under the control of MAP-kinase signaling pathways. A recent in vitro model of metabolic insulin resistance with compensatory hyperinsulinemia provides experimental support for this concept (22).

Simultaneous treatment of endothelial cells with wortmannin (PI 3-kinase inhibitor) and high insulin levels blunts PI 3-kinase-dependent effects of insulin such as induction of eNOS expression and production of NO. Of note, under these conditions, insulin signaling through Ras/MAP-kinase pathways is substantially enhanced beyond that observed in the absence of wortmannin. This leads to increased prenylation of Ras and Rho proteins via the MAP-kinase pathway and to enhanced mitogenic responsiveness of cells to insulin and VEGF that are known to contribute to proliferation of vascular smooth muscle cells. In addition, upregulation of endothelial cellular adhesion molecules VCAM-1 and E-selectin and increased rolling interactions of monocytes with endothelial cells is observed (22). Thus, compensatory hyperinsulinemia in the presence of metabolic insulin resistance with pathway-specific impairment of PI 3-kinase in endothelium and vascular smooth muscle cells can lead to enhanced mitogenic actions of insulin through MAP-kinase-dependent pathways. Unbalanced effects of insulin in states of insulin resistance and compensatory hyperinsulinemia may contribute to vascular pathogenesis via these mechanisms (Fig. 7.8). Interactions of endothelin and insulin are discussed in detail below.

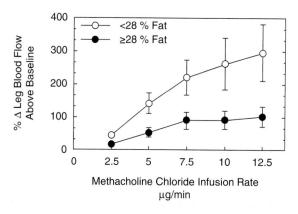

Figure 7.7. Impaired endothelium-dependent vasodilation is a feature of obesity/insulin resistance. Obesity (> 28% body fat) is associated with reduced vasodilatory responses to progressive infusions of methacholine chloride. (Reprinted with permission from ref. 27.)

Vascular and Hemodynamic Actions of Insulin

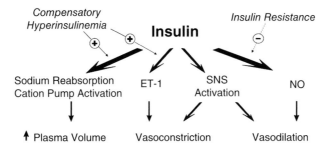

Figure 7.8. Pathway-specific insulin resistance creates imbalance between pro-hypertensive and anti-hypertensive vascular actions of insulin exacerbated by compensatory hyperinsulinemia.

EXOGENOUS INSULIN RESISTANCE INDUCES VASCULAR DYSFUNCTION

Is the vascular dysfunction observed in insulin resistance due to the insulin resistance per se, or due to some other feature of the insulin-resistant state? To address this question, studies have been undertaken employing a variety of interventions to experimentally induce insulin resistance, evaluating the effects of this intervention on vascular function. Free fatty acids are well recognized as having the capacity to induce metabolic insulin resistance. Based on in vitro data suggesting that free fatty acids (FFA) impair NO synthase activity in cultured endothelial cells (74), we tested the idea that elevated circulating FFA levels can impair endothelial cell function in vivo. Graded intrafemoral artery infusions of methacholine chloride were performed to establish the full dose-response curve for endothelium-dependent vasodilation during an infusion of either saline or two hours of a lipid emulsion in conjunction with heparin to enhance hydrolysis of the triglyceride particle and elevate circulating FFA concentrations to approximately 1200 uM. As predicted, raising FFA concentrations caused a marked impairment of endothelium-dependent vasodilation (Fig. 7.9). Similar endothelial dysfunction was also induced by inhibition of endogenous insulin secretion with somatostatin, thereby enhancing the release of endogenous FFA to achieve circulating levels approximating those achieved with exogenous infusions (75). Thus, elevating circulating FFA concentrations from endogenous or exogenous sources causes marked endothelial cell dysfunction.

Similar effects have been observed with other agents that induce insulin resistance, in particular tumor necrosis factor (TNF)-alpha (76,77). Applying the microvascular visualization technique described above, infusion of triglycerides in rats inhibited insulin-stimulated capillary recruitment and glucose uptake in skeletal muscle without affecting total limb blood flow (78). Further, TNF-alpha was able to induce impairment in insulin-induced microvascular recruitment at physiological insulin levels (79).

Insulin and Endothelin Action in the Vasculature

In 1988, Yanigasawa et al. reported the discovery of a novel, endothelium-derived vasoconstrictor that they named *endothelin* (80). The major form of endothelin in the peripheral vasculature is endothelin-1 (ET-1), which is produced directly within

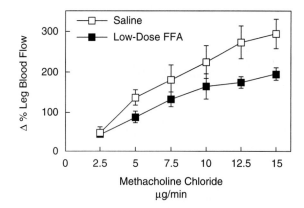

Figure 7.9. Leg blood flow increments relative to baseline in response to a graded intrafemoral artery infusion of the endothelium-dependent vasodilator, methacholine chloride, during infusion of saline of 20% intralipid emulsion (45 cc/h) plus heparin (0.2 U/kg/min) designed to increase systemic FFA level two-to threefold (–1200 uM). Elevated free fatty acids induce endothelial dysfunction in otherwise healthy, lean subjects. (Reprinted with permission from ref. 75.)

endothelial cells throughout the vascular tree (81) and acts principally on underlying vascular smooth muscle cells in a paracrine manner (82, 83). In addition to acute effects on vascular tone, endothelin exerts pro-atherosclerotic effects (81, 82). Circulating levels of endothelin are elevated across the spectrum of abnormalities in glucose metabolism, including populations with hypertension (84), obesity (85–89), impaired glucose tolerance (90), and type 2 diabetes (91–94). Interestingly, reductions in circulating ET-1 have also been reported following interventions that improve insulin sensitivity, including weight loss (89,95–97), metformin (98), and thiazolidinediones (99).

Furthermore, in vitro and in vivo studies suggest that production of endothelin by endothelial cells is regulated by a variety of metabolic factors, including stimulatory effects of insulin (100–103), triglycerides (104), inflammatory mediators such as TNF-alpha (105,106), and inhibitory effects of nitric oxide (107–109). These observations suggest that states of insulin resistance are characterized by elevated endothelin levels, which raises the question of whether this phenomenon might contribute to vascular dysfunction in states of insulin resistance.

In humans, circulating insulin levels appear to modulate endothelin levels, although the literature is inconsistent on this point (84,103,104,110–116). Given the paracrine mode of action of endothelin, it is probably more relevant to examine endothelin action rather than circulating levels. In lean healthy individuals, insulin infusions stimulate both nitric oxide and endothelin action (117). In subjects with obesity/insulin resistance (118) and type 2 diabetes (118,119), responses to antagonism of type A endothelin receptors under basal conditions is magnified relative to healthy, nonobese control subjects (Fig. 7.10). This antagonism is also sufficient to normalize impaired endothelium-dependent vasodilation observed in obesity and diabetes (118), and acutely restores nitric oxide bioavailability (Fig. 7.11) (120). Thus, increased ET-1 action in the vessels may be upstream of the well-described reductions in NO bioavailability in obesity and type 2 diabetes. This issue is unresolved, however, in part because of known reciprocal interactions of NO and ET-1. It is possible that reductions in NO bioavailability

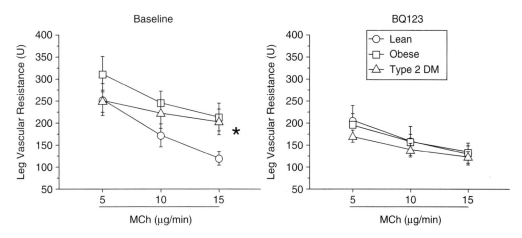

Figure 7.10. Antagonism of type A endothelin receptors with BQ123 is sufficient to correct baseline impairments in methacholine-stimulated endothelium-dependent vasodilation in subjects with obesity with or without concurrent type 2 diabetes mellitus. (Left panel) Baseline conditions. (Right panel) Infusion of BQ123 1 μmol/min. (Adapted with permission from ref. 118.)

independent of ET-1 actions result in a disinhibition of ET-1 production. Experiments designed to address this question are currently underway in our laboratory.

There is evidence that ET-1 contributes to insulin resistance. Effects of systemic infusion of ET-1 on insulin sensitivity have been examined in rats and in humans. In normal conscious rats, bolus intraperitoneal injection of ET-1 raises endogenous glucose and insulin levels and reduces whole-body responses to infused insulin (121). Sustained exposure to ET-1 (delivered continuously by osmotic minipump for five days) induces whole-body insulin resistance, and is associated with reduced skeletal muscle glucose uptake and impaired insulin signaling in muscle (122). In humans, ET-1 infusion induces insulin resistance as measured by the hyperinsulinemic/euglycemic clamp (123,124). Effects of ET-1 on splanchnic glucose production independent of glucagon

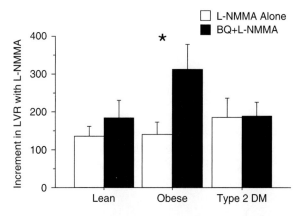

Figure 7.11. Antagonism of type A endothelin receptors with BQ123 augments the vasoconstrictor response to the nitric oxide synthase inhibitor L-NMMA in obese subjects. This suggests that endothelin antagonism can unmask an increased underlying capacity for nitric oxide production in obesity. (Reprinted with permission from ref. 120.)

or insulin appear to be a component of this response (125). These whole-body effects likely comprise responses from multiple tissues, as effects on glucagon production (126), insulin release (127,128), and splanchnic glucose production (129) have been described in addition to direct effects on the vasculature. In the Goto-Kakizaki rat, a model of type 2 diabetes mellitus, antagonism of the ET(A) receptor improves glucose metabolism and significantly reduces hyperglycemia (130). In insulin-sensitive humans, ET(A) antagonism prevents endothelin-induced insulin resistance (124). But does this specifically reflect an increase in the vascular action of endothelin? This question has been evaluated in animal models of insulin resistance as well as in humans. The fructose-fed rat is a commonly used model of acquired insulin resistance (131). Aortic rings from these rats demonstrate specific impairment in insulin-mediated vasodilation (132) that is restored by endothelin receptor antagonism (133,134). This is associated with an increase in ET-1 and ET-1 receptors in vascular tissue (132,135,136).

Observations of increased vascular actions of ET-1 have been made in other models of insulin resistance, including rats with genetic forms of insulin resistance (134,137–139) and insulin-resistant diabetes (130). Relevant human studies have not yet been published. Nevertheless, data from animal studies support the idea that increased endogenous activity of endothelin in the vasculature is a feature of vascular dysfunction and impaired vascular insulin response present in insulin resistance, obesity, and diabetes mellitus.

Emerging Metabolic Factors and the Vasculature

From the above discussion it is reasonable to conclude that impaired nitric oxide bioavailability and augmented endogenous endothelin action are characteristic features of insulin resistance. These factors represent mechanisms by which vascular function contributes to regulation of metabolism. Recent discoveries also provide mechanisms for direct effects of metabolic factors on the vasculature. Prominent among these are adipocyte products such as adiponectin, leptin, tumor necrosis factor alpha, interleukin-6, hepatic growth factor, and angiotensin II. This has been termed the *adipovascular axis*, and a more specific hypothesis of effects of local perivascular fat to regulate vascular biology (*vasocrine* signaling) has also been put forward (140). These ideas have some support from animal data, particularly as they relate to combined effects of adiponectin on both vascular and metabolic functions (32,141–148). Testing of these concepts in humans is an important area of future investigation.

CLINICAL IMPLICATIONS

The above evidence indicates a close association between insulin resistance and vascular dysfunction, with clear implications for both short-term physiology and long-term vascular health. This presents two corollary opportunities: It is possible that treating insulin resistance will produce beneficial effects on the vasculature; and conversely, treatments that improve or restore vascular health may contribute to improvements in metabolism.

Pharmacological Therapies Targeting Insulin Resistance

Nonpharmacological approaches to improving insulin sensitivity, consisting principally of exercise- and diet-induced weight loss, are effective at improving vascular and metabolic function concurrently (96,149–154). Thiazolidinediones, synthetic PPAR-γ ligands, are insulin sensitizers that also have effects to increase forearm blood flow in humans (155). Metformin, another agent that improves insulin sensitivity, also improves endothelial-dependent vasodilation in patients with type 2 diabetes (156). Thiazolidinediones have anti-atherogenic properties to inhibit vascular smooth muscle cell proliferation and decrease accumulation of lipid by macrophages that may be mediated by anti-inflammatory mechanisms (157). Moreover, administration of thiazolidinediones significantly increases adiponectin expression and plasma levels in patients with insulin resistance or type 2 diabetes without affecting body weight (158,159). Adiponectin directly stimulates production of NO from vascular endothelium using a PI 3-kinase-dependent signaling mechanism similar to that of insulin, which may explain its effects to oppose atherogenesis and improve endothelial function (32).

Taken together, these studies suggest that drugs that improve insulin sensitivity may have both direct and indirect effects to improve endothelial function and oppose atherogenesis through mechanisms that include enhancing PI 3-kinase-dependent signaling in vascular endothelium, increasing expression and plasma concentrations of adiponectin, and anti-inflammatory actions. Thus, pharmacological therapies targeting insulin resistance may be beneficial for treatment of cardiovascular disorders associated with insulin resistance. Indeed, therapy with thiazolidinediones or metformin lowers blood pressure in insulin-resistant patients who are also hypertensive (160,161) and both reduce cardiovascular events in randomized clinical trials (162).

Current thinking implicates local and/or systemic inflammation as a marker or modulator of vascular dysfunction as well as a contributor to insulin resistance (77,153,163). The natural question arising from this is whether anti-inflammatory therapy can be applied in a focused or targeted manner that improves vascular function and insulin resistance. Currently available therapeutics such as salicylic acid or pentoxyfilline may be able to provide this effect, but it appears overall that novel therapies will be required if this mechanism is to be addressed directly.

Similarly, if pro-inflammatory adipokines are involved in the pathogenesis of vascular dysfunction, antagonism of these responses may be feasible and may allow improvements in both metabolism and vascular function. However, at present it remains to be shown whether these agents are in fact pathophysiologically relevant, let alone whether effective therapeutic interventions can be found that directly target these factors. The major conceptual problem with these approaches is that the mechanism underlying the link between insulin resistance and vascular dysfunction remains incompletely understood. Therefore we cannot say whether concurrent observations of improvements in metabolism and vascular function, for example as seen with thiazolidinediones, in fact reflects a downstream effect of improved insulin resistance on vascular function or whether this is simply a concurrent beneficial effect in both systems.

Pharmacological Therapies Targeting Endothelial Dysfunction

Some drugs used for treatment of hypertension also have beneficial metabolic effects. Angiotensin converting enzyme (ACE) inhibitors reduce circulating angiotensin II levels while angiotensin receptor blockers (ARB) block actions of angiotensin II. These effects lower blood pressure, improve endothelial function, and reduce circulating markers of inflammation. In addition, treatment of patients with ACE inhibitors or ARBs results in significant increases in adiponectin levels and improvement in insulin sensitivity without changing BMI (164–166). These beneficial metabolic effects may be mediated, in part, by blocking inhibitory crosstalk between angiotensin II receptor signaling and insulin receptor signaling at the level of IRS-1 and PI 3-kinase (167). ACE inhibitors and ARBs may also have direct effects to induce PPAR-γ activity that augment insulin-stimulated glucose uptake and promote differentiation of adipocytes (168,169). Losartan (ARB) therapy significantly increases both plasma adiponectin levels and insulin sensitivity relative to baseline measurements in hypercholesterolemic, hypertensive patients (165).

Of note is that these findings are significantly correlated with improvements in endothelial function and inflammatory markers. Similar findings are observed with ramipril (ACE inhibitor) therapy in patients with type 2 diabetes (170). However, in both of these studies, treatment with simvastatin (HMG-CoA reductase inhibitor) did not increase adiponectin levels or improve insulin sensitivity. Yet, simvastatin does improve endothelial function and inflammatory markers in an additive manner when combined with losartan or ramipril. This suggests that only some mechanisms for improving endothelial function have a beneficial effect on insulin sensitivity and adiponectin levels.

Recent clinical trials demonstrate that using ACE inhibitors or ARBs to treat patients with cardiovascular disease significantly lowers the risk of developing type 2 diabetes (171,172). Conversely, using ACE inhibitors to treat patients with type 2 diabetes significantly improves cardiovascular outcomes (173). Thus, therapeutic interventions with ACE inhibitors and ARBs support the existence of reciprocal relationships between endothelial dysfunction and insulin resistance. Fibrates are synthetic PPAR-α ligands that improve the circulating lipoprotein profile, resulting in improved endothelial function, reduced vascular inflammation, and reduction in cardiovascular events in randomized clinical trials (174).

In one recent study, fenofibrate therapy (2 months) significantly increased plasma adiponectin levels and insulin sensitivity and was associated with improvements in endothelial function and inflammatory markers without changing body weight in patients with primary hypertriglyceridemia (166). The fact that body weight did not change raises the possibility that fenofibrate is directly altering adiponectin levels independent of adiposity. Thus, it is possible that increased adiponectin levels may directly contribute to improvement in insulin sensitivity and endothelial function. In another study (175), treatment with atorvastatin (HMG-CoA reductase inhibitor) as adjunctive therapy to fenofibrate did not increase adiponectin levels or improve insulin sensitivity, but was associated with improved endothelial function and reduced inflammatory markers in an additive manner. Thus, in this study, the beneficial effects of statins on endothelial function and inflammatory markers are dissociable from improvements in metabolic parameters.

Taken together, the data suggest that improvements in insulin sensitivity and metabolic parameters are closely linked to improvements in endothelial function. Indeed, some (e.g., ACE inhibitor, ARB, fenofibrate) but not all (e.g., statins) therapeutic approaches that improve endothelial function are closely linked to improvements in metabolic parameters.

FUTURE DIRECTIONS

A variety of interacting molecular, cellular, and physiological mechanisms in metabolic and vascular tissues contribute to important reciprocal relationships between insulin resistance and endothelial dysfunction. These complex relationships may underlie epidemiological data supporting associations and increased risks linking metabolic and cardiovascular disorders. Among these mechanisms, parallel insulin signaling pathways in classic target tissues and vascular tissues, coupling of blood flow with glucose metabolism, and pathophysiological crosstalk between metabolic and vascular tissues are particularly important. Recent additions to this list of mechanisms such as *pathway-specific insulin resistance* and *crosstalk between inflammatory signaling and insulin signaling* are likely to provide the foundation for the next set of advances. These numerous interacting pathways provide an opportunity to develop therapeutic approaches that target multiple mechanisms. Such combination approaches are likely to have beneficial effects on metabolic and cardiovascular health that go beyond benefits available from monotherapy alone.

The central importance of the interacting roles of nitric oxide and endothelin in the vessel wall is well established. Vascular actions of insulin to regulate tissue perfusion are now considered integral components of our understanding of insulin's overall actions on carbohydrate metabolism. Important areas for future investigations include newly discovered hormonal factors associated with obesity, insulin resistance, and endothelial dysfunction including adipokines and inflammatory markers and mediators. A deeper understanding of mechanisms underlying the coupling of metabolism and vascular function will be essential for developing novel beneficial therapeutic approaches for the metabolic syndrome and related disorders.

ACKNOWLEDGMENTS

This work was supported in part by awards from the American Diabetes Association to K.J.M (Junior Faculty and Career Development Awards) and M.J.Q (Research Award), by the Extramural Research Program of the NIH (DK42469 to A.D.B.), and by the Intramural Research Program of the NIH NCCAM (M.J.Q.). Some of the human studies described took place in the Indiana University General Clinical Research Center (NIH grant MO1RR00750).

REFERENCES

1. Vallance P, Collier JG, Moncada S. Effects of endothelium-derived nitric oxide on peripheral arteriolar tone in man. *Lancet* 1989; 160:881–886.
2. Stamler JS, Loh E, Roddy MA, Currie KE, Creager MA. Nitric oxide regulates basal systemic and pulmonary vascular resistance in healthy humans. *Circulation* 1994; 89(5):2035–2040.
3. Wu KK, Thiagarajan P. Role of endothelium in thrombosis and hemostasis. *Ann Rev Med* 1996; 47:315–331.
4. Adams MR, Jessup W, Hailstones D, Celermajer DS. L-arginine reduces human monocyte adhesion to vascular endothelium and endothelial expression of cell adhesion molecules. *Circulation* 1997; 95:662–668.
5. Lefer AM. Nitric oxide: Nature's naturally occurring leukocyte inhibitor. *Circulation* 1997; 95(3):553–554.
6. Malmstrom RE, Weitzberg E. Endothelin and nitric oxide in inflammation: could there be a need for endothelin blocking anti-inflammatory drugs? *J Hypertens* 2004; 22(1):27–29.

7. Barton M, Haudenschild CC. Endothelium and atherogenesis: Endothelial therapy revisited. *J Cardiovasc Pharmacol* 2001; 8(suppl 2):S23–25.
8. Bruckdorfer KR, Jacobs M, Rice-Evans C. Endothelium-derived relaxing factor (nitric oxide), lipoprotein oxidation and atherosclerosis. *Biochem Soc Trans* 1990; 18(6):1061–1063.
9. Hogg N, Kalyanaraman B, Joseph J, Struck A, Parthasarathy S. Inhibition of low-density lipoprotein oxidation by nitric oxide: Potential role in atherogenesis. *FEBS Lett* 1993; 334(2):170–174.
10. Jessup W, Dean RT. Autoinhibition of murine macrophage-mediated oxidation of low-density lipoprotein by nitric oxide synthesis. *Atherosclerosis* 1993; 101(2):145–155.
11. Moncada S, Higgs A. The L-arginine-nitric oxide pathway. *N Engl J Med* 1993; 329(27):2002–2012.
12. Cooke JP, Tsao PS. Endothelium-derived relaxing factor. In: *Endocrinology of the Vasculature.* Sowers JR (ed.). Humana Press, Totowa, NJ, 1996, pp. 3–20.
13. Cohen RA. The role of nitric oxide and other endothelium-derived vasoactive substances in vascular disease. *Prog Cardiovasc Dis* 1995; 38(2):105–128.
14. Lloyd-Jones DM, Bloch KD. The vascular biology of nitric oxide and its role in atherogenesis. *Ann Rev Med* 1996; 47:365–75.
15. Montagnani M, Quon MJ. Insulin action in vascular endothelium: Potential mechanisms linking insulin resistance with hypertension. *Diabetes Obes Metab* 2000; 2(5):285–292.
16. Vincent MA, Montagnani M, Quon MJ. Molecular and physiologic actions of insulin related to production of nitric oxide in vascular endothelium. *Curr Diab Rep* 2003; 3(4):279–288.
17. Michel JB, Feron O, Sacks D, Michel T. Reciprocal regulation of endothelial nitric-oxide synthase by Ca2+- calmodulin and caveolin. *J Biol Chem* 1997; 272(25):15583–15586.
18. Michel JB, Feron O, Sase K, Prabhakar P, Michel T. Caveolin versus calmodulin: Counterbalancing allosteric modulators of endothelial nitric oxide synthase. *J Biol Chem* 1997; 272(41):25907–25912.
19. Montagnani M, Chen H, Barr VA, Quon MJ. Insulin-stimulated activation of eNOS is independent of Ca2+ but requires phosphorylation by Akt at Ser(1179). *J Biol Chem* 2001; 276(32):30392–30398.
20. Zeng G, Quon MJ. Insulin-stimulated production of nitric oxide is inhibited by wortmannin: Direct measurement in vascular endothelial cells. *J Clin Investig* 1996; 98(4):894–898.
21. Zeng G, Nystrom FH, Ravichandran LV et al. Roles for insulin receptor, PI3-kinase, and Akt in insulin-signaling pathways related to production of nitric oxide in human vascular endothelial cells. *Circulation* 2000; 101(13):1539–1545.
22. Montagnani M, Golovchenko I, Kim I et al. Inhibition of phosphatidylinositol 3-kinase enhances mitogenic actions of insulin in endothelial cells. *J Biol Chem* 2002; 277(3):1794–1799.
23. Nystrom FH, Quon MJ. Insulin signalling: Metabolic pathways and mechanisms for specificity. *Cell Signal* 1999; 11(8):563–574.
24. Montagnani M, Ravichandran LV, Chen H, Esposito DL, Quon MJ. Insulin receptor substrate-1 and phosphoinositide-dependent kinase-1 are required for insulin-stimulated production of nitric oxide in endothelial cells. *Mol Endocrinol* 2002; 16(8):1931–1942.
25. Dimmeler S, Fleming I, Fisslthaler B, Hernamm C, Busse R, Zeiher AM. Activation of nitric oxide synthase in endothelial cells by Akt-dependent phosphorylation. *Nature* 1999; 399:601–605.
26. Potenza MA, Marasciulo FL, Chieppa DM et al. Insulin resistance in spontaneously hypertensive rats is associated with endothelial dysfunction characterized by imbalance between NO and ET-1 production. *Am J Physiol Heart Circ Physiol* 2005; 289(2):H813–822.
27. Steinberg HO, Chaker H, Leaming R, Johnson A, Brechtel G, Baron AD. Obesity/insulin resistance is associated with endothelial dysfunction: Implications for the syndrome of insulin resistance. *J Clin Investig* 1996; 97(11):2601–2610.
28. Ferri C, Desideri G, Valenti M et al. Early upregulation of endothelial adhesion molecules in obese hypertensive men. *Hypertension* 1999; 34(4, pt. 1):568–573.
29. Campia U, Sullivan G, Bryant MB, Waclawiw MA, Quon MJ, Panza JA. Insulin impairs endothelium-dependent vasodilation independent of insulin sensitivity or lipid profile. *Am J Physiol Heart Circ Physiol* 2004; 286(1):H76–82.
30. Cardillo C, Mettimano M, Mores N, Koh KK, Campia U, Panza JA. Plasma levels of cell adhesion molecules during hyperinsulinemia and modulation of vasoactive mediators. *Vasc Med* 2004; 9(3):185–188.

31. Vecchione C, Maffei A, Colella S et al. Leptin effect on endothelial nitric oxide is mediated through Akt-endothelial nitric oxide synthase phosphorylation pathway. *Diabetes* 2002; 51(1):168–173.
32. Chen H, Montagnani M, Funahashi T, Shimomura I, Quon MJ. Adiponectin stimulates production of nitric oxide in vascular endothelial cells. *J Biol Chem* 2003; 278(45):45021–45026.
33. Mineo C, Yuhanna IS, Quon MJ, Shaul PW. High-density lipoprotein-induced endothelial nitric-oxide synthase activation is mediated by Akt and MAP kinases. *J Biol Chem* 2003; 278(11):9142–9149.
34. Simoncini T, Hafezi-Moghadam A, Brazil DP, Ley K, Chin WW, Liao JK. Interaction of oestrogen receptor with the regulatory subunit of phosphatidylinositol-3-OH kinase. *Nature* 2000; 407(6803):538–541.
35. Hafezi-Moghadam A, Simoncini T, Yang Z et al. Acute cardiovascular protective effects of corticosteroids are mediated by non-transcriptional activation of endothelial nitric oxide synthase. *Nat Med* 2002; 8(5):473–479.
36. Formoso G, Chen H, Kim J, Montagnani M, Consoli A, Quon MJ. DHEA mimics acute actions of insulin to stimulate production of both NO and ET-1 via distinct PI 3-kinase- and MAP-kinase-dependent pathways in vascular endothelium. *Mol Endocrinol* 2006; in press.
37. Laakso M, Edelman SV, Brechtel G, Baron AD. Decreased effect of insulin to stimulate skeletal muscle blood flow in obese man: A novel mechanism for insulin resistance. *J Clin Investig* 1990; 85(6):1844–1852.
38. Laakso M, Edelman SV, Brechtel G, Baron AD. Impaired insulin-mediated skeletal muscle blood flow in patients with NIDDM. *Diabetes* 1992; 41(9):1076–1083.
39. Baron AD. Insulin and the vasculature: Old actors, new roles. *J Investig Med* 1996; 44:406–412.
40. Baron AD, Brechtel G. Insulin differentially regulates systemic and skeletal muscle vascular resistance. *Am J Physiol* 1993; 265(1, pt. 1):E61–E67.
41. Steinberg HO, Brechtel G, Johnson A, Fineberg N, Baron AD. Insulin mediated skeletal muscle vasodilation is nitric oxide dependent: A novel action of insulin to increase nitric oxide release. *J Clin Investig* 1994; 94(3):1172–1179.
42. Scherrer U, Randin D, Vollenweider P, Vollenweider L, Nicod P. Nitric oxide release accounts for insulin's vascular effects in humans. *J Clin Investig* 1994; 94(6):2511–2515.
43. Taddei S, Virdis A, Mattei P, Natali A, Ferrannini E, Salvetti A. Effect of insulin on acetylcholine-induced vasodilation in normotensive subjects and patients with essential hypertension. *Circulation* 1995; 92(10):2911–2918.
44. Nagao T, Illiano S, Vanhoutte PM. Heterogeneous distribution of endothelium-dependent relaxations resistant to NG-nitro-L-arginine in rats. *Am J Physiol* 1992; 263(4, pt. 2):H1090–1094.
45. Baron AD, Steinberg HO, Chaker H, Leaming R, Johnson A, Brechtel G. Insulin-mediated skeletal muscle vasodilation contributes to both insulin sensitivity and responsiveness in lean humans. *J Clin Investig* 1995; 96(2):786–792.
46. Trovati M, Massucco P, Mattiello L et al. Human vascular smooth muscle cells express a constitutive nitric oxide synthase that insulin rapidly activates, thus increasing guanosine $3' : 5'$-cyclic monophosphate and adenosine $3' : 5'$-cyclic monophosphate concentrations. *Diabetologia* 1999; 42(7):831–839.
47. Kim J, Montagnani M, Koh KK, Quon MJ. Reciprocal relationships between insulin resistance and endothelial dysfunction: Molecular and pathophysiological mechanisms. *Circulation* 2006; in press.
48. Renkin EM. Control of microcirculation and blood-tissue exchange. In: *Handbook of Physiology: The Cardiovascular System Microcirculation,* Am. Physiol. Soc., Bethesda, 1984, pp. 627–687.
49. Grubb B, Snarr JF. Effect of flow rate and glucose concentration on glucose uptake rate by the rat limb. *Proc Soc Exp Biol Med* 1977; 154(1):33–36.
50. Mather K, Laakso M, Edelman S, Hook G, Baron A. Evidence for physiologic coupling of limb blood flow and insulin mediated glucose metabolism. *Am J Physiol* 2000; 279:E1264–1270.
51. Rattigan S, Clark MG, Barrett EJ. Hemodynamic actions of insulin in rat skeletal muscle: Evidence for capillary recruitment. *Diabetes* 1997; 46(9):1381–1388.
52. Clark AD, Barrett EJ, Rattigan S, Wallis MG, Clark MG. Insulin stimulates laser Doppler signal by rat muscle in vivo, consistent with nutritive flow recruitment. *Clin Sci (Colch)* 2001; 100(3):283–290.

53. Vincent MA, Dawson D, Clark AD et al. Skeletal muscle microvascular recruitment by physiological hyperinsulinemia precedes increases in total blood flow. *Diabetes* 2002; 51(1):42–48.
54. Baron AD, Clark MG. Role of blood flow in the regulation of muscle glucose uptake. *Annual Review of Nutrition* 1997; 17:487–499.
55. Baron AD, Tarshoby M, Hook G et al. Interaction between insulin sensitivity and muscle perfusion on glucose uptake in human skeletal muscle: Evidence for capillary recruitment. *Diabetes* 2000; 49:768–774.
56. Bonadonna RC, Saccomani MP, Del Prato S, Bonora E, DeFronzo RA, Cobelli C. Role of tissue-specific blood flow and tissue recruitment in insulin mediated glucose uptake of human skeletal muscle. *Circulation* 1998; 98(3):234–241.
57. Serne EH, IJzerman RG, Gans RO et al. Direct evidence for insulin-induced capillary recruitment in skin of healthy subjects during physiological hyperinsulinemia. *Diabetes* 2002; 51(5):1515–1522.
58. Vincent MA, Clerk LH, Lindner JR et al. Microvascular recruitment is an early insulin effect that regulates skeletal muscle glucose uptake in vivo. *Diabetes* 2004; 53(6):1418–1423.
59. Zhang L, Vincent MA, Richards SM et al. Insulin sensitivity of muscle capillary recruitment in vivo. *Diabetes* 2004; 53(2):447–453.
60. Coggins M, Lindner J, Rattigan S et al. Physiologic hyperinsulinemia enhances human skeletal muscle perfusion by capillary recruitment. *Diabetes* 2001; 50(12):2682–2690.
61. Cusi K, Maezono K, Osman A et al. Insulin resistance differentially affects the PI 3-kinase- and MAP kinase-mediated signaling in human muscle. *J Clin Investig* 2000; 105(3):311–320.
62. Abe H, Yamada N, Kamata K et al. Hypertension, hypertriglyceridemia, and impaired endothelium-dependent vascular relaxation in mice lacking insulin receptor substrate-1. *J Clin Investig* 1998; 101(8):1784–1788.
63. Federici M, Pandolfi A, De Filippis EA et al. G972R IRS-1 variant impairs insulin regulation of endothelial nitric oxide synthase in cultured human endothelial cells. *Circulation* 2004; 109(3):399–405.
64. Laine H, Yki-Jarvinen H, Kirvela O et al. Insulin resistance of glucose uptake in skeletal muscle cannot be ameliorated by enhancing endothelium-dependent blood flow in obesity. *J Clin Investig* 1998; 101(5):1156–1162.
65. Kinoshita J, Tanaka Y, Niwa M, Yoshii H, Takagi M, Kawamori R. Impairment of insulin-induced vasodilation is associated with muscle insulin resistance in type 2 diabetes. *Diab Res Clin Pract* 2000; 47(3):185–190.
66. Cleland SJ, Petrie JR, Small M, Elliott HL, Connell JM. Insulin action is associated with endothelial function in hypertension and type 2 diabetes. *Hypertension* 2000; 35(1, pt. 2):507–511.
67. Lembo G, Iaccarino G, Vecchione C, Rendina V, Trimarco B. Insulin modulation of vascular reactivity is already impaired in prehypertensive spontaneously hypertensive rats. *Hypertension* 1995; 26(2):290–293.
68. Natali A, Taddei S, Quinones GA et al. Insulin sensitivity, vascular reactivity, and clamp-induced vasodilatation in essential hypertension. *Circulation* 1997; 96(3):849–855.
69. Steinberg HO, Paradisi G, Cronin J et al. Type II diabetes abrogates sex differences in endothelial function in premenopausal women. *Circulation* 2000; 101(17):2040–2046.
70. Bohlen HG, Lash JM. Topical hyperglycemia rapidly suppresses EDRF-mediated vasodilation of normal rat arterioles. *Am J Physiol* 1993; 265(1, pt. 2):H219–225.
71. Jin JS, Bohlen HG. Non-insulin-dependent diabetes and hyperglycemia impair rat intestinal flow-mediated regulation. *Am J Physiol* 1997; 272(2, pt. 2):H728–734.
72. Williams SB, Cusco JA, Roddy MA, Johnstone MT, Creager MA. Impaired nitric oxide-mediated vasodilation in patients with non-insulin-dependent diabetes mellitus. *J Am Coll Cardiol* 1996; 27(3):567–574.
73. Beckman JA, Goldfine AB, Gordon MB, Creager MA. Ascorbate restores endothelium-dependent vasodilation impaired by acute hyperglycemia in humans. *Circulation* 2001; 103(12):1618–1623.
74. Davda RK, Stepniakowski KT, Lu G, Ullian ME, Goodfriend TL, Egan BM. Oleic acid inhibits endothelial nitric oxide synthase by a protein-kinase-C-independent mechanism. *Hypertension* 1995; 26(5):764–770.
75. Steinberg HO, Tarshoby M, Monestel R et al. Elevated circulating free fatty acid levels impair endothelium-dependent vasodilation. *J Clin Investig* 1997; 100:1230–1239.

76. Aljada A, Ghanim H, Assian E, Dandona P. Tumor necrosis factor-alpha inhibits insulin-induced increase in endothelial nitric oxide synthase and reduces insulin receptor content and phosphorylation in human aortic endothelial cells. *Metab Clin Exp* 2002; 51(4):487–491.

77. Rask-Madsen C, Dominguez H, Ihlemann N, Hermann T, Kober L, Torp-Pedersen C. Tumor necrosis factor-alpha inhibits insulin's stimulating effect on glucose uptake and endothelium-dependent vaso-dilation in humans. *Circulation* 2003; 108(15):1815–1821.

78. Clerk LH, Rattigan S, Clark MG. Lipid infusion impairs physiologic insulin-mediated capillary recruitment and muscle glucose uptake in vivo. *Diabetes* 2002; 51(4):1138–1145.

79. Zhang L, Wheatley CM, Richards SM, Barrett EJ, Clark MG, Rattigan S. TNF-alpha acutely inhibits vascular effects of physiological but not high insulin or contraction. *Am J Physiol Endocrinol Metab* 2003; 285(3):E654–660.

80. Yanagisawa M, Kurihara H, Kimura A et al. A novel potent vasoconstrictor peptide produced by vascular endothelial cells. *Nature* 1988; 332:411–415.

81. Levin ER. Endothelins. *N Engl J Med* 1995; 333:356–363.

82. Schiffrin EL, Touyz RM. Vascular biology of endothelin. *J Cardiovasc Pharmacol* 1998; 32(suppl 3):S2–13.

83. Wagner OF, Christ G, Wojta J et al. Polar secretion of endothelin-1 by cultured endothelial cells. *J Biol Chem* 1992; 267(23):16066–16068.

84. Seljeflot I, Moan A, Aspelin T, Tonnessen T, Kjeldsen SE, Arnesen H. Circulating levels of endo-thelin-1 during acute hyperinsulinemia in patients with essential hypertension treated with type 1 angiotensin receptor antagonist or placebo. *Metab Clin Exp* 1998; 47(3):292–296.

85. Irving RJ, Noon JP, Watt GC, Webb DJ, Walker BR. Activation of the endothelin system in insulin resistance. *Qjm* 2001; 94(6):321–326.

86. Piatti P, Fragasso G, Monti LD et al. Endothelial and metabolic characteristics of patients with angina and angiographically normal coronary arteries: Comparison with subjects with insulin resistance syndrome and normal controls. *J Am Coll Cardiol* 1999; 34(5):1452–1460.

87. Piatti PM, Monti LD, Galli L et al. Relationship between endothelin-1 concentration and metabolic alterations typical of the insulin resistance syndrome. *Metab Clin Exp* 2000; 49(6):748–752.

88. Ferri C, Bellini C, Desideri G, et al. Plasma endothelin-1 levels in obese hypertensive and normo-tensive men. *Diabetes* 1995; 44(4):431–436.

89. Ferri C, Bellini C, Desideri G et al. Circulating endothelin-1 levels in obese patients with the meta-bolic syndrome. *Exper Clin Endocrinol Diab* 1997; 105(suppl 2):38–40.

90. Andronico G, Mangano M, Ferrara L, Lamanna D, Mule G, Cerasola G. In vivo relationship between insulin and endothelin role of insulin resistance. *J Hum Hypertens* 1997; 11(1):63–66.

91. Ak G, Buyukberber S, Sevinc A et al. The relation between plasma endothelin-1 levels and metabolic control, risk factors, treatment modalities, and diabetic microangiopathy in patients with type 2 dia-betes mellitus. *J Diab Complic* 2001; 15(3):150–157.

92. Caballero AE, Arora S, Saouaf R et al. Microvascular and macrovascular reactivity is reduced in subjects at risk for type 2 diabetes. *Diabetes* 1999; 48(9):1856–1862.

93. Mangiafico RA, Malatino LS, Santonocito M, Spada RS. Plasma endothelin-1 concentrations in non-insulin-dependent diabetes mellitus and nondiabetic patients with chronic arterial obstructive disease of the lower limbs. *Int Angiol* 1998; 17(2):97–102.

94. Sanchez SS, Aybar MJ, Velarde MS, Prado MM, Carrizo T. Relationship between plasma endothelin-1 and glycemic control in type 2 diabetes mellitus. *Horm Metab Res* 2001; 33(12):748–751.

95. Pontiroli AE, Pizzocri P, Koprivec D et al. Body weight and glucose metabolism have a different effect on circulating levels of ICAM-1, E-selectin, and endothelin-1 in humans. *Eur J Endocrinol* 2004; 150(2):195–200.

96. Lavrencic A, Salobir BG, Keber I. Physical training improves flow-mediated dilation in patients with the polymetabolic syndrome. *Arterioscler Thromb Vasc Biol* 2000; 20(2):551–555.

97. Wolpert HA, Steen SN, Istfan NW, Simonson DC. Insulin modulates circulating endothelin-1 levels in humans. *Metab Clin Exp* 1993; 42(8):1027–1030.

98. Diamanti-Kandarakis E, Spina G, Kouli C, Migdalis I. Increased endothelin-1 levels in women with polycystic ovary syndrome and the beneficial effect of metformin therapy. *J Clin Endocrinol Metab* 2001; 86(10):4666–4673.

99. Nakamura T, Ushiyama C, Shimada N, Hayashi K, Ebihara I, Koide H. Comparative effects of pioglitazone, glibenclamide, and voglibose on urinary endothelin-1 and albumin excretion in diabetes patients. *J Diab Complic* 2000; 14(5):250–254.

100. Anfossi G, Cavalot F, Massucco P et al. Insulin influences immunoreactive endothelin release by human vascular smooth muscle cells. *Metab Clin Exp* 1993; 42(9):1081–1083.

101. Hu RM, Levin ER, Pedram A, Frank HJ. Insulin stimulates production and secretion of endothelin from bovine endothelial cells. *Diabetes* 1993; 42(2):351–358.

102. Oliver FJ, de la Rubia G, Feener EP et al. Stimulation of endothelin-1 gene expression by insulin in endothelial cells. *J Biol Chem* 1991; 266(34):23251–23256.

103. Ferri C, Carlomagno A, Coassin S et al. Circulating endothelin-1 levels increase during euglycemic hyperinsulinemic clamp in lean NIDDM men. *Diabetes Care* 1995; 18(2):226–233.

104. Piatti PM, Monti LD, Conti M et al. Hypertriglyceridemia and hyperinsulinemia are potent inducers of endothelin-1 release in humans. *Diabetes* 1996; 45(3):316–321.

105. Kohan DE. Production of endothelin-1 by rat mesangial cells: Regulation by tumor necrosis factor. *J Lab Clin Med* 1992; 119(5):477–484.

106. Patel JN, Jager A, Schalkwijk C et al. Effects of tumour necrosis factor-alpha in the human forearm: Blood flow and endothelin-1 release. *Clin Sci (Lond)* 2002; 103(4):409–415.

107. Kourembanas S, McQuillan LP, Leung GK, Faller DV. Nitric oxide regulates the expression of vasoconstrictors and growth factors by vascular endothelium under both normoxia and hypoxia. *J Clin Investig* 1993; 92(1):99–104.

108. Flowers MA, Wang Y, Stewart RJ, Patel B, Marsden PA. Reciprocal regulation of endothelin-1 and endothelial constitutive NOS in proliferating endothelial cells. *Am J Physiol* 1995; 269(6, pt. 2): H1988–1997.

109. Li H, Wallerath T, Forstermann U. Physiological mechanisms regulating the expression of endothelial-type NO synthase. *Nitric Oxide* 2002; 7(2):132–147.

110. Wollesen F, Berglund L, Berne C. Plasma endothelin-1 and total insulin exposure in diabetes mellitus. *Clin Sci (Colch)* 1999; 97(2):149–56.

111. Leyva F, Wingrove C, Felton C, Stevenson JC. Physiological hyperinsulinemia is not associated with alterations in venous plasma levels of endothelin-1 in healthy individuals. *Metab Clin Exp* 1997; 46(10):1137–1139.

112. Metsarinne K, Saijonmaa O, Yki-Jarvinen H, Fyhrquist F. Insulin increases the release of endothelin in endothelial cell cultures in vitro but not in vivo. *Metab Clin Exp* 1994; 43(7):878–882.

113. Katsumori K, Wasada T, Saeki A, Naruse M, Omori Y. Lack of acute insulin effect on plasma endothelin-1 levels in humans. *Diab Res Clin Pract* 1996; 32(3):187–189.

114. Gottsater A, Rendell M, Anwaar I, Lindgarde F, Hulthen UL, Mattiasson I. Increasing neopterin and decreasing endothelin-1 in plasma during insulin infusion in women. *Scand J Clin Lab Invest* 1999; 59(6):417–424.

115. Polderman KH, Stehouwer CD, van Kamp GJ, Gooren LJ. Effects of insulin infusion on endothelium-derived vasoactive substances. *Diabetologia* 1996; 39(11):1284–1292.

116. Surdacki A, Nowicki M, Sandmann J et al. Effects of acute euglycemic hyperinsulinemia on urinary nitrite/nitrate excretion and plasma endothelin-1 levels in men with essential hypertension and normotensive controls. *Metab Clin Exp* 1999; 48(7):887–891.

117. Cardillo C, Nambi SS, Kilcoyne CM et al. Insulin stimulates both endothelin and nitric oxide activity in the human forearm. *Circulation* 1999; 100(8):820–825.

118. Mather K, Mirzamohammadi B, Lteif A, Steinberg H, Baron A. Endothelin contributes to basal vascular tone and endothelial dysfunction in human obesity and type 2 diabetes mellitus. *Diabetes* 2002; 51(12):3517–3523.

119. Cardillo C, Campia U, Bryant MB, Panza JA. Increased activity of endogenous endothelin in patients with type II diabetes mellitus. *Circulation* 2002; 106(14):1783–1787.

120. Mather KJ, Lteif A, Steinberg HO, Baron AD. Interactions between endothelin and nitric oxide in the regulation of vascular tone in obesity and diabetes. *Diabetes* 2004; 53(8):2060–2066.

121. Juan CC, Fang VS, Huang YJ, Kwok CF, Hsu YP, Ho LT. Endothelin-1 induces insulin resistance in conscious rats. *Biochem Biophys Res Comm* 1996; 227(3):694–699.

122. Wilkes JJ, Hevener A, Olefsky J. Chronic endothelin-1 treatment leads to insulin resistance in vivo. *Diabetes* 2003; 52(8):1904–1909.

123. Ottosson-Seeberger A, Lundberg JM, Alvestrand A, Ahlborg G. Exogenous endothelin-1 causes peripheral insulin resistance in healthy humans. *Acta Physiologica Scandinavica* 1997; 161(2):211–220.

124. Ahlborg G, Lindstrom J. Insulin sensitivity and big ET-1 conversion to ET-1 after ETA- or ETB-receptor blockade in humans. *J Appl Physiol* 2002; 93(6):2112–2121.

125. Ahlborg G, Weitzberg E, Lundberg JM. Endothelin-1 infusion reduces splanchnic glucose production in humans. *J Appl Physiol* 1994; 77(1):121–126.

126. Zimmerman RS, Maymind M. NG-methyl-L-arginine and somatostatin decrease glucose and insulin and block endothelin-1 (ET-1)-induced insulin release but not ET-1-induced hypoglycemia. *Metab Clin Exp* 1995; 44(12):1532–1535.

127. De Carlo E, Milanesi A, Martini C, Maffei P, Sicolo N, Scandellari C. Endothelin-1 and endothelin-3 stimulate insulin release by isolated rat pancreatic islets. *J Endocrinol Investig* 2000; 23(4):240–245.

128. Gregersen S, Thomsen JL, Brock B, Hermansen K. Endothelin-1 stimulates insulin secretion by direct action on the islets of Langerhans in mice. *Diabetologia* 1996; 39(9):1030–1035.

129. Roden M, Vierhapper H, Liener K, Waldhausl W. Endothelin-1-stimulated glucose production in vitro in the isolated perfused rat liver. *Metab Clin Exp* 1992; 41(3):290–295.

130. Balsiger B, Rickenbacher A, Boden PJ et al. Endothelin A-receptor blockade in experimental diabetes improves glucose balance and gastrointestinal function. *Clin Sci (Lond)* 2002; 103(suppl)48:430S–433S.

131. Verma S, Bhanot S, Yao L, McNeill JH. Vascular insulin resistance in fructose-hypertensive rats. *Eur J Pharmacol* 1997; 322(2–3):R1–R2.

132. Santure M, Pitre M, Marette A et al. Induction of insulin resistance by high-sucrose feeding does not raise mean arterial blood pressure but impairs haemodynamic responses to insulin in rats. *Br J Pharmacol* 2002; 137(2):185–196.

133. Verma S, Yao L, Stewart DJ, Dumont AS, Anderson TJ, McNeill JH. Endothelin antagonism uncovers insulin-mediated vasorelaxation in vitro and in vivo. *Hypertension* 2001; 37(2):328–333.

134. Miller AW, Tulbert C, Puskar M, Busija DW. Enhanced endothelin activity prevents vasodilation to insulin in insulin resistance. *Hypertension* 2002; 40:78–82.

135. Lee DH, Lee JU, Kang DG, Paek YW, Chung DJ, Chung MY. Increased vascular endothelin-1 gene expression with unaltered nitric oxide synthase levels in fructose-induced hypertensive rats. *Metab Clin Exp* 2001; 50(1):74–78.

136. Juan CC, Fang VS, Hsu YP et al. Overexpression of vascular endothelin-1 and endothelin-A receptors in a fructose-induced hypertensive rat model. *J Hypertens* 1998; 16(12, pt. 1):1775–1782.

137. McKendrick JD, Salas E, Dube GP, Murat J, Russell JC, Radomski MW. Inhibition of nitric oxide generation unmasks vascular dysfunction in insulin-resistant, obese JCR:LA-cp rats. *Br J Pharmacol* 1998; 124(2):361–369.

138. Katakam PV, Pollock JS, Pollock DM, Ujhelyi MR, Miller AW. Enhanced endothelin-1 response and receptor expression in small mesenteric arteries of insulin-resistant rats. *Am J Physiol Heart Circ Physiol* 2001; 280(2):H522–H527.

139. Wu J, Michel H, Rossomando A et al. Renaturation and partial peptide sequencing of mitogen-activated protein kinase (MAP kinase) activator from rabbit skeletal muscle. *Biochem J* 1992; 285(pt. 3):701–705.

140. Yudkin JS, Eringa E, Stehouwer CD. "Vasocrine" signalling from perivascular fat: A mechanism linking insulin resistance to vascular disease. *Lancet* 2005; 365(9473):1817–18120.

141. Yamauchi T, Kamon J, Waki H et al. The fat-derived hormone adiponectin reverses insulin resistance associated with both lipoatrophy and obesity. *Nat Med* 2001; 7(8):941–946.

142. Kubota N, Terauchi Y, Yamauchi T et al. Disruption of adiponectin causes insulin resistance and neointimal formation. *J Biol Chem* 2002; 277(29):25863–25866.

143. Fernandez-Real JM, Lopez-Bermejo A, Casamitjana R, Ricart W. Novel interactions of adiponectin with the endocrine system and inflammatory parameters. *J Clin Endocrinol Metab* 2003; 88(6):2714–2718.

144. Hattori Y, Suzuki M, Hattori S, Kasai K. Globular adiponectin upregulates nitric oxide production in vascular endothelial cells. *Diabetologia* 2003; 46(11):1543–1549.

145. Heilbronn LK, Smith SR, Ravussin E. The insulin-sensitizing role of the fat derived hormone adiponectin. *Curr Pharm Des* 2003; 9(17):1411–1418.

146. Kishida K, Nagaretani H, Kondo H et al. Disturbed secretion of mutant adiponectin associated with the metabolic syndrome. *Biochem Biophys Res Comm* 2003; 306(1):286–292.
147. Yamauchi T, Hara K, Kubota N et al. Dual roles of adiponectin/acrp30 in vivo as an anti-diabetic and anti-atherogenic adipokine. *Curr Drug Targets Immune Endocr Metabol Disord* 2003; 3(4):243–254.
148. Yamauchi T, Kamon J, Waki H et al. Globular adiponectin protected ob/ob mice from diabetes and ApoE-deficient mice from atherosclerosis. *J Biol Chem* 2003; 278(4):2461–2468.
149. Hambrecht R, Wolf A, Gielen S et al. Effect of exercise on coronary endothelial function in patients with coronary artery disease. *N Engl J Med* 2000; 342(7):454–460.
150. Arvola P, Wu X, Kahonen M et al. Exercise enhances vasorelaxation in experimental obesity associated hypertension. *Cardiovasc Res* 1999; 43(4):992–1002.
151. Minami A, Ishimura N, Harada N, Sakamoto S, Niwa Y, Nakaya Y. Exercise training improves acetylcholine-induced endothelium-dependent hyperpolarization in type 2 diabetic rats, Otsuka Long-Evans Tokushima fatty rats. *Atherosclerosis* 2002; 162(1):85–92.
152. Nicoletti G, Giugliano G, Pontillo A et al. Effect of a multidisciplinary program of weight reduction on endothelial functions in obese women. *J Endocrinol Investig* 2003; 26(3):RC5–8.
153. Vazquez LA, Pazos F, Berrazueta JR et al. Effects of changes in body weight and insulin resistance on inflammation and endothelial function in morbid obesity after bariatric surgery. *J Clin Endocrinol Metab* 2005; 90(1):316–322.
154. Williams IL, Chowienczyk PJ, Wheatcroft SB et al. Endothelial function and weight loss in obese humans. *Obes Surg* 2005; 15(7):1055–1060.
155. Fujishima S, Ohya Y, Nakamura Y, Onaka U, Abe I, Fujishima M. Troglitazone, an insulin sensitizer, increases forearm blood flow in humans. *Am J Hypertens* 1998; 11(9):1134–1137.
156. Mather KJ, Verma S, Anderson TJ. Improved endothelial function with metformin in type 2 diabetes mellitus. *J Am Coll Cardiol* 2001; 37(5):1344–1350.
157. Hsueh WA, Law RE. PPAR-gamma and atherosclerosis: Effects on cell growth and movement. *Arterioscler Thromb Vasc Biol* 2001; 21(12):1891–1895.
158. Maeda N, Takahashi M, Funahashi T et al. PPAR-gamma ligands increase expression and plasma concentrations of adiponectin, an adipose-derived protein. *Diabetes* 2001; 50(9):2094–2099.
159. Yu JG, Javorschi S, Hevener AL et al. The effect of thiazolidinediones on plasma adiponectin levels in normal, obese, and type 2 diabetic subjects. *Diabetes* 2002; 51(10):2968–2974.
160. Nolan JJ, Ludvik B, Beerdsen P, Joyce M, Olefsky J. Improvement in glucose tolerance and insulin resistance in obese subjects treated with troglitazone. *N Engl J Med* 1994; 331:1188–1193.
161. Giugliano D, De Rosa N, Di Maro G et al. Metformin improves glucose, lipid metabolism, and reduces blood pressure in hypertensive, obese women. *Diabetes Care* 1993; 16(10):1387–1390.
162. Panunti B, Kunhiraman B, Fonseca V. The impact of antidiabetic therapies on cardiovascular disease. *Curr Atheroscler Rep* 2005; 7(1):50–57.
163. Weyer C, Yudkin JS, Stehouwer CD, Schalkwijk CG, Pratley RE, Tataranni PA. Humoral markers of inflammation and endothelial dysfunction in relation to adiposity and in vivo insulin action in Pima Indians. *Atherosclerosis* 2002; 161(1):233–242.
164. Furuhashi M, Ura N, Higashiura K et al. Blockade of the renin-angiotensin system increases adiponectin concentrations in patients with essential hypertension. *Hypertension* 2003; 42(1):76–81.
165. Koh KK, Quon MJ, Han SH et al. Additive beneficial effects of losartan combined with simvastatin in the treatment of hypercholesterolemic, hypertensive patients. *Circulation* 2004; 110(24): 3687–3692.
166. Koh KK, Han SH, Quon MJ, Yeal Ahn J, Shin EK. Beneficial effects of fenofibrate to improve endothelial dysfunction and raise adiponectin levels in patients with primary hypertriglyceridemia. *Diabetes Care* 2005; 28(6):1419–1424.
167. Folli F, Kahn CR, Hansen H, Bouchie JL, Feener EP. Angiotensin II inhibits insulin signaling in aortic smooth muscle cells at multiple levels: A potential role for serine phosphorylation in insulin/ angiotensin II crosstalk. *J Clin Investig* 1997; 100:2158–2169.
168. Sharma AM, Janke J, Gorzelniak K, Engeli S, Luft FC. Angiotensin blockade prevents type 2 diabetes by formation of fat cells. *Hypertension* 2002; 40(5):609–611.

169. Schupp M, Janke J, Clasen R, Unger T, Kintscher U. Angiotensin type 1 receptor blockers induce peroxisome proliferator-activated receptor-gamma activity. *Circulation* 2004; 109(17):2054–2057.

170. Koh KK, Quon MJ, Han SH et al. Vascular and metabolic effects of combined therapy with ramipril and simvastatin in patients with type 2 diabetes. *Hypertension* 2005; 45(6):1088–1093.

171. Yusuf S, Gerstein H, Hoogwerf B et al. Ramipril and the development of diabetes. *JAMA* 2001; 286(15):1882–1885.

172. Yusuf S, Ostergren JB, Gerstein HC et al. Effects of candesartan on the development of a new diagnosis of diabetes mellitus in patients with heart failure. *Circulation* 2005; 112(1):48–53.

173. Heart Outcomes Prevention Evaluation Study Investigators. Effects of ramipril on cardiovascular and microvascular outcomes in people with diabetes mellitus: Results of the HOPE study and MICRO-HOPE substudy. *Lancet* 2000; 355(9200):253–259.

174. Keech A, Simes RJ, Barter P et al. Effects of long-term fenofibrate therapy on cardiovascular events in 9,795 people with type 2 diabetes mellitus (the FIELD study): Randomised controlled trial. *Lancet* 2005; 366(9500):1849–1861.

175. Koh KK, Quon MJ, Han SH et al. Additive beneficial effects of fenofibrate combined with atorvastatin in the treatment of combined hyperlipidemia. *J Am Coll Cardiol* 2005; 45(10):1649–1653.

8   Macro- and Microvascular Disease in an Insulin-Resistant Pre-Diabetic Animal Model

The JCR:LA-cp Rat

James C. Russell and Spencer D. Proctor

CONTENTS

INTRODUCTION

The metabolic syndrome is a particularly insidious disease state due to the asymptomatic character of its early stages. A typical clinical history involves a long period of increasing abdominal obesity without obvious underlying disease, followed by an apparently sudden development of frank type 2 diabetes. As the clinical diabetes becomes recognized and treated, medical follow-up reveals established cardiovascular disease (CVD). The associated significant damage to the vascular system develops steadily, beginning during the pre-diabetic period, a process that is only now becoming widely appreciated. Thus, a crucial feature of the metabolic syndrome is widespread endothelial and vascular dysfunction that develops during the pre-diabetic and early diabetic phases of type 2 diabetes. Similarly, the concomitant insulin resistance and hyperinsulinaemia appear to be major determinants of early stage vasculopathy, atherosclerosis, ischemic cardiovascular disease, and glomerular sclerosis, leading to end-stage renal complications (1,2). The metabolic syndrome thus encompasses the primary

From: *Contemporary Endocrinology: The Metabolic Syndrome: Epidemiology, Clinical Treatment, and Underlying Mechanisms*
Edited by: B.C. Hansen and G.A. Bray © Humana Press, Totowa, NJ

elements that contribute to the widespread burden of ischemic disease of the heart and brain and renal failure in prosperous societies worldwide. Recently, we have begun to appreciate that the metabolic syndrome and its pathophysiological complications are modulated by complex interactions between the environment (in the broadest sense) and the genome (3). However, prevention and even amelioration of this disease burden will require greater understanding of the underlying mechanisms. Only appropriate animal models that mimic all aspects of the disease process provide an opportunity to understand the complex pathophysiological mechanisms operating within the metabolic syndrome. In this chapter, we attempt to offer some perspective on the advances that one animal model, the JCR:LA-*cp* rat, has provided to understanding of this disease.

THE OBESE RATS

The cp *(Corpulent) Gene*

The *cp* or *corpulent gene* was first isolated by Koletsky as a mutation in a cross between an SHR rat and a Sprague Dawley (4,5). The *cp* mutation causes an absence of the transmembrane portion of the ObR leptin receptor due to a T2349A transversion, resulting in a Tyr763Stop nonsense mutation in the gene (6). Rats of the original colony, which Koletsky called the *obese SHR*, had a life span of approximately 10 months and died with a fulminant atherosclerosis, including complications such as dissecting aortic aneurisms (5). Animals from the original Koletsky strain were transferred to the Veterinary Resources Branch of the National Institutes of Health in Bethesda, Maryland, where Hansen created several congenic strains of rats incorporating the mutant gene and subsequently named the mutation *corpulent* (*cp*). The congenic strains were produced by crossing the Koletsky strain with in-house strains at NIH, and backcrossing a minimum of 12 times to the parent strain, creating inbred strains with, and without, the *cp* gene mutation. The "Hansen-derived" congenic strains were designated SHR/N-*cp* (hypertensive), the LA/N-*cp* (normotensive), and the WKY/N-*cp* (a normotensive parent strain to the SHR/N).

In 1978, at the fifth backcross in the creation of the LA/N-*cp* strain, Hansen sent a core breeding stock of three females and one male to the then-laboratories of the senior author at the University of Alberta in Edmonton, Alberta Canada. The new Edmonton LA/N-*cp*-based strain was redesignated JCR:LA-*cp* in 1989, as the colony has been maintained throughout as a closed outbred strain (unlike the NIH colonies that were maintained inbred and congenic). Recently, the JCR:LA-*cp* colony was rederived and established at Charles River Laboratories (Wilmington, MA) designated as Crl: JCR(LA)- *Lepr^cp*. At the seventh backcross, animals of the SHR/N-*cp* strain were transferred to G.D. Searle & Co. in Indianapolis, where rats bred in the colony were found to spontaneously develop a cardiomyopathy (7). These animals were then transferred to Dr. Sylvia McCune, who ultimately moved them to Ohio State University in Columbus, OH. The McCune colony has been inbred to accentuate the cardiomyopathy that culminates in congestive heart failure (8). The strain has also been established at Charles River Laboratories and designated SHHF/MccCrl-*Lepr^cp*. The original NIH Veterinary Resources Branch breeding program, which maintained an extensive range of genetic rodent models for many years, has now been effectively closed with some strains having been preserved as frozen embryos and a few others transferred to external agencies.

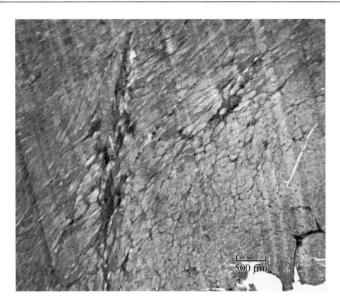

Figure 8.1 Photomicrograph of the heart of a 9-month-old WKY/N-*cp* rat fed a high-sucrose diet, showing interstitial fibrosis. Masson's trichrome, bar = 500 μm.

Collectively, the *cp* strains have provided a group of complementary small animal models that develop various aspects of the metabolic syndrome and associated pathological complications. Thus, the fully congenic LA/N-*cp* and SHR/N-*cp* strains become obese and, in the latter case, hypertensive. They exhibit hyperlipidemia and hyperinsulinemia, but like the *fa/fa* Zucker, do not progress to type 2 diabetes or cardiovascular disease (9). In contrast, the WKY/N-cp rat was shown by Michaelis to be highly sensitive to high-sugar diets, developing a striking interstitial myocardial fibrosis (O.E. Michaelis IV and J.C. Russell, unpublished observations) (Fig. 8.1). The related hypertensive SHR/N-*cp* rat responds to high sugar intake with renal damage and perivascular fibrosis (10). These differences have not been followed up by other investigators and the status of the WYK/N-*cp* strain is unclear. The SHHF strain is different again and does not appear to develop vascular disease, although it exhibits widespread diffuse damage in the myocardium (11).

The fa *(Fatty) Gene*

The *fa* mutation of the fatty Zucker rat is the other mutation that results in phenotypic obesity in the rat. The *fa* mutation consists of a glycine-to-proline substitution at position 269 of the ObR, resulting in a 10-fold reduction in binding affinity for leptin (12). The *fa/fa* Zucker rat develops a less severe variant of the metabolic syndrome with no progression to diabetes, has lower circulating levels of insulin, and does not exhibit any cardiovascular complications (13). A variant of the Zucker rat, the Zucker Diabetic Fatty (ZDF), has been developed more recently by Peterson (14). This strain, especially under challenge by a high-fat diet, progresses to overt type 2 diabetes with plasma glucose levels in the range of 700–800 mg/100 ml. While the ZDF animals have been shown to have some vascular dysfunction, they do not evidently develop atherosclerosis or the ischemic sequelae. It is noteworthy that the ZDF rat has been shown to develop

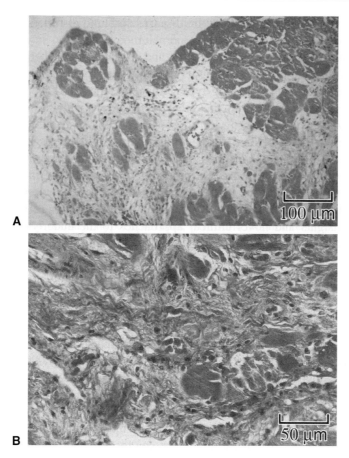

Figure 8.2 Ischemic lesions in the heart of *cp/cp* rats of the JCR:LA-*cp* strain. (A) Stage 2 early lesion with chronic inflammatory cell infiltration and cell drop out, Masson's trichrome, bar = 100 μm. (B) Stage 4 mature lesion with collagen deposition and scarring. H&E staining, bar = 100 μm.

Vasculopathy

We have shown repeatedly that hyperinsulinemia in the *cp/cp* rat is a significant factor in the development of marked vasculopathy, a process that can be modulated by reduction of circulating levels of insulin (29). Vasculopathy in the JCR:LA-*cp* rat is characterized by exaggerated aortic contractile response to noradrenergic agonists (such as phenylephrine (PE)), and impaired endothelium-dependent relaxation, which is evident in both aorta and mesenteric resistance vessels (20,30,31). In contrast, vasculopathy is not evident at all in +/? rats and is significantly less pronounced in *cp/cp* female rats (32). The *cp/cp* model has enabled us to reveal that the noradrenergic-mediated hypercontractility has two components—first, impaired endothelial nitric oxide (NO) metabolism and release, accompanied by an exaggerated vascular smooth muscle contractility, evident even in the presence of inhibition of nitric oxide synthase (NOS) by L-NAME (N^G-nitro-L-arginine methyl ester) (see Fig. 8.5). Notably, there is no impairment in relaxation of precontracted vessels in response to the direct NO donor sodium nitroprusside, indicating that the response of the vascular smooth muscle cells (VSMCs) per se is not compromised. Vascular dysfunction in the *cp/cp* male rat is also evident in the coronary circulation (33), consistent with the development of ischemic lesions of the heart, especially in older rats. We have found that coronary artery dysfunction in these animals is accompanied by significant alterations in myocardial metabolism (34). When perfused in vitro, hearts from *cp/cp* rats require high concentrations of insulin (2000 mU/l) and low concentrations of Ca^{++} (≤ 1.75 mM) in order to maintain mechanical function. In addition, the *cp/cp* heart has a specific impairment of NO-mediated relaxation of coronary resistance vessels not associated with impaired baseline myocardial contractility (35). We have not been able to detect discrepancies, either in the level of NOS activity within in the aorta or the left ventricle, or in plasma levels of biopterin between *cp/cp* and +/? male rats. However, we have been able to reverse the

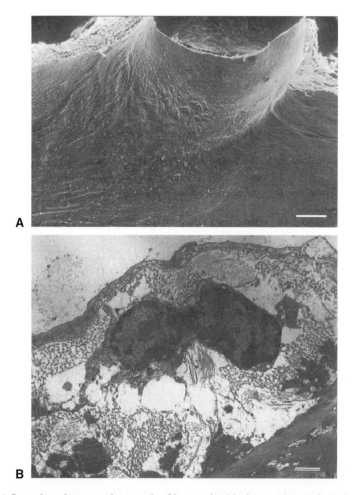

Figure 8.3 (A) Scanning electron micrograph of large raised lesion on the aortic arch of a 9-month-old *cp/cp* male rat. Bar = 0.1 mm. (B) Transmission electron micrograph of an advanced intimal lesion on the aortic arch of a 9-month-old *cp/cp* male rat showing overlying abnormal endothelial cell and necrotic smooth muscle cell, lipid, and proteoglycan in the intimal space. Bar = 1 μm.

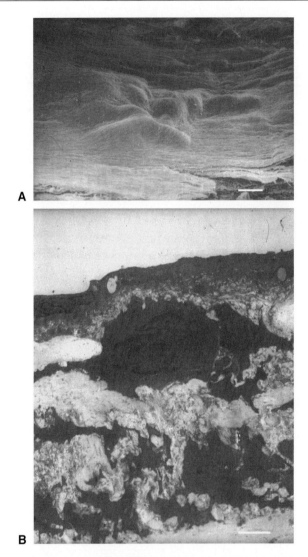

Figure 8.4 (A) Scanning electron micrograph of a large intimal lesion in a human coronary artery. Bar = 0.1 mm. (B) Transmission electron micrograph of similar lesion. Bar = 0.5 μm.

defect in endothelium-dependent relaxation in the coronary vascular system with exogenous tetrahydrobiopterin (H_4biopterin), suggesting that NO production is impaired in the *cp/cp* rat, but secondary to a defect in H_4biopterin metabolism (36). This opens up the possibility that suboptimal levels of H_4biopterin may lead to a NOS-dependent generation of superoxide anions, which in turn could result in physiologically significant endothelial damage. In any event, the vasculopathy is a strong indicator of vascular damage in the JCR:LA-*cp* rat and treatments that reduce the hyperinsulinemia consistently reduce the vascular dysfunction (37,38), consistent with a primary role for insulin in the endothelial damage.

The arterial hypercontractility in *cp/cp* male rats is sufficient to render the vasculature susceptible to vasospasm, particularly in response to neuronal or hormonal

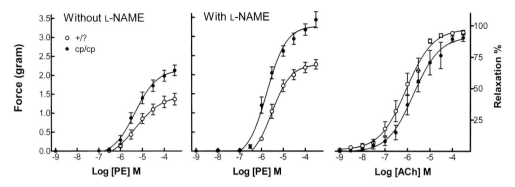

Figure 8.5. Vascular contractility/relaxation of aortic rings from JCR:LA-*cp* rats. Dose response of PE-mediated contraction in absence and presence of l-NAME, 10^{-4} mol/l to inhibit nitric oxide synthase and relaxant dose response to the endothelial-dependent NO releasing agent acetyl choline.

noradrenergic stimulus. There is evidence that significant levels of stress (restraint or anticipation of an adverse event) can lead to vasospasm, followed by cardiac arrhythmia, ischemic damage, and sudden death in the *cp/cp* animals (unpublished observations). The *cp/cp* rats also respond adversely to intravenous doses of noradrenergic or other vasoconstrictive agents with the same symptoms (see the section titled Environmental Stress and Toxic Agents, near the end of the chapter), while *+/?* animals do not. Our evidence indicates that spontaneous ischemic lesions seen in the heart of the *cp/cp* rat are probably due to a similar sequence of vasospasm and associated thrombosis (as indicated by the elevated levels of PAI-1 and occlusive thrombi in the coronary circulation).

Cerebral Vessels

To date there has been no definitive study characterizing the status of the cerebral vasculature of the *cp/cp* rat. However, the presence of advanced atherosclerosis and mural thrombi throughout the arterial system (including the major abdominal vessels and coronary arteries) (27) is suggestive of complementary cerebral artery damage. We have speculated that such damage to carotid and cerebral arteries would be expected to lead to cerebral ischemic injury. Consistent with this, we have limited preliminary evidence of atherosclerosis in the cerebral arteries (P. Redondo Saez et al., unpublished observations) and have anecdotally observed ataxia and other behavioral evidence of cerebral dysfunction in older rats.

Vascular Smooth Muscle Cells

One of the critical, yet unresolved, issues surrounding the vasculopathy associated with the metabolic syndrome is the underlying mechanism(s) leading to the enhanced vascular damage and smooth muscle dysfunction. We have reported (39) that vascular smooth muscle cells (VSMCs) grown from aortic explants from *cp/cp* male rats are more motile and have greater growth rates in culture. Interestingly, VSMCs from *cp/cp* rats show a marked growth response to a number of cytokines, including insulin itself (Fig. 8.6). In a simple experiment, *cp/cp* rats were subjected to a protocol in which mild

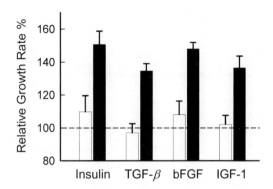

Figure 8.6 Relative growth response of VSMC isolated from JCR:LA-*cp* rats to cytokines; 100% is the growth rate in the absence of added cytokine. Open bars: +/? rats; solid bars: *cp/cp* rats. All cytokines shown gave significantly higher growth rates in the *cp/cp* rats ($p < 0.02$–0.005) at 10 ng/ml.

food restriction induces sustained wheel running with associated reduction in insulin resistance and circulating plasma insulin (40). The VSMCs from these animals exhibited growth rates in culture that were directly and strongly correlated with the plasma insulin concentration, as shown in Figure 8.7. Thus, we have concluded that high circulating levels of insulin can be responsible (at least in part) for the induction of both medial smooth muscle dysfunction and impaired endothelial NO metabolism. Whether the physiological response to insulin in the *cp/cp* rat is being driven indirectly by the cellular insulin signal transduction cascade or by direct cellular action is not yet clear.

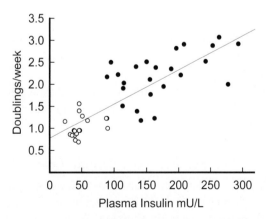

Figure 8.7 Regression analysis of the relationship of growth rate of VSMC to plasma insulin concentration. The *cp/cp* rats either were subjected to mild food restriction or were sedentary and freely fed. The +/? rats were sedentary and freely fed. Open circles: +/? rats; closed circles: *cp/cp* rats. The regression is significant ($p < 0.001$).

ABNORMAL METABOLISM

Insulin Resistance

One of the major advantages of the JCR:LA-*cp* model has been the ability to characterize the metabolic events leading to atherogenesis and the ischemic injury. The metabolism of the *cp/cp* rat has been studied extensively and essentially shown to exhibit all the principal aspects of the metabolic syndrome seen in humans. The *cp/cp* rat is, at weaning, essentially metabolically normal, with only minimal elevations in plasma triglyceride and insulin concentrations. Plasma triglyceride levels rise almost immediately after weaning in these hyperphagic animals, and after 4–5 weeks of age the insulin levels rise rapidly (see Fig. 8.8) (41). While at 4 weeks of age the rats still have normal insulin-mediated glucose uptake in the peripheral tissues, this is completely lost by 8 weeks of age. At this age, the animals are profoundly insulin resistant with no response in a euglycemic insulin clamp, even at insulin concentrations of 10,000 mU/l (41). The rise in circulating insulin concentrations (an indication of the failing insulin sensitivity) is preceded by the appearance of intracellular lipid droplets in skeletal muscle (41). Treatment of *cp/cp* rats from weaning with the powerful inhibitor of triglyceride synthesis, MEDICA16, prevents the intracellular lipid accumulation, and greatly delays and blunts the rise in plasma insulin concentrations. Collectively, these observations are consistent with the hypothesis that insulin resistance is intimately related to intracellular accumulation, storage, and utilization of triglyceride.

Despite profound peripheral insulin resistance, the *cp/cp* rat is able to maintain relative euglycemia, even in the postprandial state, albeit at the expense of very high plasma insulin levels (Fig. 8.9). The concentrations of insulin observed in the plasma of *cp/cp* male rats, following a meal challenge, is well within the pharmacological range (42), and these levels resemble those found in insulin-resistant humans following an analogous meal challenge (43). In both the *cp/cp* rat and indeed insulin-resistant human subjects, elevated insulin levels occur following each meal (some 6–8 per day in the

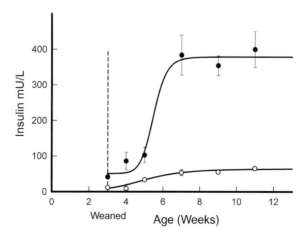

Figure 8.8 Age dependence of plasma insulin concentration of JCR:LA-*cp* rats in the fed state (3–4 hours into the dark, active, phase of the light cycle). Open circles: +/? rats; closed circles: *cp/cp* rats.

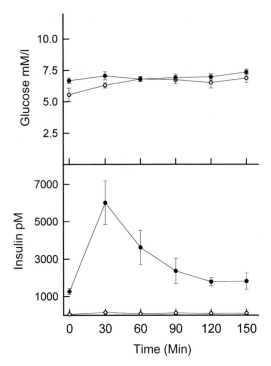

Figure 8.9 Plasma glucose and insulin response of 12-week-old JCR:LA-*cp* rats to a standard meal tolerance test. The rats were food deprived over the light portion of the diurnal cycle, a blood sample taken from conscious nonrestrained animals, a 5 g food pellet provided, and further blood samples taken at times shown.

rat). These repeated spikes in plasma insulin concentration exacerbate the pathophysiologically significant role of insulin in atherogenesis and vascular damage.

The *cp/cp* male rat has a very high rate of insulin secretion, placing extreme demands on the β-cells of the pancreas, resulting in a marked hyperplasia of the β-cell and the islets of Langerhans, with volume density of islets approaching 20% in older rats (44). Despite this, the β-cells in rats of this strain remain viable and the rats do not convert to an overtly diabetic state, as seen in the ZDF rat (45), but remain in the hyperinsulinemic and pre-diabetic state. Paradoxically, as *cp/cp* male rats age beyond 9 months, new small, morphologically normal islets appear in the pancreas (Fig. 8.10), with concomitant slowly decreasing plasma insulin concentrations. This observation is consistent with very recent reports that pancreatic ductal cells are able to differentiate into insulin-secreting β-cells in the presence of diabetes (46).

Insulin must be transported across the vascular endothelium and reach the interstitial fluid compartment in order to reach the peripheral tissue cells. This process is potentially limited by the capillary endothelial cells, which translocate insulin by a receptor-mediated saturable and unidirectional process (47). We have shown that the transfer of insulin across the coronary endothelium is substantially delayed in the *cp/cp* rat, leading to markedly lower concentrations of insulin within the interstitial space of the myocardiumal under dynamic conditions (36). These findings imply reduced uptake of insulin by peripheral tissues in the *cp/cp* rat that may well contribute to the impaired postprandial metabolism of glucose.

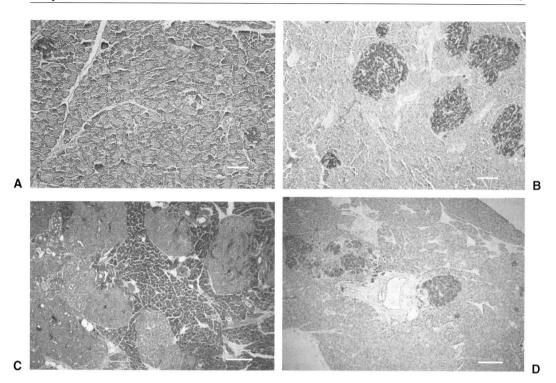

Figure 8.10 Islets of Langerhans of male JCR:LA-*cp* rats. (A) 3-month-old +/? showing two small islets in upper left and lower right. Bar = 200 μm. (B) 3-month-old *cp/cp* showing numerous enlarged islets. Bar = 400 μm. (C) 9-month-old *cp/cp* showing hyperplastic and grossly enlarged islets. Bar = 1000 μm. (D) 12-month-old *cp/cp* showing new smaller islets and involuting older islets. Bar = 400 μm.

Hyperlipdemia

The hyperlipidemia of the *cp/cp* rat is primarily due to hepatic hypersecretion of VLDL with subsequent "flow-through" effects into LDL and HDL fractions (48,49). Thus, under "normal" rodent dietary conditions, the hyperlipidemia is essentially confined to triglyceride-rich fractions and elevations of cholesterol are generally marginal. We have shown that hyper-VLDL secretion in the *cp/cp* rat is essentially a compensatory response of the liver to metabolize large amounts of glucose absorbed by the hyperphagic animals from a carbohydrate diet. In the absence of any insulin-mediated glucose uptake (42), the *cp/cp* rat can only divert excess glucose to the liver, where the high insulin levels promote upregulated fatty acid and triglyceride synthesis, leading to increased VLDL assembly and secretion (29). VLDL-associated hyperlipidemia is well recognized as an independent risk factor for CVD, consistent with the lipid effects observed in the *cp/cp* rat.

Elam et al. (50) have confirmed that the *cp/cp* rat liver secretes increased numbers of VLDL particles that are enriched in triglyceride, apoE and apoC. The greater secretion of VLDL, at least in part, results from higher endogenous fatty acid synthesis, which in turn may occur in response to increased expression of the lipogenic enzyme regulator SREBP-1c. These findings have been extended to show that expression of many peroxisomal proliferator-activated receptor-dependent enzymes mediating fatty

rat suggest that insulin resistance, from an early age, enhances susceptibility to the development of CVD, caused by associated physical and environmental risk factors, consistent with recent reports in humans. The following section summarizes a number of studies with the JCR:LA-*cp* model that have investigated the impact of physical, environmental, nutritional, and pharmaceutical treatments on the development of the metabolic syndrome, insulin resistance, and end-stage pathophysiology.

Physical/Environmental Factors

The ready availability of high-caloric-content food is a major determinant of development of the metabolic syndrome potentiating the complex interaction between the genome and environment (2,3). Reduction of food intake by the *cp/cp* rat might, thus, be expected to reduce the severity of the metabolic syndrome and the associated CVD. Severe, but not mild, food restriction does in fact result in a dramatic reduction of body weight in the *cp/cp* rat and essentially prevents the development of myocardial lesions (72). However, the restriction required (12 g/day, compared to 38 g/day for *cp/cp* controls and 21 g/day for +/? rats) over the period from weaning to 9 months of age is physiologically extreme and still does not normalize body weight to that of the +/? male rat. The *cp/cp* rat is a genetic spontaneous model that that is hyperphagous and develops obesity and the metabolic syndrome. However, the difficulty in reducing the metabolic and vascular consequences through dietary restriction alone is comparable to that seen in the clinic with obese subjects.

In the clinic, a complementary approach to reduce body weight associated with the metabolic syndrome is chronic exercise. We have induced *cp/cp* rats to run spontaneously and consistently in exercise (running) wheels (~6000 m/day) over periods ranging from 6 to 26 weeks of age (73). Exercise protocols with the *cp/cp* rat involve mild food restriction (18 g/day) and no aversive stimuli. Exercised *cp/cp* rats had lower body weights than sedentary, freely eating +/? rats and also developed a significantly smaller frame size, as indicated by shorter (11%) femurs. Fasting insulin concentrations were reduced significantly by chronic exercise (79%), virtually into the normal range for +/? rats. Exercise has also been shown to cause a major reduction in all lipid classes, especially triglycerides (~70%), primarily associated with the VLDL fraction. We have also shown that chronic exercise reduced or totally prevented the development of ischemic myocardial lesions. Rats pair-fed to the exercised animals (i.e., similar diet restriction only) showed similar, but less marked changes and a nonsignificant reduction in myocardial lesion frequency. Thus, the more extreme metabolic deprivation of the running animals appears to have been highly protective of the heart, perhaps through a combination of marked reduction in plasma insulin and atherogenic hyperlipidemia.

α-Glucosidase Inhibitors

Treatment with the α-glucosidase inhibitors acarbose and miglitol has been suggested as a method of reducing insulin resistance, and hyperinsulinemia, by reducing the postprandial rate of glucose absorption. Acarbose-treated *cp/cp* rats develop lower body weights at 3 months of age with unaltered food consumption, while miglitol-treated rats show a comparable reduction in body weight, but with reduced food consumption (74). Furthermore, *cp/cp* animals treated with either acarbose or migolitol have significantly improved fasting insulin concentrations and the rate of plasma glucose disappearance increased. The insulin response of control rats to a test meal containing miglitol was sharply reduced (75). In a meal tolerance test using control (non-miglitol-containing) food, treated rats demonstrated markedly improved insulin sensitivity, with a greatly reduced insulin response, which may reflect an improved hepatic glucose metabolism. Neither acarbose nor miglitol treatment have any effect on whole-serum triglyceride concentrations in *cp/cp* male rats. Despite this, the frequency of myocardial lesions was decreased by acarbose treatment. These results in the *cp/cp* rat support α-glucosidase inhibitors as highly effective insulin-sensitizers independent of the lipid profile.

Dietary Components and Supplements

It is well established that dietary components and micronutrients play a significant role in the susceptibility to CVD, and many of these remain understudied in the context of pre-diabetes and insulin resistance. For instance, there is an established literature demonstrating a J-shaped curve relating cardiovascular disease, and all-cause mortality, with intake of ethanol in the human population. In humans, the relative risk for CVD in moderate alcohol drinkers compared to abstainers is approximately 0.5–0.6, in epidemiological terms a substantial reduction in risk (76). However, the underlying mechanism(s) remain speculative and obscure. We have reported that long-term intake of a moderate level of ethanol (4% in drinking water) by *cp/cp* rats results in limited changes in the total lipid profile, with effects primarily on the HDL fraction (77). Ethanol consumption in *cp/cp* rats was found to induce a persistent and significant decrease in fasting insulin levels, with associated reduction in pancreatic β-cell volume density. The frequency of myocardial nodules of chronic inflammatory cells (small Stage 2 lesions) was increased in both +/? and *cp/cp* ethanol-consuming rats. In contrast, old organized scarred ischemic lesions (Stage 4) were completely absent in the hearts of *cp/cp* rats consuming ethanol.

Overall, ethanol consumption did not significantly affect serum lipids but did reduce insulin resistance and islet cell hyperplasia, together with an associated protection against large ischemic myocardial lesions. In this, the *cp/cp* rat again strongly mimics the clinical data on the metabolic syndrome in humans and confirms the epidemiological observations, including the association of higher levels of ethanol consumption with cardiomyopathy or diffuse myocardial damage and protection against CVD at moderate levels.

It is well established that dietary lipids, of various kinds, influence both lipid metabolism and CVD risk. We have studied both fatty acid and a phytosterol preparation in the *cp/cp* rat. Olive oil (oleic acid rich) supplementation in *cp/cp* rats reduces plasma triglyceride concentrations by about half (45%) without any changes in cholesterol or phospholipids (78). In contrast, an omega-3 fatty acid–rich diet (red fish oil) reduced triglycerides by more than half (65%) and further reduced plasma cholesterol concentrations by about a third (35%). Olive oil diet in the *cp/cp* rat raised the relative content of oleic acid in triglyceride fractions, while fish oil preferentially enriched the longer-chain fatty acids in the triglycerides.

More recently, we have found that diets rich in DHA and EPA omega-3 fatty acids can reduce total cholesterol by more than half and improve both VLDL and LDL fractions during cholesterol-fed conditions (Vine et al., unpublished data). While short-term dietary treatments have mild metabolic effects, we have observed that longer-term dietary studies can lead to a powerful metabolic response in the *cp/cp* rat. For example,

expression of acetyl-CoA carboxylase and acyl-CoA synthase. S15261 also reduced the expression of carnitine palmitoyltransferase I and hydroxymethyl-glutaryl-CoA synthase. S15261, but not troglitazone, reduced the exaggerated contractile response of mesenteric resistance vessels to norepinephrine, and increased the maximal nitric oxide–mediated relaxation. The suggestion of Duhault et al. (89) that the mechanism of action of S15261 also involves enhanced glucose uptake by peripheral tissues is consistent with our results. Such an effect may involve alteration of the insulin signal transduction pathway in a long-term manner. These results are encouraging in that they demonstrate the potential to ameliorate severe insulin resistance in a manner sufficient to reverse associated vasculopathy.

Hypolipidemic Agents and PPAR Agonists

The fibrate series of lipid-lowering agents have been widely used in the clinical setting. Administration of clofibrate to *cp/cp* rats reduced plasma cholesterol ester concentration by 50% compared with that of lean controls (90). Triglyceride concentrations were lowered modestly in young rats (from 282 to 220 mg/100 ml), but markedly (from 305 to 136 mg/100 ml) in 9-month-old chronically treated rats. Clofibrate treatment was also shown to reduce plasma apolipoproteins A-1 and E in *cp/cp* rats, while paradoxically apo B increased. Fasting plasma glucose and insulin concentrations in the *cp/cp* rat were not altered, nor was there any change in the impaired glucose tolerance with clofibrate treatment. The frequency of ischemic myocardial lesions was also not reduced by clofibrate treatment, an observation consistent with our other studies that showed inhibition of myocardial lesion formation only in combination with reductions in plasma insulin levels. These data further confirm that, in this strain of rats, CVD is probably dependent on the presence of hypertriglyceridemia and critically on hyperinsulinemia.

Probucol is an antihyperlipidemic agent that has been shown to have antioxidant effects and antiatherosclerotic properties, particularly under hypercholesterolemic conditions. In chow-fed *cp/cp* rats, probucol treatment did not reduce plasma lipid concentrations or hyperinsulinemia (91). The frequency of intimal lesions of the aortic arch (as assessed by scanning electron microscopy) in probucol-treated rats was not statistically different from that of controls, although the lesions appeared, qualitatively, to be more severe. However, there were significantly fewer adherent macrophages on the endothelial surface and the endothelial layer smoothly covered the vascular surface, including the intimal lesions of vessels from probucol-treated rats. Notwithstanding the extensive atherosclerotic lesions, it was striking that probucol-treated rats had markedly fewer ischemic myocardial lesions. The selective cardioprotective effect of probucol in the *cp/cp* rat, possibly due to its antioxidant properties, appears to occur at the level of the endothelium and occurs in the presence of ongoing obesity, hyperinsulinemia, hypertriglyceridemia, and atherosclerosis.

Nitric Oxide Metabolism

Given that the vascular dysfunction of the *cp/cp* rat is related to impaired NO metabolism (92), improvement in NO availability might be expected to result in functional improvement in the vascular system. Nitric oxide is derived from the precursor arginine, through the action of NOS (93), suggesting that indirect arginine administration could have protective effects against cardiovascular disease, especially in the presence of insulin resistance. Recently, we investigated the efficacy of a novel arginine silicate inositol complex that was developed to enhance the systemic bioavailability of arginine in vivo. We hypothesized that beneficial effects of arginine supplementation would occur independently of any improvement in insulin sensitivity (94). There was no change in food intake, body weight, or plasma lipid concentrations in arginine-treated *cp/cp* male rats. In contrast, fasting insulin levels increased in arginine-treated animals, probably due to the insulin secretagogue activity of arginine. Despite this, treatment of *cp/cp* rats with the arginine silicate complex normalized the hypercontractile response of the aorta to PE via a nitric oxide–dependent pathway. Coronary artery function (as indicated by reactive hyperemia to warm ischemia) was also enhanced by arginine treatment, as was coronary vasodilation to bradykinin. Moreover, glomerular sclerosis was significantly reduced in rats treated with the novel arginine silicate complex. Thus, treatment of *cp/cp* rats with exogenous arginine, in an efficiently absorbed form, improved vascular function and reduced nephropathy, via mechanism(s) independent of lipid and insulin concentrations.

Angiotensin Converting Enzyme Inhibitors

Angiotensin converting enzyme (ACE) is a critical element in the renin/angiotensin system regulation of blood pressure and thus has been a major pharmaceutical target in the context of vascular dysfunction and indeed aspects of the metabolic syndrome. Because ACE is a neutral endopeptidase, ACE inhibitors also inhibit a range of other enzymatic pathways, including those responsible for inactivation of peptides such as the vasodilatory kinin bradykinin (95). These combined physiological effects are likely responsible for the cardioprotective effects of ACE inhibitors, such as captopril and ramipril, both in experimental models of myocardial infarct and in acute coronary events in humans (96). Consistent with this, captopril has antiatherogenic and cardio-protective effects in the *cp/cp* rat that are not accompanied by improvement in insulin sensitivity and are probably related to bradykinin metabolism (97). In contrast, ramipril and the new neutral endopeptidase inhibitor AVE7688 reduce the postprandial insulin response of the *cp/cp* rat by 50%, indicating a significant improvement in insulin sensitivity. Both agents enhanced endothelial NO-mediated aortic relaxation and coronary artery relaxant response to bradykinin (98).

The well-documented sodium-hydrogen exchanger (NHE) plays a major role in post-ischemic and post-infarct myocyte damage and necrosis through the induction of intra-cellular Na^+ and Ca^{++} overload and ATP depletion (99). Cariporide (HOE642), a recently developed inhibitor of the NHE, has been found to have significant insulin-sensitizing effects in the *cp/cp* rat, reducing both fasting and postprandial insulin levels by some 50% (100). Cariporide was also shown to normalize the relaxant EC_{50} of the aorta to ACh and the response of the coronary circulation to bradykinin in *cp/cp* rats, consistent with the cardioprotective effects seen in humans (101,102).

Calcium Channel Antagonists

Calcium channel antagonists have been widely used to inhibit smooth muscle contraction, especially in treatment of hypertension and vasospasm (103). These agents have also been shown to lower plasma triglyceride concentrations (confined to the longer-chain fatty acids), effects that occur in the absence of any significant change in insulin/glucose metabolism (104). Treatment of *cp/cp* male rats with the dihydropyridine calcium channel antagonist nifedipine also prevented the development of large ischemic myocardial lesions (105). Nisoldipine treatment also ameliorated atherosclerotic damage and caused a major reduction in the incidence of ischemic myocardial lesions (106). In our hands, these protective effects occurred in the absence of any improvement in the impaired endothelium-dependent (NO-mediated) vascular relaxation and in the presence of ongoing gross obesity, hyperinsulinemia, and significant hyperlipidemia (106). We concluded that these effects appear to involve protection of the vascular wall from atherogenesis and probably anti-vasocontractile effects at the level of the vascular smooth muscle. Clearly, the calcium channel agonists have complex metabolic effects, and we have also studied the effects of two members of the second class of calcium channel antagonists, the benzothiazepines diltiazem and clentiazem, in both male and female JCR:LA-*cp* rats (104). In male *cp/cp* rats, diltiazem caused a 50% decrease in triglycerides (confined essentially to the VLDL fraction), with a corresponding decrease in the VLDL particle diameter. The closely related clentiazem gave similar decreases in VLDL levels, but without a change in the particle diameter. Most striking was that neither agent caused any change in the VLDL or LDL fractions in *cp/cp* female rats, but did result in an approximately 50% increase in the cholesterol esters in the HDL fraction. The marked sexual dimorphism in the lipid metabolism and response to the calcium channel antagonists may reflect a significant role of calcium in the regulation of lipid metabolism in the insulin-resistant state. It is noteworthy that our observations are also consistent with the fact that *cp/cp* females are at significantly less risk of developing CVD relative to *cp/cp* male rats. These later observations provide further evidence that in many respects, both the male and female rats of the JCR:LA-*cp* strain are very similar in the CVD risk–sex relationship to that observed in the human population.

Environmental Stress and Toxic Agents

End-stage CVD in the *cp/cp* rat appears to be related to both a pro-thrombotic and vasospastic status, secondary to vascular dysfunction and atherosclerosis. We have conducted preliminary studies with interventions that exacerbate, rather than minimize, the disease processes. The *cp/cp* rat is hypersensitive to an intravenous infusion of the noradrenergic agonist PE, with resultant cardiac arrhythmias and ischemic myocardial lesions. These effects are seen acutely with a dose of PE of 1 mg/kg in *cp/cp* male rats (unpublished observations), while +/? rats or Sprague Dawley rats tolerate a dose of 25 mg/kg (107). The *cp/cp* rat also shows similar cardiovascular responses (including fatal arrhythmias) to agents that are known to bind NO. The mechanism of damage, in this case, appears to be coronary artery vasospasm, with resultant ischemia, ensuing myocardial infarct, arrhythmia, and occasional cardiac arrest. We have used a protocol wherein isofluorane-anesthetized *cp/cp* rats are infused with the vasoactive agents, and blood pressure and ECG monitored for 3 hours, and the animal allowed to recover. After 3 days, the rat is sacrificed and the heart examined histologically for ischemic lesions (108). This technique has allowed us to assess modifications of intravenous preparations and the development of nonvasoconstricting preparations and generation of new analogs, much of which is work in progress.

There is a growing body of epidemiological evidence showing a significant association between ambient airborne particulate matter exposure and adverse cardiovascular events within susceptible subpopulations, particularly those with preexisting cardiovascular disease and type 2 diabetes (109,110). The diabetes/cardiovascular–environmental risk relationship has not been widely recognized, yet the environmentally induced disease burden has major implications for public policy and health care. The epidemiological studies show statistical associations between specific particulate matter (PM) emission sources, particularly of particles less than 2.5 μm aerodynamic size ($PM_{2.5}$), and mortality and morbidity (111,112). However, these associations do not permit unequivocal identification of the mechanisms of injury or the pathophysiological mechanisms involved.

We have recently studied the effects of residual oil fly ash (ROFA, a $PM_{2.5}$ material) from a large U.S. power plant on vascular function in the JCR:LA-*cp* rat (113). The effects of ROFA leachate (ROFA-L) on vascular function were studied in vitro using aortic rings from 12-week-old +/? and *cp/cp* male rats. ROFA-L (12.5 μg/ml) increased PE-mediated contraction in *cp/cp*, but not in +/?, rat aortae, with the effect being exacerbated by L-NAME, and reduced acetylcholine-mediated relaxation of both *cp/cp* and +/? aortae. Initial exposure of aortae to ROFA-L caused a small contractile response (<0.05 g), which was markedly greater on second exposure in the *cp/cp* (~0.6 g), but marginal in +/? (~0.1 g) aortae. The data demonstrate that bioavailable constituents of oil combustion particles enhance noradrenergic-mediated vascular contraction, impair endothelium-mediated relaxation, and induce direct vasocontraction in the presence of the metabolic syndrome. These observations provide the first direct evidence of the causal properties of $PM_{2.5}$ and identify the pathophysiological role of the insulin-resistant or early pre-diabetic state in susceptibility to environmentally induced cardiovascular disease.

SUMMARY

The *cp/cp* rat exhibits the range of metabolic and pathological abnormalities seen in humans with the metabolic or pre-diabetic insulin-resistant syndrome. Unlike other rodent models, the *cp/cp* rat develops the sequelae of end-stage complications of atherosclerosis, vasculopathy, myocardial infarct, and glomerular sclerosis. The initial cardiovascular mechanisms appear to involve endothelial damage by high circulating levels of insulin, and perhaps other cytokines. In the presence of the accompanying hyperlipidemia and postprandial dyslipidemia, damage occurs to the VSMC and ensuing atherosclerotic lesions develop. The compromised endothelium may also be responsible for contractile dysfunction and elevated levels of PAI-1, leading to the pro-thrombotic status. The resultant ischemic damage occurs through a combination of vasospasm and thrombus formation, triggered by neurogenic and external factors. Importantly, this animal model responds to a variety of stimuli, including both nutritional and pharmaceutical interventions, in a manner that is highly comparable to humans with this disease. To date it has provided a unique tool for the exploration of the underlying mechanisms and the advancement of preclinical therapies for both early insulin resistance and the more complexed pathologies of the metabolic syndrome.

REFERENCES

1. Steiner G. Hyperinsulinemia and hypertriglyceridemia. *J Int Med* 1994; 736(suppl):23–26.
2. Després J-P, Lamarche B, Mauriège P, Cantin B, Dagenais GR, Moorjani S, Lupien PJ. Hyperinsulinemia as an independent risk factor for ischemic heart disease. *N Engl J Med* 1996; 334:952–957.

3. Hegele RA, Zinman B, Hanley AJ, Harris SB, Barrett PH, Cao H. Genes, environment and Oji-Cree type 2 diabetes. *Clin Biochem* 2003; 36:163–170.
4. Koletsky S. Obese spontaneously hypertensive rats: A model for the study of atherosclerosis. *Exp Mol Pathol* 1973; 19:53–60.
5. Koletsky S. Pathologic findings and laboratory data in a new strain of obese hypertensive rats. *Am J Pathol* 1975; 80:129–142.
6. Wu-Peng XS, Chua SC Jr, Okada N, Liu S-M, Nicolson M, Leibel RL. Phenotype of the obese Koletsky (f) rat due to Tyr763Stop mutation in the extracellular domain of the leptin receptor: Evidence for deficient plasma-to-CSF transport of leptin in both the Zucker and Koletsky obese rat. *Diabetes* 1997; 46:513–518.
7. Ruben Z, Miller JE, Rohrbacher E, Walsh GM. A potential model for a human disease: Spontaneous cardiomyopathy–congestive heart failure in SHR/N-cp rats. *Hum Pathol* 1984; 15:902–903.
8. McCune S, Park S, Radin MJ, Jurin RR. The SHHF/Mcc-fa^{cp}: A genetic model of congestive heart failure. In: *Mechanisms of Heart Failure*, Singal PK, Beamish RE, Dhalla NS (eds.), Kluwer Academic, Boston, 1995, pp. 91–106.
9. Russell JC, Amy RM, Michaelis OE, McCune SM, Abraham AA. Myocardial disease in the corpulent strains of rats. In: *Frontiers in Diabetes Research: Lessons from Animal Diabetes III*, Shafrir E. (ed.), Smith-Gordon, London, 1990, pp. 402–407.
10. Velasquez MT, Abraham AA, Kimmel PL, Farkas-Szallasi T, Michaelis OE. Diabetic glomerulopathy in the SHR/N-corpulent rat: Role of dietary carbohydrate in a model of NIDDM. *Diabetologia* 1995; 38:31–38.
11. Hohl CM, Hu B, Fertel RH, Russell JC, McCune SA, Altschuld RA. Effects of obesity and hypertension on ventricular myocytes: Comparison of cells from adult SHHF/Mcc-cp and JCR:LA-cp rats. *Cardiovasc Res* 1993; 27:238–242.
12. Chua SC Jr, White DW, Wu-Peng XS, Liu SM, Okada N, Kershaw EE, Chung WK, Power-Kehoe L, Chua M, Tartaglia LA, Leibel RL. Phenotype of fatty due to Gln269Pro mutation in the leptin receptor (Lepr). *Diabetes* 1996; 45:1141–1143.
13. Amy RM, Dolphin PJ, Pederson RA, Russell JC. Atherogenesis in two strains of obese rats: The fatty Zucker and LA/N-corpulent. *Atherosclerosis* 1988; 69:199–209.
14. Orci L, Ravazzola M, Baetens D, Inman L, Amherdt M, Peterson RG, Newgard CB, Johnson JH, Unger RH. Evidence that downregulation of beta-cell glucose transporters in non-insulin-dependent diabetes may be the cause of diabetic hyperglycemia. *Proc Natl Acad Sci USA* 1990; 87:9953–9957.
15. Schäfer S, Steioff K, Linz W, Bleich M, Busch AE, Löhn M. Chronic vasopeptidase inhibition normalizes diabetic endothelial dysfunction. *Euro J Pharmacol* 2004; 484:361–362.
16. Russell JC, Graham SE, Dolphin PJ. Glucose tolerance and insulin resistance in the JCR:LA-cp rat: Effect of miglitol (Bay m1099). *Metabolism* 1999; 48:701–706.
17. Russell JC, Bar-Tana J, Shillabeer G, Lau DCW, Richardson M, Wenzel LM, Graham SE, Dolphin PJ. Development of insulin resistance in the JCR:LA-cp rat: Role of triacylglycerols and effects of MEDICA 16. *Diabetes* 1998; 47:770–778.
18. Vance JE, Russell JC. Hypersecretion of VLDL, but not HDL, by hepatocytes from the JCR:LA-corpulent rat. *J Lipid Res* 1990; 31:1491–1501.
19. Russell JC, Graham SE, Richardson M. Cardiovascular disease in the JCR:LA-cp rat. *Mol Cell Biochem* 1998; 188:113–126.
20. O'Brien SF, Russell JC, Davidge ST. Vascular wall dysfunction in JCR:LA-cp rats: Effects of age and insulin resistance. *Am J Physiol* 1999; 277:C987–993.
21. Proctor SD, Kelly SE and Russell JC. A novel complex of arginine–silicate improves micro- and macrovascular function and inhibits glomerular sclerosis in insulin-resistant JCR:LA-cp rats. *Diabetologia* 2005; 48:1925–1932.
22. Davignon J. Beneficial cardiovascular pleiotropic effects of statins. *Circulation* 2004; 109(suppl 1): III39–43.
23. Brown MS, Goldstein, JL. Heart attacks: Gone with the century? *Science* 1996; 372:629.
24. Proctor SD, Mamo JC. Arterial fatty lesions have increased uptake of chylomicron remnants but not low-density lipoproteins. *Coron Artery Dis* 1996; 7:239–245.
25. Russell JC, Amy RM. Early atherosclerotic lesions in a susceptible rat model: The LA/N-corpulent rat. *Atherosclerosis* 1986; 60:119–129.

26. Russell JC, Amy RM. Myocardial and vascular lesions in the LA/N-corpulent rat. *Can J Physiol Pharmacol* 1986; 64:1272–1280.

27. Richardson M, Schmidt AM, Graham SE, Achen B, DeReske M, Russell JC. Vasculopathy and insulin resistance in the JCR:LA-cp rat. *Atherosclerosis* 1998; 138:135–146.

28. Schneider DJ, Absher PM, Neimane D, Russell JC, Sobel BE. Fibrinolysis and atherogenesis in the JCR:LA-cp rat in relation to insulin and triglyceride concentrations in blood. *Diabetologia* 1998; 41:141–147.

29. Brindley DN, Russell JC. Animal models of insulin resistance and cardiovascular disease: Some therapeutic approaches using the JCR:LA-cp rat. *Diab Obes Metab* 2002; 4:1–10.

30. O'Brien SF, McKendrick JD, Radomski MW, Davidge ST, Russell JC. Vascular wall reactivity in conductance and resistance arteries: Differential effects of insulin resistance. *Can J Physiol Pharmacol* 1998; 76:72–76.

31. O'Brien SF, Russell JC. Insulin resistance and vascular wall function: Lessons from animal models. *Endocrinol Metab* 1997; 4:155–162.

32. O'Brien SF, Russell JC, Dolphin PJ, Davidge ST. Vascular wall function in insulin-resistant JCR:LA-cp rats: Role of male and female sex. *J Cardiovasc Pharmacol* 2000; 36:176–181.

33. Russell JC, Kelly SE, Schäfer S. Vasopeptidase inhibition improves insulin sensitivity and endothelial function in the JCR:LA-cp Rat. *J Cardiovasc Pharmacol* 2004; 44:258–265.

34. Lopaschuk GD, Russell JC. Myocardial function and energy substrate metabolism in the insulin-resistant JCR:LA-corpulent rat. *J Appl Physiol* 1991; 71:1302–1308.

35. Brunner F, Wölkart G, Russell JC, Wascher T. Vascular dysfunction and myocardial contractility in the JCR:LA-corpulent rat. *Cardiovasc Res* 2000; 47:150–158.

36. Wascher TC, Wölkart G, Russell JC, Brunner F. Delayed insulin transport across endothelium in insulin resistant JCR:LA-cp rats. *Diabetes* 2000; 49:803–809.

37. Russell JC, Graham SE, Dolphin PJ, Amy RM, Wood GO, Brindley DN. Antiatherogenic effects of long-term benfluorex treatment in male insulin resistant JCR:LA-cp rats. *Atherosclerosis* 1997; 132:187–197.

38. Russell JC, Dolphin PJ, Graham SE, Amy RM, Brindley DN. Improvement of insulin sensitivity and cardiovascular outcomes in the JCR:LA-cp rat by D–fenfluramine. *Diabetologia* 1998; 41:380–389.

39. Absher PM, Schneider DJ, Russell JC, Sobel BE. Increased proliferation of explanted vascular smooth muscle cells: A marker presaging atherogenesis. *Atherosclerosis* 1997; 131:187–194.

40. Absher PM, Schneider DJ, Baldor LC, Russell JC, Sobel BE. The retardation of vasculopathy induced by attenuation of insulin resistance in the corpulent JCR:LA-cp rat is reflected by decreased vascular smooth muscle cell proliferation in vivo. *Atherosclerosis* 1999; 143:245–251.

41. Russell JC, Bar-Tana J, Shillabeer G, Lau DCW, Richardson M, Wenzel LM, Graham SE, Dolphin PJ. Development of insulin resistance in the JCR:LA-cp rat: Role of triacylglycerols and effects of MEDICA 16. *Diabetes* 1998; 47:770–778.

42. Russell JC, Graham S, Hameed M. Abnormal insulin and glucose metabolism in the JCR:LA-corpulent rat. *Metabolism* 1994; 43:538–543.

43. Couillard C, Bergeron N, Pascot A, Almeras N, Bergeron J, Tremblay A, Prud'homme D, Despres JP. Evidence for impaired lipolysis in abdominally obese men: Postprandial study of apolipoprotein B-48- and B-100-containing lipoproteins. *Am J Clin Nutr* 2002; 76:311–318.

44. Russell JC, Ahuja SK, Manickavel V, Rajotte RV, Amy RM. Insulin resistance and impaired glucose tolerance in the atherosclerosis-prone LA/N corpulent rat. *Arteriosclerosis* 1987; 7:620–626.

45. Friedman JE, de Vente JE, Peterson RG, Dohm GL. Altered expression of muscle glucose transporter GLUT-4 in diabetic fatty Zucker rats (ZDF/Drt-fa). *Am J Physiol* 1991; 261:E782–788.

46. Suarez-Pinzon WL, Yan Y, Power R, Brand SJ, Rabinovitch A. Combination therapy with epidermal growth factor and gastrin increases beta-cell mass and reverses hyperglycemia in diabetic NOD mice. *Diabetes* 2005; 54:2596–2601.

47. King GL, Johnson SM. Receptor-mediated transport of insulin across endothelial cells. *Science* 1985; 227:1583–1586.

48. Russell JC, Koeslag DG, Amy RM, Dolphin PJ. Plasma lipid secretion and clearance in the hyperlipidemic JCR:LA-corpulent rat. *Arteriosclerosis* 1989; 9:869–876.

49. Vance JE, Russell JC. Hypersecretion of VLDL, but not HDL, by hepatocytes from the JCR:LA-corpulent rat. *J Lipid Res* 1990; 31:1491–1501.

50. Elam MB, Wilcox HG, Cagen LM, Deng X, Raghow R, Kumar P, Heimberg M, Russell JC. Increased hepatic VLDL secretion, lipogenesis, and SREBP-1 expression in the corpulent JCR:LA-cp rat. *J Lipid Res* 2001; 42:2039–2048.
51. Deng X, Elam MB, Wilcox HG, Cagen LM, Park E, Raghow R, Patel D, Kumar P, Sheybani A, Russell JC. Dietary olive oil and menhaden oil mitigate induction of lipogenesis in hyperinsulinemic corpulent JCR:LA-cp rats: Microarray analysis of lipid-related gene expression. *Endocrinology* 2004; 145:5847–5861.
52. Proctor SD, Vine DF, Mamo JCL. Arterial retention of apolipoprotein-B48 and B100-containing lipoproteins in atherogenesis. *Curr Opin Lipidol* 2002; 13:461–470.
53. Proctor SD, Vine DF, Mamo JC. Arterial permeability and efflux of apolipoprotein B-containing lipoproteins assessed by in-situ perfusion and three-dimensional quantitative confocal microscopy. *Arterioscler Thromb Vasc Biol* 2004; 24:2162–2167.
54. Proctor SD, Mamo JC. Intimal retention of cholesterol derived from apolipoprotein B100- and apolipoprotein B48-containing lipoproteins in carotid arteries of Watanabe heritable hyperlipidemic rabbits. *Arterioscler Thromb Vasc Biol* 2003; 23:1595–600.
55. Taggart C, Gibney J, Owens D, Collins P, Johnson A, Tomkin GH. The role of dietary cholesterol in the regulation of postprandial apolipoprotein B48 levels in diabetes. *Diabet Med* 1997; 14:1051–1058.
56. Schaefer EJ, McNamara JR, Shah PK, Nakajima K, Cupples LA, Ordovas JM, Wilson PW, Framingham Offspring Study Group. Elevated remnant-like particle cholesterol and triglyceride levels in diabetic men and women in the Framingham Offspring Study. *Diabetes Care* 2002; 25:989–994.
57. Chan DC, Watts GF, Barrett PH, O'Neill FH, Redgrave TG, Thompson GR. Relationships between cholesterol homoeostasis and triacylglycerol-rich lipoprotein remnant metabolism in the metabolic syndrome. *Clin Sci (Lond)* 2003; 104:383–388.
58. Mamo JC, Watts GF, Barrett PH, Smith D, James AP, Pal S. Postprandial dyslipidemia in men with visceral obesity: An effect of reduced LDL receptor expression? *Am J Physiol Endocrinol Metab* 2001; 281:E626–632.
59. Vine DF, Russell JC, Proctor SD. Impaired metabolism of chylomicrons and corresponding postprandial response can contribute to accelerated vascular disease in the JCR:LA cp/cp rat model of obesity and insulin resistance. *Can J Cardiol* 2005; 21(suppl C):A677.
60. Lewis GF, Murdoch S, Uffelman K, Naples M, Szeto L, Albers A, Adeli K, Brunzell JD. Hepatic lipase mRNA, protein, and plasma enzyme activity is increased in the insulin-resistant, fructose-fed Syrian golden hamster and is partially normalized by the insulin sensitizer rosiglitazone. *Diabetes* 2004; 53:2893–2900.
61. Kobayashi K, Inoguchi T, Sonoda N, Sekiguchi N, Nawata H. Adiponectin inhibits the binding of low-density lipoprotein to biglycan, a vascular proteoglycan. *BBRC* 2005; 335:66–70.
62. Okamoto Y, Kihara S, Ouchi N. Adiponectin reduces atherosclerosis in apolipoprotein E-deficient mice. *Circulation* 2002; 106:2767–2770.
63. Alemzadeh R, Tushaus KM. Modulation of adipoinsular axis in prediabetic Zucker diabetic fatty rats by diazoxide. *Endocrinology* 2004; 145:5476–5484.
64. Altomonte J, Harbaran S, Richter A, Dong H. Fat depot–specific expression of adiponectin is impaired in Zucker fatty rats. *Metabolism* 2003; 52:958–963.
65. Tannock LR, Little PJ, Wight TN, Chait A. Arterial smooth muscle cell proteoglycans synthesized in the presence of glucosamine demonstrate reduced binding to LDL. *J Lipid Res* 2002; 43:149–157.
66. Little PJ, Tannock L, Olin KL, Chait A, Wight TN. Proteoglycans synthesized by arterial smooth muscle cells in the presence of transforming growth factor–beta1 exhibit increased binding to LDLs. *Arterioscler Thromb Vasc Biol* 2002; 22:55–60.
67. Pandey M, Loskutoff DJ, Samad F. Molecular mechanisms of tumor necrosis factor-alpha-mediated plasminogen activator inhibitor-1 expression in adipocytes. *FASEB J* 2005; 19:1317–1319.
68. Bauer BS, Ghahary A, Scott PG, Iwashina T, Demare J, Russell JC, Tredget EE. The JCR:LA:cp rat: A novel model for impaired wound healing. *Wound Repair Regen* 2004; 12:86–92.
69. Russell JC, Amy RM, Graham S, Dolphin PJ. Effect of castration on hyperlipidemic, insulin6 resistant JCR:LA-corpulent rats. *Atherosclerosis* 1993; 100:113–122.
70. Cussons AJ, Stuckey BGA, Watts GF. Cardiovascular disease in the polycystic ovary syndrome: New insights and perspectives. *Athersclerosis* 2005; epub: doi:10.1016.

71. Kafali H, Iradam M, Ozaardah I, Demir N. Letrozole-induced polycystic ovaries in the rat: A new model for cystic ovarian disease. *Arch Med Res* 2004; 35:103–108.
72. Russell JC, Amy RM. Plasma lipids and other factors in the LA/N-corpulent rat in the presence of chronic exercise and food restriction. *Can J Physiol Pharmacol* 1986; 64:750–756.
73. Russell JC, Amy RM, Manickavel V, Dolphin PJ, Epling WF, Pierce D, Boer D. Prevention of myocardial disease in the JCR:LA-corpulent rat by running. *J Appl Physiol* 1989; 66:1649–1655.
74. Russell JC, Koeslag DG, Dolphin PJ, Amy RM. Beneficial effects of acarbose in the atherosclerosis prone JCR:LA-corpulent rat. *Metabolism* 1993; 42:218–223.
75. Russell JC, Graham SE, Dolphin PJ. Glucose tolerance and insulin resistance in the JCR:LA-cp rat: Effect of miglitol (Bay m1099). *Metabolism* 1999; 48:701–706.
76. Lucas DL, Brown RA, Wassef M, Giles TD. Alcohol and the cardiovascular system: Research challenges and opportunities. *J Am Coll Cardiol* 2005; 45:1916–1924.
77. Russell JC, Amy RM, Manickavel V, Dolphin PJ. Effects of chronic ethanol consumption in atherosclerosis-prone JCR:LA-corpulent rat. *Arteriosclerosis* 1989; 9:122–128.
78. Russell JC, Amy RM, Dolphin PJ. Effect of n-3 fatty acids on atherosclerosis prone JCR:LA-corpulent rats. *Exp Mol Pathol* 1991; 55:285–293.
79. Russell JC, Ewart HS, Kelly SE, Kralovec J, Wright JLC, Dolphin PJ. Improvement of vascular dysfunction in insulin resistance by a marine oil–based phytosterol compound. *Lipids* 2002; 37:147–152.
80. Vaskonen T, Mervaala E, Sumuvuori V, Seppanen-Laakso T, Karppanen H. Effects of calcium and plant sterols on serum lipids in obese Zucker rats on a low-fat diet. *Br J Nutr* 2002; 87:239–245.
81. Law M. Plant sterol and stanol margarines and health. *BMJ* 2000; 320:861–864.
82. Proctor SD, Kelly SE, Stanhope KL, Havel PJ, Russell JC. Synergistic effects of conjugated linoleic acid and chromium picolinate improve vascular function and renal pathophysiology in the insulin-resistant JCR:LA-cp rat. *Diab Obesity Metab* (in press).
83. Cefalu WT, Wang ZQ, Zhang XH, Baldor LC, Russell JC. Oral chromium picolinate improves carbohydrate and lipid metabolism and enhances skeletal muscle Glut-4 translocation in obese, hyperinsulinemic (JCR-LA corpulent) rats. *J Nutr* 2002; 132:1107–1114.
84. Wang ZQ, Zhang XH, Russell JC, Hulver M, Cefalu WT. Chromium picolinate enhances skeletal muscle cellular insulin signaling *in vivo* in obese, insulin resistant JCR-LA-cp rats. *J Nutr* (in press).
85. Colman E. Anorectics on trial: A half century of federal regulation of prescription appetite suppressants. *Ann Intern Med* 2005; 143:380–385.
86. Rubin LJ. Primary pulmonary hypertension. *N Engl J Med* 1997; 336:111–117.
87. Mitani Y, Mutlu A, Russell JC, Brindley DN, DeAlmeida J, Rabinovitch M. Dexfenfluramine protects against pulmonary hypertension in rats. *J Appl Physiol* 2002; 93:1770–1778.
88. Russell JC, Ravel D, Pégorier J-P, Delrat P, Jochemsen R, O'Brien SF, Kelly SE, Davidge ST, Brindley DN. Beneficial insulin-sensitizing and vascular effects of S15261 in the insulin-resistant JCR:LA-cp rat. *J Pharmacol Exp Ther* 2000; 295:753–760.
89. Duhault J, Berger S, Boulanger M, Zuana OD, Lacour F, Wierzbicki M. General pharmacology of S15261, a new concept for treatment of diabetes. *Arzneim-Forsch* 1998; 48:734–744
90. Russell JC, Amy RM, Koeslag DG, Dolphin PJ. Independence of myocardial disease in the JCR: LA-corpulent rat of plasma cholesterol concentration. *Clin Invest Med* 1991; 14:288–295.
91. Russell JC, Graham SE, Amy RM, Dolphin PJ. Cardioprotective effect of probucol in the atherosclerosis-prone JCR:LA-cp rat. *Eur J Pharmacol* 1998; 350:203–210.
92. O'Brien SF, Russell JC, Davidge ST. Vascular wall dysfunction in JCR:LA-cp rats: Effects of age and insulin resistance. *Am J Physiol* 1999; 277:C987–993.
93. Radomski MW, Salas E. Nitric oxide—biological mediator, modulator and factor of injury: Its role in the pathogenesis of atherosclerosis. *Atherosclerosis* 1995; 118:S69–80.
94. Proctor SD, Kelly SE, Russell JC. A novel complex of arginine–silicate improves micro- and macrovascular function and inhibits glomerular sclerosis in insulin-resistant JCR:LA-cp rats. *Diabetologia* 2005; 48:1925–1932.
95. Linz W, Martorana PA, Schölkens BA. Local inhibition of bradykinin degradation in ischemic hearts. *J Cardiovasc Pharmacol* 1990; 15:S99–109.
96. Linz W, Schölkens BA, Han YF. Beneficial effects of converting enzyme inhibitor, ramipril, in ischemic rat hearts. *J Cardiovasc Pharmacol* 1986; 8:S91–99.

C-REACTIVE PROTEIN (CRP): BIOLOGICAL PROPERTIES AND CLINICAL USE

C-reactive protein (CRP) is a member of the pentraxin family of calcium-dependent ligand-binding plasma proteins, which appears to be a phylogenetically highly conserved protein (1,2). CRP is a 115-kDa acute-phase reaction protein that consists of five identical, noncovalently associated 23-kDa protomers arranged symmetrically around a central pore (1,2). CRP was first identified by Tillett and Francis in 1930 and was named for its capacity to precipitate the C-polysaccharide derived from the cell wall of *Streptococccus pneumoniae* (3). In humans, CRP induction in the liver is part of the nonspecific acute-phase response to most forms of inflammation, infection, and tissue damage (1,2,4). CRP is primarily synthesized by hepatocytes and regulated by inflammatory cytokines, mostly tumor necrosis factor (TNF)-α, and interleukin (IL)-6 (1,2,4). Plasma levels of CRP in the human body may rise rapidly and markedly, as much as 100- or 1,000-fold or more, during the acute phase of infection or injury response (1,2,4). Recent evidence suggests that genetic heritability may be an important determinant of human CRP levels (5,6). However, common genetic variation in the human CRP gene appears to explain a much smaller proportion of the variance in plasma levels of CRP (2–5%) than environmental and lifestyle factors (7).

There is increasing evidence that chronic inflammation plays a key role in the pathophysiology of atherosclerosis (8,9). Chronic systemic inflammation is known to be proatherogenic and/or predispose to atherothrombotic events, but the mechanisms responsible for the low-grade upregulation of CRP production that predicts coronary events as well as the development of diabetes in general populations are unknown. In vitro studies have shown that CRP has a direct effect on promoting atherosclerotic processes via endothelial, inflammatory, and smooth muscle cell activation (10–21). CRP potently downregulates endothelial biosynthesis of nitric oxide synthase and thereby reduce bioactivity of endothelial nitric oxide (NO), a key endothelium-derived relaxing factor (15,19). CRP has also been shown to upregulate the expression of endothelial cell surface adhesion molecules (14), stimulate the release of endothelin-1 (18) and endothelial plasminogen activator inhibitor-1 (12), and upregulate nuclear factor-κB in endothelial cells, which facilitates the transcription of numerous proatherosclerotic genes (16). CRP potently stimulates monocytes to express chemoattractant protein-1 (13) and tissue factors (11) while facilitating LDL uptake by macrophages (21). CRP also upregulates angiotensin type 1 receptor expression in smooth muscle cells (20). Additionally, CRP may inhibit endothelial progenitor cell differentiation, survival, and function, key components of angiogenesis and the response to chronic ischemia (17). Recent in vivo studies (22,23), though not all (24,25), have suggested that CRP may have potential proatherogenic effects by promoting thrombotic occlusion after arterial injury (22) and accelerating aortic atherosclerosis (23) in human CRP-transgenic mouse models.

In epidemiological studies, CRP levels, even within the range previously considered normal (1–10 mg/L), have consistently been predictive of cardiovascular disease (26,27) and type 2 diabetes in various populations (28–31). The "high sensitivity" refers to the lower detection limit of the assay procedures being used than previous commercial assays routinely used for clinical measurements (32). High-sensitivity assays for CRP are widely used in epidemiological studies to precisely measure values within the range less than 10 mg/L and high-sensitivity CRP; thus, CRP has become a clinically useful marker of low-grade chronic inflammation. Although debate persists regarding the etiological role of CRP in the development of atherosclerosis, the prognostic value of high-sensitivity CRP as a sensitive marker of cardiovascular risk is now firmly established. CRP has a long plasma half-life of 18 to 20 hours, allowing measures to be made accurately in fresh or frozen blood without requirements for special collection procedures (33). CRP exhibits a relatively low degree of intraindividual variability (32). Importantly, CRP levels are unaffected by food intake and show almost no circadian variation (34,35), so there is no need for considering fasting status or time of day for clinical testing for CRP. The Centers for Disease Control and Prevention (CDC) and the American Heart Association (AHA) issued the first set of guidelines for the screening of high-sensitivity CRP for global cardiovascular risk assessment among selected patients; this occurs because CRP is considered the only inflammatory biomarker currently available with adequate standardization and predictive value to justify its use in traditional cardiovascular disease (CVD) risk factor screening (36). Ranges of <1, 1 to 3, and >3 mg/L, which correspond to approximate tertiles of the CRP distribution in healthy U.S. adults, are used to denote low-, moderate-, and high-risk cardiovascular groups (32,37). Although the CDC/AHA joint statement recommends that the mean of two CRP measures taken two weeks apart should be averaged to provide a clinically useful value (36), one single CRP measurement was widely used in almost all epidemiological studies and appeared to be a strong predictor of CVD and type 2 diabetes (26–31).

CRP AND INDIVIDUAL METABOLIC SYNDROME COMPONENTS

Low-grade chronic inflammation has been postulated to be one integral component of the metabolic syndrome (Fig. 9.1) (38,39). There is increasing evidence supporting the link between CRP and metabolic disorders. As a reliable marker of systemic inflammation, CRP levels have been observed to be associated with all features of the metabolic syndrome including abdominal obesity, hypertension, hyperglycemia and/or hyperinsulinemia, and dyslipidemia (high triglyceride–low HDL cholesterol). The relationship between CRP and each of these components, as well as with the overall entity of metabolic syndrome, will be discussed.

CRP and Obesity

The relationships between CRP levels and adiposity are consistent with a growing body of evidence implicating adipose tissue, especially visceral adiposity, as a source for the production and release of proinflammatory cytokines (40). Two earlier cross-sectional studies reported a significant association between body mass index (BMI), waist girth, waist-to-hip ratio (WHR), and CRP levels in healthy middle-aged men (41) and elderly men and women (42). Subsequently, numerous cross-sectional studies consistently showed similar associations in Europeans (43–47), American Caucasians (48–52), American blacks and Hispanics (48), Japanese (53,54), Koreans (55), Chinese (46), and South Asians (43). Taken together, these studies have specifically examined the associations of CRP with various indirect measures of adiposity such as BMI, waist circumference, and WHR. It was demonstrated that CRP levels are strongly related to overall adiposity and abdominal obesity in healthy individuals (41–44,46–53,56,57).

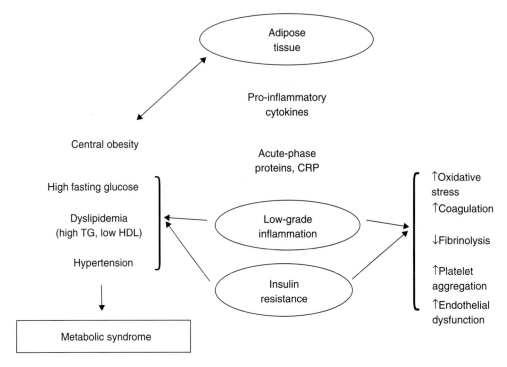

Figure 9.1 Integrated scheme for metabolic abnormalities correlated with pro-inflammatory state as reflected by elevated CRP.

Consistently, several large population-based studies have also confirmed the associations between elevated CRP and adiposity (58–61). For example, in the Third National Health and Nutrition Examination Survey (NHANES III) (1988–1994), elevated CRP levels were significantly associated with BMI in a large representative sample of U.S. children ($n = 5,305$) aged 6 to 18 years (59) and U.S. adults aged ≥ 20 years ($n = 16,573$) (58,60). Furthermore, a high waist-to-hip ratio, indicative of abdominal visceral fat, was associated with CRP in men and women independent of BMI (60). The associations of CRP levels with BMI and waist were consistent across different ethnic groups (58,59,62). Such associations are also evident in individuals with newly diagnosed diabetes or impaired glucose tolerance, although the magnitude of the association tends to be weak compared with those with normal glucose tolerance (56,63).

Elevated levels of CRP are also associated with various direct measures of adiposity, such as total fat mass as measured by bioelectric impedance analysis (44,48,53,63) or dual energy X-ray absorptiometry (43,51), or direct measurement of visceral adipose tissue using computed tomography (43,49,51). For example, in 159 healthy middle-aged men with a wide range of adiposity (BMI from 21 to 41 kg/m²), Lemieux et al. found all indexes of adiposity, such as BMI, total body fat mass, waist girth, subcutaneous and visceral adipose tissue area, and waist girth, were significantly correlated with CRP (49). Body fatness measured by hydrostatic weighing and abdominal adipose tissue accumulation assessed by computed X-ray tomography were strong correlates of elevated plasma CRP levels (49). Similarly, high levels of CRP are related to increased accumulation of visceral and subcutaneous fat depots measured by computerized tomography scan in a total of 113 healthy South Asian and European men and women aged 40–55 years (43). Regardless of hormone replacement therapy (HRT) use, CRP levels are strongly positively correlated with measures of both central adiposity (waist girth, waist-to-hip ratio, and visceral fat) and overall adiposity (BMI, subcutaneous fat, and percent body fat) among healthy postmenopausal women (51). In a small sample of nonobese, middle-aged premenopausal ($n = 45$) and early postmenopausal women ($n = 44$) without HRT, CRP was observed to be positively associated with total adiposity (measured by dual-energy X-ray absorptiometry) in both premenopausal and postmenopausal women, while relating to visceral fat (measured by computed tomography) only in postmenopausal women (64).

The associations of CRP and adiposity do not differ significantly by age or race (58,59,61); however, sex appears to modify the relation of body composition and CRP in racially diverse populations, including a representative American population (60), a triethnic population of non-Hispanic whites, African Americans, and Mexican Americans (48), European whites (46,63), Chinese (46), and Oji-Cree population (56). Stronger associations between measures of overall body fatness and CRP are observed in women compared to men, whereas the association of fat distribution and CRP is stronger in men than in women (46,48,56,60,63). Similar findings are evident for other inflammatory biomarkers including IL-6, serum amyloid A, and fibrinogen (63). There are several explanations for the observed sex differences. First, men and women have different body composition. Women have larger total and subcutaneous fat deposits, whereas men have larger intraabdominal fat deposits. Intraabdominal or visceral fat depots have the strongest impact on inflammatory markers (40,65,66). Second, it is likely that indirect measures of obesity may not reflect intraabdominal fat area for men as well as for women. Third, sex hormones could affect body fat distribution and thereby influence levels of inflammatory markers (67,68).

These results underscore the importance of adipose tissue, especially visceral adiposity, as a source for the production and release of proinflammatory cytokines such as TNF-α and IL-6. As compared to subcutaneous adipose tissue, abdominal visceral adipose tissue has been reported to release more IL-6 and TNF-α, which in turn induce hepatic synthesis of CRP (40,65,66). Adipose tissue, as an active endocrine organ, also secretes a variety of other metabolically important adipocytokines such as adiponectin and resistin (69). Adiponectin can exhibit anti-inflammatory effects while resistin possesses some inflammatory properties. Emerging evidence has suggested that CRP levels are inversely associated with adiponectin (70–78) and positively associated with resistin (77,79,80). These cross-sectional observations suggest that CRP may be a marker of increased production of obesity-related proinflammatory cytokines. In agreement with the presumed relation of adipose tissue and CRP, interventions that target weight loss have been observed to decrease CRP levels (81,82). In a group of healthy obese women with an average BMI of 34 (28–44), a very-low-fat diet for 12 weeks resulted in an average weight loss of 8 kg and a reduction in CRP levels by 26% (81). In a sample of 61 obese, postmenopausal women with an average BMI of 35.6 kg/m^2, plasma CRP levels were reduced on average by 32.3% in response to an average weight loss of 14.5 kg (82). These small intervention trials lend further support to the concept that body adipose tissue plays a pivotal role in systemic inflammation.

CRP and Glucose Homeostasis

The role of insulin resistance as a common antecedent of impaired glucose tolerance, type 2 diabetes, and cardiovascular disease is well accepted. CRP may have an indirect influence on insulin resistance and insulin secretion through altered innate immune response, although the biological mechanisms through which CRP promotes insulin resistance are not well understood.

Many cross-sectional studies have specifically examined the associations of CRP with various indirect measures of insulin resistance and/or glucose intolerance such as fasting glucose, fasting insulin, hemoglobin A1c (HbA1c), and HOMA-IR, an indirect surrogate for insulin resistance derived from both measures of fasting insulin and glucose. Overall, several cross-sectional studies in nondiabetic individuals or the general population have shown a strong positive relationship between CRP and insulin resistance and/or glucose intolerance (41,42,83,84). CRP was independently associated with fasting insulin levels independent of BMI (83). Strong associations of CRP with fasting insulin levels were also observed among the 3 ethnic groups in the Insulin Resistance Atherosclerosis Study (IRAS) of 1,008 nondiabetic and healthy individuals aged 40 to 69 years; correlation coefficients were 0.35 for non-Hispanic whites, 0.29 for blacks, and 0.36 for Hispanics. (62).

The association between CRP and insulin resistance has been confirmed by additional cross-sectional studies that provided an accurate assessment of insulin sensitivity and/or secretion using some physiological protocols, such as the hyperinsulinemic-euglycemic clamp or the intravenous glucose tolerance test. In the Insulin Resistance Atherosclerosis Study (IRAS), insulin sensitivity was measured by a frequently sampled intravenous glucose tolerance test in 1,008 nondiabetic individuals aged 40 to 69 years (62). An elevation in CRP was independently related to low insulin sensitivity among three ethnic groups. Correlation coefficients were −0.41 for non-Hispanic whites, −0.33 for blacks, and −0.38 for Hispanics (all $P < 0.0001$) (62).

There may be sex-differences in the associations between CRP and markers of insulin resistance. Among 2,466 men and 2,876 women who were nondiabetic and aged ≥17 years from the NHANES III, elevated CRP was associated with higher insulin and HbA1c among men and women but with higher glucose levels among women only (84). In a population-based cross-sectional analysis in the Mexico City Diabetes Study, CRP significantly correlated with HOMA-IR ($r = 0.22$ for women and $r = 0.12$ for men) and fasting glucose only in women ($r = 0.11$) (61).

The association between CRP and obesity may explain, at least in part, the association between CRP and insulin resistance. However, the evidence from observational studies has been inconsistent (43,57,85). It has been hypothesized that CRP levels may be highly correlated with insulin resistance, which is linked to underlying total fatness and body fat distribution in prediabetic individuals. CRP levels were observed to be elevated predominantly in obese individuals who were also insulin resistant (57,85), but not in those with a primary defect in β-cell function (57), in some studies that directly measured insulin sensitivity using more invasive physiological tools. Such associations were not independent of visceral fatness assessed using dual-energy X-ray absorptiometry and abdominal CT scan (85).

Thus, it seems biologically plausible that an important link between CRP and insulin resistance may simply be the detrimental effects of proinflammatory cytokines produced by adipose tissue (such as TNF-α and IL-6) on insulin resistance or glucose uptake. Adipose tissue is a major source of endogenous TNF-α and IL-6 production (40,65,66). TNF-α and IL-6 appear to elicit elevations in CRP levels and are highly correlated with obesity. Alternatively, reverse causation may be possible. Insulin resistance may elicit enhanced hepatic CRP production because insulin has a physiological effect in raising hepatic albumin synthesis and decreasing fibrinogen synthesis (86). Resistance to this effect would then lead to increased synthesis of acute-phase proteins, such as fibrinogen and CRP.

CRP and Hypertension

There is growing recognition that hypertension has an inflammatory component (87,88). Previous cross-sectional studies have shown that CRP levels are positively associated with systolic blood pressure (BP) (50,89–92), pulse pressure (91–94), and hypertension (62,91,92,95–98). Similar findings are also evident for IL-6 and TNF-α with either BP or hypertension (87,90). A qualitative review of 13 independent cross-sectional studies showed that five of the six studies with no adjustment for confounders reported a positive association between CRP and BP, while only four of seven studies, with adjustment for potential confounders, reported a statistically significant association between CRP and BP (87). This indicates that risk factors such as age, sex, and BMI might partially explain these observed associations. Such cross-sectional evidence, mostly from Caucasian populations, is also confirmed by a recent study in a multiethnic cohort of men and women aged 45 to 84 years old recruited in six U.S. communities, the Multi-Ethnic Study of Atherosclerosis (MESA) (92). In this study, Lakoski et al. observed higher CRP in individuals with hypertension; CRP was associated with systolic BP and pulse pressure but not with diastolic BP, and significant ethnic differences were present (92). The largest difference in CRP by hypertension status was observed among Chinese participants (24%), followed by African Americans (15%), and Caucasians (10%), whereas there were no significant differences in CRP levels between hypertensive patients and normotensive participants in Hispanics (92). Of note, the lack of association between inflammation and hypertension in Hispanics was also seen in two previous studies in a Spanish (99) and a Colombian population (100). The mechanisms of such ethnic differences in the relation of CRP and hypertension are uncertain and require further evaluation.

However, results from the cross-sectional studies need to be interpreted cautiously. The cross-sectional evidence does not necessarily imply that CRP is a cause or a consequence of raised BP. First, reverse causality is possible. There is evidence to indicate that both systolic BP and pulse pressure could promote oscillatory shear stress to stimulate the expression of endothelial adhesion molecules and the release of proinflammatory cytokines (101). Pulse pressure is also positively associated with increased production of reactive oxygen species (ROS), which in turn can stimulate inflammatory response (102). In addition, inadequate statistical adjustment and residual confounding in many studies may have distorted the association between CRP and BP (103). Note that CRP levels highly correlate with many metabolic disorders, including obesity and impaired glucose tolerance, that may potentially influence BP. The possibility of statistical collinearity does not allow us to fully address an independent effect of CRP on BP.

The evidence that CRP levels are strongly associated with systolic BP and pulse pressure may have important implications, because systolic BP (104) and pulse pressure (105,106) have been shown to be important predictors of cardiovascular risk.

Subclinical inflammation, as indicated by elevated CRP levels, may be one of the causal mechanisms contributing to the development of hypertension. To date, one prospective study from the Women's Health Study indicated that elevated levels of CRP predict the risk of incident hypertension (107). A total of 20,525 women were followed up for a median of 7.8 years and the multivariate-adjusted RRs of incident hypertension for increasing CRP quintiles were 1.00 (referent), 1.07 (95% CI, 0.95–1.20), 1.17 (95% CI, 1.04–1.31), 1.30 (95% CI, 1.17–1.45), and 1.52 (95% CI, 1.36–1.69), respectively (P for trend <.001) (107). The analysis controlled for multiple covariates including BMI, exercise, smoking, alcohol intake, and HRT use. Moreover, an elevated CRP level was associated with an increased risk of incident hypertension at all baseline BP levels. Despite sparse prospective data, it has been hypothesized that CRP may play a causative role in the pathogenesis of hypertension. Recently, whether BP reduction leads to decreased levels of CRP has been tested in a randomized clinical trial, Preterax in Regression of Arterial Stiffness—the Controlled Double-Blind Study (REASON). Antihypertensive combination therapy with an angiotensin converting enzyme (ACE) inhibitor, perindopril, and a diuretic, indapamide, was effective in reducing pulse pressure and lowering CRP levels over 1 year (108). Whether CRP reduction is due to a direct drug effect requires further evaluation. Additionally, there is no evidence yet that lowering CRP will necessarily lower BP.

The causative role of CRP in the development of hypertension has yet to be fully elucidated, but several mechanisms have been proposed. First, inflammatory cytokines from obesity, insulin resistance, or both could promote arterial inflammation (88). A possible effect of systemic inflammation on BP may be mediated through alteration in the synthesis and degradation of vasodilating and vasoconstricting factors (87). The inflammatory state itself may promote production of free radicals and could increase the NO degradation rate and lower its availability (109). CRP directly downregulates the expression of endothelial nitric oxide (NO) synthase and therefore reduces NO release and bioactivity (15,19). CRP has also been reported to upregulate the expression of endothelial cell surface adhesion molecules (14) and angiotensin type 1 receptor expression in smooth muscle cells (20), thus affecting endothelial function and the renin-angiotensin system. CRP increases plasminogen activator inhibitor 1 (PAI-1) expression and activity in endothelial cells, which in turn could aggravate prothrombotic state (12). PAI-1, as a marker of impaired fibrinolysis and atherothrombosis, has been positively associated with both systolic and diastolic BP (110,111). Conversely, elevated CRP levels may be a consequence of hypertension because the hypertensive status itself can stimulate the release of inflammatory cytokines (112), upregulation of monocyte chemoattractant protein-1(112), and generation of reactive oxygen species (113).

CRP and Lipid Metabolism

Systemic inflammation is closely associated with an atherogenic lipoprotein profile, characterized by elevated triglyceride, lower HDL, and small LDL particles. Although the mechanism has not been firmly established, a large number of studies have shown that higher levels of circulating CRP are correlated with dyslipidemia, in particular elevated triglycerides and low HDL levels (41,42,51,61). However, it is difficult to assess whether a cause-and-effect relationship between CRP and dyslipidemia is present, because most studies have been cross-sectional. Almost all the observed associations are attributable to the high correlation between CRP levels and central obesity and/or insulin resistance. Many metabolic correlates of CRP levels may themselves influence lipid levels. There is a general consensus that the relation between CRP levels and the atherogenic lipid profile of metabolic syndrome is a direct manifestation of excess adiposity or is due to metabolic changes frequently associated with obesity. The observed associations between CRP levels and plasma lipid levels may also reflect residual confounding because of inadequate statistical control for such factors.

Systemic inflammation may also have some direct effects on triglyceride metabolism via cytokines (114). A variety of cytokines acting at different receptors can affect multiple processes that can alter lipid metabolism and increase serum lipid levels. Despite different pathways or mechanisms of cytokine activation, systemic inflammation results in potentially proatherogenic lipid profiles. TNF-α has been implicated in the pathogenesis of insulin resistance (115). TNF-α induces hypertriglyceridemia by stimulating hepatic de novo fatty acid synthesis and an increase in lipolysis. TNF-α decreases the activity of lipoprotein lipase, an enzyme responsible for clearance of triglyceride-rich lipoproteins (114). IL-6 can increase hepatic gluconeogenesis and triglyceride synthesis, resulting in increased VLDL production and hypertriglyceridemia (114). In addition to changes in circulating levels of lipids and lipoproteins, the lipid and protein composition of the lipoprotein particles may be also altered (86). However, there is no generally consistent pattern of other lipid profiles related to systemic inflammation.

CRP AND THE PREVALENCE AND INCIDENCE OF METABOLIC SYNDROME: EPIDEMIOLOGICAL EVIDENCE

Elevated levels of CRP are associated with all the features of the metabolic syndrome. Regardless of diverse definitions used for the metabolic syndrome in different studies, there is an emerging consensus that CRP levels are also associated with the presence of the metabolic syndrome itself as an entity. Earlier cross-sectional studies reported elevated levels of various inflammatory markers in diabetic patients with features of the metabolic syndrome (116,117). These findings are supported by several cross-sectional studies in nondiabetic populations that utilized variable definitions of the metabolic syndrome (summarized in Table 9.1) (62,98,118). In the Insulin Resistance Atherosclerosis Study (IRAS), insulin sensitivity was directly measured by a frequently sampled intravenous glucose tolerance test (62). Festa et al. first reported a linear increase in CRP levels with an increase in the number of metabolic disorders including dyslipidemia (high triglyceride >200 mg/dl and/or low HDL: men $\leq$ 35 mg/dl and women $\leq$ 45 mg/dl), upper body adiposity ($\geq$75th percentile for waist), insulin resistance (<25th percentile for insulin sensitivity) and hypertension (BP $\geq$ 140/90 mmHg or current use of antihypertensive medication) (62). After adjustment for age, sex, ethnicity, clinic, and smoking status, the mean log of CRP levels were 0.075, 0.511, 0.845, 1.34, and 1.39 in the presence of 0, 1, 2, 3, or 4 metabolic disorders (62). Similar associations are also observed in two recent small studies using the National Cholesterol Education Program (NCEP) Adult Treatment Panel III (ATP III) criteria to define the metabolic syndrome (119,120).

Table 9.1

Cross-sectional Evidence for the Relationship Between CRP and the Metabolic Syndrome

Study (Reference)	Participants	Age (mean or range)	MetS Definition	MetS Prevalence *	CRP Levels	Adjusted variables
Festa et al. 2000 [62]	1,088 nondiabetic participants in the IRAS (non-Hispanic whites, blacks, and Hispanic)	54.7	Insulin resistance syndrome (without diabetes)	14.4%	# metabolic disorders, CRP levels: 0, 1.08 mg/L; 1, 1.67 mg/L; 2, 2.33 mg/L; 3, 3.82 mg/L; 4, 4.01 mg/L	Age, sex, ethnicity, clinic, and smoking status
Frohlich et al. 2000[†] [121]	1,703 Germans (747 men and 956 women)	18–89	Metabolic syndrome defined using BMI, total cholesterol, HDL, triglyceride, fasting glucose, uric acid levels, and hypertension.	21.4%	# metabolic disorders, CRP levels: 0, 1.15 mg/L; 1, 1.08 mg/L; 2, 1.14 mg/L; 3, 1.50 mg/L; 4, 1.94 mg/L; 5, 2.73 mg/L; 6, 3.28 mg/L	Age, sex, smoking status
Ridker et al. 2003[‡] [98]	14,719 U.S. women (mostly Caucasian)	≥45	Modified NCEP ATP III criteria (excluding prevalent diabetes)	24.4%	MetS component #, CRP levels: 0, 0.68 mg/L; 1, 1.09 mg/L; 2, 1.93 mg/L; 3, 3.01 mg/L; 4, 3.88 mg/L; 5, 5.75 mg/L (P for trend < 0.0001)	None
Rutter et al. 2004 [118]	3,037 Americans (1,681 women and 1,356 men)	26–82	NCEP ATP III criteria (excluding diabetes)	24%	MetS component #, CRP levels: 0, 2.2 mg/L; 1, 3.5 mg/L; 2, 4.2 mg/L; 3, 6.0 mg/L; 4, 6.6 mg/L (P for trend < 0.0001) Aged-adjusted CRP higher in women than men with MetS (≥3): 7.8 versus 4.6 mg/L	Age
Florez et al. 2005 [119]	190 (83 men and 107 women) (96% Hispanic)	25–75	NCEP ATP III criteria (including diabetic cases)	36.8%	# MetS components, CRP levels: For women: 0, 2.7 mg/L; 1–2, 4.9 mg/L; 3–5, 6.3 mg/L For men: 0, 2.4 mg/L; 1–2, 2.3 mg/L; 3–5, 3.5 mg/L	Age, Hispanic ethnicity, and glucose tolerance status.

Study	N	Age	MetS definition	Prevalence	Results	Adjustments
Lamonte et al. 2005 [120]	135 (44 African American, 45 Native American, and 46 American Caucasian)	55	NCEP ATP III criteria (without diabetes)	22.6% (African American, 29.5%; Native American, 28.8%; Caucasian, 8.9%)	# MetS component, CRP levels: 0, 1.6 mg/L; 1, 3.8 mg/L; 2, 3.7 mg/L; 3, 4.5 mg/L; 4, 4.7 mg/L (P for trend <0.0001)	Race
Lim et al. 2005 [55]	9,773 Koreans (4,611 men and 5,162 women)	40–69	NCEP ATP III criteria (including diabetic cases)	26%	# MetS component, CRP levels: 0, 1.4 mg/L; 1, 1.6 mg/L; 2, 1.9 mg/L; 3, 2.1 mg/L; 4, 2.4 mg/L; 5, 2.9 mg/L (P for trend <0.0001)	None
Nakanishi et al. 2005 [54]	1,715 Japanese (723 men and 992 women)	40–69	Modified NCEP criteria (including diabetic cases)	12.2% (nonobese men, 5.53%; obese men, 57.8%; nonobese women, 2.58%; obese women, 30.9%)	# MetS components, CRP levels: For nonobese men: 0, 0.39 mg/L; 1, 0.55 mg/L; 2, 0.54 mg/L; ≥3, 0.77 mg/L. For obese men: 1, 0.44 mg/L; 2, 0.83 mg/L; ≥3, 0.81 mg/L. For nonobese women: 0, 0.28 mg/L; 1, 0.33 mg/L; 2, 0.47 mg/L; ≥3, 0.61 mg/L. For obese women: 1, 0.58 mg/L; 2, 0.63 mg/L; ≥3, 0.93 mg/L	Age, smoking status, drinking status.
Santos et al. 2005 [45]	957 participants from Portugal (358 men and 599 women for analysis)	18–92	NCEP ATP III criteria (without excluding diabetic cases)	16.7% (men, 16%; women, 17.2%)	MetS (≥3) (no versus yes): CRP 0.97 vs. 3.18 mg/L	Age, sex, alcohol consumption, and smoking status

IRAS: The Insulin Resistance Atherosclerosis Study; MetS: the metabolic syndrome; NCEP ATP III: the National Cholesterol Education Program (NCEP) Adult Treatment Panel III.

*The MetS was considered when having at least 3 components.

†The MetS definition: BMI ≥26 for women and ≥27 for men; TC ≥ 5.2 mmol/l; TG ≥ 1.7 mmol/l for men and <1.1 mmol/l for women; TG ≥ 1.7 mmol/l; HDL < 0.9 mmol/l for men and <1.1 mmol/l for women; uric acid ≥ 400 umol/l; prevalent diabetes (fasting glucose ≥ 7.0 mmol/l and/or self-reported diabetes and/or antidiabetic treatments); and hypertension (self-reported hypertension and/or antihypertensive treatments).

‡In their MetS definition, obesity was defined by a BMI > 26.7 kg/m2, a value corresponding to the same percentile BMI cutpoint as did a waist of 88 cm measured at year 6, and the diagnosis of incident type 2 diabetes was considered as an alternative.

Such a positive linear relationship between CRP and the number of metabolic syndrome components is also clearly shown in one small German population (121) and two large American populations that are predominantly Caucasian (98,118). In the Women's Health Study, which included 14,179 women aged 45 or older and not using postmenopausal hormone, CRP levels for women with 0, 1, 2, 3, 4, or 5 metabolic syndrome components were 0.68, 1.09, 1.93, 3.01, 3.88 and 5.75 mg/L, respectively. Because baseline fasting glucose levels were not available, the metabolic syndrome was defined in this study according to a modified NCEP ATP III definition using the diagnosis of incident type 2 diabetes during follow-up as an alternative measure of baseline abnormal glucose metabolism. However, the prevalence of the metabolic syndrome was 24.4 %, which was comparable to 23.4% reported in a nationally representative population of women from the NHANES study (98). The Framingham Offspring Study reported similar associations based on 3,037 U.S. men and women (mean age = 54 years). Mean age-adjusted CRP levels for those with 1, 2, 3, 4, or 5 metabolic syndrome components were 2.2, 3.5, 4.2, 6.0, or 6.6 mg/L, respectively (118). However, residual confounding by adiposity is possible in any studies of the metabolic syndrome, which was a binary classification for obesity.

One controversy is whether low-grade chronic inflammation, as indicated by CRP levels, contributes to the development of the metabolic syndrome or is just a consequence. The Mexico City Diabetes Study was the first prospective study showing that CRP predicted the development of the metabolic syndrome (61). In this population-based study of 515 men and 729 women aged 35–64 years who were free of diabetes at baseline, information on hypertension (BP $\geq$ 140/90 mmHg), dyslipidemia (hypertriglyceridemia $\geq$200 mg/dl and low HDL levels $\leq$ 35 mg/dl in men and $\leq$40 mg/dl in women), and hyperglycemia (fasting plasma glucose $\geq$126 mg/dl or a 2-h glucose level $\geq$200 mg/dl) were collected in both baseline and after 6 years. The metabolic syndrome was defined as two or more metabolic disorders (dyslipidemia, hypertension, or diabetes). After 6 years of follow-up, among those who were free of diabetes and had one or none of the other metabolic disorders (hypertension or dyslipidemia), 14.2% of men and 16% of women developed incident metabolic syndrome. After adjustment for age, cigarette smoking, alcohol consumption, and physical activity, the incidence of the metabolic syndrome was significantly higher in women with higher levels of CRP (7.5, 18.1, and 23.8% across increasing tertiles of CRP; P for trend <0.01), but was not significant in men (14.2, 11.9, and 14.1%, P for trend =0.54). After further controlling for BMI, waist circumference, WHR, or insulin resistance (HOMA-IR), elevated CRP remained a significant predictor of the development of the metabolic syndrome in women, independent of postmenopausal hormone use (61). In line with these findings, several cross-sectional studies had observed gender-specific association between CRP levels and the metabolic syndrome (118). The Framingham Offspring Study showed that age-adjusted CRP levels was more strongly related to the individual components of the metabolic syndrome in women than in men (118). Such gender-based differences may indicate an underlying interrelationship between sex hormones and the proinflammatory response, although greater adiposity and larger sample size in women than men could, at least in part, explain such sex differences.

Taken together, cross-sectional analyses suggest that elevated CRP levels correlate significantly with features of the metabolic syndrome using either strict NCEP-ATP III criteria or modified NCEP-based definitions. Although prospective data are limited, the available evidence parallels the findings from cross-sectional studies.

COMPARISON OF THE PREDICTIVE VALUES OF CRP AND THE METABOLIC SYNDROME ON CARDIOVASCULAR AND DIABETES RISK

CVD and type 2 diabetes are the major sequelae of the metabolic syndrome. CRP independently predicts both CVD and type 2 diabetes, but it is unknown whether CRP evaluation is a valuable addition to the metabolic syndrome for risk assessment of CVD and diabetes.

Whether elevated CRP levels improve the ability of the metabolic syndrome to predict prevalent risk of CVD was cross-sectionally examined in a representative sample of U.S. adults (122). Among 3,873 participants aged ≥18 years from NHANES 1999–2000, CRP levels were 3.36 mg/L for individuals with neither metabolic syndrome nor diabetes, 5.97 mg/L for those with metabolic syndrome, and 6.77 mg/L for those with prevalent diabetes. Stratification by CRP seemed to add prognostic information for people with metabolic syndrome or diabetes. As compared with those with neither metabolic syndrome nor diabetes and low CRP levels (<1 mg/L), those with no diabetes and high CRP levels had an OR of 1.99 (95% CI, 1.10–3.59) for CVD risk. Those with metabolic syndrome and high CRP (>3 mg/L) are more likely to have CVD (OR, 3.33; 95% CI, 1.80–6.16) but have a similar CVD risk as those with diabetes and low CRP (OR, 3.21; 95% CI, 1.27–8.09) (122).

Beyond the assessment of the metabolic syndrome, CRP has been explored in prospective observational studies with the hope that CRP might improve our ability to predict future risk of developing CVD and type 2 diabetes. These studies are summarized in Table 9.1. In the Women's Health Study, Ridker et al. studied whether CRP status improves cardiovascular risk prediction beyond that of the metabolic syndrome status as assessed using a modified NCEP definition (98). Within the WHS population, 14,719 initially healthy middle-aged U.S. women were prospectively followed up over an 8-year period for cardiovascular events. Cardiovascular event-free survival among women with the metabolic syndrome was markedly different across different levels of CRP. Baseline CRP levels were categorized as <1, 1 to 3, and >3 mg/L, corresponding to low-, moderate-, and high-risk groups. Levels of CRP were shown to correlate with the major components of the metabolic syndrome (98). In univariate analyses, those who had CRP levels <3 mg/L without metabolic syndrome had the lowest cardiac risk, whereas those who had CRP levels >3 mg/L with the metabolic syndrome had the highest vascular risk. Beyond LDL cholesterol and the Framingham risk score, the addition of CRP to the conventional definition of the metabolic syndrome provided the best predictive algorithm (98).

A similar pattern of results was observed in the West of Scotland Coronary Prevention Study (WOSCOPS), which followed 6,447 moderately hypercholesterolemic men (LDL cholesterol, 174–232 mg/dL; triglycerides, <530 mg/dL) for 4.9 years (123). In the WOSCOPS Study, CRP was higher in the 26% of men with the metabolic syndrome defined using a modified NCEP definition compared with those without. In the multivariate analyses that adjusted for conventional risk factors, the metabolic syndrome increased the risk for CHD but not risk of diabetes while CRP levels remained a significant predictor of both CHD and diabetes (123). They also found that a CRP cutoff of 3 mg/L enhanced prognostic information for CHD and especially diabetes in men with or without the metabolic syndrome. CRP, coded as $\geq$3 mg/L versus <3 mg/L, was stratified by metabolic syndrome status. Among men in the "low-CRP/metabolic syndrome absent," "high-CRP/metabolic syndrome absent," "low-CRP/metabolic syndrome present," and "high-CRP/metabolic syndrome present" groups, the RRs for incident CHD were 1.0 (referent), 1.6 (95% CI, 1.3–2.1), 1.6 (95% CI, 1.2–2.1), and 2.75 (95% CI, 2.1–3.6), respectively, for CHD, and 1.0 (referent), 1.8 (95% CI, 1.1–3.0), 3.6 (95% CI, 2.3–5.6), and 5.3 (95% CI, 3.3–8.3) for incident diabetes (123).

Using standardized NCEP ATP III definition, the Framingham Offspring Study had similar results in a population-based cohort of men and women from the United States (118). Rutter et al. found that both CRP and metabolic syndrome were independent predictors of new CVD events among 3,037 initially healthy men and women (mean age, 54 years) over 7 years of follow-up. However, using both CRP and the metabolic syndrome in the age- and sex-adjusted model was not better than using either CRP or the metabolic syndrome; the c-statistic associated with the age- and sex-adjusted model including CRP was 0.72; including the metabolic syndrome, 0.74; and including CRP and metabolic syndrome, 0.74 (118). In women, increased risk of CVD was observed for both CRP and the metabolic syndrome in age-adjusted models (RR, 1.9, 95% CI, 1.1–3.1 for the metabolic syndrome; and RR, 2.4, 95% CI, 1.1–5.4 for CRP). However, the metabolic syndrome was significantly related to CVD risk in men whereas CRP was not (RR, 1.6, 95% CI, 0.9–2.7 for CRP; and RR, 1.8, 95% CI, 1.2–2.6 for the metabolic syndrome).

Collectively, these data provide a clear message that the addition of CRP as a criterion for the diagnosis of metabolic syndrome may add more prognostic information. Adding it formally to the metabolic syndrome definition could improve our ability to identify high-risk patients in both primary and secondary prevention. However, these referenced studies were not able to fully account for residual confounding, particularly from obesity or insulin resistance, leaving unresolved the independent values of CRP measurement for predicting CVD and type 2 diabetes.

IMPLICATIONS AND FUTURE RESEARCH

In summary, biological and epidemiological evidence suggest that systemic inflammation may be an integral part of the metabolic syndrome. A large body of evidence has shown strong correlations of CRP levels with the features of the metabolic syndrome as defined by different criteria, individually or overall. Prospective data, mostly from Caucasian populations, are consistent with the findings from cross-sectional studies and further demonstrate that CRP measurement adds clinically significant prognostic information at all levels of the metabolic syndrome in predicting future risk of CVD and type 2 diabetes.

However, there are still many important questions that require answers before we add CRP into the metabolic syndrome to improve our ability to identify high-risk patients in both primary and secondary prevention.

First, biological plausibility requires consideration. The available evidence, mostly from cross-sectional studies, cannot help us to tease out causes and consequences among highly correlated biological variables. Whether CRP plays a direct role in the multifactorial etiology of CVD and diabetes remains elusive. The nonspecific nature of the acute-phase response makes CRP less than ideal as a marker of CVD and diabetes. An elevated plasma CRP level may be a marker of an inflammatory component associated with a cluster of metabolic risk factors.

Given the fact that there is no evidence that interventions to treat the entire metabolic syndrome are more efficacious than treating its individual components, the question of whether CRP-lowering therapy may carry an additional risk reduction is uncertain. If subclinical inflammation as reflected by CRP levels is causally related to any of the metabolic syndrome components, anti-inflammatory treatment may be potentially beneficial. Alternatively, if elevated CRP levels were merely a marker of clustered metabolic disorders, treatment aiming at improving inflammatory status would not provide additional therapeutic effects beyond traditional treatment of individual risk factors. However, the potential benefits of targeting the metabolic syndrome with and without CRP measurements have not yet been specifically investigated in terms of clinical therapy.

There is considerable controversy about the validity of the metabolic syndrome construct (124,125). One may question how CRP could be incorporated into the metabolic syndrome as conventionally defined. Specifically, it is important to decide appropriate clinical cut points for CRP, as well as the optimal cut points for each of the five elements of the metabolic syndrome. Moreover, individual syndrome components do not have equal predictive weights for specific outcomes. It remains controversial whether simply counting the number of components is "good enough" or whether the components should be weighted or grouped in clusters. Previous studies have also shown that CRP levels are positively correlated with many correlated metabolic components that are not incorporated into the metabolic syndrome definitions being used, such as endothelial adhesion molecules (47,87), microalbuminuria (126), and impaired fibrinolysis (127). It is unclear whether or to what extent these variables confer additional prognostic values for the metabolic syndrome. Additionally, the interrelationships between CRP and other adipokines such as adiponectin and resistin are less well studied.

Finally, as documented above, almost all prospective studies demonstrating value from the addition of CRP into the metabolic syndrome in predicting future risk of CVD have relied on the NCEP ATP III diagnostic criteria (10). There are no data available addressing similar issues using other commonly used diagnostic criteria, specifically those of the World Health Organization (128), the European Group on Insulin Resistance (EGIR) (129), the American Association of Clinical Endocrinologists (AACE) (130), or the International Diabetes Federation (IDF) (131). In addition to CVD and type 2 diabetes, individuals with the metabolic syndrome are at increased risk of developing essential hypertension (132), nonalcoholic fatty liver diseases (133–136), polycystic ovary syndrome (137–139), certain forms of cancer (140), and sleep apnea (141,142). There is no prospective data that evaluate the clinical values of CRP as a criterion for the diagnosis of metabolic syndrome for prediction of these chronic disorders other than CVD and type 2 diabetes.

Thus, epidemiological evidence for a relationship between CRP and the metabolic syndrome has been substantial but most studies have been cross-sectional. There is a notable lack of data from prospective studies regarding the practical clinical and public health significance of incorporating CRP measurements into the metabolic syndrome definition. Although careful consideration should be given to the incremental value of adding CRP, more research in this area is needed. From a clinical perspective, physicians should continue to focus on evaluating and treating individual and traditional risk factors.

REFERENCES

1. Black S, Kushner I, Samols D. C-reactive Protein. *J Biol Chem* 2004; 279:48487–48490.
2. Volanakis JE. Human C-reactive protein: expression, structure, and function. *Mol Immunol* 2001; 38:189–197.
3. Tillett WS, Francis T. Serological reactions in pneumonia with a non-protein somatic fraction of pneumococcus. *J Exp Med* 1930; 52:561–571.
4. Pepys MB, Hirschfield GM. C-reactive protein: A critical update. *J Clin Invest* 2003; 111:1805–1812.
5. Pankow JS, Folsom AR, Cushman M, Borecki IB, Hopkins PN, Eckfeldt JH, Tracy RP. Familial and genetic determinants of systemic markers of inflammation: The NHLBI family heart study. *Atherosclerosis* 2001; 154:681–689.
6. Vickers MA, Green FR, Terry C, Mayosi BM, Julier C, Lathrop M, Ratcliffe PJ, Watkins HC, Keavney B. Genotype at a promoter polymorphism of the interleukin-6 gene is associated with baseline levels of plasma C-reactive protein. *Cardiovasc Res* 2002; 53:1029–1034.
7. Miller DT, Zee RY, Suk Danik J, Kozlowski P, Chasman DI, Lazarus R, Cook NR, Ridker PM, Kwiatkowski DJ. Association of common CRP gene variants with CRP levels and cardiovascular events. *Ann Hum Genet* 2005; 69:623–638.
8. Libby P, Ridker PM, Maseri A. Inflammation and atherosclerosis. *Circulation* 2002; 105: 1135–1143.
9. Ross R. Atherosclerosis: An inflammatory disease. *N Engl J Med* 1999; 340:115–126.
10. Executive Summary of the Third Report of the National Cholesterol Education Program (NCEP) Expert Panel on Detection, Evaluation, and Treatment of High Blood Cholesterol in Adults (Adult Treatment Panel III). *JAMA* 2001; 285:2486–2497.
11. Cermak J, Key NS, Bach RR, Balla J, Jacob HS, Vercellotti GM. C-reactive protein induces human peripheral blood monocytes to synthesize tissue factor. *Blood* 1993; 82:513–520.
12. Devaraj S, Xu DY, Jialal I. C-reactive protein increases plasminogen activator inhibitor-1 expression and activity in human aortic endothelial cells: Implications for the metabolic syndrome and athero-thrombosis. *Circulation* 2003; 107:398–404.
13. Pasceri V, Cheng JS, Willerson JT, Yeh ET. Modulation of C-reactive protein-mediated monocyte chemoattractant protein-1 induction in human endothelial cells by anti-atherosclerosis drugs. *Circulation* 2001; 103:2531–2534.
14. Pasceri V, Willerson JT, Yeh ET. Direct proinflammatory effect of C-reactive protein on human endothelial cells. *Circulation* 2000; 102:2165–2168.
15. Venugopal SK, Devaraj S, Yuhanna I, Shaul P, Jialal I. Demonstration that C-reactive protein decreases eNOS expression and bioactivity in human aortic endothelial cells. *Circulation* 2002; 106:1439–1441.
16. Verma S, Badiwala MV, Weisel RD, Li SH, Wang CH, Fedak PW, Li RK, Mickle DA. C-reactive protein activates the nuclear factor-kappaB signal transduction pathway in saphenous vein endothelial cells: Implications for atherosclerosis and restenosis. *J Thorac Cardiovasc Surg* 2003; 126: 1886–1891.
17. Verma S, Kuliszewski MA, Li SH, Szmitko PE, Zucco L, Wang CH, Badiwala MV, Mickle DA, Weisel RD, Fedak PW, Stewart DJ, Kutryk MJ. C-reactive protein attenuates endothelial progenitor cell survival, differentiation, and function: Further evidence of a mechanistic link between C-reactive protein and cardiovascular disease. *Circulation* 2004; 109:2058–2067.
18. Verma S, Li SH, Badiwala MV, Weisel RD, Fedak PW, Li RK, Dhillon B, Mickle DA. Endothelin antagonism and interleukin-6 inhibition attenuate the proatherogenic effects of C-reactive protein. *Circulation* 2002; 105:1890–1896.
19. Verma S, Wang CH, Li SH, Dumont AS, Fedak PW, Badiwala MV, Dhillon B, Weisel RD, Li RK, Mickle DA, Stewart DJ. A self-fulfilling prophecy: C-reactive protein attenuates nitric oxide production and inhibits angiogenesis. *Circulation* 2002; 106:913–919.

20. Wang CH, Li SH, Weisel RD, Fedak PW, Dumont AS, Szmitko P, Li RK, Mickle DA, Verma S. C-reactive protein upregulates angiotensin type 1 receptors in vascular smooth muscle. *Circulation* 2003; 107:1783–1790.
21. Zwaka TP, Hombach V, Torzewski J. C-reactive protein-mediated low density lipoprotein uptake by macrophages: Implications for atherosclerosis. *Circulation* 2001; 103:1194–1197.
22. Danenberg HD, Szalai AJ, Swaminathan RV, Peng L, Chen Z, Seifert P, Fay WP, Simon DI, Edelman ER. Increased thrombosis after arterial injury in human C-reactive protein-transgenic mice. *Circulation* 2003; 108:512–515.
23. Paul A, Ko KW, Li L, Yechoor V, McCrory MA, Szalai AJ, Chan L. C-reactive protein accelerates the progression of atherosclerosis in apolipoprotein E-deficient mice. *Circulation* 2004; 109:647–655.
24. Trion A, de Maat MP, Jukema JW, van der Laarse A, Maas MC, Offerman EH, Havekes LM, Szalai AJ, Princen HM, Emeis JJ. No effect of C-reactive protein on early atherosclerosis development in apolipoprotein E*3-leiden/human C-reactive protein transgenic mice. *Arterioscler Thromb Vasc Biol* 2005; 25:1635–1640.
25. Hirschfield GM, Gallimore JR, Kahan MC, Hutchinson WL, Sabin CA, Benson GM, Dhillon AP, Tennent GA, Pepys MB. Transgenic human C-reactive protein is not proatherogenic in apolipoprotein E-deficient mice. *Proc Natl Acad Sci USA* 2005; 102:8309–8314.
26. Danesh J, Collins R, Appleby P, Peto R. Association of fibrinogen, C-reactive protein, albumin, or leukocyte count with coronary heart disease: Meta-analyses of prospective studies. *JAMA* 1998; 279:1477–1482.
27. Ridker PM, Hennekens CH, Buring JE, Rifai N. C-reactive protein and other markers of inflammation in the prediction of cardiovascular disease in women. *N Engl J Med* 2000; 342:836–843.
28. Festa A, D'Agostino R, Jr., Tracy RP, Haffner SM. Elevated levels of acute-phase proteins and plasminogen activator inhibitor-1 predict the development of type 2 diabetes: The insulin resistance atherosclerosis study. *Diabetes* 2002; 51:1131–1137.
29. Pradhan AD, Manson JE, Rifai N, Buring JE, Ridker PM. C-reactive protein, interleukin 6, and risk of developing type 2 diabetes mellitus. *JAMA* 2001; 286:327–334.
30. Schmidt MI, Duncan BB, Sharrett AR, Lindberg G, Savage PJ, Offenbacher S, Azambuja MI, Tracy RP, Heiss G. Markers of inflammation and prediction of diabetes mellitus in adults (Atherosclerosis Risk in Communities study): A cohort study. *Lancet* 1999; 353:1649–1652.
31. Thorand B, Lowel H, Schneider A, Kolb H, Meisinger C, Frohlich M, Koenig W. C-reactive protein as a predictor for incident diabetes mellitus among middle-aged men: Results from the MONICA Augsburg cohort study, 1984–1998. *Arch Intern Med* 2003; 163:93–99.
32. Ridker PM. High-sensitivity C-reactive protein: Potential adjunct for global risk assessment in the primary prevention of cardiovascular disease. *Circulation* 2001; 103:1813–1818.
33. Rifai N, Ridker PM. High-sensitivity C-reactive protein: A novel and promising marker of coronary heart disease. *Clin Chem* 2001; 47:403–411.
34. Meier-Ewert HK, Ridker PM, Rifai N, Price N, Dinges DF, Mullington JM. Absence of diurnal variation of C-reactive protein concentrations in healthy human subjects. *Clin Chem* 2001; 47:426–430.
35. Ockene IS, Matthews CE, Rifai N, Ridker PM, Reed G, Stanek E. Variability and classification accuracy of serial high-sensitivity C-reactive protein measurements in healthy adults. *Clin Chem* 2001; 47:444–450.
36. Pearson TA, Mensah GA, Alexander RW, Anderson JL, Cannon RO, 3rd, Criqui M, Fadl YY, Fortmann SP, Hong Y, Myers GL, Rifai N, Smith SC, Jr., Taubert K, Tracy RP, Vinicor F. Markers of inflammation and cardiovascular disease—application to clinical and public health practice: A statement for healthcare professionals from the Centers for Disease Control and Prevention and the American Heart Association. *Circulation* 2003; 107:499–511.
37. Rifai N, Ridker PM. Population distributions of C-reactive protein in apparently healthy men and women in the United States: Implication for clinical interpretation. *Clin Chem* 2003; 49:666–669.
38. Dandona P, Aljada A, Chaudhuri A, Mohanty P, Garg R. Metabolic syndrome: A comprehensive perspective based on interactions between obesity, diabetes, and inflammation. *Circulation* 2005; 111:1448–1454.
39. Ridker PM, Wilson PW, Grundy SM. Should C-reactive protein be added to metabolic syndrome and to assessment of global cardiovascular risk? *Circulation* 2004; 109:2818–2825.

40. Mohamed-Ali V, Pinkney JH, Coppack SW. Adipose tissue as an endocrine and paracrine organ. *Int J Obes Relat Metab Disord* 1998; 22:1145–1158.
41. Mendall MA, Patel P, Asante M, Ballam L, Morris J, Strachan DP, Camm AJ, Northfield TC. Relation of serum cytokine concentrations to cardiovascular risk factors and coronary heart disease. *Heart* 1997; 78:273–277.
42. Tracy RP, Psaty BM, Macy E, Bovill EG, Cushman M, Cornell ES, Kuller LH. Lifetime smoking exposure affects the association of C-reactive protein with cardiovascular disease risk factors and subclinical disease in healthy elderly subjects. *Arterioscler Thromb Vasc Biol* 1997; 17:2167–2176.
43. Forouhi NG, Sattar N, McKeigue PM. Relation of C-reactive protein to body fat distribution and features of the metabolic syndrome in Europeans and South Asians. *Int J Obes Relat Metab Disord* 2001; 25:1327–1331.
44. Pannacciulli N, Cantatore FP, Minenna A, Bellacicco M, Giorgino R, De Pergola G. C-reactive protein is independently associated with total body fat, central fat, and insulin resistance in adult women. *Int J Obes Relat Metab Disord* 2001; 25:1416–1420.
45. Santos AC, Lopes C, Guimaraes JT, Barros H. Central obesity as a major determinant of increased high-sensitivity C-reactive protein in metabolic syndrome. *Int J Obes (Lond)* 2005; 29:1452–1456.
46. Lear SA, Chen MM, Birmingham CL, Frohlich JJ. The relationship between simple anthropometric indices and C-reactive protein: ethnic and gender differences. *Metabolism* 2003; 52:1542–1546.
47. Yudkin JS, Stehouwer CD, Emeis JJ, Coppack SW. C-reactive protein in healthy subject—associations with obesity, insulin resistance, and endothelial dysfunction: A potential role for cytokines originating from adipose tissue? *Arterioscler Thromb Vasc Biol* 1999; 19:972–978.
48. Festa A, D'Agostino R, Jr., Williams K, Karter AJ, Mayer-Davis EJ, Tracy RP, Haffner SM. The relation of body fat mass and distribution to markers of chronic inflammation. *Int J Obes Relat Metab Disord* 2001; 25:1407–1415.
49. Lemieux I, Pascot A, Prud'homme D, Almeras N, Bogaty P, Nadeau A, Bergeron J, Despres JP. Elevated C-reactive protein: Another component of the atherothrombotic profile of abdominal obesity. *Arterioscler Thromb Vasc Biol* 2001; 21:961–967.
50. Bermudez EA, Rifai N, Buring J, Manson JE, Ridker PM. Interrelationships among circulating interleukin-6, C-reactive protein, and traditional cardiovascular risk factors in women. *Arterioscler Thromb Vasc Biol* 2002; 22:1668–1673.
51. Barinas-Mitchell E, Cushman M, Meilahn EN, Tracy RP, Kuller LH. Serum levels of C-reactive protein are associated with obesity, weight gain, and hormone replacement therapy in healthy postmenopausal women. *Am J Epidemiol* 2001; 153:1094–1101.
52. Rexrode KM, Pradhan A, Manson JE, Buring JE, Ridker PM. Relationship of total and abdominal adiposity with CRP and IL-6 in women. *Ann Epidemiol* 2003; 13:674–682.
53. Saito I, Yonemasu K, Inami F. Association of body mass index, body fat, and weight gain with inflammation markers among rural residents in Japan. *Circ J* 2003; 67:323–329.
54. Nakanishi N, Shiraishi T, Wada M. Association between fasting glucose and C-reactive protein in a Japanese population: The Minoh study. *Diabetes Res Clin Pract* 2005; 69:88–98.
55. Lim S, Lee HK, Kimm KC, Park C, Shin C, Cho NH. C-reactive protein level as an independent risk factor of metabolic syndrome in the Korean population: CRP as risk factor of metabolic syndrome. *Diabetes Res Clin Pract* 2005; 70:126–133.
56. Connelly PW, Hanley AJ, Harris SB, Hegele RA, Zinman B. Relation of waist circumference and glycemic status to C-reactive protein in the Sandy Lake Oji-Cree. *Int J Obes Relat Metab Disord* 2003; 27:347–354.
57. Festa A, Hanley AJ, Tracy RP, D'Agostino R Jr, Haffner SM. Inflammation in the prediabetic state is related to increased insulin resistance rather than decreased insulin secretion. *Circulation* 2003; 108:1822–1830.
58. Ford ES. Body mass index, diabetes, and C-reactive protein among U.S. adults. *Diabetes Care* 1999; 22:1971–1977.
59. Ford ES, Galuska DA, Gillespie C, Will JC, Giles WH, Dietz WH. C-reactive protein and body mass index in children: Findings from the Third National Health and Nutrition Examination Survey, 1988–1994. *J Pediatr* 2001; 138:486–492.
60. Visser M, Bouter LM, McQuillan GM, Wener MH, Harris TB. Elevated C-reactive protein levels in overweight and obese adults. *JAMA* 1999; 282:2131–2135.

61. Han TS, Sattar N, Williams K, Gonzalez-Villalpando C, Lean ME, Haffner SM. Prospective study of C-reactive protein in relation to the development of diabetes and metabolic syndrome in the Mexico City Diabetes Study. *Diabetes Care* 2002; 25:2016–2021.

62. Festa A, D'Agostino R Jr, Howard G, Mykkanen L, Tracy RP, Haffner SM. Chronic subclinical inflammation as part of the insulin resistance syndrome: The Insulin Resistance Atherosclerosis Study (IRAS). *Circulation* 2000; 102:42–47.

63. Thorand B, Baumert J, Doring A, Herder C, Kolb H, Rathmann W, Giani G, Koenig W. Sex differences in the relation of body composition to markers of inflammation. *Atherosclerosis* 2006; 184:216–224.

64. Sites CK, Toth MJ, Cushman M, L'Hommedieu GD, Tchernof A, Tracy RP, Poehlman ET. Menopause-related differences in inflammation markers and their relationship to body fat distribution and insulin-stimulated glucose disposal. *Fertil Steril* 2002; 77:128–135.

65. Kershaw EE, Flier JS. Adipose tissue as an endocrine organ. *J Clin Endocrinol Metab* 2004; 89:2548–2556.

66. Wajchenberg BL. Subcutaneous and visceral adipose tissue: their relation to the metabolic syndrome. *Endocr Rev* 2000; 21:697–738.

67. Mayes JS, Watson GH. Direct effects of sex steroid hormones on adipose tissues and obesity. *Obes Rev* 2004; 5:197–216.

68. Pfeilschifter J, Koditz R, Pfohl M, Schatz H. Changes in proinflammatory cytokine activity after menopause. *Endocr Rev* 2002; 23:90–119.

69. Shuldiner AR, Yang R, Gong DW. Resistin, obesity and insulin resistance: The emerging role of the adipocyte as an endocrine organ. *N Engl J Med* 2001; 345:1345–1346.

70. Engeli S, Feldpausch M, Gorzelniak K, Hartwig F, Heintze U, Janke J, Mohlig M, Pfeiffer AF, Luft FC, Sharma AM. Association between adiponectin and mediators of inflammation in obese women. *Diabetes* 2003; 52:942–947.

71. Krakoff J, Funahashi T, Stehouwer CD, Schalkwijk CG, Tanaka S, Matsuzawa Y, Kobes S, Tataranni PA, Hanson RL, Knowler WC, Lindsay RS. Inflammatory markers, adiponectin, and risk of type 2 diabetes in the Pima Indian. *Diabetes Care* 2003; 26:1745–1751.

72. Mantzoros CS, Li T, Manson JE, Meigs JB, Hu FB. Circulating adiponectin levels are associated with better glycemic control, more favorable lipid profile, and reduced inflammation in women with type 2 diabetes. *J Clin Endocrinol Metab* 2005; 90:4542–4548.

73. Matsushita K, Yatsuya H, Tamakoshi K, Wada K, Otsuka R, Zhang H, Sugiura K, Kondo T, Murohara T, Toyoshima H. Inverse association between adiponectin and C-reactive protein in substantially healthy Japanese men. *Atherosclerosis* 2006; 188:184–189.

74. Ouchi N, Kihara S, Funahashi T, Nakamura T, Nishida M, Kumada M, Okamoto Y, Ohashi K, Nagaretani H, Kishida K, Nishizawa H, Maeda N, Kobayashi H, Hiraoka H, Matsuzawa Y. Reciprocal association of C-reactive protein with adiponectin in blood stream and adipose tissue. *Circulation* 2003; 107:671–674.

75. Rothenbacher D, Brenner H, Marz W, Koenig W. Adiponectin, risk of coronary heart disease and correlations with cardiovascular risk markers. *Eur Heart J* 2005; 26:1640–1646.

76. Schulze MB, Rimm EB, Shai I, Rifai N, Hu FB. Relationship between adiponectin and glycemic control, blood lipids, and inflammatory markers in men with type 2 diabetes. *Diabetes Care* 2004; 27:1680–1687.

77. Shetty GK, Economides PA, Horton ES, Mantzoros CS, Veves A. Circulating adiponectin and resistin levels in relation to metabolic factors, inflammatory markers, and vascular reactivity in diabetic patients and subjects at risk for diabetes. *Diabetes Care* 2004; 27:2450–2457.

78. Winzer C, Wagner O, Festa A, Schneider B, Roden M, Bancher-Todesca D, Pacini G, Funahashi T, Kautzky-Willer A. Plasma adiponectin, insulin sensitivity, and subclinical inflammation in women with prior gestational diabetes mellitus. *Diabetes Care* 2004; 27:1721–1727.

79. Al-Daghri N, Chetty R, McTernan PG, Al-Rubean K, Al-Attas O, Jones AF, Kumar S. Serum resistin is associated with c-reactive protein & ldl cholesterol in type 2 diabetes and coronary artery disease in a Saudi population. *Cardiovasc Diabetol* 2005; 4:10.

80. Bo S, Gambino R, Pagani A, Guidi S, Gentile L, Cassader M, Pagano GF. Relationships between human serum resistin, inflammatory markers and insulin resistance. *Int J Obes (Lond)* 2005; 29:1315–1320.

81. Heilbronn LK, Noakes M, Clifton PM. Energy restriction and weight loss on very-low-fat diets reduce C-reactive protein concentrations in obese, healthy women. *Arterioscler Thromb Vasc Biol* 2001; 21:968–970.

82. Tchernof A, Nolan A, Sites CK, Ades PA, Poehlman ET. Weight loss reduces C-reactive protein levels in obese postmenopausal women. *Circulation* 2002; 105:564–569.

83. Pradhan AD, Cook NR, Buring JE, Manson JE, Ridker PM. C-reactive protein is independently associated with fasting insulin in nondiabetic women. *Arterioscler Thromb Vasc Biol* 2003; 23:650–655.

84. Wu T, Dorn JP, Donahue RP, Sempos CT, Trevisan M. Associations of serum C-reactive protein with fasting insulin, glucose, and glycosylated hemoglobin: The Third National Health and Nutrition Examination Survey, 1988–1994. *Am J Epidemiol* 2002; 155:65–71.

85. McLaughlin T, Abbasi F, Lamendola C, Liang L, Reaven G, Schaaf P, Reaven P. Differentiation between obesity and insulin resistance in the association with C-reactive protein. *Circulation* 2002; 106:2908–2912.

86. Bloomgarden ZT. Inflammation, atherosclerosis, and aspects of insulin action. *Diabetes Care* 2005; 28:2312–2319.

87. Bautista LE. Inflammation, endothelial dysfunction, and the risk of high blood pressure: epidemiologic and biological evidence. *J Hum Hypertens* 2003; 17:223–230.

88. Grundy SM. Inflammation, hypertension, and the metabolic syndrome. *JAMA* 2003; 290:3000–3002.

89. Yamada S, Gotoh T, Nakashima Y, Kayaba K, Ishikawa S, Nago N, Nakamura Y, Itoh Y, Kajii E. Distribution of serum C-reactive protein and its association with atherosclerotic risk factors in a Japanese population: Jichi Medical School Cohort Study. *Am J Epidemiol* 2001; 153:1183–1190.

90. Chae CU, Lee RT, Rifai N, Ridker PM. Blood pressure and inflammation in apparently healthy men. *Hypertension* 2001; 38:399–403.

91. Schillaci G, Pirro M, Gemelli F, Pasqualini L, Vaudo G, Marchesi S, Siepi D, Bagaglia F, Mannarino E. Increased C-reactive protein concentrations in never-treated hypertension: The role of systolic and pulse pressures. *J Hypertens* 2003; 21:1841–1846.

92. Lakoski SG, Cushman M, Palmas W, Blumenthal R, D'Agostino RB, Jr., Herrington DM. The relationship between blood pressure and C-reactive protein in the Multi-Ethnic Study of Atherosclerosis (MESA). *J Am Coll Cardiol* 2005; 46:1869–1874.

93. Abramson JL, Weintraub WS, Vaccarino V. Association between pulse pressure and C-reactive protein among apparently healthy U.S. adults. *Hypertension* 2002; 39:197–202.

94. Amar J, Ruidavets JB, Sollier CB, Bongard V, Boccalon H, Chamontin B, Drouet L, Ferrieres J. Relationship between C reactive protein and pulse pressure is not mediated by atherosclerosis or aortic stiffness. *J Hypertens* 2004; 22:349–355.

95. Bautista LE, Atwood JE, O'Malley PG, Taylor AJ. Association between C-reactive protein and hypertension in healthy middle-aged men and women. *Coron Artery Dis* 2004; 15:331–336.

96. Bautista LE, Lopez-Jaramillo P, Vera LM, Casas JP, Otero AP, Guaracao AI. Is C-reactive protein an independent risk factor for essential hypertension? *J Hypertens* 2001; 19:857–861.

97. Chrysohoou C, Pitsavos C, Panagiotakos DB, Skoumas J, Stefanadis C. Association between prehypertension status and inflammatory markers related to atherosclerotic disease: The ATTICA Study. *Am J Hypertens* 2004; 17:568–573.

98. Ridker PM, Buring JE, Cook NR, Rifai N. C-reactive protein, the metabolic syndrome, and risk of incident cardiovascular events: An 8-year follow-up of 14,719 initially healthy American women. *Circulation* 2003; 107:391–397.

99. Fernandez-Real JM, Vayreda M, Richart C, Gutierrez C, Broch M, Vendrell J, Ricart W. Circulating interleukin 6 levels, blood pressure, and insulin sensitivity in apparently healthy men and women. *J Clin Endocrinol Metab* 2001; 86:1154–1159.

100. Bautista LE, Vera LM, Arenas IA, Gamarra G. Independent association between inflammatory markers (C-reactive protein, interleukin-6, and TNF-alpha) and essential hypertension. *J Hum Hypertens* 2005; 19:149–154.

101. Chappell DC, Varner SE, Nerem RM, Medford RM, Alexander RW. Oscillatory shear stress stimulates adhesion molecule expression in cultured human endothelium. *Circ Res* 1998; 82:532–539.

102. Ryan SM, Waack BJ, Weno BL, Heistad DD. Increases in pulse pressure impair acetylcholine-induced vascular relaxation. *Am J Physiol* 1995; 268:H359–363.

103. Davey Smith G, Lawlor DA, Harbord R, Timpson N, Rumley A, Lowe GD, Day IN, Ebrahim S. Association of C-reactive protein with blood pressure and hypertension: Life course confounding and mendelian randomization tests of causality. *Arterioscler Thromb Vasc Biol* 2005; 25:1051–1056.

104. Kannel WB. Elevated systolic blood pressure as a cardiovascular risk factor. *Am J Cardiol* 2000; 85:251–255.
105. Franklin SS, Khan SA, Wong ND, Larson MG, Levy D. Is pulse pressure useful in predicting risk for coronary heart Disease? The Framingham Heart Study. *Circulation* 1999; 100:354–360.
106. Benetos A, Rudnichi A, Safar M, Guize L. Pulse pressure and cardiovascular mortality in normotensive and hypertensive subjects. *Hypertension* 1998; 32:560–564.
107. Sesso HD, Buring JE, Rifai N, Blake GJ, Gaziano JM, Ridker PM. C-reactive protein and the risk of developing hypertension. *JAMA* 2003; 290:2945–2951.
108. Amar J, Ruidavets JB, Peyrieux JC, Mallion JM, Ferrieres J, Safar ME, Chamontin B. C-reactive protein elevation predicts pulse pressure reduction in hypertensive subjects. *Hypertension* 2005; 46:151–155.
109. Bouloumie A, Bauersachs J, Linz W, Scholkens BA, Wiemer G, Fleming I, Busse R. Endothelial dysfunction coincides with an enhanced nitric oxide synthase expression and superoxide anion production. *Hypertension* 1997; 30:934–941.
110. Srikumar N, Brown NJ, Hopkins PN, Jeunemaitre X, Hunt SC, Vaughan DE, Williams GH. PAI-1 in human hypertension: Relation to hypertensive groups. *Am J Hypertens* 2002; 15:683–690.
111. Poli KA, Tofler GH, Larson MG, Evans JC, Sutherland PA, Lipinska I, Mittleman MA, Muller JE, D'Agostino RB, Wilson PW, Levy D. Association of blood pressure with fibrinolytic potential in the Framingham offspring population. *Circulation* 2002; 101:264–269.
112. Capers QT, Alexander RW, Lou P, De Leon H, Wilcox JN, Ishizaka N, Howard AB, Taylor WR. Monocyte chemoattractant protein-1 expression in aortic tissues of hypertensive rats. *Hypertension* 1997; 30:1397–1402.
113. Crawford DW, Blankenhorn DH. Arterial wall oxygenation, oxyradicals, and atherosclerosis. *Atherosclerosis* 1991; 89:97–108.
114. Feingold KR, Grunfeld C. Role of cytokines in inducing hyperlipidemia. *Diabetes* 1992; 4(suppl 2):97–101.
115. Hotamisligil GS, Peraldi P, Budavari A, Ellis R, White MF, Spiegelman BM. IRS-1-mediated inhibition of insulin receptor tyrosine kinase activity in TNF-alpha- and obesity-induced insulin resistance. *Science* 1996; 271:665–668.
116. Pickup JC, Mattock MB, Chusney GD, Burt D. NIDDM as a disease of the innate immune system: Association of acute-phase reactants and interleukin-6 with metabolic syndrome X. *Diabetologia* 1997; 40:1286–1292.
117. Saito I, Folsom AR, Brancati FL, Duncan BB, Chambless LE, McGovern PG. Nontraditional risk factors for coronary heart disease incidence among persons with diabetes: The Atherosclerosis Risk in Communities (ARIC) Study. *Ann Intern Med* 2000; 133:81–91.
118. Rutter MK, Meigs JB, Sullivan LM, D'Agostino RB, Sr., Wilson PW. C-reactive protein, the metabolic syndrome, and prediction of cardiovascular events in the Framingham Offspring Study. *Circulation* 2004; 110:380–385.
119. Florez H, Castillo-Florez S, Mendez A, Casanova-Romero P, Larreal-Urdaneta C, Lee D, Goldberg R. C-reactive protein is elevated in obese patients with the metabolic syndrome. *Diabetes Res Clin Pract* 2006; 71:92–100.
120. LaMonte MJ, Ainsworth BE, Durstine JL. Influence of cardiorespiratory fitness on the association between C-reactive protein and metabolic syndrome prevalence in racially diverse women. *J Womens Health (Larchmt)* 2005; 14:233–239.
121. Frohlich M, Imhof A, Berg G, Hutchinson WL, Pepys MB, Boeing H, Muche R, Brenner H, Koenig W. Association between C-reactive protein and features of the metabolic syndrome: A population-based study. *Diabetes Care* 2000; 23:1835–1839.
122. Malik S, Wong ND, Franklin S, Pio J, Fairchild C, Chen R. Cardiovascular disease in U.S. patients with metabolic syndrome, diabetes, and elevated C-reactive protein. *Diabetes Care* 2005; 28:690–693.
123. Sattar N, Gaw A, Scherbakova O, Ford I, O'Reilly DS, Haffner SM, Isles C, Macfarlane PW, Packard CJ, Cobbe SM, Shepherd J. Metabolic syndrome with and without C-reactive protein as a predictor of coronary heart disease and diabetes in the West of Scotland Coronary Prevention Study. *Circulation* 2003; 108:414–419.
124. Grundy SM, Cleeman JI, Daniels SR, Donato KA, Eckel RH, Franklin BA, Gordon DJ, Krauss RM, Savage PJ, Smith SC, Jr., Spertus JA, Costa F. Diagnosis and management of the metabolic

syndrome: An American Heart Association/National Heart, Lung, and Blood Institute Scientific Statement. *Circulation* 2005; 112:2735–2752.

125. Kahn R, Buse J, Ferrannini E, Stern M. The metabolic syndrome: time for a critical appraisal: Joint statement from the American Diabetes Association and the European Association for the Study of Diabetes. *Diabetes Care* 2005; 28:2289–2304.

126. Bakker SJ, Gansevoort RT, Stuveling EM, Gans RO, de Zeeuw D. Microalbuminuria and C-reactive protein: Similar messengers of cardiovascular risk? *Curr Hypertens Rep* 2005; 7:379–384.

127. Lipid, lipoproteins, C-reactive protein, and hemostatic factors at baseline in the diabetes prevention program. *Diabetes Care* 2005; 28:2472–2479.

128. Alberti KG, Zimmet PZ: Definition, diagnosis and classification of diabetes mellitus and its complications. Part 1: Diagnosis and classification of diabetes mellitus provisional report of a WHO consultation. *Diabet Med* 1998; 15:539–553.

129. Balkau B, Charles MA. Comment on the provisional report from the WHO consultation: European Group for the Study of Insulin Resistance (EGIR). *Diabet Med* 1999; 16:442–443.

130. Einhorn D, Reaven GM, Cobin RH, Ford E, Ganda OP, Handelsman Y, Hellman R, Jellinger PS, Kendall D, Krauss RM, Neufeld ND, Petak SM, Rodbard HW, Seibel JA, Smith DA, Wilson PW. American College of Endocrinology position statement on the insulin resistance syndrome. *Endocr Pract* 2003; 9:237–252.

131. Alberti KG, Zimmet P, Shaw J. The metabolic syndrome: A new worldwide definition. *Lancet* 2005; 366:1059–1062.

132. Schillaci G, Pirro M, Vaudo G, Gemelli F, Marchesi S, Porcellati C, Mannarino E. Prognostic value of the metabolic syndrome in essential hypertension. *J Am Coll Cardiol* 2004; 43:1817–1822.

133. Angelico F, Del Ben M, Conti R, Francioso S, Feole K, Fiorello S, Cavallo MG, Zalunardo B, Lirussi F, Alessandri C, Violi F. Insulin resistance, the metabolic syndrome, and nonalcoholic fatty liver disease. *J Clin Endocrinol Metab* 2005; 90:1578–1582.

134. Hamaguchi M, Kojima T, Takeda N, Nakagawa T, Taniguchi H, Fujii K, Omatsu T, Nakajima T, Sarui H, Shimazaki M, Kato T, Okuda J, Ida K. The metabolic syndrome as a predictor of nonalcoholic fatty liver disease. *Ann Intern Med* 2005; 143:722–728.

135. Marchesini G, Brizi M, Bianchi G, Tomassetti S, Bugianesi E, Lenzi M, McCullough AJ, Natale S, Forlani G, Melchionda N. Nonalcoholic fatty liver disease: A feature of the metabolic syndrome. *Diabetes* 2001; 50:1844–1850.

136. Marchesini G, Marzocchi R, Agostini F, Bugianesi E. Nonalcoholic fatty liver disease and the metabolic syndrome. *Curr Opin Lipidol* 2005; 16:421–427.

137. Ehrmann DA, Liljenquist DR, Kasza K, Azziz R, Legro RS, Ghazzi MN. Prevalence and predictors of the metabolic syndrome in women with polycystic ovary syndrome. *J Clin Endocrinol Metab* 2006; 91:48–53.

138. Rabelo Acevedo M, Vick MR. Association between the polycystic ovary syndrome and the metabolic syndrome in Puerto Rico. *P R Health Sci J* 2005; 24:203–206.

139. Vrbikova J, Vondra K, Cibula D, Dvorakova K, Stanicka S, Sramkova D, Sindelka G, Hill M, Bendlova B, Skrha J. Metabolic syndrome in young Czech women with polycystic ovary syndrome. *Hum Reprod* 2005; 20:3328–3332.

140. Bugianesi E. Review article: Steatosis, the metabolic syndrome and cancer. *Aliment Pharmacol Ther* 2005; 22(suppl 2):40–43.

141. Vgontzas AN, Bixler EO, Chrousos GP. Sleep apnea is a manifestation of the metabolic syndrome. *Sleep Med Rev* 2005; 9:211–224.

142. Svatikova A, Wolk R, Gami AS, Pohanka M, Somers VK. Interactions between obstructive sleep apnea and the metabolic syndrome. *Curr Diab Rep* 2005; 5:53–58.

10 Insulin Signaling in Adipocytes and the Role of Inflammation

Christian X. Andersson, Ann Hammarstedt, Per-Anders Jansson, and Ulf Smith

CONTENTS

Type 2 diabetes has during the last 20 years increased dramatically and taken epidemic-like proportions. One major cause is the highly increased incidence of obesity, which in turn is caused by a sedentary lifestyle as well as an increased consumption of a more energy-dense diet containing high levels of sugar and saturated fats. Obesity is associated with insulin resistance and an impaired intracellular insulin signaling. Current knowledge about the adipose cells and the role of inflammation are reviewed in this chapter.

FIRST-DEGREE RELATIVES OF TYPE 2 DIABETIC PATIENTS AND RISK OF DIABETES

Prospective studies of first-degree relatives of type 2 diabetic patients have shown during 25 years a cumulative incidence of type 2 diabetes as high as 76% if the first-degree relatives exhibited values below the group median of insulin sensitivity and insulin-independent glucose removal rate (1). There are also reports estimating the lifetime risk of developing type 2 diabetes as high as 40–80% in this cohort (2). Thus, this is an excellent group of individuals for studying the pre-diabetic condition without the confounding secondary effect induced by diabetes per se.

From: *Contemporary Endocrinology: The Metabolic Syndrome: Epidemiology, Clinical Treatment, and Underlying Mechanisms*
Edited by: B.C. Hansen and G.A. Bray © Humana Press, Totowa, NJ

Facets of the Insulin-Resistance (or Metabolic) Syndrome (IRS) in First-Degree Relatives

The key feature in the development of type 2 diabetes (T2D), insulin resistance, has been repeatedly shown to characterize first-degree relatives (FDRs) (3–6). While no defect in insulin secretion was apparent in an early study (4), this is in contrast to recent findings when, appropriately, beta-cell function was related to degree of insulin resistance (7,8).

Reports in the literature suggest that the first-degree relatives have an increased abdominal obesity measured as waist circumference or waist–hip ratio (WHR), both considered to be cardinal symptoms for the definition of the insulin resistance syndrome (IRS) (9). However, in a recent study we could show that first-degree relatives, carefully matched with healthy control subjects for age, gender, BMI, and WHR, still were insulin resistant (10), thus challenging the concept that increased abdominal obesity is a prerequisite for insulin resistance. This study, in agreement with the results from a prospective study of first-degree relatives of T2D at the Joslin Clinic (11), demonstrates that the genetic predisposition harbors factor(s) that are of major importance for developing type 2 diabetes also in the absence of abdominal obesity. However, first-degree relatives also have an increased risk to develop type 2 diabetes following weight gain (12), supporting a prominent role of obesity and adipose tissue.

Dyslipidemia with elevated fasting triglyceride levels and reduced HDL-cholesterol, other facets of IRS, have also been shown in first-degree relatives (9,13). Importantly, however, also normotriglyceridemic first-degree relatives are lipid-intolerant following a standardized meal (14), a defect related to risk of developing atherosclerosis. VLDL1 was the major lipid fraction that was increased postprandially in first-degree relatives (15). Improved insulin secretion induced by an acute administration of the insulin secretagogue, nateglinide, was unable to reverse this defect (16).

In recent years, liver steatosis has been suggested to be a component of the IRS. Nonalcoholic fatty liver disease (NFLD) is also frequently found in first-degree relatives (17) and the mechanism behind such ectopic lipid accumulation and its relation to insulin resistance has gained much interest in recent years. The most abundant gene transcript in adipose cells, adiponectin, seems to prevent the development of NFLD, and thus this adipokine is a current focus of interest (18,19). We have also found that degree of liver steatosis in non-alcohol-abusing first-degree relatives and others was correlated with insulin sensitivity and adiponectin levels (10).

Evidence of Dysregulated Adipose Tissue in First-Degree Relatives and Insulin Resistance

There is an intricate interplay between adipose tissue, muscle, liver, and pancreas, even in the early course of development of diabetes and atherosclerosis. A number of studies performed in our laboratory have led to the conclusion that there is a dysregulation of the adipose tissue long before type 2 diabetes develops (20). Low adipocyte IRS-1 protein (and gene) expression (LIRS) is present in ≈30% of normoglycemic first-degree relatives compared to ≈5% in healthy control subjects without a known genetic predisposition (21). Interestingly, low IRS-1 is also accompanied by low GLUT-4 expression in the adipose cells as well as insulin resistance (22). This cannot be accounted for by concomitant hyperglycemia, obesity, or hyperinsulinemia per se (22).

Multiple signaling defects were also found in low adipocyte IRS-1 protein as reviewed below. Interestingly, mice with an adipose-specific disruption of the GLUT-4 gene are insulin resistant, and this has recently been related to an increased secretion of the retinol binding protein 4 (23,24).

Studies of the metabolic phenotype in low adipocyte IRS-1 protein subjects demonstrate a profile consistent with a high risk of conversion to type 2 diabetes and propensity for macrovascular complications (25). The low adipocyte IRS-1 protein group showed insulin resistance, hyperleptinemia, hypoadiponectinemia, and increased inflammation as indicated by higher circulating CRP levels (25). Thiazolidinedione (TZD) treatment for three weeks in LIRS subjects improved insulin sensitivity and increased the expression of genes important for function of the adipose cells, such as GLUT-4 and adiponectin (26). However, IRS-1 expression was not restored (26). One cornerstone in insulin resistance may thus be an impaired ability to store fat in the adipose cells, which in turn leads to ectopic lipid accumulation in the liver and the skeletal muscles. In addition, the dysregulated adipose tissue is associated with increased expression of cytokines and reduced secretion of beneficial adipokines like adiponectin. These aspects are further discussed below.

ADIPOSE TISSUE AND INSULIN RESISTANCE

Adipose tissue, in contrast to skeletal muscle, accounts for a small part of the insulin-stimulated glucose disposal in vivo. While skeletal muscle has been the focus of most researchers in order to define mechanisms for peripheral insulin resistance, adipose tissue has long been neglected. However, recent studies have clearly shown that adipose tissue not only stores and releases energy as lipids, but it is also the largest endocrine organ of the body. Several factors secreted from adipose tissue, such as free fatty acids (FFA), cytokines, adiponectin, resistin, and the recently identified visfatin (27–29), have been shown to affect insulin sensitivity and action not only in adipose tissue but also in other tissues. Many of these factors are altered in both the pre-diabetic and diabetic state, and they are likely to play an important role for the development of insulin resistance and type 2 diabetes.

Our research has mainly focused on adipose tissue and its involvement in insulin resistance and type 2 diabetes—not only in terms of glucose uptake but also its role as an endocrine organ. During recent years, the concept of dysregulated adipose tissue playing a major role in the development of insulin resistance and type 2 diabetes has become more evident. Future studies must therefore address the underlying mechanisms that result in dysregulated adipose tissue. An important factor will most likely involve the early steps of adipogenesis (i.e., the commitment and development of adipocyte precursor cells).

Insulin Signaling Leading to Glucose Uptake and Other Effects in Adipose Cells

Insulin is the key anabolic and anti-catabolic hormone. It binds to specific surface receptors, which in turn leads to the activation of a complex intracellular signaling cascade (Fig. 10.1). Ligation of insulin to the insulin receptor leads to activation of the intracellular domain and autophosphorylation of several sites in the receptor that creates binding sites for members of the insulin receptor substrate (IRS) family of proteins (30).

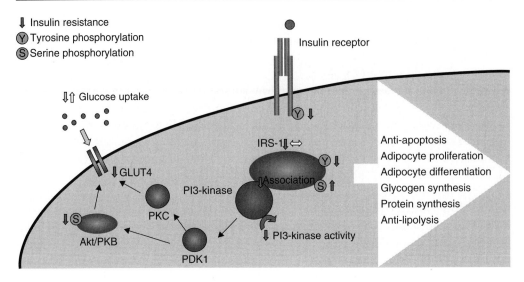

Figure 10.1. Insulin signaling in the adipose tissue. Alterations seen in insulin resistance and type 2 diabetes are also indicated.

The most prominent of the IRS members are IRS-1 and IRS-2; they have partly over-lapping but also distinct functions in different tissues. IRS-1 is the predominantly expressed isoform in the adipose tissue. A pleckstrin homology (PH) domain in the N-terminal domain of the IRSs targets the molecules to the plasma membrane and the vicinity of the insulin receptor. The IRS proteins do not contain catalytic activity but relay the insulin signal to downstream adaptor molecules. Phosphorylation of the IRS proteins by the insulin receptor creates phospho-tyrosine binding (PTB) domains that are recognized by Src homology 2 (SH2) domains of adaptor proteins, such as the regulatory subunit, p85, of the dual lipid and serine kinase phosphatidylinositol (PI) 3 kinase (31).

PI3kinase is an important signaling intermediate between the insulin receptor/IRS-1 and the activation of glucose transporter (GLUT) 4 translocation to the plasma membrane. The use of PI3kinase inhibitors and molecular biology approaches has provided evidence that PI3kinase is necessary for insulin-stimulated glucose uptake (32). The protein kinase activity of the catalytic subunit of PI3kinase (p110) seems to primarily serve an autoregulatory role since the main substrate is the regulatory subunit (p85), but it also plays a role in the regulation of downstream targets (33). The lipid products of PI3kinase, particularly PI(3,4)P$_2$ and PI(3,4,5)P$_3$, interact with PH domains in target proteins to modulate activity and/or localization. The downstream serine kinases, 3-phosphoinositide dependent kinase-1 (PDK1) and protein kinase B (PKB)/Akt, have been shown to contain PH domains that are necessary for their sequential activation by PI3kinase (34,35). Activation of the atypical protein kinase C (PKC) ζ by PDK1 is an additional pathway emanating from PI3kinase that appears to be important for the insulin-stimulated glucose uptake (36). Although the insulin signaling and GLUT4 trafficking have been intensively studied, the events linking PDK1, PKB/Akt, and PKCζ to GLUT4 translocation and glucose uptake are still far from fully elucidated. Recent findings by Cushman and co-workers have shown that in the basal and nonstimulated state, GLUT4 vesicles are constantly moving along common microtubule-based pathways to the plasma membrane where they transiently stop and loosely tether. Insulin inhibits this movement, tightly tethering the vesicles to the plasma membrane where they form clusters and fuse with the membrane. Still, the molecular mechanisms providing the specificity of insulin action on the GLUT4 vesicles remain to be established (37).

The IRS-1/PI3kinase pathway is not only involved in insulin-stimulated glucose uptake; it is also involved in signaling pathways leading to other effects of insulin such as anti-lipolysis, glycogen synthesis, protein synthesis, and, importantly, cell proliferation and differentiation. Proliferation, commitment, and finally differentiation of adipocyte precursor cells are complex processes involving tightly regulated signaling pathways. The IRS-1/PI3kinase pathway is essential for both adipocyte differentiation and the development of an insulin-sensitive phenotype. This pathway is upstream of the transcription factors PPARγ and C/EBPα (38,39), the master regulators of adipocyte differentiation (40,41).

Adipose Tissue Is Dysregulated in Insulin Resistance and Type 2 Diabetes—Effects on Insulin Signaling and Adipocyte Function

Perturbations in the intracellular insulin-signaling cascade are associated with insulin resistance. Several impairments in the insulin signaling cascade have also been found in the adipose cells, as well as in skeletal muscle, of insulin-resistant and diabetic individuals. In skeletal muscle, most studies have shown that in nonobese but diabetic individuals there are no consistent changes in the expression of either the insulin receptor, IRS-1, PI3kinase, PKB/Akt, or GLUT4. However, several impairments are seen in the signal transduction as well as in GLUT4 translocation (42).

We and others have sought to uncover the impairments of the insulin-signaling cascade in the adipose cells in insulin resistance and diabetes, and a different picture emerges as compared to that seen in skeletal muscle (summarized in Table 10.1).

Most studies have reported no clear differences of the insulin receptor protein or tyrosine phosphorylation in the adipose tissue of diabetic or insulin-resistant individuals. However, the major substrate for the insulin receptor in adipose tissue, IRS-1, is commonly reduced in type 2 diabetic patients, while the expression of IRS-2 is unchanged (43). IRS-1 is the main docking protein for PI3kinase in healthy individuals and, thus, the downstream activation of PI3kinase is also reduced in diabetic subjects. Although

Table 10.1
Alterations in Insulin Signaling in Insulin Resistance

Signaling Molecules	Adipose Tissue	
	Protein	*Phosphorylation/Activity*
Insulin receptor	⇔	⇓⇔
IRS-1	⇓	⇓
PI3-kinase	⇔	⇓
PKB/Akt	⇔	⇓
GLUT4	⇓	⇓

IRS-2 can partially compensate for IRS-1 in the activation of PI3kinase, activation of this pathway requires much higher insulin concentrations (43).

The insulin signaling is not only (positively) regulated by tyrosine phosphorylation. Normal IRS-1 signaling can also be inhibited by serine phosphorylation induced by cytokines or fatty acid metabolites. This in turn leads to an increased degradation of IRS-1 and impaired downstream insulin signaling (44,45). The serine kinase activity is enhanced in the adipose tissue from animal models of insulin resistance or human type 2 diabetes (46,47). However, no data are yet available on the serine phosphorylation of IRS-1 in the adipose tissue of diabetic or insulin-resistant subjects.

As expected, downstream insulin signaling is impaired in adipose cells from type 2 diabetic subjects (48). Although the amount of PKB/Akt protein is unchanged, both the sensitivity to insulin and insulin-stimulated serine phosphorylation of PKB/Akt are decreased, and this is associated with an impaired GLUT4 translocation. PKB/Akt is, however, normally phosphorylated by agents that bypass the upstream defects in the insulin-signaling pathway (48). Experiments with human adipose cells from healthy and type 2 diabetic subjects have shown that the subcellular distribution of PKB/Akt in response to insulin is impaired in diabetes—a partial explanation for the impaired serine phosphorylation of the protein (49).

We have also studied the insulin-signaling pathway in individuals who are prone to develop type 2 diabetes (i.e., first-degree relatives of type 2 diabetic patients). IRS-1 protein expression was found to be more commonly (~1:6 relation) reduced in these individuals compared to a healthy control group (21). Furthermore, the insulin-resistant individuals were characterized by impairments in the downstream insulin-signaling pathway in the absence of any changes in the protein levels of IRS-2, PI3kinase, or PKB/Akt. However, the activation of PI3kinase and PKB/Akt in response to insulin was substantially reduced (22). Several studies have also shown that not only is the translocation of GLUT4 impaired, but the protein expression of GLUT4 is also markedly reduced in the adipose cells from insulin-resistant subjects (22,50).

In addition to the impairments of the insulin-signaling pathway in adipose cells from insulin-resistant and type 2 diabetic individuals, we subsequently identified a number of alterations related to adipocyte differentiation, regulation, and function. Several genes involved in, or reflecting degree of, adipocyte differentiation such as PPARγ, C/EBPα, aP2, and adiponectin are reduced in insulin-resistant individuals (25). Furthermore, genes important for energy-generating processes as well as production of metabolites necessary for triglyceride storage are also altered in the adipose cells from insulin-resistant individuals (51–53). In addition, gene profiling implicated an impaired precursor cell development in the adipose tissue of insulin-resistant subjects (54).

Identification of the molecular basis of dysregulated adipose tissue may provide new insight into the causes of insulin resistance and type 2 diabetes and the associated complications.

ADIPOSE TISSUE AND INFLAMMATION

Molecules secreted by the adipose tissue are commonly referred to as *adipokines* and include several cytokines, hormones, and growth factors. Obesity frequently alters the adipokine efflux in association with the increased fat cell size (55), and this is associated with a pro-inflammatory state in the adipose tissue and increased circulating levels of inflammatory cytokines and markers such as interleukin-6 (IL-6), C-reactive protein

(CRP), and serum amyloid A (SAA). Conversely, a decreased adipose tissue mass by weight loss (e.g., through decreased dietary intake, exercise, or liposuction) reduces the circulating levels of inflammatory markers (56–60).

In addition to the increased expression of certain cytokines by the adipose cells, the adipose tissue in obese individuals becomes inflamed as a consequence of macrophage infiltration. Upon weight gain, the adipocytes increase in size and this is associated with an enhanced secretion of cytokines. This in turn stimulates the preadipocytes and the endothelial cells in the adipose tissue to secrete chemokines, such as the monocyte chemotactic protein-1 (MCP-1), which recruits macrophages. In the adipose tissue, the recruited macrophages further increase the cytokine production and trigger inflammatory signals (e.g., activation of NF-κB pathway), eventually leading to a dysregulated adipose tissue and pronounced insulin resistance (61–63).

TNF-α and IL-6 are the two most studied cytokines that are expressed in adipose tissue. In 1993, Hotamisligil et al. reported that TNF-α was induced at both protein and mRNA levels in the adipose tissue of obese rodents (64). The same results were soon also shown in humans and, in addition, that weight loss decreased the TNF-α expression in the adipose tissue. TNF-α expression was found to be associated with hyperinsulinemia, thus providing a link between inflammation and insulin resistance (65,66). However, the increased expression of TNF-α in adipocytes in obesity was not accompanied by an increased circulating level of TNF-α, probably due to an impaired proteolytic cleavage and release of membrane-bound TNF-α. It was, therefore, suggested that TNF-α induced insulin resistance in obesity through its membrane-bound activity (67).

Increased serum levels of IL-6 and upregulated IL-6 expression in adipose tissue have also been found in obesity and insulin resistance (68–70). IL-6 is likely to be a paracrine regulator in human adipose tissue as the interstitial IL-6 concentrations in vivo in human beings are 50–100 times higher than the circulating levels. In addition, IL-6 mRNA levels, secretion by the adipose tissue, and the interstitial IL-6 concentrations in situ are correlated with the size of the adipocytes (71). Interestingly, several steps of the insulin-signaling pathway are negatively affected by an increased cytokine production. For example, both IL-6 and TNF-α were shown to have negative effects on the transcription and translation of GLUT-4 and IRS-1 (70).

In addition to pro-inflammatory molecules, the adipocytes also produce and secrete anti-inflammatory molecules, like adiponectin. This molecule is markedly reduced in obese and insulin-resistant subjects, and the adipose cell size is inversely correlated with adiponectin gene expression (18,54). Both TNF-α and IL-6 reduce the expression and protein secretion of adiponectin by adipose cells (71–73). In contrast, the suppressor of cytokine signaling-3 (SOCS-3) is upregulated by IL-6. SOCS3 is a feedback regulator of IL-6 signaling but, interestingly, it can also induce an inhibitory effect on insulin signaling by impairing the interaction between IRS-1 and the insulin receptor and reducing the insulin-stimulated glucose transport (74,75). In addition, TNF-α (but not IL-6) induces serine-phosphorylation of IRS-1 through an activated Janus kinase (JNK) pathway, and this inhibits the interaction between the insulin receptor and IRS-1 (70,76). Notably, short-term in vivo studies in Sprague-Dawley rats showed no acute effect of IL-6 on insulin sensitivity, indicating that IL-6 is a chronic modulator of insulin signaling (77). Moreover, a recent study has shown that the IL-6 promoter polymorphism (−174 G/C) is associated with an increased expression of IL-6 in the adipose tissue as well as insulin resistance in vivo (78).

One of the important inflammatory effects of TNF-α is to activate the NF-κB pathway, which in turn regulates many genes related to inflammation and insulin resistance. Inhibition of NF-κB restores many genes that would normally be altered in the presence of TNF-α (79). Transgenic mice lacking expression of either TNF-α or the TNF-α receptors maintained their insulin sensitivity when becoming obese, and inhibition of NF-κB activation was also found to decrease the development of insulin resistance in vivo (80–82). Apart from NF-κB, TNF-α also regulates the expression of several other genes, notably other cytokines. Explants of human adipose tissue exposed to TNF-α showed a strong induction of both gene expression and secretion of cytokines such as IL-6, IL-8, and TNF-α itself (83).

In addition to cytokines, other pro-inflammatory molecules have been described in the adipose tissue. Interleukin-8 (IL-8), macrophage inflammatory protein-1α (MIF-1α), and monocyte chemotactic protein-1 (MCP-1) belong to the chemokine family. They are all constitutively expressed by preadipocytes and TNF-α increases their expression (83,84). Resistin is another molecule described to be associated with inflammation, obesity, and insulin resistance (hence the name—resistance to insulin). Pro-inflammatory properties of resistin were recently reported as it induced expression and secretion of TNF-α, IL-6, and IL-1β in human peripheral blood mononuclear cells. High levels of resistin were found in the synovial fluid of patients with rheumatoid arthritis, and intraarticular injection of resistin into the knee joint of healthy mice was shown to induce arthritis (85). Although resistin is a clear pro-inflammatory cytokine, the role of resistin in obesity-induced insulin resistance is still unclear and seems to differ between species (86). Resistin is, for example, expressed in mature rodent, but not human, adipose cells (87,88). This discrepancy is probably due to the low degree of sequence homology between species (e.g., the homology between mouse and human resistin is only 53%). This indicates a possible variation both in expression and function of resistin analogs among species (86).

Taken together, pro-inflammatory molecules are important links between obesity and insulin resistance, and the pro-inflammatory state in adipose tissue is further augmented by the recruitment of inflammatory cells into adipose tissue in obesity.

Inflammatory Markers CRP and SAA

Both CRP and SAA are inflammatory serum markers secreted upon cytokine induction, most prominently by TNF-α and IL-6 (89–91). CRP is a conserved protein of the pentraxin family and is expressed in both vertebrates and invertebrates. It was described already in 1930 and in 1954 CRP was related to myocardial infarction and that high circulating levels implied a poor prognosis (92,93). CRP binds to phosphorylcholine on certain bacterial and fungal surfaces and thereby functions as an alarm mechanism for the host-defense system. It has been reported that the phosphorylcholine-binding site can also interact with oxidized lipids in the LDL particle, cholesterol, and additionally complement factors and initiate their activation (94–97). These molecules are all present and involved in the formation of atherosclerotic plaques and lesions. Whether CRP itself has a pro- or an antiatherogenic effect is a matter of debate. Apolipoprotein E (apoE)-deficient mice, known to be atherogenic, crossed with CRP-overexpressing mice were shown to develop an increased atherosclerosis (98), but when the apoE-knockout mice were crossed with transgenic mice expressing human CRP, no induction

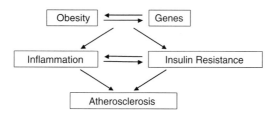

Figure 10.2. Schematic figure of the putative relationship among inflammation, insulin resistance, and atherosclerosis.

of atherosclerosis was found (99). Nevertheless, CRP is widely used as an indicator of inflammation, infection, and future cardiovascular risk.

As CRP is highly induced by IL-6 (89) and the IL-6 expression is increased in fat cells from insulin-resistant subjects (70), associations among CRP, obesity, and type 2 diabetes are evident. An extensive study of 14,719 apparently healthy women followed over an 8-year period showed that the serum level of CRP increased with the number of components of the metabolic syndrome (100).

The serum amyloid A (SAA) family consists of apolipoproteins involved in the host-defense alarm system. Upon inflammation, tissue damage, or bacterial infection, the serum level of SAA may increase 1,000-fold compared to normal levels, and the plasma concentration of SAA can then exceed 1 mg/ml. There are four human and five mouse SAA family members. SAAs are mainly synthesized by the liver, but they are also expressed in adipocytes and macrophages. Notably, SAA3 differs from the other SAA family members in terms of homology, and the human SAA3 is a pseudogene (101–103). One of the suggested functions of SAA is to associate with high-density lipoprotein (HDL) and regulate the HDL function and thus cholesterol transport. HDL prevents atherosclerosis by mediating reverse cholesterol transport from the macrophages to the HDL particle, thereby facilitating cholesterol removal from sites of tissue damage during inflammation (e.g. the atherosclerotic plaque) (101). Recently, SAAs have been reported to bind to the HDL receptor, scavenger receptor BI (SR-BI), and to compete with the HDL function to reduce cellular cholesterol levels (104).

In addition to playing a potentially important role in atherosclerosis, high levels of SAA are also seen in obese individuals, probably due to the increased levels of cytokines (e.g., IL-6) inducing SAA production by both the liver and the adipose cells (56,91). Additionally, adipose tissue from diabetic *ob/ob* and *db/db* mice expresses high levels of SAA3 compared to wild-type mice, and hyperglycemia has been found to induce SAA3 secretion (103). Taken together, obesity is associated with low-grade inflammation, which in turn also is likely to contribute to the insulin resistance and propensity for atherosclerosis (Fig. 10.2).

THIAZOLIDINEDIONES

Thiazolidinediones (TZDs) is a recently discovered group of PPARγ agonists that have been shown to improve insulin resistance in the liver, skeletal muscle, and adipose tissue without primarily affecting insulin secretion from the beta-cells. These agents markedly decrease plasma glucose, insulin, and triglyceride levels in animal models of insulin resistance and obesity (105). Studies in type 2 diabetic patients have also shown that TZDs have beneficial effects on many of the metabolic abnormalities seen in these patients. Most, but not all individuals, respond with increased glucose disposal, reduced hepatic glucose production, and improvements in HbA_{1c}, triglycerides, and HDL-cholesterol levels. Studies in nondiabetic subjects with impaired glucose tolerance have shown that TZDs have similar beneficial effects in this pre-diabetic group (106). Although functional PPAR response elements have not been found in the regulatory region of the key insulin-signaling proteins, TZD treatment has been reported to have several beneficial effects on both insulin signaling and insulin-stimulated glucose uptake. Studies in isolated adipocytes from type 2 diabetic individuals treated for three months with troglitazone showed no effect on the expression of IRS-1, PI3kinase, or PKB/Akt. However, insulin-stimulated serine phosphorylation of PKB/Akt and expression of GLUT4 were improved as well as the insulin-stimulated glucose uptake in vivo (107). We have recently obtained similar results in insulin-resistant but nondiabetic individuals (26). Furthermore, TZD treatment has been reported to reduce the inhibitory serine phosphorylation of IRS-1 (108).

Treatment with TZDs not only enhances insulin signaling, but it is also thought to improve the insulin sensitivity of adipose tissue by recruiting new, and more insulin-sensitive, adipocytes and to drive the terminal differentiation of preexisting adipocytes (109). One consequence of this is the increased expression of adiponectin, which in turn is considered to be an important mechanism for the improved insulin sensitivity following TZD treatment.

In addition to improving insulin signaling and action, TZDs also have an anti-inflammatory effect. Plasma levels of TNF-α, CRP, and SAA are all reduced following treatment of obese patients with TZD (110,111). Less is known about potential effects on the level of IL-6 or other cytokines. However, one study has shown that serum levels of IL-6 in diabetic patients were not significantly reduced following treatment with TZDs for three months (112), whereas LPS-induced IL-6 and TNF-α expression in the adipose tissue of mice were reduced (113). Furthermore, TZDs can efficiently prevent the negative effect of TNF-α and IL-6 on insulin signaling in 3T3-L1 cells. TZDs not only cause a reduction of the mRNA expression of both TNF-α and IL-6, but they also reduce the induction of NF-κB-regulated genes (55,73,114,115).

Thus, TZDs can both improve insulin sensitivity and reduce different markers of inflammation. It is likely that the anti-inflammatory effect of TZD also plays a role for the insulin-sensitizing action.

In conclusion, we have here reviewed evidence strongly implicating the early development of a dysregulated adipose tissue in insulin resistance and type 2 diabetes. Although this can have negative consequences for lipid storage in the adipose tissue and lead to the accumulation of ectopic fat in other tissues, a major effect is probably the concomitant alteration in the secretion of adipokines like adiponectin, cytokines, and RBP-4. These and other adipokines crosstalk with the skeletal muscles and liver, leading to an impaired effect of insulin as well as an increased systemic inflammation and propensity for the development of atherosclerosis.

REFERENCES

1. Martin BC, Warram JH, Krolewski AS, Bergman RN, Soeldner JS, Kahn CR. Role of glucose and insulin resistance in development of type 2 diabetes mellitus: Results of a 25-year follow-up study. *Lancet* 1992; 340:925–929.

2. Köbberling J, Tillil H. Empirical risk figures for first-degree relatives of non-insulin-dependent diabetics. In: *The Genetics of Diabetes Mellitus,* Köbberling J, Tattersall R (eds.), Academic Press, London, 1982, pp. 201–209.

3. Haffner SM, Stern MP, Hazuda HP, Mitchell BD, Patterson JK. Increased insulin concentrations in nondiabetic offspring of diabetic parents. *N Engl J Med* 1988; 319:1297–1301.

4. Eriksson J, Franssila-Kallunki A, Ekstrand A, Saloranta C, Widen E, Schalin C, Groop L. Early metabolic defects in persons at increased risk for non-insulin-dependent diabetes mellitus. *N Engl J Med* 1989; 321:337–343.

5. Eriksson JW, Smith U, Waagstein F, Wysocki M, Jansson PA. Glucose turnover and adipose tissue lipolysis are insulin-resistant in healthy relatives of type 2 diabetes patients: Is cellular insulin resistance a secondary phenomenon? *Diabetes* 1999; 48:1572–1578.

6. Vaag A, Henriksen JE, Beck-Nielsen H. Decreased insulin activation of glycogen synthase in skeletal muscles in young nonobese Caucasian first-degree relatives of patients with non-insulin-dependent diabetes mellitus. *J Clin Invest* 1992; 89:782–788.

7. Henriksen JE, Alford F, Handberg A, Vaag A, Ward GM, Kalfas A, Beck-Nielsen H. Increased glucose effectiveness in normoglycemic but insulin-resistant relatives of patients with non-insulin-dependent diabetes mellitus: A novel compensatory mechanism. *J Clin Invest* 1994; 94: 1196–1204.

8. Perseghin G, Ghosh S, Gerow K, Shulman GI. Metabolic defects in lean nondiabetic offspring of NIDDM parents: A cross-sectional study. *Diabetes* 1997; 46:1001–1009.

9. Groop L, Forsblom C, Lehtovirta M, Tuomi T, Karanko S, Nissen M, Ehrnstrom BO, Forsen B, Isomaa B, Snickars B, Taskinen MR. Metabolic consequences of a family history of NIDDM (the Botnia study): Evidence for sex-specific parental effects. *Diabetes* 1996; 45: 1585–1593.

10. Johanson EH, Jansson PA, Lonn L, Matsuzawa Y, Funahashi T, Taskinen MR, Smith U, Axelsen M. Fat distribution, lipid accumulation in the liver, and exercise capacity do not explain the insulin resistance in healthy males with a family history for type 2 diabetes. *J Clin Endocrinol Metab* 2003; 88:4232–4238.

11. Goldfine AB, Bouche C, Parker RA, Kim C, Kerivan A, Soeldner JS, Martin BC, Warram JH, Kahn CR. Insulin resistance is a poor predictor of type 2 diabetes in individuals with no family history of disease. *Proc Natl Acad Sci USA* 2003; 100:2724–2729.

12. Grill V, Persson G, Carlsson S, Norman A, Alvarsson M, Ostensson CG, Svanstrom L, Efendic S. Family history of diabetes in middle-aged Swedish men is a gender unrelated factor which associates with insulinopenia in newly diagnosed diabetic subjects. *Diabetologia* 1999; 42:15–23.

13. Laws A, Stefanick ML, Reaven GM. Insulin resistance and hypertriglyceridemia in nondiabetic relatives of patients with noninsulin-dependent diabetes mellitus. *J Clin Endocrinol Metab* 1989; 69: 343–347.

14. Axelsen M, Smith U, Eriksson JW, Taskinen MR, Jansson PA. Postprandial hypertriglyceridemia and insulin resistance in normoglycemic first-degree relatives of patients with type 2 diabetes. *Ann Intern Med* 1999; 131:27–31.

15. Johanson EH, Jansson PA, Gustafson B, Lonn L, Smith U, Taskinen MR, Axelsen M. Early alterations in the postprandial VLDL1 apoB-100 and apoB-48 metabolism in men with strong heredity for type 2 diabetes. *J Intern Med* 2004; 255:273–279.

16. Johanson EH, Jansson PA, Gustafson B, Sandqvist M, Taskinen MR, Smith U, Axelsen M. No acute effect of nateglinide on postprandial lipid and lipoprotein responses in subjects at risk for type 2 diabetes. *Diabetes Metab Res Rev* 2005; 21:376–381.

17. Marchesini G, Brizi M, Bianchi G, Tomassetti S, Bugianesi E, Lenzi M, McCullough AJ, Natale S, Forlani G, Melchionda N. Nonalcoholic fatty liver disease: A feature of the metabolic syndrome. *Diabetes* 2001; 50:1844–1850.

18. Yamauchi T, Kamon J, Waki H, Terauchi Y, Kubota N, Hara K, Mori Y, Ide T, Murakami K, Tsuboyama-Kasaoka N, Ezaki O, Akanuma Y, Gavrilova O, Vinson C, Reitman ML, Kagechika H, Shudo K, Yoda M, Nakano Y, Tobe K, Nagai R, Kimura S, Tomita M, Froguel P, Kadowaki T. The fat-derived hormone adiponectin reverses insulin resistance associated with both lipoatrophy and obesity. *Nat Med* 2001; 7:941–946.

19. Pellme F, Smith U, Funahashi T, Matsuzawa Y, Brekke H, Wiklund O, Taskinen MR, Jansson PA. Circulating adiponectin levels are reduced in nonobese but insulin-resistant first-degree relatives of type 2 diabetic patients. *Diabetes* 2003; 52:1182–1186.

20. Smith U. Impaired ("diabetic") insulin signaling and action occur in fat cells long before glucose intolerance: Is insulin resistance initiated in the adipose tissue? *Int J Obes Relat Metab Disord* 2002; 26:897–904.

21. Carvalho E, Jansson PA, Axelsen M, Eriksson JW, Huang X, Groop L, Rondinone C, Sjostrom L, Smith U. Low cellular IRS 1 gene and protein expression predict insulin resistance and NIDDM. *Faseb J* 1999; 13:2173–2178.

22. Carvalho E, Jansson PA, Nagaev I, Wenthzel AM, Smith U. Insulin resistance with low cellular IRS-1 expression is also associated with low GLUT4 expression and impaired insulin-stimulated glucose transport. *Faseb J* 2001; 15:1101–1103.

23. Abel ED, Peroni O, Kim JK, Kim YB, Boss O, Hadro E, Minnemann T, Shulman GI, Kahn BB. Adipose-selective targeting of the GLUT4 gene impairs insulin action in muscle and liver. *Nature* 2001; 409:729–733.

24. Yang Q, Graham TE, Mody N, Preitner F, Peroni OD, Zabolotny JM, Kotani K, Quadro L, Kahn BB. Serum retinol binding protein 4 contributes to insulin resistance in obesity and type 2 diabetes. *Nature* 2005; 436:356–362.

25. Jansson PA, Pellme F, Hammarstedt A, Sandqvist M, Brekke H, Caidahl K, Forsberg M, Volkmann R, Carvalho E, Funahashi T, Matsuzawa Y, Wiklund O, Yang X, Taskinen MR, Smith U. A novel cellular marker of insulin resistance and early atherosclerosis in humans is related to impaired fat cell differentiation and low adiponectin. *Faseb J* 2003; 17:1434–1440.

26. Hammarstedt A, Sopasakis VR, Gogg S, Jansson PA, Smith U. Improved insulin sensitivity and adipose tissue dysregulation after short-term treatment with pioglitazone in non-diabetic, insulin-resistant subjects. *Diabetologia* 2005; 48:96–104.

27. Faraj M, Lu HL, Cianflone K. Diabetes, lipids, and adipocyte secretagogues. *Biochem Cell Biol* 2004; 82:170–190.

28. Meier U, Gressner AM. Endocrine regulation of energy metabolism: review of pathobiochemical and clinical chemical aspects of leptin, ghrelin, adiponectin, and resistin. *Clin Chem* 2004; 50:1511–1525.

29. Fukuhara A, Matsuda M, Nishizawa M, Segawa K, Tanaka M, Kishimoto K, Matsuki Y, Murakami M, Ichisaka T, Murakami H, Watanabe E, Takagi T, Akiyoshi M, Ohtsubo T, Kihara S, Yamashita S, Makishima M, Funahashi T, Yamanaka S, Hiramatsu R, Matsuzawa Y, Shimomura I. Visfatin: A protein secreted by visceral fat that mimics the effects of insulin. *Science* 2005; 307:426–430.

30. Giovannone B, Scaldaferri ML, Federici M, Porzio O, Lauro D, Fusco A, Sbraccia P, Borboni P, Lauro R, Sesti G. Insulin receptor substrate (IRS) transduction system: Distinct and overlapping signaling potential. *Diabetes Metab Res Rev* 2000; 16:434–441.

31. Backer JM, Myers MG, Jr., Shoelson SE, Chin DJ, Sun XJ, Miralpeix M, Hu P, Margolis B, Skolnik EY, Schlessinger J et al. Phosphatidylinositol 3′-kinase is activated by association with IRS-1 during insulin stimulation. *Embo J* 1992; 11:3469–3479.

32. Cheatham B, Vlahos CJ, Cheatham L, Wang L, Blenis J, Kahn CR. Phosphatidylinositol 3-kinase activation is required for insulin stimulation of pp70 S6 kinase, DNA synthesis, and glucose transporter translocation. *Mol Cell Biol* 1994; 14:4902–4911.

33. Dhand R, Hiles I, Panayotou G, Roche S, Fry MJ, Gout I, Totty NF, Truong O, Vicendo P, Yonezawa K et al. PI 3-kinase is a dual specificity enzyme: Autoregulation by an intrinsic protein-serine kinase activity. *Embo J* 1994; 13:522–533.

34. Alessi DR, Deak M, Casamayor A, Caudwell FB, Morrice N, Norman DG, Gaffney P, Reese CB, MacDougall CN, Harbison D, Ashworth A, Bownes M. 3-Phosphoinositide-dependent protein kinase-1 (PDK1): Structural and functional homology with the Drosophila DSTPK61 kinase. *Curr Biol* 1997; 7:776–789.

35. Downward J. Mechanisms and consequences of activation of protein kinase B/Akt. *Curr Opin Cell Biol* 1998; 10:262–267.

36. Standaert ML, Galloway L, Karnam P, Bandyopadhyay G, Moscat J, Farese RV. Protein kinase C-zeta as a downstream effector of phosphatidylinositol 3-kinase during insulin stimulation in rat adipocytes: Potential role in glucose transport. *J Biol Chem* 1997; 272:30075–30082.

37. Lizunov VA, Matsumoto H, Zimmerberg J, Cushman SW, Frolov VA. Insulin stimulates the halting, tethering, and fusion of mobile GLUT4 vesicles in rat adipose cells. *J Cell Biol* 2005; 169:481–489.

38. Fasshauer M, Klein J, Kriauciunas KM, Ueki K, Benito M, Kahn CR. Essential role of insulin receptor substrate 1 in differentiation of brown adipocytes. *Mol Cell Biol* 2001; 21:319–329.

39. Miki H, Yamauchi T, Suzuki R, Komeda K, Tsuchida A, Kubota N, Terauchi Y, Kamon J, Kaburagi Y, Matsui J, Akanuma Y, Nagai R, Kimura S, Tobe K, Kadowaki T. Essential role of insulin receptor substrate 1 (IRS-1) and IRS-2 in adipocyte differentiation. *Mol Cell Biol* 2001; 21:2521–2532.
40. El-Jack AK, Hamm JK, Pilch PF, Farmer SR. Reconstitution of insulin-sensitive glucose transport in fibroblasts requires expression of both PPARgamma and C/EBPalpha. *J Biol Chem* 1999; 274:7946–7951.
41. Wu Z, Rosen ED, Brun R, Hauser S, Adelmant G, Troy AE, McKeon C, Darlington GJ, Spiegelman BM. Cross-regulation of C/EBP alpha and PPAR gamma controls the transcriptional pathway of adipogenesis and insulin sensitivity. *Mol Cell* 1999; 3:151–158.
42. Zierath JR, Krook A, Wallberg-Henriksson H. Insulin action and insulin resistance in human skeletal muscle. *Diabetologia* 2000; 43:821–835.
43. Rondinone CM, Wang LM, Lonnroth P, Wesslau C, Pierce JH, Smith U. Insulin receptor substrate (IRS) 1 is reduced and IRS-2 is the main docking protein for phosphatidylinositol 3-kinase in adipocytes from subjects with non-insulin-dependent diabetes mellitus. *Proc Natl Acad Sci USA* 1997; 94:4171–4175.
44. Aguirre V, Werner ED, Giraud J, Lee YH, Shoelson SE, White MF. Phosphorylation of Ser307 in insulin receptor substrate-1 blocks interactions with the insulin receptor and inhibits insulin action. *J Biol Chem* 2002; 277:1531–1537.
45. Greene MW, Sakaue H, Wang L, Alessi DR, Roth RA. Modulation of insulin-stimulated degradation of human insulin receptor substrate-1 by Serine 312 phosphorylation. *J Biol Chem* 2003; 278:8199–8211.
46. Gao Z, Zhang X, Zuberi A, Hwang D, Quon MJ, Lefevre M, Ye J. Inhibition of insulin sensitivity by free fatty acids requires activation of multiple serine kinases in 3T3-L1 adipocytes. *Mol Endocrinol* 2004; 18:2024–2034.
47. Carlson CJ, Koterski S, Sciotti RJ, Poccard GB, Rondinone CM. Enhanced basal activation of mitogen-activated protein kinases in adipocytes from type 2 diabetes: Potential role of p38 in the downregulation of GLUT4 expression. *Diabetes* 2003; 52:634–641.
48. Rondinone CM, Carvalho E, Wesslau C, Smith UP. Impaired glucose transport and protein kinase B activation by insulin, but not okadaic acid, in adipocytes from subjects with type II diabetes mellitus. *Diabetologia* 1999; 42:819–825.
49. Carvalho E, Eliasson B, Wesslau C, Smith U. Impaired phosphorylation and insulin-stimulated translocation to the plasma membrane of protein kinase B/Akt in adipocytes from type II diabetic subjects. *Diabetologia* 2000; 43:1107–1115.
50. Ducluzeau PH, Perretti N, Laville M, Andreelli F, Vega N, Riou JP, Vidal H. Regulation by insulin of gene expression in human skeletal muscle and adipose tissue: Evidence for specific defects in type 2 diabetes. *Diabetes* 2001; 50:1134–1142.
51. Hammarstedt A, Jansson PA, Wesslau C, Yang X, Smith U. Reduced expression of PGC-1 and insulin-signaling molecules in adipose tissue is associated with insulin resistance. *Biochem Biophys Res Commun* 2003; 301:578–582.
52. Semple RK, Crowley VC, Sewter CP, Laudes M, Christodoulides C, Considine RV, Vidal-Puig A, O'Rahilly S. Expression of the thermogenic nuclear hormone receptor coactivator PGC-1alpha is reduced in the adipose tissue of morbidly obese subjects. *Int J Obes Relat Metab Disord* 2004; 8:176–179.
53. Yang X, Enerback S, Smith U. Reduced expression of FOXC2 and brown adipogenic genes in human subjects with insulin resistance. *Obes Res* 2003; 11:1182–1191.
54. Yang X, Jansson PA, Nagaev I, Jack MM, Carvalho E, Sunnerhagen KS, Cam MC, Cushman SW, Smith U. Evidence of impaired adipogenesis in insulin resistance. *Biochem Biophys Res Commun* 2004; 317:1045–1051.
55. Hammarstedt A, Andersson CX, Rotter Sopasakis V, Smith U. The effect of PPARgamma ligands on the adipose tissue in insulin resistance. *Prostaglandins Leukot Essent Fatty Acids* 2005; 73:65–75.
56. O'Brien KD, Brehm BJ, Seeley RJ, Bean J, Wener MH, Daniels S, D'Alessio DA. Diet-induced weight loss is associated with decreases in plasma serum amyloid a and C-reactive protein independent of dietary macronutrient composition in obese subjects. *J Clin Endocrinol Metab* 2005; 90:2244–2249.
57. Park HS, Park JY, Yu R. Relationship of obesity and visceral adiposity with serum concentrations of CRP, TNF-alpha and IL-6. *Diabetes Res Clin Pract* 2005; 69:29–35.

58. Pai JK, Pischon T, Ma J, Manson JE, Hankinson SE, Joshipura K, Curhan GC, Rifai N, Cannuscio CC, Stampfer MJ, Rimm EB. Inflammatory markers and the risk of coronary heart disease in men and women. *N Engl J Med* 2004; 351:2599–2610.
59. Giugliano G, Nicoletti G, Grella E, Giugliano F, Esposito K, Scuderi N, D'Andrea F. Effect of liposuction on insulin resistance and vascular inflammatory markers in obese women. *Br J Plast Surg* 2004; 57:190–194.
60. Ziccardi P, Nappo F, Giugliano G, Esposito K, Marfella R, Cioffi M, D'Andrea F, Molinari AM, Giugliano D. Reduction of inflammatory cytokine concentrations and improvement of endothelial functions in obese women after weight loss over one year. *Circulation* 2002; 105:804–809.
61. Xu H, Barnes GT, Yang Q, Tan G, Yang D, Chou CJ, Sole J, Nichols A, Ross JS, Tartaglia LA, Chen H. Chronic inflammation in fat plays a crucial role in the development of obesity-related insulin resistance. *J Clin Invest* 2003; 112:1821–1830.
62. Wellen KE, Hotamisligil GS. Obesity-induced inflammatory changes in adipose tissue. *J Clin Invest* 2003; 112:1785–1788.
63. Weisberg SP, McCann D, Desai M, Rosenbaum M, Leibel RL, Ferrante AW, Jr. Obesity is associated with macrophage accumulation in adipose tissue. *J Clin Invest* 2003; 112:1796–1808.
64. Hotamisligil GS, Shargill NS, Spiegelman BM. Adipose expression of tumor necrosis factor-alpha: direct role in obesity-linked insulin resistance. *Science* 1993; 259:87–91.
65. Hotamisligil GS, Arner P, Caro JF, Atkinson RL, Spiegelman BM. Increased adipose tissue expression of tumor necrosis factor-alpha in human obesity and insulin resistance. *J Clin Invest* 1995; 95:2409–2415.
66. Kern PA, Saghizadeh M, Ong JM, Bosch RJ, Deem R, Simsolo RB. The expression of tumor necrosis factor in human adipose tissue: Regulation by obesity, weight loss, and relationship to lipoprotein lipase. *J Clin Invest* 1995; 95:2111–2119.
67. Xu H, Uysal KT, Becherer JD, Arner P, Hotamisligil GS. Altered tumor necrosis factor-alpha (TNF-alpha) processing in adipocytes and increased expression of transmembrane TNF-alpha in obesity. *Diabetes* 2002; 51:1876–1883.
68. Kern PA, Ranganathan S, Li C, Wood L, Ranganathan G. Adipose tissue tumor necrosis factor and interleukin-6 expression in human obesity and insulin resistance. *Am J Physiol Endocrinol Metab* 2001; 280:E745–751.
69. Kado S, Nagase T, Nagata N. Circulating levels of interleukin-6, its soluble receptor and interleukin-6/interleukin-6 receptor complexes in patients with type 2 diabetes mellitus. *Acta Diabetol* 1999; 36:67–72.
70. Rotter V, Nagaev I, Smith U. Interleukin-6 (IL-6) induces insulin resistance in 3T3-L1 adipocytes and is, like IL-8 and tumor necrosis factor-alpha, overexpressed in human fat cells from insulin-resistant subjects. *J Biol Chem* 2003; 278:45777–45784.
71. Sopasakis VR, Sandqvist M, Gustafson B, Hammarstedt A, Schmelz M, Yang X, Jansson PA, Smith U. High local concentrations and effects on differentiation implicate interleukin-6 as a paracrine regulator. *Obes Res* 2004; 12:454–460.
72. Fasshauer M, Kralisch S, Klier M, Lossner U, Bluher M, Klein J, Paschke R. Adiponectin gene expression and secretion is inhibited by interleukin-6 in 3T3-L1 adipocytes. *Biochem Biophys Res Commun* 2003; 301:1045–1050.
73. Gustafson B, Jack MM, Cushman SW, Smith U. Adiponectin gene activation by thiazolidinediones requires PPAR gamma 2, but not C/EBP alpha: Evidence for differential regulation of the aP2 and adiponectin genes. *Biochem Biophys Res Commun* 2003; 308:933–939.
74. Starr R, Willson TA, Viney EM, Murray LJ, Rayner JR, Jenkins BJ, Gonda TJ, Alexander WS, Metcalf D, Nicola NA, Hilton DJ. A family of cytokine-inducible inhibitors of signalling. *Nature* 1997; 387:917–921.
75. Ueki K, Kondo T, Kahn CR. Suppressor of cytokine signaling 1 (SOCS-1) and SOCS-3 cause insulin resistance through inhibition of tyrosine phosphorylation of insulin receptor substrate proteins by discrete mechanisms. *Mol Cell Biol* 2004; 24:5434–5446.
76. Lee YH, Giraud J, Davis RJ, White MF. c-Jun N-terminal kinase (JNK) mediates feedback inhibition of the insulin signaling cascade. *J Biol Chem* 2003; 278:2896–2902.
77. Rotter Sopasakis V, Larsson BM, Johansson A, Holmang A, Smith U. Short-term infusion of interleukin-6 does not induce insulin resistance in vivo or impair insulin signalling in rats. *Diabetologia* 2004; 47:1879–1887.

78. Yang X, Jansson PA, Pellme F, Laakso M, Smith U. Effect of the interleukin-6 (-174) g/c promoter polymorphism on adiponectin and insulin sensitivity. *Obes Res* 2005; 13:813–817.
79. Ruan H, Hacohen N, Golub TR, Van Parijs L, Lodish HF. Tumor necrosis factor-alpha suppresses adipocyte-specific genes and activates expression of preadipocyte genes in 3T3-L1 adipocytes: Nuclear factor-kappaB activation by TNF-alpha is obligatory. *Diabetes* 2002; 51:1319–1336.
80. Uysal KT, Wiesbrock SM, Hotamisligil GS. Functional analysis of tumor necrosis factor (TNF) receptors in TNF-alpha-mediated insulin resistance in genetic obesity. *Endocrinology* 1998; 139:4832–4838.
81. Uysal KT, Wiesbrock SM, Marino MW, Hotamisligil GS. Protection from obesity-induced insulin resistance in mice lacking TNF-alpha function. *Nature* 1997; 389:610–614.
82. Arkan MC, Hevener AL, Greten FR, Maeda S, Li ZW, Long JM, Wynshaw-Boris A, Poli G, Olefsky J, Karin M. IKK-beta links inflammation to obesity-induced insulin resistance. *Nat Med* 2005; 11:191–198.
83. Sopasakis VR, Nagaev I, Smith U. Cytokine release from adipose tissue of nonobese individuals. *Int J Obes Relat Metab Disord* 2005; 29:1144–1147
84. Gerhardt CC, Romero IA, Cancello R, Camoin L, Strosberg AD. Chemokines control fat accumulation and leptin secretion by cultured human adipocytes. *Mol Cell Endocrinol* 2001; 175:81–92.
85. Bokarewa M, Nagaev I, Dahlberg L, Smith U, Tarkowski A. Resistin, an adipokine with potent pro-inflammatory properties. *J Immunol* 2005; 174:5789–5795.
86. Banerjee RR, Lazar MA. Resistin: molecular history and prognosis. *J Mol Med* 2003; 81:218–226.
87. Steppan CM, Bailey ST, Bhat S, Brown EJ, Banerjee RR, Wright CM, Patel HR, Ahima RS, Lazar MA. The hormone resistin links obesity to diabetes. *Nature* 2001; 409:307–312.
88. Nagaev I, Smith U. Insulin resistance and type 2 diabetes are not related to resistin expression in human fat cells or skeletal muscle. *Biochem Biophys Res Commun* 2001; 285:561–564.
89. Li SP, Liu TY, Goldman ND. Cis-acting elements responsible for interleukin-6 inducible C-reactive protein gene expression. *J Biol Chem* 1990; 265:4136–4142.
90. Ramadori G, Van Damme J, Rieder H, Meyer zum Buschenfelde KH. Interleukin 6, the third mediator of acute-phase reaction, modulates hepatic protein synthesis in human and mouse: Comparison with interleukin 1 beta and tumor necrosis factor-alpha. *Eur J Immunol* 1988; 18:1259–1264.
91. Benigni F, Fantuzzi G, Sacco S, Sironi M, Pozzi P, Dinarello CA, Sipe JD, Poli V, Cappelletti M, Paonessa G, Pennica D, Panayotatos N, Ghezzi P. Six different cytokines that share GP130 as a receptor subunit, induce serum amyloid A and potentiate the induction of interleukin-6 and the activation of the hypothalamus-pituitary-adrenal axis by interleukin-1. *Blood* 1996; 87:1851–1854.
92. Tillett WS, Francis T. Serological reactions in pneumonia with a nonprotein somatic fraction of pneumococcus. *J Exp Med* 1930; 52:561–585.
93. Kroop IG, Shackman NH. Level of C-reactive protein as a measure of acute myocardial infarction. *Proc Soc Exp Biol Med* 1954; 86:95–97.
94. Chang MK, Binder CJ, Torzewski M, Witztum JL. C-reactive protein binds to both oxidized LDL and apoptotic cells through recognition of a common ligand: Phosphorylcholine of oxidized phospholipids. *Proc Natl Acad Sci USA* 2002; 99:13043–13048.
95. Torzewski J, Torzewski M, Bowyer DE, Frohlich M, Koenig W, Waltenberger J, Fitzsimmons C, Hombach V. C-reactive protein frequently colocalizes with the terminal complement complex in the intima of early atherosclerotic lesions of human coronary arteries. *Arterioscler Thromb Vasc Biol* 1998; 18:1386–1392.
96. Agrawal A. CRP after 2004. *Mol Immunol* 2005; 42:927–930.
97. Taskinen S, Hyvonen M, Kovanen PT, Meri S, Pentikainen MO. C-reactive protein binds to the 3beta-OH group of cholesterol in LDL particles. *Biochem Biophys Res Commun* 2005; 329:1208–1216.
98. Paul A, Ko KW, Li L, Yechoor V, McCrory MA, Szalai AJ, Chan L. C-reactive protein accelerates the progression of atherosclerosis in apolipoprotein E-deficient mice. *Circulation* 2004; 109:647–655.
99. Hirschfield GM, Gallimore JR, Kahan MC, Hutchinson WL, Sabin CA, Benson GM, Dhillon AP, Tennent GA, Pepys MB. Transgenic human C-reactive protein is not proatherogenic in apolipoprotein E-deficient mice. *Proc Natl Acad Sci USA* 2005; 102:8309–8314.
100. Ridker PM, Buring JE, Cook NR, Rifai N. C-reactive protein, the metabolic syndrome, and risk of incident cardiovascular events: An 8-year follow-up of 14,719 initially healthy American women. *Circulation* 2003; 107:391–397.

101. Uhlar CM, Whitehead AS. Serum amyloid A: The major vertebrate acute-phase reactant. *Eur J Biochem* 1999; 265:501–523.

102. Meek RL, Eriksen N, Benditt EP. Murine serum amyloid A3 is a high density apolipoprotein and is secreted by macrophages. *Proc Natl Acad Sci USA* 1992; 89:7949–7952.

103. Lin Y, Rajala MW, Berger JP, Moller DE, Barzilai N, Scherer PE. Hyperglycemia-induced production of acute phase reactants in adipose tissue. *J Biol Chem* 2001; 276:42077–42083.

104. Cai L, de Beer MC, de Beer FC, van der Westhuyzen DR. Serum amyloid A is a ligand for scavenger receptor class B type I and inhibits high density lipoprotein binding and selective lipid uptake. *J Biol Chem* 2005; 280:2954–2961.

105. Fujiwara T, Yoshioka S, Yoshioka T, Ushiyama I, Horikoshi H. Characterization of new oral antidiabetic agent CS-045: Studies in KK and ob/ob mice and Zucker fatty rats. *Diabetes* 1988; 37: 1549–1558.

106. Yki-Jarvinen H. Thiazolidinediones. *N Engl J Med* 2004; 351:1106–1118.

107. Ciaraldi TP, Kong AP, Chu NV, Kim DD, Baxi S, Loviscach M, Plodkowski R, Reitz R, Caulfield M, Mudaliar S, Henry RR. Regulation of glucose transport and insulin signaling by troglitazone or metformin in adipose tissue of type 2 diabetic subjects. *Diabetes* 2002; 51:30–36.

108. Jiang G, Dallas-Yang Q, Biswas S, Li Z, Zhang BB. Rosiglitazone, an agonist of peroxisome-proliferator-activated receptor gamma (PPARgamma), decreases inhibitory serine phosphorylation of IRS1 in vitro and in vivo. *Biochem J* 2004; 377:339–346.

109. Okuno A, Tamemoto H, Tobe K, Ueki K, Mori Y, Iwamoto K, Umesono K, Akanuma Y, Fujiwara T, Horikoshi H, Yazaki Y, Kadowaki T. Troglitazone increases the number of small adipocytes without the change of white adipose tissue mass in obese Zucker rats. *J Clin Invest* 1998; 101: 1354–1361.

110. Mohanty P, Aljada A, Ghanim H, Hofmeyer D, Tripathy D, Syed T, Al-Haddad W, Dhindsa S, Dandona P. Evidence for a potent antiinflammatory effect of rosiglitazone. *J Clin Endocrinol Metab* 2004; 89:2728–2735.

111. Katsuki A, Sumida Y, Murata K, Furuta M, Araki-Sasaki R, Tsuchihashi K, Hori Y, Yano Y, Gabazza EC, Adachi Y. Troglitazone reduces plasma levels of tumour necrosis factor-alpha in obese patients with type 2 diabetes. *Diabetes Obes Metab* 2000; 2:189–191.

112. Haffner SM, Greenberg AS, Weston WM, Chen H, Williams K, Freed MI. Effect of rosiglitazone treatment on nontraditional markers of cardiovascular disease in patients with type 2 diabetes mellitus. *Circulation* 2002; 106:679–684.

113. Sigrist S, Bedoucha M, Boelsterli UA. Down-regulation by troglitazone of hepatic tumor necrosis factor-alpha and interleukin-6 mRNA expression in a murine model of non-insulin-dependent diabetes. *Biochem Pharmacol* 2000; 60:67–75.

114. Peraldi P, Xu M, Spiegelman BM. Thiazolidinediones block tumor necrosis factor-alpha-induced inhibition of insulin signaling. *J Clin Invest* 1997; 100:1863–1869.

115. Lagathu C, Bastard JP, Auclair M, Maachi M, Capeau J, Caron M. Chronic interleukin-6 (IL-6) treatment increased IL-6 secretion and induced insulin resistance in adipocyte: Prevention by rosiglitazone. *Biochem Biophys Res Commun* 2003; 311:372–379.

11 Insulin Resistance and Dyslipidemia

Tina J. Chahil, Gissette Reyes, and Henry N. Ginsberg

Contents

INTRODUCTION

During the past two decades, there has been an increasing recognition of the significance of a clustering of cardiovascular disease (CVD) risk factors, leading expert panels to formally link them as the *metabolic syndrome* (1,2). Although there has been controversy regarding the criteria to be used in defining the metabolic syndrome, and the utility of the term itself (3–5), it is clear that the featured components of central obesity, hypertension, dyslipidemia, and abnormal glucose metabolism commonly coexist in individuals at high risk for CVD and type 2 diabetes mellitus (T2DM). It has been widely recognized that insulin resistance (IR) plays a central, unifying role in the pathophysiology of this syndrome. In this chapter, we will focus on the associations between IR and the dyslipidemia characterized by high plasma triglyceride (TG) levels, reduced plasma high-density lipoprotein (HDL) cholesterol concentrations, and abnormalities in low-density lipoprotein (LDL) composition and size in the face of relatively normal plasma LDL cholesterol (LDL-C) levels.

EPIDEMIOLOGY OF DYSLIPIDEMIA AND INSULIN RESISTANCE

It has been clear for many years that individuals with T2DM have increased plasma TG and decreased plasma HDL cholesterol (HDL-C) levels compared with their counterparts without diabetes (6–8). However, it is also well recognized that IR is associated

Supported by NIH grants from NHLBI: R01 HL69190, R01 HL55638, R01 HL73030, T32 HL07343

From: *Contemporary Endocrinology: The Metabolic Syndrome: Epidemiology, Clinical Treatment, and Underlying Mechanisms*
Edited by: B.C. Hansen and G.A. Bray © Humana Press, Totowa, NJ

with increased plasma TG levels and increased rates of very-low-density lipoprotein (VLDL) production, even in the absence of diabetes (9,10). More recently, the role of IR in determining levels of HDL-C and both the size and composition of LDL has also been demonstrated (11). Thus, IR has been associated with the pattern B profile of LDL in which LDL-C cholesterol levels that are normal or slightly elevated are associated with increased numbers of small, dense LDL particles that are depleted of cholesteryl esters (CE) (12). This lipoprotein pattern was first called *hyperapobetalipoproteinemia*, a disorder noted to be present in many individuals with premature coronary heart disease (CHD) (13).

As noted above, much of the literature to date has examined dyslipidemia seen in the setting of T2DM (8,10). However, the Insulin Resistance Atherosclerosis Study demonstrated the progressive changes in lipoprotein composition among study subjects with normal glucose tolerance, impaired glucose tolerance, and T2DM. In that study, worsening glucose tolerance was correlated with a progressively more unfavorable lipoprotein profile, both in terms of concentrations and compositional abnormalities (14,15). Furthermore, the relationship between insulin-mediated glucose disposal and dyslipidemia was consistent and did not differ by gender or ethnicity (16). Interestingly, an analysis of those study subjects who did not have diabetes at baseline demonstrated more unfavorable baseline metabolic characteristics among those individuals who eventually developed T2DM ("converters") compared to those who remained diabetes-free at follow-up ("nonconverters") over a mean period of 5.2 years (17). Thus, converters to T2DM had higher baseline levels of fasting insulin and glucose and decreased insulin sensitivity compared to their counterparts who did not develop diabetes. Additionally, converters were noted to have worse lipoprotein concentrations and compositional changes at baseline compared to nonconverters. Chief among these differences were higher baseline TG and lower baseline HDL-C concentrations as well as larger VLDL particle size and higher concentrations of small HDL particles seen among converters. As expected, LDL-C concentrations at baseline were similar between both groups; in fact, they were similar to those of individuals with preexisting diabetes at baseline. These results support previous findings of an increased prevalence of risk factors for CVD in individuals with *pre-diabetes* (18).

In addition to derangements in fasting plasma lipoprotein levels and composition, postprandial lipoprotein abnormalities have been closely linked to IR. Postprandial dyslipidemia is primarily characterized by an increase in chylomicrons and their remnant particles, although VLDL can also accumulate. There is a strong correlation between fasting and postprandial TG levels, but increased postprandial lipemia has been shown to occur even in the setting of normal fasting TG levels and satisfactory glycemic control among individuals with T2DM (19,20). The importance of abnormalities in postprandial lipid metabolism is underscored by their association with the presence of atherosclerotic CVD (19,21,22).

NORMAL LIPID AND LIPOPROTEIN PHYSIOLOGY

The association of IR with dyslipidemia is multifactorial and complex, but a better understanding of the lipid abnormalities present in individuals with IR can be gained through an understanding of normal lipoprotein physiology. Lipoproteins are macromolecular complexes composed of varying amounts of lipids and proteins. The hydrophobic lipid core consists of TG and CE. This is surrounded by an amphipathic monolayer of phospholipids, free cholesterol, and surface proteins called *apolipoproteins*. Lipoproteins can be classified according to their physical characteristics and lipid composition. Additionally, their surface proteins play critical roles in metabolic regulation (23–25). Two key apolipoproteins are apolipoprotein B (apo B) and apolipoprotein A-I (apo A-I). Apo B is synthesized in two forms: a full-length form, apo B-100, which is made in the liver, and a truncated form resulting from messenger RNA (mRNA) editing, apo B-48, which is produced in the small intestine. Apo B-100 is the necessary component of VLDL, intermediate density lipoproteins (IDL), and LDL, while apo B-48 is necessary for the assembly and secretion of chylomicrons. Apo A-I, made in the liver and small intestine, is the critical structural protein for HDL. As described below, physiological interactions between the apo B-lipoprotein family and the apo A-I-lipoprotein family are central to the generation of the dyslipidemia present in individuals with IR and T2DM.

Each of the apolipoprotein-specific families must be viewed in the context of the fasted and postprandial states. Indeed, we can consider lipoprotein metabolism as occurring in two parallel but interconnected physiological pathways: fasting lipoprotein metabolism and postprandial lipoprotein metabolism. In the fasting state, apo B-100-containing lipoproteins, primarily VLDL, are assembled and secreted by the liver. The assembly of VLDL is determined in large part by the availability of its major lipid components, TG, cholesterol, and phospholipids, the presence of microsomal triglyceride transfer protein (MPT) activity, and hormonal influences, particularly insulin (26). Of importance is the relatively stable expression of the apo B gene; although there are some situations in which the levels of apo B mRNA are altered, the majority of the regulation of apo B-lipoprotein assembly and secretion occurs co- and posttranslationally (26,27). Cotranslational degradation of apo B occurs via the proteasome, after ubiquitinylation of the nascent protein. Posttranslational degradation can occur either in the endoplasmic reticulum (ER) or post-ER. The latter includes degradation in lysosomes, possibly after reuptake of nascent VLDL from the cell surface or by recognition of a defective lipoprotein in the Golgi apparatus (28). Insulin can target apo B for post-ER degradation (28,29). Insulin-mediated targeting of apo B for degradation appears to require the involvement of the phosphoinositide 3-kinase pathway.

Hepatic TG appears to be particularly important as a signal for the targeting of apo B for VLDL assembly and secretion, and there are three main sources of hepatic TG: hepatic uptake of plasma albumin-bound fatty acids (FA), hepatic uptake of TG-FA in remnant lipoproteins, and hepatic de novo synthesis of FA (lipogenesis) (Fig. 11.1). Abnormalities in insulin sensitivity can affect each of these processes to ultimately create the dyslipidemia associated with IR (see below) (11,25).

In addition to the requisite apo B-100, VLDL may be secreted with other apolipoproteins, including alpolipoproteins E, C-I, C-II, and C-III (apo E, apo C-I, apo C-II, and apo C-III). VLDL can also acquire these proteins in the circulation, along with alpolipoprotein A-V (apo A-V). Circulating VLDL normally interacts with lipoprotein lipase (LpL). LpL is synthesized in adipose tissue and muscle (30), secreted by those tissues, and stabilized on the surface of capillary endothelial cells through its binding to heparan sulfate proteoglycans. Endothelial cell surface-bound LpL interacts with circulating lipoprotein particles to initiate lipolysis of lipoprotein TG. The interaction of LpL and VLDL is facilitated by VLDL apo E, which also binds to cell surface pro-

Substrate Driving Forces for the Assembly and Secretion of Apo B-Lipoproteins

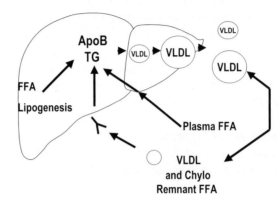

Figure 11.1. VLDL secretion is dependent on hepatic lipid availability, with TG being the major lipid component secreted with apo B in VLDL. There are three sources of hepatic TG. The most important is plasma albumin–bound FA derived from lipolysis of adipose tissue TG (and to a much lesser extent, LpL-mediated lipolysis of plasma VLDL and chylomicron TG). In IR and T2DM, lipolysis of TG in adipocytes can be increased, with increased FA flux to the liver. Plasma remnant lipoprotein TG-FA, remaining after LpL-mediated lipolysis of VLDL and chylomicron TG in adipose tissue and muscle, is a second source of hepatic TG. In IR, LpL-mediated lipolysis may be modestly reduced, leading to hepatic uptake of remnants carrying more TG than normal. The third source of hepatic TG is from de novo lipogenesis of FA from glucose in the liver. This is usually a small source of hepatic TG, but can become more significant in IR and T2DM.

teoglycans, and by apo C-II, an activator of LpL. Apo C-III, also found on the surface of VLDL particles, inhibits LpL activity (31,32); the balance between apo C-II and apo C-III determines in part the efficiency with which lipolysis occurs. The recent discovery of apo A-V (33) has revealed another player in VLDL catabolism; this protein appears to be involved in LpL-mediated lipolysis of VLDL TG (34,35). Insulin is a major regulator of LpL synthesis and activity and, under normal circumstances, stimulates the synthesis and secretion of LpL (36).

Lipolysis of VLDL TG results in remnant particles, some of which are in the denser range of VLDL and others that are IDL. Both VLDL remnants and IDL can be removed by the liver via apo B-100 or apo E binding to the hepatic LDL receptor. There are three isoforms of apo E: apo E2, apo E3, and apo E4, which differ in their affinity for the LDL receptor; apo E2 is defective as a ligand, and if only apo E2 is present, remnant uptake will be impaired. All of the apo E isoforms can bind to the LDL receptor–related protein (LRP) (37), although remnant removal via this pathway appears to play a minor role in most instances. Hepatocyte cell surface proteoglycans can facilitate the uptake of remnants by both the LDL and LRP receptors. Despite their different roles in lipolysis, all of the apo C apolipoproteins can inhibit remnant uptake by the liver (32,38), probably by interfering with interactions between remnant lipoproteins and hepatocyte cell surface proteoglycans. Hepatic lipase (HL), secreted from hepatocytes, also plays a role in remnant uptake through both lipolytic and lipoprotein-binding pathways. Between 25 and 75% of VLDL remnants and IDL are not removed by the liver but are converted to LDL. Larger, more TG-enriched remnant lipoproteins containing more apo

E may be better substrates for removal, while smaller remnant lipoproteins are further lipolyzed in the hepatic circulation, yielding LDL. Clearance of LDL is primarily via LDL receptor–mediated pathways; about one-half of LDL uptake is by the liver. LDL size and composition can be modified in plasma by interactions with VLDL (and chylomicrons; see below) via the action of cholesteryl ester transfer protein (CETP) (39).

HDL are perhaps the most heterogeneous lipoprotein class; depending on the methods used, more than ten lipoprotein classes, differing by size, charge, and lipid and apolipoprotein composition, have been identified. Much of this heterogeneity derives from the participation of HDL in the reverse cholesterol transport system. In the fasting state, cells in the liver and small intestine synthesize and secrete precursor forms of HDL called pre-α and pre-β HDL, which very likely represent newly secreted phospholipid discs with apo A-I on the surface. The ATP-binding cassette transporter A1 (ABCA1) is a cellular transport protein that plays a critical role in transferring intracellular or plasma membrane–associated cholesterol to these nascent lipid-poor forms of HDL (40). Transfer (possibly co-secretory) of cholesterol from hepatocytes and intestinal mucosal cells to newly secreted apo A-I/phospholipid discs stabilizes the apo A-I and prolongs its lifespan in the circulation. This allows repetitive cycles of ABCA1-mediated cholesterol efflux to occur not only from the liver and intestine, but also from tissues throughout the body, including macrophages containing CE derived from apo B-lipoproteins. Repeated transfer of cholesterol to the surface of the apo A-I/phospholipid disc is coupled with cholesterol esterification by the enzyme, lecithin cholesterol acyl transferase (LCAT), which is activated by apo A-I. Esterification allows newly generated CE to move from the surface to the core of what then becomes a spherical HDL$_3$ particle. Further accumulation of CE in the core of HDL$_3$ leads to the generation of HDL$_2$, which in turn can take on additional cholesterol through interactions with the scavenger receptor class B, type 1 (SRB1) and a second ATP-binding cassette transporter: ABCG1 (41). The mature CE-rich HDL$_2$ particles are capable of delivering their free and esterified cholesterol to the liver through additional interactions with hepatic SRB1. Of note, apo A-I can return to the circulation after interacting with SRB1 and as a "reincarnated" nascent HDL can take part in another cycle of reverse cholesterol transport. HDL$_2$ particles can also participate in the CETP-mediated exchange of their CE for TG in VLDL and VLDL remnants. The impact of the CETP-mediated exchange of core lipids between HDL and both VLDL and their remnants was clarified after the discovery of individuals lacking CETP who had extraordinarily high plasma HDL-C and apo A-I levels in plasma (39). The role of CETP in the dyslipidemia of IR will be discussed further below.

Postprandial lipoprotein metabolism, which is characterized by dramatic increases in chylomicrons and chylomicron remnants in plasma, also has significant effects on the composition and metabolism of all the circulating lipoproteins, including VLDL, LDL, and HDL. After ingestion of a meal, nutrients are digested and eventually absorbed in the small intestine. The enterocytes subsequently assemble and secrete chylomicrons, lipoproteins that are uniquely characterized by the presence of apo B-48 (42). In addition to apo B-48, the chylomicron surface is characterized by the presence of apo A-I, apo A-II, and apo A-IV. Composed primarily of TG derived from dietary fat, these lipoproteins also function in the transport of cholesterol and fat-soluble nutrients. Upon entry into the lymphatic system and, eventually, the circulation, chylomicrons acquire apo C-I, apo C-II, apo C-III, apo A-V, and apo E. As they circulate through the microvasculature, chylomicrons are lipolyzed by LpL in a process analogous to the lipolysis of circulating VLDL particles in the fasting state. As noted above, apo C-II, apo C-III, and apo A-V play key roles in LpL-mediated lipolysis. The products of this catabolism are chylomicron remnants, which are eventually removed by the liver via several pathways that are also involved in VLDL remnant removal by the liver (see above) (37). Of note, while VLDL removal from the liver can vary widely, with some to most of the VLDL converted to LDL, essentially all of the chylomicron remnants are removed by the liver under normal conditions.

Circulating LDL and HDL are also typically altered after a meal, mainly through interactions with chylomicrons and CETP (39). Thus, circulating chylomicrons interact with LDL and HDL in the presence of CETP, and there is an exchange of TG (from the chylomicrons) and CE (from LDL and HDL), leading to a transient reductions in both LDL and HDL cholesterol levels during the postprandial period. The TG-enriched LDL and HDL are substrates for LpL and HL, which remove the TG and shrink the lipoproteins. The degree to which LDL and HDL cholesterol levels fall during the postprandial period will be determined by the duration and extent of the hypertriglyceridemia.

ABNORMALITIES OF LIPID AND LIPOPROTEIN METABOLISM IN INSULIN RESISTANCE

Overproduction of VLDL

As noted earlier, there are three major sources of hepatic TG that can stimulate VLDL assembly and secretion (Fig. 11.1). Uptake of plasma albumin–bound FA is one source, and this pathway is typically increased in individuals with IR. This process begins at the level of the adipocyte, which can liberate FA through lipolysis of its stored TG. Adipose TG lipase (ATGL), a recently discovered lipase, is thought to initiate lipolysis in the adipocyte by hydrolyzing adipose TG to diacylglycerol (DAG) and FA. This provides substrate for hormone-sensitive lipase (HSL), which functions primarily to catalyze the conversion of DAG to monoglyceride (MG) and FA. The final step in this process involves the conversion of MG to glycerol and FA by monoglyceride lipase (MGL). While the effects of insulin on ATGL remain to be elucidated, insulin is known to inhibit HSL-mediated lipolysis through inhibition of phosphorylation of HSL, thereby inactivating it. However, with IR, there is ineffective inhibition of HSL in the adipocyte, leading to intracellular lipolysis of stored TG and increased release of FA (43,44). Increased delivery of plasma FA to the liver stimulates the assembly and secretion of VLDL (11,45,46). The exact mechanism whereby plasma FAs target nascent apo B away from degradation and toward lipoprotein assembly and secretion is not fully defined (26), and may be dependent on FA acting both as a substrate for TG synthesis and as a signaling molecule (47).

VLDL and chylomicron remnants are a second source of substrate for VLDL assembly and secretion. Remnant lipoprotein removal by the liver under normal conditions has been described earlier (37), and the delivery of remnant TG-FA to the liver can stimulate the assembly and secretion of VLDL (47). In the setting of IR or T2DM, even mild reductions of LpL-mediated lipolysis of VLDL or chylomicrons can result in TG-enriched remnant lipoprotein particles (see below). Hepatic uptake of these TG-rich VLDL and chylomicron remnants results in increased availability of FA substrate, which can stimulate VLDL assembly and secretion. This is, in a sense, an energy-dissipating cycle for energy transfer between the liver and the plasma and back again to the liver.

The third major source of hepatic TG for VLDL secretion is de novo lipogenesis. Normally, insulin stimulates lipogenesis through its activation of the transcription factor, liver X receptor (LXR). LXR binds to the promoter of sterol response element-binding protein isoform 1c (SREBP-1c), the major lipogenic transcription factor, and increases SREBP-1c mRNA levels. LXR also has direct effects on the expression of fatty acid synthase (FAS), a key lipogenic enzyme, and on the transcription factor, carbohydrate-responsive element binding protein (ChREBP). Both SREBP-1c and ChREBP are activated posttranscriptionally, in processes that include translocation from cytosolic sites to the nucleus (48,49). Importantly, insulin can stimulate hepatic de novo FA synthesis even when there is resistance to insulin's actions on carbohydrate metabolism (50). In addition to the regulation of lipogenesis by SREBP-1c and ChREBP, recent studies by several other groups indicate that peroxisome proliferator–activated receptor gamma (PPARγ) can also regulate lipogenesis: Increased expression of PPARγ2 in livers of several mouse models of IR, fatty liver, and dyslipidemia have been linked to increased lipogenesis (5,52). We have unpublished data supporting the importance of PPARγ2 in lipogenesis.

As noted earlier in the discussion of normal lipoprotein metabolism, insulin is another key modifier of the link between substrate availability and VLDL secretion, because it can target apo B for post-ER degradation (28,29). In individuals or animals with IR, plasma insulin levels are commonly elevated, and this would seemingly predict increased apo B degradation and, therefore, decreased VLDL secretion. On the other hand, if the liver is significantly resistant to the action of insulin, even hyperinsulinemia might not be adequate to target apo B for degradation and increased VLDL secretion might result. It may be that the development of fatty liver is determined in part by the relative degrees of hepatic IR and hyperinsulinemia.

Defective VLDL, Remnant, and LDL Catabolism

Although overproduction of VLDL, both in terms of the number of apo B-lipoproteins secreted and the quantity of TG carried on those particles, is characteristic of IR and T2DM, the efficiency with which VLDL TG is cleared by tissues will certainly play a role in determining the plasma concentration of TG. VLDL catabolism is influenced by LpL, apo C-III, and possibly apo A-V. Apo C-II, the required cofactor for LpL activity, does not seem to be rate limiting for lipolysis unless completely absent, and is not altered in IR. However, modest reductions in LpL in individuals with IR (36), coupled with increased production of apo C-III (53), will reduce the efficiency of lipolysis, particularly when there is increased VLDL secretion into plasma. Recent studies have advanced our understanding of the dysregulation of apo C-III metabolism in IR. Thus, experiments in cell culture systems and in rodents suggest that apo C-III gene expression is regulated by insulin, possibly via actions of the forkhead transcription factor, O1 (Foxo1) (54), with increased apo C-III production in insulin-deficient or -resistant states. As noted above, suboptimal lipolysis of VLDL in IR and T2DM will result in TG-enriched VLDL remnants returning to the liver where they will provide substrate for enhanced VLDL secretion. Whether apo A-V regulation is altered in IR and T2DM (55) remains to be determined.

Because apo C-III can also inhibit hepatic removal of VLDL and remnants, increased apo C-III production could have a negative impact on remnant clearance (53). The apo E isoform pattern of any individual with diabetes can impact on VLDL remnant removal; however, there are no studies implicating specific defects in apo E metabolism in IR. LDL receptors themselves are highly regulated at the gene-expression level, in part by insulin. Studies of humans suggest that severe diabetes, with significant relative or absolute insulin deficiency, is accompanied by decreased clearance of LDL; whether this extends to VLDL remnant clearance is unknown. Additionally, the synthesis and maturation of cell-surface proteoglycans, carbohydrate-rich proteins that allow remnants to associate with hepatocyte plasma membranes, may be defective when insulin action is significantly reduced (56); that could impair remnant removal. Deficiency of HL could also lead to reduced remnant clearance. However, HL is elevated in individuals with IR with or without diabetes. Defects in any of these pathways would contribute to the elevated plasma TG levels seen in individuals with IR and T2DM.

Generation of Small, Dense LDL

In people with IR and T2DM, regulation of plasma levels of LDL, like that of the precursor, VLDL, is complex (57). As noted earlier, the pattern B profile of LDL, which features small, dense, CE-depleted, TG-enriched LDL, is a common characteristic of the dyslipidemia of IR (12). Although CETP clearly plays a key role in the generation of small dense LDL (Fig. 11.2), the finding that small, dense LDL particles are present in individuals with IR or T2DM even when they have relatively normal TG levels suggests that other factors are involved. One such factor is HL, which, as noted earlier, is

VLDL and LDL Metabolism in Insulin Resistance and T2DM

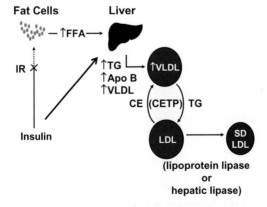

Figure 11.2. Increased VLDL secretion and hypertriglyceridemia lead to the generation of smaller, denser, cholesteryl ester depleted LDL. Generation of small, dense LDL results from the CETP-mediated exchange of LDL CEs for TG from VLDL, followed by lipolysis (mediated by either LpL or HL). The same sequence of events can occur during the postprandial period, particularly when postprandial levels of chylomicron TG remain high for prolonged periods of time. Increased HL, which is common in IR, can exacerbate the effects of CETP-mediated transfer of core lipids between VLDL (or chylomicrons) and LDL.

VLDL and HDL Metabolism in Insulin Resistance and T2DM

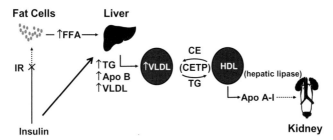

Figure 11.3. Increased VLDL secretion and hypertriglyceridemia can also lead to reduced levels of HDL. This is mainly the result of CETP-mediated core lipid exchange between VLDL and HDL, followed by HL-mediated lipolysis of HDL TG. In addition, when the HDL become smaller and lipid-poor, apo A-I dissociates more readily and, as a small protein, can be cleared rapidly from the circulation by a number of organs, including the kidneys. The same series of reactions can occur with prolonged postprandial elevations of chylomicron TG. The result is that in IR and T2DM, reverse cholesterol transport is disrupted in two ways: HDL CEs are transferred to apo B-lipoproteins, and there are fewer apo A-I lipoproteins. Other effects of IR on HDL metabolism must be invoked to explain low HDL even when TG levels are relatively normal.

increased in IR and can therefore more effectively hydrolyze TG in LDL. Another factor is the plasma FA concentration, which is elevated in individuals with the dyslipidemia of IR. Increased levels of plasma FA can stimulate exchange of CE and TG between LDL (or HDL; see below) and VLDL, even when plasma TG is "normal." A third factor is the postprandial lipemia commonly present in IR: Even when fasting TG levels are normal, elevated postprandial levels of chylomicrons can, via CETP-mediated exchange of core lipids, stimulate the production of small, dense LDL. Finally, individuals with IR secrete larger, more buoyant TG-enriched VLDL, and studies suggest that because of a higher TG content, these VLDL particles are more likely to become triglyceride-enriched LDL, which will then generate small, dense LDL (25). Whether smaller, CE-depleted LDL particles are more atherogenic than other apo B-lipoproteins is still debated. However, it is important to note that for any plasma LDL-C concentration, the presence of small, dense LDL reflects a greater number of LDL particles, and it is ultimately the number of apo B-lipoprotein particles that is critical in terms of atherogenic risk.

Increased Catabolism of HDL

The complexity of HDL, in terms of both composition and metabolism, is striking. It is clear, however, that low HDL-C levels are a very common characteristic of the dyslipidemia of IR and T2DM. In fact, it may be the most common finding; HDL-C and apo A-I levels in plasma can be low even when plasma TG levels are normal.

Why are HDL-C and apo A-I levels reduced in individuals with IR and T2DM? As was the case for LDL, the answer lies mainly, but not completely, with CETP (Fig. 11.3). As described earlier in this chapter, the reverse cholesterol transport system moves cholesterol from tissues to nascent, cholesterol-poor apo A-I/phospholipid discs, where the cholesterol is esterified. Progressive accumulation of CE leads to the maturation of the HDL into a spherical lipoprotein that delivers the CE and some of the unesterified cholesterol to the liver. Alternatively, HDL_2 particles can participate in the CETP-mediated exchange of their CE for TG in VLDL, VLDL remnants, and chylomicron remnants (58). The impact of this exchange on reverse cholesterol transport is unclear: If the TG-rich lipoproteins that receive the CE from HDL are removed by the liver, there may be no effect on reverse cholesterol transport, assuming that delivery of CE via uptake of apo B-lipoproteins results in delivery of the lipid to the biliary tract with the same efficiency as does delivery via SRB1. Unfortunately, increased CETP-mediated exchange of HDL CE for TGs is associated with lipolysis of HDL TG by HL, and this produces a small, lipid-depleted HDL that resembles nascent particles. Apo A-I binding to this HDL particle is diminished, causing apo A-I to dissociate from the particle and be cleared more rapidly from the plasma (59). Thus, fractional catabolism of apo A-I is increased in patients with T2DM, reducing the number of HDL particles in the circulation. Additionally, if the CE-enriched apo B-lipoproteins are not removed by the liver, but rather find their way into the artery wall, then reverse cholesterol transport will have been "short-circuited" and atherogenesis may be accelerated.

There are other metabolic pathways that can also generate low HDL in IR and T2DM. IR is associated with increased HL activity, which can increase hydrolysis of HDL TG and generate smaller HDL. The potential roles of defective ABCA1-mediated efflux of cellular free cholesterol, defective LCAT activity, or increased selective delivery of HDL CE to hepatocytes as causes of the low HDL levels present in IR are under investigation. However, the observation that low HDL-C and apo A-I are frequently present even when TG levels are relatively normal suggests that non-CETP mechanisms are clearly important in the pathogenesis of low HDL-C concentrations in IR.

Postprandial Hyperlipidemia

As described above, the postprandial period is characterized by the absorption of dietary TG and cholesterol, the assembly and secretion of chylomicrons, the delivery of TG to adipose and muscle tissue, and the delivery of cholesterol to the liver. Importantly, IR plays a major role in the regulation of postprandial chylomicron metabolism (e.g., increased postprandial levels of TG-rich lipoproteins, both chylomicrons and VLDL, are commonly observed in individuals with IR or T2DM). (19). In a study of normal individuals, insulin-mediated glucose disposal was an independent predictor of postprandial TG excursion (60). Furthermore, in a large population-based cohort study, the best predictor of postprandial TG levels was fasting TG, and the latter was related to obesity, diabetes, and markers of IR (59). Studies have also demonstrated correlations between visceral fat and postprandial lipemia; whether this is a mechanism-based association or simply visceral fat acting as a marker of IR is not clear (60). However, although several groups have demonstrated an association between postprandial hyperlipidemia and the presence of CHD in individuals without diabetes (19), this association has not been demonstrated in patients with T2DM. The lack of an association between CHD and postprandial lipemia in patients with T2DM may derive from the fact that all individuals with IR have postprandial hyperlipidemia.

A complete characterization of the effects of IR and T2DM on postprandial lipemia has not been reported. Although studies of normal intracellular assembly of chylomicrons have found many similarities to the assembly of VLDL (see above), including the potential targeting of nascent apo B-48 for degradation (42), few studies have examined the effect of IR on chylomicron formation. Recent studies, however, suggest that IR may lead to increased chylomicron formation in the enterocyte (61,62) and further work is needed in this area. By contrast, much work has been done on the effect of IR on the blood levels and clearance of lipids and lipoproteins during the postprandial period. As described earlier, LpL activity is diminished in the setting of IR, resulting in reduced rates of lipolysis of both chylomicron and VLDL TG. In addition, modest reductions in post-heparin LpL levels have been associated with T2DM. Correspondingly, reduced partitioning of TG-FA from chylomicron TG to adipose tissue is seen in the fed state, resulting in TG-enriched remnant lipoproteins (43).

All of the apolipoproteins that play roles in VLDL TG catabolism are active in the postprandial removal of chylomicron TG, and the same potential impacts of IR on their functions (see above) are relevant to postprandial lipemia. This is particularly true for apo C-III. Importantly, increased secretion of VLDL in states of IR leads to increased levels of VLDL TGs that compete with chylomicrons for LpL-mediated lipolysis, irrespective of the level of LpL activity (63).

Chylomicron remnants are removed from the circulation by the liver via the same pathways as are VLDL remnants. There are two important differences: First, chylomicrons carry apo B-48, which lacks the LDL receptor-binding domain of apo B-100. As a result, chylomicrons utilize apo E as the ligand for the LDL receptor. Second, essentially all chylomicron remnants are removed by the liver compared with removal of 25–75% of VLDL remnants. However, all of the defects present in IR can affect chylomicron remnant removal in a manner similar to their effects on VLDL remnant catabolism.

The impact of postprandial lipemia on the composition and metabolism of LDL and HDL in the insulin-resistant state has been described earlier in conjunction with the description of VLDL metabolism. Thus, CETP-mediated exchange of core lipids between chylomicrons or their remnant particles and either LDL or HDL will result in CE depletion of the latter two lipoproteins; TG-enriched LDL and HDL will, after lipolytic remodeling, become small, dense LDL and HDL, respectively. The generation of small HDL will in turn accelerate the catabolism of apo A-I, thus impeding the process of reverse cholesterol transport.

SUMMARY

States of IR, with or without T2DM, are characterized by multiple abnormalities in the levels, composition, and metabolism of the apo B-containing and apo A-I-containing lipoprotein families. The characteristic fasting dyslipidemia of hypertriglyceridemia, decreased HDL-C levels, and small, dense LDL particles can be considered a "group defect" largely resulting from increased hepatic secretion of TG-rich VLDL coupled with CETP-mediated exchange of core lipids between lipoprotein particles. However, it is also clear that inefficient peripheral tissue lipolysis is a key contributor to elevated plasma TG levels and that other, less well-characterized abnormalities associated with IR play important roles in regulating LDL and HDL composition and concentration.

The metabolic derangements apparent in the fasting state also characterize the postprandial period, when, in fact, they may be magnified. Indeed, the dysregulation of postprandial lipid metabolism parallels and is, for the most part, an exaggeration of the defects present during the fasting state. Improvements in insulin sensitivity, particularly by improving the body's energy balance, will reverse many of the lipid and lipoprotein abnormalities present in the dyslipidemia.

REFERENCES

1. Alberti KGMM, Zimmet PZ. Definition, diagnosis and classification of diabetes mellitus and its complications. Part 1: Diagnosis and classification of diabetes mellitus. Provisional Report of a WHO Consultation. *Diab Med* 1998; 15:539–553.
2. Executive summary of the third report of the National Cholesterol Education Program (NCEP) expert panel on detection, evaluation, and treatment of high blood cholesterol in adults (adult treatment panel III). *JAMA* 2001; 285(19):2486–2497.
3. Eckel RH, Grundy SM, Zimmet PZ. The metabolic syndrome. *Lancet* 2005; 365:1415–1428.
4. Kahn R, Buse J, Ferrannini E, Stern M, American Diabetes Association, European Association for the Study of Diabetes. The metabolic syndrome: time for a critical appraisal: Joint statement from the American Diabetes Association and the European Association for the Study of Diabetes. *Diabetes Care* 2005; 28:2289–2304.
5. Alberti KG, Zimmet P, Shaw J, IDF Epidemiology Task Force Consensus Group. The metabolic syndrome: A new worldwide definition. *Lancet* 2005; 366:1059–1062.
6. Albrink MJ, Man EB. Serum triglycerides in health and diabetes. *Diabetes* 1958; 7:194–201.
7. Lopes-Virella MF, Stone PG, Colwell JA. Serum high density lipoprotein in diabetic patients. *Diabetologia* 1977; 13:285–291.
8. Ginsberg HN. Lipoprotein physiology in nondiabetic and diabetes states. *Diabetes Care* 1991; 14:839–855.
9. Reaven GM, Lerner RL, Stern MP, Farquhar JW. Role of insulin in endogenous hypertriglyceridemia. *J Clin Invest* 1967; 46:1756–1767.
10. Reaven GM, Chen Y-D. Role of insulin in regulation of lipoprotein metabolism in diabetes. *Diabetes Metab Rev* 1988; 4:639–652.
11. Ginsberg HN, Zhang YL, Hernandez-Ono A. Regulation of plasma triglycerides in insulin resistance and diabetes. *Arch Med Res* 2005; 36:232–240.
12. Austin MA, King MD, Vranizan KM, Krauss RM. Atherogenic lipoprotein phenotype: A proposed genetic marker for coronary heart disease risk. *Circulation* 1990; 82:495–506.
13. Sniderman AD, Wolfson C, Teng B, Franklin FA, Bachorik PS, Kwiterowovich PO. Association of hyperapobetalipoproteinemia with endogenous hypertriglyceridemia and atherosclerosis. *Ann Int Med* 1982; 97:833–839.
14. Goff DC Jr, D'Agostino RB Jr, Haffner SM, Saad MF, Wagenknecht LE. Lipoprotein concentrations and carotid atherosclerosis by diabetes status: Results from the Insulin Resistance Atherosclerosis Study. *Diabetes Care* 2000; 23:1006–1011.
15. Goff DC Jr, D'Agostino RB Jr, Haffner SM, Otvos JD. Insulin resistance and adiposity influence lipoprotein size and subclass concentrations: Results from the Insulin Resistance Atherosclerosis Study. *Metabolism* 2005; 54:264–270.
16. Howard BV, Mayer-Davis EJ, Goff D et al. Relationships between insulin resistance and lipoproteins in nondiabetic African Americans, Hispanics, and non-Hispanic whites: The Insulin Resistance Atherosclerosis Study. *Metabolism* 1998; 47:1174–1179.
17. Festa A, Williams K, Hanley AJ et al. Nuclear magnetic resonance lipoprotein abnormalities in prediabetic subjects in the Insulin Resistance Atherosclerosis Study. *Circulation* 2005; 111:3465–3472.
18. Haffner SM, Stern MP, Hazuda HP, Mitchell BD, Patterson JK. Cardiovascular risk factors in confirmed prediabetic individuals: Does the clock for coronary heart disease start ticking before the onset of clinical diabetes? *JAMA* 1990; 263:2893–2898.
19. Ginsberg HN, Illingworth DR. Postprandial dyslipidemia: An atherogenic disorder common in patients with diabetes. *Am J Cardiol* 2001; 88:9H–15H.

20. Annuzzi G, De Natale C, Iovine C et al. Insulin resistance is independently associated with postprandial alterations of triglyceride-rich lipoproteins in type 2 diabetes mellitus. *Arterio Thromb Vasc Biol* 2004; 24:2397.

21. Ginsberg HN. Association of postprandial triglyceride and Retinyl Palmitate responses with newly diagnosed exercise-induced myocardial ischemia in middle aged men and women. *Arterio Thromb Vasc Biol* 1995; 15:1829–1838.

22. Sharret AR, Chambless LE, Heiss G, Paton CC, Patsch W. Association of postprandial triglyceride and retinyl palmitate responses with asymptomatic carotid artery atherosclerosis in middle-aged men and women. *Arterio Thromb Vasc Biol* 1995; 15:2122–2129.

23. Ginsberg HN. New perspectives on atherogenesis: Role of abnormal triglyceride rich lipoprotein metabolism. *Circulation* 2002; 106:2137–2142.

24. Ginsberg HN. Hypertriglyceridemia: New insights and new approaches to pharmacologic therapy. *Am J Cardiol* 2001; 87:1174–1180.

25. Krauss RM, Siri PW. Metabolic abnormalities: Triglyceride and low-density lipoprotein. *Endocrinol Metab Clinic NA* 2004; 33:405–415.

26. Fisher EA, Ginsberg HN. Complexity in the secretory pathway: The assembly and secretion of apolipoprotein B-containing lipoproteins. *J Biol Chem* 2002; 277:17377–17380.

27. Yao Z, Tran K, McLeod RS. Intracellular degradation of newly synthesized apolipoprotein B. *J Lipid Res* 1997; 38(10):1937–1953.

28. Fisher EA, Pan M, Chen X et al. The triple threat to nascent apolipoprotein B: Evidence for multiple, distinct degradative pathways. *J Biol Chem* 2001; 276:27855–27863.

29. Sparks JD, Sparks CE. Insulin regulation of triacylglycerol-rich lipoprotein synthesis and secretion. *Biochim Biophys Acta* 1994; 1215:9–32.

30. Otarod JK, Goldberg IJ. Lipoprotein lipase and its role in regulation of plasma lipoproteins and cardiac risk. *Curr Atheroscler Rep* 2004; 6:335–342.

31. Ginsberg HN, Le N-A, Goldberg IJ et al. Apolipoprotein B metabolism in subjects with deficiency of apolipoprotein C-III and A-I: Evidence that apolipoprotein C-III inhibits lipoprotein lipase in vivo. *J Clin Invest* 1986; 78:1287–1295.

32. Shachter NS. Apolipoproteins C-I and C-III as important modulators of lipoprotein metabolism. *Curr Opin Lipidol* 2001; 12:297–304.

33. Pennacchio LA, Olivier M, Hubacek JA et al. An apolipoprotein influencing triglycerides in humans and mice revealed by comparative sequencing. *Science* 2001; 294:169–172.

34. van Dijk KW, Rensen PC, Voshol PJ, Havekes LM. The role and mode of action of apolipoproteins CIII and AV: Synergistic actors in triglyceride metabolism? *Curr Opin Lipidol* 2004; 15:239–246.

35. Merkel M, Loeffler B, Kluger M et al. Apolipoprotein AV accelerates plasma hydrolysis of triglyceride-rich lipoproteins by interaction with proteoglycan-bound lipoprotein lipase. *J Biol Chem* 2005; 280:21553–21560.

36. Goldberg IJ. Lipoprotein lipase and lipolysis: Central roles in lipoprotein metabolism and atherosclerosis. *J Lipid Res* 1996; 37:693–707.

37. Cooper AD. Hepatic uptake of chylomicron remnants. *J Lipid Res* 1997; 38(11):2173–2192.

38. Windler E, Chao Y, Havel RJ. Determinants of hepatic uptake of triglyceride-rich lipoproteins and their remnants in the rat. *J Biol Chem* 1980; 255:5475–5480.

39. Bruce C, Chouinard RA Jr, Tall AR. Plasma lipid transfer proteins, high-density lipoproteins, and reverse cholesterol transport. *Annu Rev Nutr* 1998; 18:297–330.

40. Oram JF, Heinecke JW. ATP-binding cassette transporter A1: A cell cholesterol exporter that protects against cardiovascular disease. *Physiol Rev* 2005; 85:1343–1372.

41. Wang N, Lan D, Chen W, Matsuura F, Tall AR. ATP-binding cassette transporters G1 and G4 mediate cellular cholesterol efflux to high-density lipoproteins. *Proc Natl Acad Sci USA* 2004; 101:9774–9779.

42. Hussain MM, Kedees MH, Singh K, Athar H, Jamali NZ. Signposts in the assembly of chylomicrons. *Frontiers Biosci* 2001; 6:d320–d331.

43. Yu Y, Ginsberg HN. Adipocyte signaling and lipid homeostasis: Sequelae of insulin-resistant adipose tissue. *Circ Res* 2005; 96:1042–1052.

44. Zechner R, Strauss JG, Haemmerle G, Lass A, Zimmermann R. Lipolysis: Pathway under construction. *Curr Op Lipidol* 2005; 16:333–340.

45. Kissebah AH, Alfarsi S, Adams PW, Seed M, Folkard J, Wynn V. Transport kinetics of plasma free fatty acid, very low density lipoprotein triglycerides and apoprotein in patients with endogenous hypertriglycerideaemia. *Atherosclerosis* 1976; 24:199–218.

46. Ginsberg HN. Very low density lipoprotein metabolism in diabetes mellitus. *Diab/Metab Rev* 1987; 3:571–589.
47. Zhang Y-L, Hernandez-Ono A, Ko C, Yasunaga K, Huang L-S, Ginsberg HN. Regulation of hepatic apolipoprotein B-lipoprotein assembly and secretion by the availability of fatty acids 1: Differential effects of delivering fatty acids via albumin or remnant-like emulsion particles. *J Biol Chem* 2004; 279:19362–19374.
48. Horton JD, Goldstein JL, Brown MS. SREBPs: Activators of the complete program of cholesterol and fatty acid synthesis in the liver. *J Clin Invest* 2002; 109:1125–1131.
49. Kabashima T, Kawaguchi T, Wadzinski BE, Uyeda K. Xylulose 5-phosphate mediates glucose-induced lipogenesis by xylulose 5-phosphate-activated protein phosphatase in rat liver. *PNAS* 2003; 100:5107–5112.
50. Chen G, Liang G, Ou J, Goldstein JL, Brown MS. Central role for liver X receptor in insulin-mediated activation of Srebp-1c transcription and stimulation of fatty acid synthesis in liver. *PNAS* 2004; 101:11245–11250.
51. Gavrilova O, Haluzik M, Matsusue K et al. Liver peroxisome proliferator-activated receptor gamma contributes to hepatic steatosis, triglyceride clearance, and regulation of body fat mass. *J Biol Chem* 2003; 278:34268–34276.
52. Herzig S, Hedrick S, Morantte I, Koo S-H, Galimi F, Montminy M. CREB controls hepatic lipid metabolism through nuclear hormone receptor PPAR-. *Nature* 2003; 426:190–193.
53. Cohn JS, Patterson BW, Uffelman KD, Davignon J, Steiner G. Rate of production of plasma and very-low-density lipoprotein (VLDL) apolipoprotein C-III is strongly related to the concentration and level of production of VLDL triglyceride in male subjects with different body weights and levels of insulin sensitivity. *J Clin Endocrinol Metab* 2004; 89:3949–3955.
54. Altomonte J, Cong L, Harbaran S et al. Foxo1 mediates insulin action on apoC-III and triglyceride metabolism. *J Clin Invest* 2004; 114:1493–1503.
55. Nowak M, Helleboid-Champman A, Jakel H et al. Insulin-mediated down-regulation of apolipoprotein A5 gene expression through the phosphatidylinositol 3-kinase pathway: Role of upstream stimulatory factor. *Mol Cell Biol* 2005; 25:1537–1548.
56. Ebara T, Conde K, Kako Y et al. Delayed catabolism of apoB-48 lipoproteins due to decreased heparan sulfate proteoglycan production in diabetic mice. *J Clin Invest* 2000; 105(12):1807–1818.
57. Kissebah AH, Alfarsi S, Evans DJ, Adams PW. Integrated regulation of very-low-density lipoprotein triglyceride and apolipoprotein-B kinetics in non-insulin-dependent diabetes mellitus. *Diabetes* 1982; 31:217–225.
58. Stein O, Stein Y. Lipid transfer proteins (LTP) and atherosclerosis. *Atherosclerosis* 2005; 178:217–230.
59. Sharret AR, Heiss G, Chambless LE et al. Metabolic and lifestyle determinants of postprandial lipemia differ from those of fasting triglycerides: The Atherosclerosis Risk in Communities (ARIC) Study. *Arterio Thromb Vasc Biol* 2001; 21:275–281.
60. Despres JP. Gender difference in postprandial lipemia: Importance of visceral adipose tissue accumulation. *Arterio Thromb Vasc Biol* 1999.
61. Avramoglu RK, Qiu W, Adeli K. Mechanisms of metabolic dyslipidemia in insulin resistant states: Deregulation of hepatic and intestinal lipoprotein secretion. *Frontiers Biosci* 2003; 8:464–476.
62. Guo Q, Avramoglu RK, Adeli K. Intestinal assembly and secretion of highly dense/lipid-poor apolipoprotein B48-containing lipoprotein particles in the fasting state: Evidence for induction by insulin resistance and exogenous fatty acids. *Metabolism* 2005; 54:689–697.
63. Brunzell JD, Hazzard WR, Porte DJ, Bierman EL. Evidence for a common saturable triglyceride removal mechanism for chylomicrons and very low density lipoprotein in man. *J Clin Invest* 1973; 52:1578.

III

INSULIN—SECRETION AND ACTION: UNDERLYING MECHANISMS OF THE METABOLIC SYNDROME

12 Pancreatic Islet Pathophysiology and Pathology in Obesity

Anne Clark, Jenni Moffitt,
Lianne van de Laar, Katherine Pinnick,
and Farhina Sayyed

CONTENTS

ABSTRACT

The term *metabolic syndrome* embraces a complex array of metabolic in-balances that are all interrelated (1,2). This includes abnormal insulin secretion that, in obesity, is usually in the form of hypersecretion of insulin associated with increased insulin resistance. Whether the association of all of the metabolic defects represents a true clinical syndrome remains controversial (3). However, the disturbances in the circulating and local concentrations of cellular fuels, hormones, and metabolic intermediates have a significant impact on pancreatic islet function and pathology. In many susceptible individuals, the resulting deteriorating pancreatic function results in type 2 diabetes. This chapter describes some of the pathological features present in the pancreas in obese individuals, the roles of lipids in islet cell function and survival, and the potential consequences of sustained increased insulin resistance and hyperlipidemia for islet cell function.

OBESITY AND PANCREATIC FAT

Increased insulin resistance correlates with increases in ectopically deposited triglycerides (4). Obesity results in both metabolic and morphological changes in the pancreas, both of which have profound effects on pancreatic islet function. In obese human

From: *Contemporary Endocrinology: The Metabolic Syndrome: Epidemiology, Clinical Treatment, and Underlying Mechanisms*
Edited by: B.C. Hansen and G.A. Bray © Humana Press, Totowa, NJ

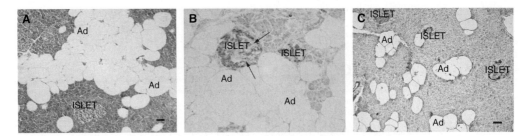

Figure 12.1 Swollen adipocytes in the pancreas. (A) Pancreatic tissue from an obese human showing swollen adipocytes (Ad) within the exocrine tissue situated close to a pancreatic islet (islet). (B) Islets can be very close to adipocytes (Ad) in human pancreas and islet capillaries (arrows) pass adjacent to adipocytes. (C) Pancreas from an obese diabetic Macaca mulatta monkey showing adipocytes (Ad) within the exocrine tissue. Scale bars = 50 microns.

subjects and animals, visceral fat in the form of swollen adipocytes in the omentum, pancreas, and peri-renal areas surrounds all organs in the abdomen. Increased storage of nutrients at these sites is a response to the increased availability of nonesterified fatty acids (NEFAs), and these adipocytes act both as depots for metabolic fuels and organs for secretion of a large number of endocrine factors (5). The extent of adipocyte mass at these different sites varies among individuals and among species; humans and monkeys accumulate fat in the pancreas in parallel with other visceral sites, but obese rodents appear to have less fat in the pancreas compared to peri-renal and epididymal areas. In general, ectopic fat deposition can have a deleterious impact on local organ function but also can be considered to provide systemic protection by removal of elevated concentrations of circulating NEFAs. The role of pancreatic adipocytes in exocrine tissue is largely unknown and could be different from islet triglyceride storage and metabolism. The locality of the storage site determines the contribution to systemic metabolism; lipid metabolism in human gluteal adipose tissue has been shown to differ from that of abdominal subcutaneous deposits (6).

An increase in swollen adipocytes in the pancreas results either in an increase in the size of the pancreas or, in extreme cases, in more than 50% exocrine tissue being replaced by adipocytes and the organ appearing macroscopically to consist of a high proportion of lipid (Fig. 12.1A). This condition has been termed *lipomatosis of the pancreas* (7). In humans, the degree of lipomatosis reflects the degree of obesity, is loosely correlated with the BMI, and is also related to age (7,8). Under extreme conditions of pancreatic lipomatosis, both exocrine and endocrine function is decreased and many subjects become diabetic. Whether this is as a result of systemic defects in metabolism or more localized disruption of the exocrine/endocrine axis is unclear. However, moderate pancreatic fat deposition is reversible with weight loss (7).

Primates kept in captivity develop obesity and many features of the metabolic syndrome in common with humans (9). Rhesus monkeys (*Macaca mulatta*) with *ad libitum* access to food frequently and spontaneously develop obesity with increased insulin resistance. There are variable degrees of exocrine tissue replacement with swollen adipocytes (Fig. 12.1C).

Exocrine tissue replacement with adipocytes and fibrotic material is a characteristic of cystic fibrosis (CF) (10). In this genetically determined condition of defective chloride channels (11), increased viscosity of exocrine secretions leads to exocrine degeneration and islets become suspended in a matrix of small adipocytes and connective tissue. Patients with CF have abnormal lipid metabolism as a result of defective pancreatic lipase production but do not have features of the metabolic syndrome such as insulin resistance (12) and develop diabetes only as adolescents or adults (13). Hence fatty material in the pancreas in this condition does not appear to be associated per se with a major defect in insulin secretion or insulin action. However, it is possible that the relatively small adipocytes that replace the pancreas in CF are metabolically dissimilar from those appearing in the viscera in obesity.

OBESITY AND PANCREATIC ISLET FUNCTION

In all laboratory animal species, including monkeys, islet size is increased with increasing body mass as a result of increased demand for insulin secretion arising from increased insulin resistance (14). The larger islet size is very marked in rodents where obesity is genetically determined such as in fatty Zucker rats (15) and ob/ob mice (16) and in high-fat fed animals (17). Plasticity of the population of differentiated beta-cells has been proposed to account for these changes; both cell division (18) and increased cellular size (hyperplasia and hypertrophy) have been identified (17). In obese monkeys, the islet size can increase to be more than double with increased obesity (Fig. 12.2). However, there is no increase in islet number with obesity, suggesting that, as in ob/ob mice (16), the response to increasing insulin demand involves hyperplasia and/or hypertrophy of cells within existing islets and not production of new islets from ductal precursor cells (19). The capacity for insulin secretion is large in these obese primates; the concentrations of circulating insulin rise to more than nine times that of lean animals with an increase of ×3 in body weight (9). This is a greater degree of compensation than would be expected in humans. Data from postmortem specimens of human pancreas suggest that, in some populations, islet size is larger in obese compared to lean subjects, both with and without type 2 diabetes, but the effects are less dramatic than for the small animal models (20–22).

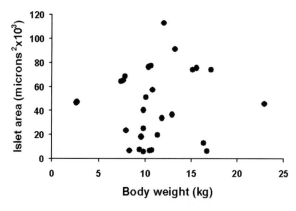

Figure 12.2 Body weight and islet size in Macaca mulatta monkeys. Mean islet area in postmortem pancreatic samples from nondiabetic animals can vary by more than 10 times but there is no clear relationship of islet size and body weight.

Effects of Sustained Hyperlipidemia on Insulin Secretion

In obesity, the physiological consequence of increased numbers of enlarged adipocytes in the pancreas is likely to be increased levels of intermediates of lipid metabolism; both delivery of lipids to the adipocytes via the circulation and subsequent release of nonesterified fatty acids (NEFAs) following lipolysis will increase the concentration of triglyceride-rich lipoproteins and NEFAs in the extracellular spaces and some of the capillary networks. When adipocytes are close to the islets (Fig. 12.1B), the concentrations of extracellular lipids adjacent to islet cells will be high. In this way, in obesity, pancreatic islets would be chronically exposed to higher-than-normal levels of triglycerides (TGs) and NEFAs. These could therefore have profound effects on beta-cell metabolism and insulin secretory responses.

The role of lipids in insulin secretion is complicated and dependent on the prevailing conditions. Acute exposure to NEFAs has been shown to increase glucose-stimulated insulin secretion (GSIS) in humans (23), animals (24), and under experimental conditions (25,26); provision of lipid-derived, intracellular metabolic fuels will promote intracellular ATP and facilitate the effects of glucose on insulin release (27,28). Sustained elevations of lipids reduce GSIS (29,30), decrease insulin gene expression, and alter cellular metabolism (31,32). Furthermore, lipids are considered to be toxic to many cells (so-called *lipotoxicity*) (33). The mechanisms of these effects of lipids on insulin secretion are largely unknown and could involve several aspects of stimulus-secretion coupling in the beta-cell.

Under normal circumstances, NEFAs provide an essential substrate for energy production in the beta-cell via beta-oxidation (34, 35). It is likely when glucose concentrations are relatively low (e.g., during fasting or overnight) that NEFAs provide essential substrates for maintenance of cellular metabolism. However, prolonged exposure of beta-cells to high levels of NEFA results in increased accumulation of triglycerides (36, 37), which can provide an energy store for later hydrolysis by lipases such as hormone-sensitive lipase (HSL) (38). The intracellular accumulations of TG per se are not toxic (39) and it is likely that relatively low concentrations of TG accumulate in beta-cells under normal conditions; lipid droplets are visible in rodent isolated islets under experimental conditions of NEFA exposure (Fig. 12.3A), but such lipid accumulations are not apparent in obese human islets (Fig. 12.3B). HSL knockout mice show no evidence of abnormal islet function or increased TG accumulation that would be consistent with defective lipolysis (40), although recent findings suggest that other lipases in beta-cells could also be important (41,42).

Prolonged exposure of islets to lipids results in decreased expression of some beta-cell genes including that of proinsulin (32,43), increased activity of uncoupling protein 2 (UCP2), and decreased production of ATP (44,45), resulting in the decline of glucose-stimulated insulin secretion. It is probable that it is not NEFAs but the intermediates of lipid metabolism, including long-chain CoA (46), which are the effectors of these changes, since NEFAs are rapidly metabolized once inside the cell (47). The mechanisms for insulin granule exocytosis are not affected by long-term exposure to NEFA (48). There is evidence for increased expression of genes responding to ER stress (49), suggesting that lipid exposure (at least in the conditions created in experiments) activates responses designed to protect beta-cells from potential damage.

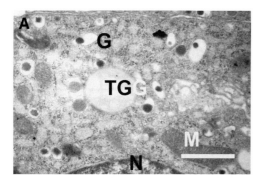
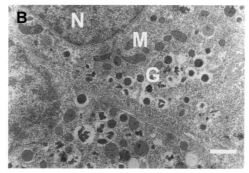

Figure 12.3 Triglyceride storage in pancreatic islets. (A) Mouse isolated islet beta-cell visualized by electron microscopy following incubation for 72 hours with 0.5 mM oleic acid. Lipid droplets (TG) formed within the cytoplasm adjacent to insulin secretory granules (G). There is no evidence of apoptotic changes in the nucleus (N) and the mitochondria (M) look normal, suggesting that lipo-apoptosis is not occurring. (B) Human islet from an obese subject. No lipid droplets could be detected, insulin secretory granules (G) are present, and mitochondria (M) are normal, indicating no lipotoxic effects of hyperlipidemia in vivo. Scale bars = 1 micron.

Beta Cell Lipoapoptosis and the Role of Saturated NEFAs

Saturated NEFAs such as palmitic and stearic acids have more pronounced effects on beta-cell function (25,50). Lipid-induced cellular toxicity (so-called *lipoapoptosis*) is more pronounced in the presence of saturated NEFAs (51). Indeed, it is proposed that lipid-induced death of beta-cells is a causal factor for islet dysfunction and decreased insulin secretion of type 2 diabetes (52). Furthermore the concept of *glucolipotoxicity* (50) proposes that concurrent elevation of glucose and NEFA, as occurs in hyperlipidemia and diabetes, is even more cytotoxic for beta-cells.

However, clinical evidence indicates that elevated lipid concentrations in obese subjects and in subjects with genetically determined hyperlipidemia do not inevitably lead to diabetes as would be expected as a result of lipid-induced beta-cell death—*lipoapoptosis*. Obesity and hyperlipidemia are usually associated with increased insulin resistance (increased insulin demand and secretion), and it is difficult to reconcile this with the hypothesis of lipoapoptosis of the beta-cells (52). Less than 12% of obese subjects with elevated lipid profiles have type 2 diabetes (53,54), suggesting that increased circulating lipids and high insulin resistance cannot be the only predisposing factors for onset of the disease. Changes in insulin secretion in response to changes in obesity are largely reversible such that loss of weight can reduce insulin resistance and insulin secretion except in extreme obesity and in subjects predisposed to develop diabetes.

Viability of all types of tissue, including cardiac (55), vascular smooth muscle (56), and kidney cells (37), is reduced by saturated NEFAs in vitro as a result of activation of signaling cascades that are associated with apoptotic cell death (57). However, palmitic acid is a normal component of lipid fractions in vivo in healthy subjects without any deleterious effects. It is now apparent from in vitro experimental observations that exposure to saturated NEFAs results in formation of TGs containing only saturated fatty acids; for example, tripalmitin is formed from palmitic acid (37). Tripalmitin is a waxy solid at body temperature (melting temperature 65°C) and would never be found in vivo; derivatives of palmitic acid are usually associated with oleic acid in vivo. Thus, so-called rescue of viability with unsaturated NEFAs (58) and decreased toxicity in the presence of increased concentrations of the desaturase enzyme, SCD-1 (59), is due to formation of triglycerides containing mixed species of fatty acids and reduced amounts of insoluble tripalmitin. Although beta-cell death is unlikely to occur in vivo, the functional changes on insulin secretion elicited by increased circulating lipids remains a problem.

LIPIDS, INSULIN RESISTANCE, AND ISLET AMYLOID FORMATION

Hyperlipidemia and increased insulin resistance are likely to play a role in islet pathology and loss of beta-cell in type 2 diabetes as a result of islet amyloidosis. Islet amyloid formation is associated with diabetes in humans, nonhuman primates, and cats (60). This pathophysiogical feature is a characteristic of pancreatic islets in type 2 diabetes in humans (61,62), where islet amyloid deposits are found in at least one islet in 90% of type 2 diabetic subjects at postmortem (63). Islet amyloid fibrils are formed from the 37 amino-acid polypeptide, islet amyloid polypeptide (IAPP, amylin), which is a normal component of beta-cells (64,65) and is co-secreted with insulin (66). The factors that are responsible for refolding of the normally soluble peptide to form insoluble fibrils remain largely undetermined. Fibrils are deposited in extracellular spaces adjacent to islet capillaries but the deposits progressively expand to occupy more of the islet space with reduction of islet cell mass (Fig. 12.4A,B) (67–70). This reduction of beta-cells in diabetes results from the cytotoxic properties of amyloid fibrils or small oligomeric molecular assemblies (71,72).

The degree of islet amyloidosis is highly variable in humans and in animal models. In humans, the number of islets affected varies between < 1% and > 80%; the extent of islet cell replacement is also variable (65,73,74). Islet amyloidosis is found in < 10% of nondiabetic individuals; interestingly, more than 50% of diabetic subjects have low

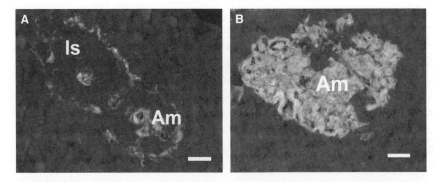

Figure 12.4 Islet amyloid deposits in Macaca mulatta monkeys. Islet amyloid labeled with thioflavin S (fluorescent marker) in (A) an islet (Is) in a hyperinsulinemic nondiabetic animal and (B) diabetic animal. Islet amyloid (Am) is deposited initially (A) in perivascular spaces adjacent to islet capillaries that are situated at the islet perimeter and penetrate the central islet core. (B) As the deposits become more extensive, cells are destroyed and amyloid occupies more than 80% of the islet mass in diabetes. Scale bars = 50 microns.

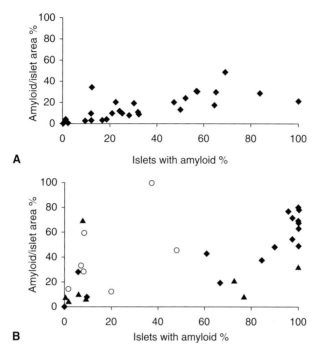

Figure 12.5 The relationship of the number of islets affected with amyloid and the degree of the islet occupied by fibrils in humans (panel A) and Macaca mulatta monkeys (panel B). In humans with established diabetes, more than 50% of subjects have less than 20% of islets affected and less than 10% of islet space is occupied with amyloid. This suggests that amyloid-induced islet cell death is unlikely to be a major cause of hyperinsulinemia or diabetes. In monkeys, most diabetic animals (diamonds) have more than 80% of islets affected with large deposits. Obese, hyperinsulinemic, normoglycemic animals (open circles) have variable degrees of islets affected. Normoglycemic animals without extreme levels of insulin resistance (triangles) have low degrees of islet amyloidosis.

numbers of islets affected with amyloid deposition (Fig. 12.5A). This suggests that in humans islet amyloid is not a causal factor for diabetes but results from beta-cell dysfunction (68). In type 2 diabetes in humans, the degree of amyloidosis (both numbers of islets affected and islet mass of amyloid) is unrelated to the duration of diabetes but an increased degree of islet amyloidosis at postmortem is related to the previous requirement for insulin replacement therapy (62,63). In animal models such as cats, monkeys, and transgenic mice expressing the gene for human islet amyloid polypeptide, the degree of amyloidosis is also variable (69,75–77) and is related to the degree of hyperglycemia (Fig. 12.5B) (77,78). This implicates amyloid formation and the associated loss of beta-cells with onset of hyperglycemia. A direct association of islet amyloid with increased insulin resistance has been described; in Rabson–Mendenhall syndrome, a disease resulting from mutations in insulin receptor gene (79), severe islet amyloidosis was found (80), suggesting that hypersecretion of IAPP with insulin promotes fibril formation. Obese monkeys with hyperinsulinemia have increased degrees of islet amyloidosis (Fig. 12.5B) (69) compared to lean animals; however, its extent is mild prior to overt diabetes and of variable extent after diabetes onset.

IAPP is derived from a larger precursor, proIAPP (67 amino acids in humans), which is proteolytically cleaved by the same convertase enzymes in secretory granules that process proinsulin (81,82). Partially processed proIAPP has been shown to have a higher susceptibility to form fibrils in animals deficient in prohormone convertase 2 (PC2) (83). It is likely therefore that, in diabetes, where the proportion of incompletely processed proinsulin is increased (84), proIAPP secretion would be similarly increased, contributing to refolding of the peptide and fibril formation. This could form a nidus, which, once established, forms a site for deposition of secreted IAPP.

The role of lipids in fibril formation is unclear. In vitro, lipids increase fibril formation from synthetic IAPP (85). Since assembly of amyloid fibrils from the monomeric peptide is associated with hydrophobic conditions, it is possible that increased extracellular lipids (especially in the basement membrane, where fibril formation commences) could provide appropriate conditions for the fibril formation. Fibril formation is likely to result from a combination of diabetes-related changes in the islet. Production of incompletely processed proIAPP, increased insulin granule secretion as a result of increased insulin resistance, and reduced clearance from the extracellular space could all contribute. Once fibrils are formed between the basement membrane and islet beta-cells, this is likely to compromise the function of the cell (e.g., signaling across the membrane and exocytosis of granules). As the deposition progresses, the fibrils replace insulin-secreting cells and contribute to an irreversible loss of insulin secretory capacity.

SUMMARY

Components of the metabolic syndrome, including hyperlipidemia and increased demand for insulin, alter pancreatic islet function and morphology. Increased expansion of adipocytes in the pancreas can affect exocrine function and increase the ambient concentrations of extracellular triglyceride and NEFAs adjacent to pancreatic islets. Sustained exposure of beta-cells to lipids affects glucose-stimulated insulin secretion due to changes in the balance of glucose and lipid metabolic pathways concerned with insulin granule release. Lipid-induced beta-cell death in vivo is unlikely since lipoapoptosis is largely an artefact created by nonphysiological conditions in vitro. Islet amyloid formation and the associated reduction in beta-cell mass could be influenced by aberrant peptide secretion and clearance and elevated pancreatic concentrations of extracellular lipids in susceptible individuals.

ACKNOWLEDGMENTS

We are grateful to Professor Barbara Hansen (University of South Florida) for providing monkey tissue and to Professors John Morris, Keith Frayn, and Dr Fredrik Karpe (Oxford University) for continuing support. We thank the Wellcome Trust (AC, JHM) and Medical Research Council (KP) for financial support.

REFERENCES

1. Reaven G. Role of insulin resistance in human disease. *Diabetes* 1998; 37:1595–1607.
2. Moller DE, Kaufman KD. Metabolic syndrome: A clinical and molecular perspective. *Annu Rev Med* 2005; 56:45–62.
3. Gale EA. The myth of the metabolic syndrome. *Diabetologia* 2005; 48:1679–1683.

4. Goodpaster BH, Wolf D. Skeletal muscle lipid accumulation in obesity, insulin resistance, and type 2 diabetes. *Pediatr Diabetes* 2004; 5:219–226.

5. Frayn KN, Karpe F, Fielding BA, Macdonald IA, Coppack SW. Integrative physiology of human adipose tissue. *Int J Obes Relat Metab Disord* 2003; 27:875–888.

6. Tan GD, Goossens GH, Humphreys SM, Vidal H, Karpe F. Upper and lower body adipose tissue function: A direct comparison of fat mobilization in humans. *Obes Res* 2004; 12:114–118.

7. Olsen TS. Lipomatosis of the pancreas in autopsy material and its relation to age and overweight. *Acta Pathol Microbiol Scand [A]* 1978; 86A:367–373.

8. Kloppel G, Drenck CR, Oberholzer M, Heitz PU. Morphometric evidence for a striking B-cell reduction at the clinical onset of type 1 diabetes. *Virchows Arch A Pathol Anat Histopathol* 1984; 403:441–452.

9. Hansen BC, Bodkin NL. Heterogeneity of insulin responses: Phases leading to type 2 (non-insulin-dependent) diabetes mellitus in the rhesus monkey. *Diabetologia* 1986; 29:713–719.

10. Lohr M, Goertchen P, Nizze H et al. Cystic fibrosis associated islet changes may provide a basis for diabetes: An immunocytochemical and morphometrical study. *Virchows Arch A Pathol Anat Histopathol* 1989; 414:179–185.

11. Riordan JR, Rommens JM, Kerem B et al. Identification of the cystic fibrosis gene: Cloning and characterization of complementary DNA. *Science* 1989; 245:1066–1073.

12. Yung B, Noormohamed FH, Kemp M, Hooper J, Lant AF, Hodson ME. Cystic fibrosis-related diabetes: The role of peripheral insulin resistance and beta-cell dysfunction. *Diabet Med* 2002; 19:221–226.

13. Lombardo F, De Luca F, Rosano M et al. Natural history of glucose tolerance, beta-cell function and peripheral insulin sensitivity in cystic fibrosis patients with fasting euglycemia. *Eur J Endocrinol* 2003; 149:53–59.

14. Bock T, Pakkenberg B, Buschard K. Genetic background determines the size and structure of the endocrine pancreas. *Diabetes* 2005; 54:133–137.

15. Tse EO, Gregoire FM, Reusens B et al. Changes of islet size and islet size distribution resulting from protein-malnutrition in lean (Fa/Fa) and obese (fa/fa) Zucker rats. *Obes Res* 1997; 5:563–571.

16. Bock T, Pakkenberg B, Buschard K. Increased islet volume but unchanged islet number in ob/ob mice. *Diabetes* 2003; 52:1716–1722.

17. Milburn JL, Jr., Hirose H, Lee YH et al. Pancreatic beta-cells in obesity: Evidence for induction of functional, morphologic, and metabolic abnormalities by increased long chain fatty acids. *J Biol Chem* 1995; 270:1295–1299.

18. Dor Y, Brown J, Martinez OI, Melton DA. Adult pancreatic beta-cells are formed by self-duplication rather than stem-cell differentiation. *Nature* 2004; 429:41–46.

19. Bonner-Weir S. Islet growth and development in the adult. *J Mol Endocrinol* 2000; 24:297–302.

20. Kloppel G, Lohr M, Habich K, Oberholtzer M, Heitz PU. Islet pathology and the pathogenesis of type 1 and type 2 diabetes mellitus revisited. *Surv Synth Pathol Res* 1985; 4:110–125.

21. Butler AE, Janson J, Bonner-Weir S, Ritzel R, Rizza RA, Butler PC. Beta-cell deficit and increased beta-cell apoptosis in humans with type 2 diabetes. *Diabetes* 2003; 52:102–110.

22. Yoon KH, Ko SH, Cho JH et al. Selective beta-cell loss and alpha-cell expansion in patients with type 2 diabetes mellitus in Korea. *J Clin Endocrinol Metab* 2003; 88:2300–2308.

23. Beysen C, Karpe F, Fielding BA, Clark A, Levy JC, Frayn KN. Interaction between specific fatty acids, GLP-1 and insulin secretion in humans. *Diabetologia* 2002; 45:1533–1541.

24. Dobbins RL, Szczepaniak LS, Myhill J et al. The composition of dietary fat directly influences glucose-stimulated insulin secretion in rats. *Diabetes* 2002; 51:1825–1833.

25. Gravena C, Mathias PC, Ashcroft SJ. Acute effects of fatty acids on insulin secretion from rat and human islets of Langerhans. *J Endocrinol* 2002; 173:73–80.

26. Stein DT, Stevenson BE, Chester MW et al. The insulinotropic potency of fatty acids is influenced profoundly by their chain length and degree of saturation. *J Clin Invest* 1997; 100:398–403.

27. Prentki M, Vischer S, Glennon MC, Regazzi R, Deeney JT, Corkey BE. Malonyl-CoA and long chain acyl-CoA esters as metabolic coupling factors in nutrient-induced insulin secretion. *J Biol Chem* 1992; 267:5802–5810.

28. Clayton PT, Eaton S, Aynsley-Green A et al. Hyperinsulinism in short-chain L-3-hydroxyacyl-CoA dehydrogenase deficiency reveals the importance of beta-oxidation in insulin secretion. *J Clin Invest* 2001; 108:457–465.

29. Sako Y, Grill VE. A 48-hour lipid infusion in the rat time-dependently inhibits glucose-induced insulin secretion and B cell oxidation through a process likely coupled to fatty acid oxidation. *Endocrinology* 1990; 127:1580–1589.

30. Zhou YP, Grill VE. Long-term exposure of rat pancreatic islets to fatty acids inhibits glucose-induced insulin secretion and biosynthesis through a glucose fatty acid cycle. *J Clin Invest* 1994; 93:870–876.

31. Xiao J, Gregersen S, Kruhoffer M, Pedersen SB, Orntoft TF, Hermansen K. The effect of chronic exposure to fatty acids on gene expression in clonal insulin-producing cells: Studies using high density oligonucleotide microarray. *Endocrinology* 2001; 142:4777–4784.

32. Bollheimer LC, Skelly RH, Chester MW, McGarry JD, Rhodes CJ. Chronic exposure to free fatty acid reduces pancreatic beta cell insulin content by increasing basal insulin secretion that is not compensated for by a corresponding increase in proinsulin biosynthesis translation. *J Clin Invest* 1998; 101:1094–1101.

33. Unger RH, Zhou YT. Lipotoxicity of beta-cells in obesity and in other causes of fatty acid spillover. *Diabetes* 2001; 50 Suppl 1:S118–121.

34. Stein DT, Esser V, Stevenson BE et al. Essentiality of circulating fatty acids for glucose-stimulated insulin secretion in the fasted rat. *J Clin Invest* 1996; 97:2728–2735.

35. Yaney GC, Corkey BE. Fatty acid metabolism and insulin secretion in pancreatic beta cells. *Diabetologia* 2003; 46:1297–1312.

36. Segall L, Lameloise N, Assimacopoulos-Jeannet F et al. Lipid rather than glucose metabolism is implicated in altered insulin secretion caused by oleate in INS-1 cells. *Am J Physiol* 1999; 277: E521–528.

37. Moffitt JH, Fielding BA, Evershed R, Berstan R, Currie JM, Clark A. Adverse physicochemical properties of tripalmitin in beta cells lead to morphological changes and lipotoxicity in vitro. *Diabetologia* 2005; 48:1819–1829.

38. Mulder H, Holst LS, Svensson H et al. Hormone-sensitive lipase, the rate-limiting enzyme in triglyceride hydrolysis, is expressed and active in beta-cells. *Diabetes* 1999; 48:228–232.

39. Cnop M, Hannaert JC, Hoorens A, Eizirik DL, Pipeleers DG. Inverse relationship between cytotoxicity of free fatty acids in pancreatic islet cells and cellular triglyceride accumulation. *Diabetes* 2001; 50:1771–1777.

40. Fex M, Olofsson CS, Fransson U et al. Hormone-sensitive lipase deficiency in mouse islets abolishes neutral cholesterol ester hydrolase activity but leaves lipolysis, acylglycerides, fat oxidation, and insulin secretion intact. *Endocrinology* 2004; 145:3746–3753.

41. Villena JA, Roy S, Sarkadi-Nagy E, Kim KH, Sul HS. Desnutrin, an adipocyte gene encoding a novel patatin domain-containing protein, is induced by fasting and glucocorticoids: Ectopic expression of desnutrin increases triglyceride hydrolysis. *J Biol Chem* 2004; 279:47066–47075.

42. Hu L, Deeney JT, Nolan CJ et al. Regulation of lipolytic activity by long-chain acyl-coenzyme A in islets and adipocytes. *Am J Physiol Endocrinol Metab* 2005; 289:E1085–1092.

43. Gremlich S, Bonny C, Waeber G, Thorens B. Fatty acids decrease IDX-1 expression in rat pancreatic islets and reduce GLUT2, glucokinase, insulin, and somatostatin levels. *J Biol Chem* 1997; 272:30261–30269.

44. Patane G, Anello M, Piro S, Vigneri R, Purrello F, Rabuazzo AM. Role of ATP production and uncoupling protein-2 in the insulin secretory defect induced by chronic exposure to high glucose or free fatty acids and effects of peroxisome proliferator-activated receptor-gamma inhibition. *Diabetes* 2002; 51:2749–2756.

45. Chan CB, Saleh MC, Koshkin V, Wheeler MB. Uncoupling protein 2 and islet function. *Diabetes* 2004; 53 Suppl 1:S136–142.

46. Corkey BE, Deeney JT, Yaney GC, Tornheim K, Prentki M. The role of long-chain fatty acyl-CoA esters in beta-cell signal transduction. *J Nutr* 2000; 130:299S–304S.

47. Kamp F, Hamilton JA, Westerhoff HV. Movement of fatty acids, fatty acid analogues, and bile acids across phospholipid bilayers. *Biochemistry* 1993; 32:11074–11086.

48. Olofsson CS, Salehi A, Holm C, Rorsman P. Palmitate increases L-type Ca2+ currents and the size of the readily releasable granule pool in mouse pancreatic beta-cells. *J Physiol* 2004; 557:935–948.

49. Kharroubi I, Ladriere L, Cardozo AK, Dogusan Z, Cnop M, Eizirik DL. Free fatty acids and cytokines induce pancreatic (beta)-cell apoptosis by different mechanisms: Role of NF-(kappa)B and endoplasmic reticulum stress. *Endocrinology* 2004; 145:5087–5096.

50. El-Assaad W, Buteau J, Peyot ML et al. Saturated fatty acids synergize with elevated glucose to cause pancreatic beta-cell death. *Endocrinology* 2003; 144:4154–4163.
51. Maedler K, Spinas GA, Dyntar D, Moritz W, Kaiser N, Donath MY. Distinct effects of saturated and monounsaturated fatty acids on beta-cell turnover and function. *Diabetes* 2001; 50:69–76.
52. Unger RH, Orci L. Lipoapoptosis: Its mechanism and its diseases. *Biochim Biophys Acta* 2002; 1585:202–212.
53. Agren G, Narbro K, Naslund I, Sjostrom L, Peltonen M. Long-term effects of weight loss on pharmaceutical costs in obese subjects: A report from the SOS intervention study. *Int J Obes Relat Metab Disord* 2002; 26:184–192.
54. Ford ES, Giles WH, Dietz WH. Prevalence of the metabolic syndrome among US adults: Findings from the third National Health and Nutrition Examination Survey. *JAMA* 2002; 287:356–359.
55. Weigert C, Brodbeck K, Staiger H et al. Palmitate, but not unsaturated fatty acids, induces the expression of interleukin-6 in human myotubes through proteasome-dependent activation of nuclear factor-kappaB. *J Biol Chem* 2004; 279:23942–23952.
56. Mattern HM, Hardin CD. Vascular metabolic dysfunction and lipotoxicity. *Physiol Res* 2007; 56:149–158.
57. Lupi R, Dotta F, Marselli L et al. Prolonged exposure to free fatty acids has cytostatic and pro-apoptotic effects on human pancreatic islets: Evidence that beta-cell death is caspase mediated, partially dependent on ceramide pathway, and Bcl-2 regulated. *Diabetes* 2002; 51:1437–1442.
58. Maedler K, Oberholzer J, Bucher P, Spinas GA, Donath MY. Monounsaturated fatty acids prevent the deleterious effects of palmitate and high glucose on human pancreatic beta-cell turnover and function. *Diabetes* 2003; 52:726–733.
59. Busch AK, Gurisik E, Cordery DV et al. Increased fatty acid desaturation and enhanced expression of stearoyl coenzyme A desaturase protects pancreatic beta-cells from lipoapoptosis. *Diabetes* 2005; 54:2917–2924.
60. Westermark P, Wilander E, Johnson KH. Islet amyloid polypeptide. *Lancet* 1987; 2:623.
61. Clark A, Wells CA, Buley ID et al. Islet amyloid, increased A-cells, reduced B-cells and exocrine fibrosis: Quantitative changes in the pancreas in type 2 diabetes. *Diabetes Res* 1988; 9:151–159.
62. Röcken C, Linke RP, Saeger W. Immunohistology of islet amyloid polypeptide in diabetes mellitus: Semi-quantitative studies in a post-mortem series. *Virchows Arch A Pathol Anat Histopathol* 1992; 421:339–344.
63. Westermark P. Amyloid and polypeptide hormones: What is their interrelationship? *Amyloid: Int J Exper Clin Invest* 1994; 1:47–57.
64. Westermark P, Wernstedt C, O'Brien TD, Hayden DW, Johnson KH. Islet amyloid in type 2 human diabetes mellitus and adult diabetic cats contains a novel putative polypeptide hormone. *Am J Pathol* 1987; 127:414–417.
65. Clark A, Cooper GJ, Lewis CE et al. Islet amyloid formed from diabetes-associated peptide may be pathogenic in type-2 diabetes. *Lancet* 1987; 2:231–234.
66. Butler PC, Chou J, Carter WB et al. Effects of meal ingestion on plasma amylin concentration in NIDDM and nondiabetic humans. *Diabetes* 1990; 39:752–756.
67. Jaikaran ETAS, Clark A. Islet amyloid and type 2 diabetes: From molecular misfolding to islet pathophysiology. *Biochim. Biophys. Acta* 2001; 1537:179–203.
68. Clark A, Nilsson MR. Islet amyloid: A complication of islet dysfunction or an aetiological factor in type 2 diabetes? *Diabetologia* 2004; 47:157–169.
69. de Koning EJ, Bodkin NL, Hansen BC, Clark A. Diabetes mellitus in Macaca mulatta monkeys is characterised by islet amyloidosis and reduction in beta-cell population. *Diabetologia* 1993; 36:378–384.
70. Hull RL, Westermark GT, Westermark P, Kahn SE. Islet amyloid: A critical entity in the pathogenesis of type 2 diabetes. *J Clin Endocrinol Metab* 2004; 89:3629–3643.
71. Kapurniotu A. Amyloidogenicity and cytotoxicity of islet amyloid polypeptide. *Biopolymers* 2001; 60:438–459.
72. Demuro A, Mina E, Kayed R, Milton SC, Parker I, Glabe CG. Calcium dysregulation and membrane disruption as a ubiquitous neurotoxic mechanism of soluble amyloid oligomers. *J Biol Chem* 2005; 280:17294–17300.
73. Westermark P, Grimelius L. The pancreatic islet cells in insular amyloidosis in human diabetic and non-diabetic adults. *Acta Pathol Microbiol Scand A* 1973; 81:291–300.

74. Maloy AL, Longnecker DS, Greenberg ER. The relation of islet amyloid to the clinical type of diabetes. *Hum Pathol* 1981; 12:917–922.
75. O'Brien TD, Hayden DW, Johnson KH, Fletcher TF. Immunohistochemical morphometry of pancreatic endocrine cells in diabetic, normoglycaemic glucose-intolerant and normal cats. *J Comp Pathol* 1986; 96:357–369.
76. Howard CF Jr. Longitudinal studies on the development of diabetes in individual Macaca nigra. *Diabetologia* 1986; 29:301–306.
77. Wang F, Hull RL, Vidal J, Cnop M, Kahn SE. Islet amyloid develops diffusely throughout the pancreas before becoming severe and replacing endocrine cells. *Diabetes* 2001; 50:2514–2520.
78. Hull RL, Andrikopoulos S, Verchere CB et al. Increased dietary fat promotes islet amyloid formation and beta-cell secretory dysfunction in a transgenic mouse model of islet amyloid. *Diabetes* 2003; 52:372–379.
79. Krook A, Kumar S, Laing I, Boulton AJ, Wass JA, O'Rahilly S. Molecular scanning of the insulin receptor gene in syndromes of insulin resistance. *Diabetes* 1994; 43:357–368.
80. O'Brien TD, Rizza RA, Carney JA, Butler PC. Islet amyloidosis in a patient with chronic massive insulin resistance due to antiinsulin receptor antibodies. *J Clin Endocrinol Metab* 1994; 79:290–292.
81. Badman MK, Shennan KI, Jermany JL, Docherty K, Clark A. Processing of pro-islet amyloid polypeptide (proIAPP) by the prohormone convertase PC2. *FEBS Lett* 1996; 378:227–331.
82. Higham. CE, Hull RL, Lawrie L et al. Processing os synthetic pro-islet amyloid polypeptide (proIAPP) "amylin" by recombinant prohormone convertase enzymes, PC2 and PC3, in vitro. *Eur J Biochem* 2000; 267:4998–5004.
83. Marzban L, Trigo-Gonzalez G, Zhu X et al. Role of beta-cell prohormone convertase (PC)1/3 in processing of pro-islet amyloid polypeptide. *Diabetes* 2004; 53:141–148.
84. Halban PA, Kahn SE. Release of incompletely processed proinsulin is the cause of the disproportionate proinsulineamia of NIDDM. *Diabetes* 1997; 46:1725–1732.
85. Ma Z, Westermark GT. Effects of free fatty acid on polymerization of islet amyloid polypeptide (IAPP) in vitro and on amyloid fibril formation in cultivated isolated islets of transgenic mice overexpressing human IAPP. *Mol Med* 2002; 8:863–868.

13 Glucagon-like Peptides and Insulin Sensitivity

Jens Juul Holst and Filip Krag Knop

CONTENTS

ABSTRACT

The glucagon gene is expressed not only in the pancreas but also in endocrine cells of the gut and in the brain stem. Here the precursor, proglucagon, gives rise to the peptides glicentin, oxyntomodulin, and glucagon-like peptides 1 and 2 (GLP-1 and 2). Whereas the physiological role of the former is unclear, the glucagon-like peptides appear to be important hormones—GLP-1 as an incretin hormone stimulating insulin release and as an enterogastrone, inhibiting appetite and gastrointestinal secretion and motility, and GLP-2 as an intestinotrophic factor regulating gut mucosal growth. GLP-1 has shown great promise as a therapeutic for type 2 diabetes, because of effects on insulin and glucagon secretion, as well as inhibition of gastric emptying and appetite, leading to weight loss. In several studies, GLP-1 has been reported to influence peripheral or hepatic glucose metabolism and to augment or mimic insulin actions, but the evidence that such actions contribute to the antidiabetogenic effects of the peptide and its analogs in type 2 diabetic patients is weak.

From: *Contemporary Endocrinology: The Metabolic Syndrome: Epidemiology, Clinical Treatment, and Underlying Mechanisms*
Edited by: B.C. Hansen and G.A. Bray © Humana Press, Totowa, NJ

species, including humans, and provided evidence that keratinocyte growth factor (KGF) produced by these cells could explain some of the growth effects of GLP-2.

BIOLOGICAL ACTIONS

Glicentin has been reported to influence gastric acid secretion (53) and single reports on growth effects and other effects have been published, but most investigators have found the peptide to be inactive. Thus, in unpublished studies from the author's laboratory, synthetic glicentin was without effects on gastric acid secretion and insulin secretion in humans. Oxyntomodulin mimics most of the actions of glucagon (39), but is less potent and probably does not act as a glucagon-like agonist physiologically. Like glucagon, it inhibits gastric acid secretion (54), but by an action that appears to be mediated by GLP-1 receptors (although their exact location is uncertain). However, it is doubtful whether the circulating concentrations of oxyntomodulin under normal circumstances reach sufficient levels to activate the receptors (55). Recently, intracerebrovascular administration of oxyntomodulin was shown to powerfully inhibit food intake in rats, by actions that did not appear to be mediated via the GLP-1 receptor (56). It is possible that oxyntomodulin released from the fibers arising from the proglucagon-producing neurons in the nucleus of the solitary tract in parallel with GLP-1 (in agreement with the gut-like processing pattern of proglucagon in these cells (16)) may contribute to the inhibitory effect on appetite and food intake apparently resulting from activation of these neurons, together with GLP-1 and GLP-2 (57).

ACTIONS OF GLP-1

The most conspicuous effect of GLP-1 is stimulation of glucose-induced insulin secretion (58). Thus, GLP-1 is considered to be one of the incretin hormones, the gut hormones that increase insulin secretion upon oral as opposed to intravenous administration of glucose (59). GLP-1 and GIP (gastric inhibitory polypeptide, also called glucose-dependent polypeptide) are thought to be responsible for the incretin effect, which may account for as much as 70% of the insulin secreted after carbohydrate intake. Indeed, glucose tolerance and insulin secretion is impaired in mice with deletions of both the GLP-1 and the GIP receptor and more so in animals with knockout of both receptors (60). However, GLP-1 has numerous other actions and its physiologically most important role may be to act as an enterogastrone hormone, inhibiting gastrointestinal motility and secretion and reducing appetite and food intake, and to enhance peripheral deposition of already-absorbed nutrients by stimulation of insulin secretion (61).

Effects on the Islets

Not only does GLP-1 stimulate insulin secretion in a glucose-dependent manner, it also enhances all steps of insulin biosynthesis as well as insulin gene transcription (62), thereby providing continued and augmented supplies of insulin for secretion. Important steps in the GLP-1 receptor signaling include activation of adenylate cyclase with subsequent accumulation of cAMP as well as increases in intracellular calcium levels. However, many of the subsequent changes that occur in the beta-cells are protein kinase A (PKA) independent. Thus cAMP-regulated guanine nucleotide exchange factors (in particular, Epac 2) appear to act as downstream mediators (63). Also the actions of

GLP-1 on the insulin gene promoter appear to be mediated by both PKA-dependent and -independent mechanisms, the latter possibly involving the MAP kinase pathway (64). The transcription factor PDX-1, a key regulator of islet growth and insulin gene transcription, appears to be essential for the most of the glucoregulatory, proliferative, and cytoprotective actions of GLP-1 (65). In addition, GLP-1 upregulates the genes for the cellular machinery involved in insulin secretion, such as the glucokinase and GLUT-2 genes (66). Much attention was aroused by the finding that GLP-1 appeared to be essential for conveying *glucose competence* to the beta-cells (i.e., that without GLP-1 signaling, beta-cells would not be responsive to glucose) (67,68). However, the beta-cells of mice with disruption of the GLP-1 receptor gene show preserved glucose competence (69).

Finally, GLP-1 also has trophic effects on beta-cells (70). Not only does it stimulate beta-cell proliferation (71,72), it also enhances the differentiation of new beta-cells from progenitor cells in the pancreatic duct epithelium (73). Moreover, GLP-1 has been shown to be capable of inhibiting apoptosis of beta-cells, including human beta-cells (74). Since the normal number of beta-cells is maintained in a balance between apoptosis and proliferation, this observation is of considerable interest, and also raises the possibility that GLP-1 could be useful in conditions with increased beta-cell apoptosis. The complicated mechanisms whereby GLP-1 may exert these effects on the beta-cells were reviewed recently (75,76).

GLP-1 also strongly inhibits glucagon secretion from the alpha-cells (77). The mechanism is still unclear, but may involve interaction with the alpha-cells directly (although in isolated alpha-cells secretion has been reported to be stimulated by GLP-1) or a paracrine action by neighboring D-cells whose secretion of somatostatin-14 is potently stimulated by GLP-1. Alternatively, it may be due to inhibitory effects of insulin or other beta-cell products whose release is stimulated by GLP-1 (78).

Effects on the Gastrointestinal Tract

Further important effects of GLP-1 include inhibition of gastrointestinal secretion and motility, notably gastric emptying (79,80). Physiologically, it may be that these effects of GLP-1 are more important than the insulinotropic activity. Thus, when GLP-1 is infused intravenously during ingestion of a meal, the insulin responses are diminished dose-dependently, rather than being enhanced (81). At the same time, gastric emptying is being progressively retarded, so that the explanation of the reduced insulin secretion is the reduced gastric emptying of and reduced subsequent absorption of insulinotropic nutrients. Thus the physiological role of GLP-1 may be to adjust the delivery of chyme to the digestive and absorptive capacity of the gut by retarding propulsion and digestion of the gastric contents (79,81,82). Most recently, Schirra et al. (83) have probed the physiological actions of GLP-1 on gastric motility in humans using the GLP-1 receptor antagonist, exendin 9-39. The antagonist both increased fasting antral motility and meal-induced gastric and duodenal motility and decreased pyloric tone. This strongly suggests that endogenous GLP-1 is a physiological regulator of antroduodenal motility. The mechanism whereby GLP-1 exerts these actions appears to involve the nervous system. As described above, GLP-1 is degraded extensively in the gut before it reaches the systemic circulation. This has led to the hypothesis that GLP-1 must act locally in the lamina propria before it gets degraded. Thus, on its way to the capillary, while still in the intact form, GLP-1 may interact with afferent sensory nerve fibers arising from the nodose ganglion, causing them to send impulses to the nucleus of the solitary tract and onward to the hypothalamus (45). It has been demonstrated that intraportal administration of GLP-1 causes increased impulse activity in the vagal trunks (84). These impulses may be reflexively transmitted to the pancreas (85). Studies employing ganglionic blockers have shown that the insulin response to intraportal administration of GLP-1 and glucose may be reduced to that elicited by glucose alone after ganglionic blockade (86). Thus, regarding the mechanism of GLP-1-stimulated insulin secretion under physiological circumstances, the neural pathway may be more important than the endocrine route. However, the concentration of intact GLP-1 *does* rise after meal intake and rises the more the larger the meal is (25). Thus, it is possible that the endocrine route becomes more prominent after extensive L-cell stimulation. Also the inhibition of gastric motility and acid secretion and emptying seems to involve regulation of efferent vagal activity via activation of vagal sensory afferents (87,88).

Effects on Appetite and Food Intake

Nutrients in the ileum are thought to have a satiating effect, curtailing food intake (89) and also cause a release of GLP-1. Infusions of slightly supraphysiological amounts of GLP-1 significantly enhance satiety and reduce food intake in normal subjects (90,91). The effect on food intake and satiety is preserved in obese subjects also (92) as well as in obese subjects with type 2 diabetes (93,94). Furthermore, direct injections of GLP-1 into the cerebral ventricles also inhibit food intake in rats (95,96). Here, the peptide presumably interacts with the cerebral GLP-1 receptors described above, likely to be targets for GLP-1 released from nerve fibres ascending from cell bodies in the nucleus of the solitary tract in the brain stem (16). The question arises whether these neurons are linked to meal-induced satiety. Rinaman et al. (97) analyzed the neurons of the nucleus of the brain stem that were activated by various procedures designed to model enteroceptive stress (lithium chloride administration, CCK injection, lipopolysaccharide) and observed c-fos expression in cell bodies that also stained for GLP-1, whereas neurons showing c-fos expression after meal ingestion were distinct from the GLP-1 neurons. In further experiments, they administered the GLP-1 receptor antagonist, exendin 9-39, intracerebroventricularly to rats given lithium chloride as above, and found that the antagonist could completely reverse the anorexigenic effect of systemic lithium chloride (98). Thus, it seems clear that GLP-1 from the brain stem functions as a mediator of the anorexic effects of enteroceptive stress, whereas its role in meal-induced satiety is less clear. However, the same group recently reported divergent results in mice, suggesting that differences between species may be of importance (99).

It should be noted, though, that GLP-1 receptor knockout mice do not become obese (100), but this may reflect the redundancy of the appetite-regulating mechanisms rather than ineffectiveness of the signal.

Other Actions

As mentioned above, there are GLP-1 receptors in the heart (43). A physiological function for these receptors was indicated in recent studies in mice lacking the GLP-1 receptor, which exhibit impaired left ventricular contractility and diastolic functions as well as impaired responses to exogenous epinephrine (101). Recent studies in rats showed that GLP-1 protects the ischemic and reperfused myocardium in rats by mechanisms independent of insulin (102). These findings may have important clinical implications. Thus Nikolaidis et al. studied patients treated with angioplasty after acute myocardial infarction, but with postoperative left ventricular ejection fractions as low as 29%. In these patients, GLP-1 administration significantly improved the ejection fraction to 39% and improved both global and regional wall motion indexes (103). Recently, GLP-1 was reported to dramatically improve left ventricular and systemic hemodynamics in dogs with induced dilated cardiomyopathy, and it was suggested that GLP-1 may be a useful metabolic adjuvant in decompensated heart failure (104). Finally, GLP-1 was recently found to improve endothelial dysfunction in patients with type 2 diabetes and coronary heart disease, again a finding with interesting therapeutic perspectives (105).

It has been reported that cerebral GLP-1 receptor stimulation increases blood pressure and heart rate and activates autonomic regulatory neurons in rats, leading to downstream activation of cardiovascular responses (106). Furthermore, it has been suggested that catecholaminergic neurons in the area postrema expressing the GLP-1 receptor may link peripheral GLP-1 and central autonomic control sites that mediate the diverse neuroendocrine and autonomic actions of peripheral GLP-1 (107). However, peripheral administration of GLP-1 in humans is not associated with changes in blood pressure or heart rate (108). Recent studies showed that intracerebroventricular GLP-1 administration was associated with improved learning in rats and also displayed neuroprotective effects (109,110), and GLP-1 has been proposed as a new therapeutic agent for neuro-degenerative diseases, including Alzheimer's disease (111).

The functions of GLP-1 in the lungs are unclear, although it has been reported to increase the secretion of macromolecules from the neuroendocrine cells (112).

ACTIONS OF GLP-2

The actions of GLP-2 remained elusive for some time until Drucker et al. (113) observed mucosal hypertrophy in mice carrying proglucagon-producing tumors with an intestinal processing pattern. In a subsequent systematic study of the effects of the various proglucagon products, GLP-2 was found to be capable of producing a similar mucosal growth. GLP-2 presumably activates its receptor on either neuronal cells (51) or subepithelial myofibroblast (52), which in turn produce growth factors that cause mucosal growth. GLP-2 enhances enterocyte proliferation as well as inhibits enterocyte apoptosis and thereby produces a pronounced growth of the epithelium (75). In addition, it may increase the expression of nutrient transporters and thereby augment the absorptive capacity of the gut (114). GLP-2 is currently thought be an important regulatory factor for adaptive intestinal growth (115). Recently, GLP-2 was also found to increase intestinal blood flow (116). The mechanism is unknown, but may be related to an increased intestinal metabolic rate. GLP-2 may also act as an enterogastrone hormone. Thus GLP-2 inhibits sham-feeding-induced acid secretion and may inhibit gastric emptying (117), but is not as potent as GLP-1 (118). Furthermore, as mentioned earlier, it may act to inhibit appetite and food intake upon release from brain stem neurons projecting to the ventromedial nuclei of the hypothalamus (49). Finally, recent studies have suggested that GLP-2 may be one of possibly several intestinal signals responsible for meal-induced regulation of bone resorption. In studies, where bone resorption was monitored by measurements of cross-linked fragments of collagen-1, the secretion of

GLP-1 and 2 was well correlated to meal-induced inhibition of resorption (119), and upon subcutaneous administration GLP-2 caused a similar reduction of bone resorption (120).

EFFECTS OF GLP-1 ON INSULIN ACTION

After the incretin functions of GLP-1 were established in humans (121) and the hormone was demonstrated to be capable of normalizing the elevated plasma glucose levels in patients with type 2 diabetes (122), several studies were carried out to elucidate in more detail its mechanisms of action. Hvidberg et al. (123) studied glucose turnover in fasting healthy subjects in response to physiological and supraphysiological infusions of GLP-1 and found that insulin secretion was enhanced and glucagon secretion inhibited. Concomitantly, hepatic glucose production was inhibited, and therefore the plasma glucose concentration fell by about 1 mmol/l. Glucose clearance was also increased, but this was interpreted to be a consequence of the increased insulin concentrations.

The role of glucagon was studied further in subjects with type 1 diabetes and no residual beta-cell function (124). In these subjects, an infusion of GLP-1 significantly lowered fasting glucose levels, concurrently with a marked lowering of plasma glucagon concentrations. It was concluded that the glucose-lowering action in this case was due to a decreased hepatic glucose production resulting from decreased glucagon secretion. D'Alessio et al. (125) found in a study involving the minimal model approach that GLP-1 was capable of increasing glucose effectiveness (glucose-mediated glucose-uptake) in healthy subjects by a mechanism independent of insulin secretion. However, the validity of the chosen approach has been questioned because insulin secretion was markedly stimulated in the GLP-1 experiment, but not in the control experiment. A valid control experiment would involve infusion of insulin to similar levels as those obtained during GLP-1 infusion (ideally identical intraportal concentrations).

In further studies, Toft-Nielsen et al. (126) administered GLP-1 to healthy subjects with or without concomitant infusion of 500 ug/h somatostatin. Glucose elimination was then studied by an intravenous glucose tolerance test. It turned out that, even with this dose of somatostatin, insulin (and C-peptide) was still slightly stimulated by GLP-1. In agreement with this, the glucose elimination rate, Kg, was increased by GLP-1. Fortuitously, the results of this experiment documented the exquisite sensitivity of the approach. The somatostatin infusion rate was then increased to 1,000 ug/h, and now insulin secretion remained constant. In this case, there was no change of Kg during GLP-1 administration, and it was concluded that GLP-1 had no direct effect on glucose uptake by the peripheral tissues (or at least that the effect must be quantitatively very small).

Subsequently, the effects of physiological elevations of GLP-1 or saline infusions on insulin-stimulated glucose uptake were studied in human volunteers by the euglycemic hyperinsulinemic clamp technique (127). In addition, somatostatin was administered to lock insulin secretion, whereas basal glucagon and growth hormone levels were maintained by intravenous infusion. Furthermore, glucose turnover rates were evaluated by a tracer technique. However, there were no differences between GLP-1 and saline infusions with respect to any parameter studied, including glucose infusion rate, glucose appearance and disappearance rates, and forearm arteriovenous glucose differences.

Vella et al. studied the effects of pharmacological doses of both the GLP-1 receptor agonist, exendin 4, and the native peptide in healthy subjects in three-step hyperinsulinemic clamp experiments. Both peptides increased cortisol secretion, but neither influenced insulin action (128). In further studies, GLP-1 was infused in supraphysiological amounts to patients with type 2 diabetes, and insulin sensitivity was estimated using clamp techniques (129). However, also in these experiments, there was no effect of GLP-1 on insulin sensitivity. In further studies, Vella et al. (130) infused pharmacological (treatment-relevant) doses of GLP-1 or saline to subjects with type 2 diabetes while at the same time infusing glucose to typical postprandial glucose concentrations and clamping insulin and glucagon levels at basal or postprandial levels. Under these conditions, GLP-1 had no influence on glucose disappearance or suppression of endogenous glucose production. On the basis of all these studies, it seems justified to conclude that GLP-1 has very little acute effect on insulin-dependent and -independent glucose turnover when its effects on the endocrine pancreas are prevented.

Zander et al. (108) infused GLP-1 or saline continuously for 6 weeks to patients with type 2 diabetes and determined insulin sensitivity by hyperinsulinemic euglycemic clamps before and after the treatment. Insulin sensitivity was unchanged in the saline-treated group, but was almost doubled in the GLP-1-treated group. The study was not designed to elucidate the underlying mechanisms, but it should be noted that GLP-1 was administered during the clamp (and actually resulted in a slightly higher insulin level), and that the GLP-1-treated subjects experienced markedly improved glycemic control as well as lower FFA levels and also lost about 2 kg of body weight. The weight loss as well as decreased gluco- and lipotoxicity induced by GLP-1 were considered likely explanations for the improved insulin sensitivity.

Similar findings were made in a study involving three months of continuous subcutaneous infusion of GLP-1 to diabetic subjects (131). However, the same group reported acute augmentation by GLP-1 of insulin-mediated glucose uptake in elderly patients with diabetes (132) and also reported insulin-mimetic effects of GLP-1 in obese subjects compared to nonobese matched controls (133). Nevertheless, the same group was unable to identify effects of GLP-1 on insulin-mediated glucose uptake in patients with type 1 diabetes (134).

D'Alessio et al., who were the first to suggest extrapancreatic metabolic effects of GLP-1 in humans (125), later studied eight healthy subjects using somatostatin clamp and tracer techniques similar to those employed by Orskov et al. (127) and reported a 17% decrease in the rate of glucose appearance, resulting in a lower blood glucose, and concluded that GLP-1 had extrapancreatic metabolic effects, possibly mediated via intraportal GLP-1 receptors (see below). As already discussed, it may be difficult to control GLP-1-stimulated insulin secretion with somatostatin, and the significance of these findings cannot be settled presently.

However, in contrast to the human studies, several mainly in vitro studies support that GLP-1 may have effects on peripheral tissues and/or the liver that are independent of its effects on the islet hormones. Thus, it has been claimed that membranes from human adipose tissue express GLP-1 receptors (135), and similar findings have been reported for rats (136). GLP-1 was also reported to enhance fatty acid synthesis in explants of rat adipose tissue (137) and was reported to enhance insulin-stimulated glucose uptake in 3T3-L1 adipocytes (138,139). The same group provided evidence that the responsible receptor differed from the GLP-1 receptor (140).

Nevertheless, in careful studies involving direct determination of lipolysis rates in human subcutaneous tissue, Bertin et al. were unable to find any effects of GLP-1 (141). GLP-1 receptors have also been claimed to be present in rat skeletal muscle (142), and were reported to stimulate glucose metabolism in human myocytes (143). Similar observations were made in studies of L6 myotubes, and again there was evidence that the effects were transmitted via receptors distinct from the classical GLP-1 receptor (144). Most recently, GLP-1 was again reported to enhance glucose uptake in human myocytes, and evidence for the involved signaling pathways was provided (145).

It should be mentioned that other studies failed to identify actions of GLP-1 on glucose metabolism in muscle tissue (146). Some of the cited studies suggested that GLP-1 may activate more than one receptor. Additional evidence includes a study of the enterogastrone of effects of GLP-1 and PYY in dogs, where the GLP-1 receptor antagonist, exendin 9-39, was incapable of blocking the inhibitory actions of GLP-1 (147), suggesting that another receptor was involved. Furthermore, the local paracrine actions of GLP-1 in the canine ileum could not be blocked by exendin 9-39 (148). The effects of intraportal GLP-1 on impulse traffic in vagal afferent sensory nerve fibers were also resistant to exendin 9-39 (149).

The liver has repeatedly been reported to be a target for GLP-1, although initial careful studies indicated that hepatocytes did not express GLP-1 receptor (150). Thus, GLP-1 has been reported to bind to rat hepatic membranes but without influencing adenylate cyclase activity, as expected from the classical GLP-1 receptor (151). Rather, inositolphosphoglycans were thought to act as mediators (152). Subsequently, the same group described activation of PI3K/PKB, PKC, and PP-1 pathways to transmit the actions on glycogen synthase in rat hepatocytes (153). A Japanese group reported inhibition of glucagon-induced glycogenolysis in isolated perivenous rat hepatocytes (154). Along the same lines, some studies have reported effects of exendin 4 that are not shared by GLP-1. Thus, exendin 4, but not GLP-1, was reported to enhance insulin sensitivity in 3T3 adipocytes (155). The two peptides were also reported to activate different signaling pathways in human myotubes (145). Again, it should be noted that these in vitro studies are in sharp contrast to the in vivo studies, particularly in humans, as discussed earlier.

Several reports have suggested that GLP-1 may interact with a portal GLP-1 sensor, which in turn may reflexively influence glucose metabolism. As mentioned, intraportal administration of GLP-1 to rats increases impulse traffic in sensory vagal afferents (84), and may reflexively activate efferent vagal fibers to the pancreas (85). Similarly, administration of a ganglionic blocker completely abolished the augmenting effect on insulin secretion of intraportal GLP-1 given together with glucose to levels corresponding to those obtained with glucose alone (86). In mice, a hepatoportal glucose sensor has been described that, when activated, influences peripheral glucose disposal (156). This sensing mechanism appears to involve a functional GLP-1 receptor, since its effects on peripheral glucose disposal are abrogated by exendin 9-39 and cannot be demonstrated in GLP-1 receptor knockout mice. Similarly, intraportal GLP-1 administration to dogs was reported to increase nonhepatic glucose disposal (157), but subsequent studies by the same group indicated that both intraportally and peripherally administered GLP-1 increased glucose disposal in the liver independent of insulin secretion (158). Similar to the findings in mice, intraportal GLP-1 and glucose infusions in dogs were found to decrease peripheral glucose levels independently of hyperinsulinemia (159). However, it should be noted that peripheral administration of GLP-1 to dogs at a similar rate is claimed not to enhance glucose-induced insulin secretion in this species (R.N. Bergman, personal communication). This is again in sharp contrast to very consistent findings in humans (121,123), and therefore suggests that dogs (and possibly mice) differ radically from humans in this respect.

PATHOPHYSIOLOGICAL IMPLICATIONS

Disturbances in L-Cell Secretion

Meal-induced secretion of GLP-1 is clearly decreased in patients with type 2 diabetes (160) and it is likely that this decrease contributes to the severely impaired incretin effect seen in these patients and thereby also to their impaired insulin secretion (59). Part of the reason why GLP-1 secretion is decreased may be the lower secretion often seen in obesity (160). In patients with severe obesity, GLP-1 responses to meal ingestion may be almost eliminated (161). Since GLP-1 inhibits appetite, the impaired secretion may contribute to or aggravate the development of obesity. As discussed above, GLP-1 secretion is related to gastric emptying rate, and in patients with accelerated gastric emptying, GLP-1 secretion may be excessive (26). Several lines of evidence suggest that excessive GLP-1 secretion may be responsible for the occurrence of postprandial reactive hypoglycemia in such patients (162,163). Thus, accelerated gastric emptying causes high postprandial glucose concentrations coinciding with high GLP-1 concentrations, resulting in exaggerated insulin secretion, which in turn causes hypoglycemia. Inhibition of glucagon secretion may contribute (163). Most recently, patients have been reported with severe hypoglycemia after Roux-en-Y gastric bypass operations for obesity. These patients had very high postprandial levels of GLP-1 (164).

Tumors producing proglucagon products generally exhibit a pancreatic processing pattern, and the resulting glucagonoma syndrome is due to the excessive secretion of glucagon (165). However, in some cases an intestinal processing pattern is observed and in these patients the most dramatic clinical symptoms (intestinal obstruction) are due to intestinal mucosal hyperplasia, likely to be a consequence of increased secretion of GLP-2.

Therapeutic Application of Proglucagon-Derived Peptides

The actions of GLP-1 have attracted great interest, because almost all of them are considered to be beneficial in patients with type 2 diabetes (166). Indeed, infusions of GLP-1 completely normalize fasting blood glucose concentrations in virtually all patients with type 2 diabetes investigated (167). In clinical studies where GLP-1 was administered by continuous subcutaneous infusion for six weeks, blood glucose levels were greatly reduced, blood lipids improved, body weight was reduced, and beta-cell secretory capacity and insulin sensitivity increased (168). Single subcutaneous injections, however, are ineffective because of rapid degradation of the peptide by DPP-IV. In order to exploit the effects of GLP-1 receptor activation, several pharmaceutical companies have developed resistant analogs of GLP-1 or activators of the receptor. One of these is exendin-4, a peptide of 39 amino acids isolated from the salivary secretions of the lizard, *Heloderma suspectum*, which is 53% homologous with GLP-1 (with respect to the sequence of the first 30 amino acids) and is a full agonist of the GLP-1 receptor (169). This peptide is resistant to the actions of DPP-IV and is cleared by the kidneys by glomerular filtration, resulting in a plasma half-life of about 30 min (170). Single subcutaneous injections, therefore, result in a plasma exposure lasting 6–8 hours. Patients with type 2 diabetes have now been treated for more than two years with exendin-4 (designated *exenatide* in its synthetic form, and now registered as a drug for diabetes treatment under the name of Byetta by the Amylin Corporation and Eli Lilly in collaboration), and the most conspicuous effects are a sustained reduction of glycated hemoglobinA1c levels (a measure of the average blood glucose levels) to about 7%, a recommended target, and a continued weight loss amounting to 8 kg on average (www. amylin.com). Other preparations, currently under clinical development, generally show similar effects although not yet documented for a similar time span.

An alternative approach is inhibition of the enzyme DPP-IV (171). Unlike the GLP-1 agonists or analogs, DPP-IV inhibitors are small molecules that are orally available. DPP-IV inhibition increases the levels of intact GLP-1 and thereby amplifies the action of the endogenous hormone, presumably with respect to both insulin and glucagon secretion. DPP-IV inhibitors are currently in late-stage clinical development. One of them, Vildagliptin (developed by Novartis), has been given for 52 weeks to patients failing on their usual therapy with metformin, a biguanide (172). This resulted in reductions of hemoglobinA1c levels to about 7% (whereas levels increased in a placebo-treated control group), and meal-stimulated insulin secretion increased in the treated group but fell in the control group, suggesting a protective effect on beta-cell function of the inhibitor. The first inhibitor (Sitagliptin or Januvia from Merck) has just been filed for registration at the FDA. It is of interest that both beta-cell function and insulin sensitivity were progressively improved by the treatment (173).

Because of its intestinotrophic activities, GLP-2 is currently being investigated as a therapy for intestinal insufficiency. Because of its much slower metabolism compared to GLP-1, GLP-2 can be used in its natural form and has been demonstrated to enhance intestinal absorption and increase lean body weight in patients with short-bowel syndrome in the course of a five-week study with two daily subcutaneous injections (174). A DPP-IV-resistant analog may be produced by substitution of amino acid residue number 2 (with Gly) and has been shown to have similar but prolonged effects (175). Studies in experimental animals have supported that GLP-2 may also be effective in the therapy of intestinal atrophy after parenteral nutrition, and in intestinal failure after experimental enteritis and after radiation and chemotherapy (176). GLP-2 is also currently investigated as a therapy for osteoporosis, and was most recently demonstrated to be able to strongly reduce the nightly increase in bone resorption in postmenopausal women (120). GLP-2 has no known effects on insulin action or insulin sensitivity.

REFERENCES

1. Holst JJ. Gut glucagon, enteroglucagon, gut glucagonlike immunoreactivity, glicentin: Current status. *Gastroenterology* 1983; 84(6):1602–1613.
2. Thim L, Moody AJ. The primary structure of porcine glicentin (proglucagon). *Regul Pept* 1981 May; 2(2):139–150.
3. Bataille D, Tatemoto K, Gespach C, Jornvall H, Rosselin G, Mutt V. Isolation of glucagon-37 (bioactive enteroglucagon/oxyntomodulin) from porcine jejuno-ileum: Characterization of the peptide. *FEBS Lett* 1982 Sep 6; 146(1):79–86.
4. Moody AJ, Holst JJ, Thim L, Jensen SL. Relationship of glicentin to proglucagon and glucagon in the porcine pancreas. *Nature* 1981; 289(5797):514–516.

5. Lund PK, Goodman RH, Dee PC, Habener JF. Pancreatic preproglucagon cDNA contains two glucagon-related coding sequences arranged in tandem. *Proc Natl Acad Sci USA* 1982; 79(2):345–349.

6. Bell GI, Sanchez-Pescador R, Laybourn PJ, Najarian RC. Exon duplication and divergence in the human preproglucagon gene. *Nature* 1983; 304(5924):368–371.

7. Irwin DM, Wong J. Trout and chicken proglucagon: Alternative splicing generates mRNA transcripts encoding glucagon-like peptide 2. *Mol Endocrinol* 1995 Mar; 9(3):267–277.

8. Mojsov S, Heinrich G, Wilson IB, Ravazzola M, Orci L, Habener JF. Preproglucagon gene expression in pancreas and intestine diversifies at the level of post-translational processing. *J Biol Chem* 1986; 261(25):11880–11889.

9. Orskov C, Holst JJ, Knuhtsen S, Baldissera FG, Poulsen SS, Nielsen OV. Glucagon-like peptides GLP-1 and GLP-2, predicted products of the glucagon gene, are secreted separately from pig small intestine but not pancreas. *Endocrinology* 1986 Oct; 119(4):1467–1475.

10. Holst JJ, Bersani M, Johnsen AH, Kofod H, Hartmann B, Orskov C. Proglucagon processing in porcine and human pancreas. *J Biol Chem* 1994; 269(29):18827–18833.

11. Orskov C, Bersani M, Johnsen AH, Hojrup P, Holst JJ. Complete sequences of glucagon-like peptide-1 from human and pig small intestine. *J Biol Chem* 1989 Aug 5; 264(22):12826–12829.

12. Hartmann B, Johnsen AH, Orskov C, Adelhorst K, Thim L, Holst JJ. Structure, measurement, and secretion of human glucagon-like peptide-2. *Peptides* 2000 Jan; 21(1):73–80.

13. Ugleholdt R, Zhu X, Deacon CF, Orskov C, Steiner DF, Holst JJ. Impaired intestinal proglucagon processing in mice lacking prohormone convertase 1. *Endocrinology* 2004 Mar; 145(3): 1349–1355.

14. Furuta M, Yano H, Zhou A, Rouille Y, Holst JJ, Carroll R et al. Defective prohormone processing and altered pancreatic islet morphology in mice lacking active SPC2. *Proc Natl Acad Sci USA* 1997 Jun 24; 94(13):6646–6651.

15. Holst JJ, Orskov C, Nielsen OV, Schwartz TW. Truncated glucagon-like peptide I: An insulin-releasing hormone from the distal gut. *FEBS Lett* 1987; 211(2):169–174.

16. Larsen PJ, Tang-Christensen M, Holst JJ, Orskov C. Distribution of glucagon-like peptide-1 and other preproglucagon-derived peptides in the rat hypothalamus and brainstem. *Neuroscience* 1997 Mar; 77(1):257–270.

17. Eissele R, Goke R, Willemer S, Harthus HP, Vermeer H, Arnold R et al. Glucagon-like peptide-1 cells in the gastrointestinal tract and pancreas of rat, pig and man. *Eur J Clin Invest* 1992; 22(4):283–291.

18. Sundler F, Alumets J, Holst J, Larsson LI, Hakanson R. Ultrastructural identification of cells storing pancreatic-type glucagon in dog stomach. *Histochemistry* 1976; 50(1):33–37.

19. Larsson LI, Holst J, Hakanson R, Sundler F. Distribution and properties of glucagon immunoreactivity in the digestive tract of various mammals: An immunohistochemical and immunochemical study. *Histochemistry* 1975; 44(4):281–290.

20. Mortensen K, Christensen LL, Holst JJ, Orskov C. GLP-1 and GIP are colocalized in a subset of endocrine cells in the small intestine. *Regul Pept* 2003 Jul 15; 114(2–3):189–196.

21. Knudsen JB, Holst JJ, Asnaes S, Johansen A. Identification of cells with pancreatic-type and gut-type glucagon immunoreactivity in the human colon. *Acta Pathol Microbiol Scand [A]* 1975; 83(6):741–743.

22. Holst JJ. Enteroglucagon. *Annu Rev Physiol* 1997; 59:257–271.

23. Gribble FM, Williams L, Simpson AK, Reimann F. A novel glucose-sensing mechanism contributing to glucagon-like peptide-1 secretion from the GLUTag cell line. *Diabetes* 2003 May; 52(5):1147–1154.

24. Hirasawa A, Tsumaya K, Awaji T, Katsuma S, Adachi T, Yamada M et al. Free fatty acids regulate gut incretin glucagon-like peptide-1 secretion through GPR120. *Nat Med* 2005 Jan; 11(1):90–94.

25. Vilsboll T, Krarup T, Sonne J, Madsbad S, Volund A, Juul AG et al. Incretin secretion in relation to meal size and body weight in healthy subjects and people with type 1 and type 2 diabetes mellitus. *J Clin Endocrinol Metab* 2003 Jun; 88(6):2706–2713.

26. Miholic J, Orskov C, Holst JJ, Kotzerke J, Meyer HJ. Emptying of the gastric substitute, glucagon-like peptide-1 (GLP-1), and reactive hypoglycemia after total gastrectomy. *Dig Dis Sci* 1991; 36(10):1361–1370.

27. Hansen L, Holst JJ. The effects of duodenal peptides on glucagon-like peptide-1 secretion from the ileum: A duodeno-ileal loop? *Regul Pept* 2002 Dec 31; 110(1):39–45.

28. Hansen L, Lampert S, Mineo H, Holst JJ. Neural regulation of glucagon-like peptide-1 secretion in pigs. *Am J Physiol Endocrinol Metab* 2004 Nov; 287(5):E939–E947.

29. Hansen L, Hartmann B, Bisgaard T, Mineo H, Jørgensen PN, Holst JJ. Somatostatin restrains the secretion of glucagon-like peptide-1 and 2 from isolated perfused porcine ileum. *Am J Physiol* 2000; 278(6):E1010–E1018.

30. Hansen L, Hartmann B, Mineo H, Holst JJ. Glucagon-like peptide-1 secretion is influenced by perfusate glucose concentration and by a feedback mechanism involving somatostatin in isolated perfused porcine ileum. *Regul Pept* 2004 Apr 15; 118(1–2):11–18.

31. Deacon CF, Pridal L, Klarskov L, Olesen M, Holst JJ. Glucagon-like peptide 1 undergoes differential tissue-specific metabolism in the anesthetized pig. *Am J Physiol* 1996 Sep; 271(3, pt. 1): E458–E464.

32. Trebbien R, Klarskov L, Olesen M, Holst JJ, Carr RD, Deacon CF. Neutral endopeptidase 24.11 is important for the degradation of both endogenous and exogenous glucagon in anesthetized pigs. *Am J Physiol Endocrinol Metab* 2004 Sep; 287(3):E431–E438.

33. Deacon CF, Johnsen AH, Holst JJ. Degradation of glucagon-like peptide-1 by human plasma in vitro yields an N-terminally truncated peptide that is a major endogenous metabolite in vivo. *J Clin Endocrinol Metab* 1995; 80(3):952–957.

34. Hartmann B, Harr MB, Jeppesen PB, Wojdemann M, Deacon CF, Mortensen PB et al. In vivo and in vitro degradation of glucagon-like peptide-2 in humans. *J Clin Endocrinol Metab* 2000 Aug; 85(8):2884–2888.

35. Vilsboll T, Agerso H, Krarup T, Holst JJ. Similar elimination rates of glucagon-like peptide-1 in obese type 2 diabetic patients and healthy subjects. *J Clin Endocrinol Metab* 2003 Jan; 88(1): 220–224.

36. Hansen L, Deacon CF, Orskov C, Holst JJ. Glucagon-like peptide-1-(7-36)amide is transformed to glucagon-like peptide-1-(9-36)amide by dipeptidyl peptidase IV in the capillaries supplying the L cells of the porcine intestine. *Endocrinology* 1999 Nov; 140(11):5356–5363.

37. Meier JJ, Nauck MA, Kranz D, Holst JJ, Deacon CF, Gaeckler D et al. Secretion, degradation, and elimination of glucagon-like peptide 1 and gastric inhibitory polypeptide in patients with chronic renal insufficiency and healthy control subjects. *Diabetes* 2004 Mar; 53(3):654–662.

38. Plamboeck A, Holst JJ, Carr RD, Deacon CF. Neutral endopeptidase 24.11 and dipeptidyl peptidase IV are both mediators of the degradation of glucagon-like peptide 1 in the anaesthetised pig. *Diabetologia* 2005 Sep; 48(9):1882–1890.

39. Baldissera FG, Holst JJ, Knuhtsen S, Hilsted L, Nielsen OV. Oxyntomodulin (glicentin-(33-69)): Pharmacokinetics, binding to liver cell membranes, effects on isolated perfused pig pancreas, and secretion from isolated perfused lower small intestine of pigs. *Regul Pept* 1988; 21(1–2):151–166.

40. Gros L, Hollande F, Thorens B, Kervran A, Bataille D. Comparative effects of GLP-1-(7-36) amide, oxyntomodulin and glucagon on rabbit gastric parietal cell function. *Eur J Pharmacol* 1995; 288(3):319–327.

41. Thorens B. Expression cloning of the pancreatic beta cell receptor for the gluco-incretin hormone glucagon-like peptide 1. *Proc Natl Acad Sci USA* 1992 Sep 15; 89(18):8641–8645.

42. Mayo KE, Miller LJ, Bataille D, Dalle S, Goke B, Thorens B et al. International Union of Pharmacology: XXXV. The glucagon receptor family. *Pharmacol Rev* 2003 Mar; 55(1):167–194.

43. Bullock BP, Heller RS, Habener JF. Tissue distribution of messenger ribonucleic acid encoding the rat glucagon-like peptide-1 receptor. *Endocrinology* 1996; 137(7):2968–2978.

44. Heller RS, Kieffer TJ, Habener JF. Insulinotropic glucagon-like peptide I receptor expression in glucagon-producing alpha-cells of the rat endocrine pancreas. *Diabetes* 1997; 46(5):785–791.

45. Nakagawa A, Satake H, Nakabayashi H, Nishizawa M, Furuya K, Nakano S et al. Receptor gene expression of glucagon-like peptide-1, but not glucose-dependent insulinotropic polypeptide, in rat nodose ganglion cells. *Auton Neurosci* 2004 Jan 30; 110(1):36–43.

46. Goke R, Larsen PJ, Mikkelsen JD, Sheikh SP. Distribution of GLP-1 binding sites in the rat brain: Evidence that exendin-4 is a ligand of brain GLP-1 binding sites. *Eur J Neurosci* 1995; 7(11):2294–2300.

47. Orskov C, Poulsen SS, Moller M, Holst JJ. Glucagon-like peptide I receptors in the subfornical organ and the area postrema are accessible to circulating glucagon-like peptide I. *Diabetes* 1996 Jun; 45(6):832–835.

48. Munroe DG, Gupta AK, Kooshesh F, Vyas TB, Rizkalla G, Wang H et al. Prototypic G protein-coupled receptor for the intestinotrophic factor glucagon-like peptide 2. *Proc Natl Acad Sci USA* 1999 Feb 16; 96(4):1569–1573.
49. Tang-Christensen M, Larsen PJ, Thulesen J, Romer J, Vrang N. The proglucagon-derived peptide, glucagon-like peptide-2, is a neurotransmitter involved in the regulation of food intake. *Nat Med* 2000 Jul; 6(7):802–807.
50. Yusta B, Huang L, Munroe D, Wolff G, Fantaske R, Sharma S et al. Enteroendocrine localization of GLP-2 receptor expression in humans and rodents. *Gastroenterology* 2000 Sep; 119(3):744–755.
51. Bjerknes M, Cheng H. Modulation of specific intestinal epithelial progenitors by enteric neurons. *Proc Natl Acad Sci USA* 2001 Oct 23; 98(22):12497–12502.
52. Orskov C, Hartmann B, Poulsen SS, Thulesen J, Hare KJ, Holst JJ. GLP-2 stimulates colonic growth via KGF, released by subepithelial myofibroblasts with GLP-2 receptors. *Regul Pept* 2005 Jan 15; 124(1–3):105–112.
53. Kirkegaard P, Moody AJ, Holst JJ, Loud FB, Olsen PS, Christiansen J. Glicentin inhibits gastric acid secretion in the rat. *Nature* 1982; 297(5862):156–157.
54. Schjoldager B, Mortensen PE, Myhre J, Christiansen J, Holst JJ. Oxyntomodulin from distal gut: Role in regulation of gastric and pancreatic functions. *Dig Dis Sci* 1989; 34(9):1411–1419.
55. Holst JJ. Molecular heterogeneity of glucagon in normal subjects and in patients with glucagon-producing tumours. *Diabetologia* 1983; 24(5):359–365.
56. Dakin CL, Gunn I, Small CJ, Edwards CM, Hay DL, Smith DM et al. Oxyntomodulin inhibits food intake in the rat. *Endocrinology* 2001 Oct; 142(10):4244–4250.
57. Dakin CL, Small CJ, Park AJ, Seth A, Ghatei MA, Bloom SR. Repeated ICV administration of oxyntomodulin causes a greater reduction in body weight gain than in pair-fed rats. *Am J Physiol Endocrinol Metab* 2002 Dec; 283(6):E1173–E1177.
58. Holst JJ, Gromada J. Role of incretin hormones in the regulation of insulin secretion in diabetic and nondiabetic humans. *Am J Physiol Endocrinol Metab* 2004 Aug; 287(2):E199–E206.
59. Vilsboll T, Holst JJ. Incretins, insulin secretion and Type 2 diabetes mellitus. *Diabetologia* 2004 Mar; 47(3):357–366.
60. Hansotia T, Baggio LL, Delmeire D, Hinke SA, Yamada Y, Tsukiyama K et al. Double incretin receptor knockout (DIRKO) mice reveal an essential role for the enteroinsular axis in transducing the glucoregulatory actions of DPP-IV inhibitors. *Diabetes* 2004 May; 53(5):1326–1335.
61. Holst JJ. Glucagon-like peptide 1(GLP-1): An intestinal hormone signalling nutritional abundance, with an unusual therapeutic potential. *Trends Endocrinol Metab* 1999; 10(6):229–234.
62. Fehmann HC, Habener JF. Insulinotropic hormone glucagon-like peptide-I(7-37) stimulation of proinsulin gene expression and proinsulin biosynthesis in insulinoma beta TC-1 cells. *Endocrinology* 1992; 130(1):159–166.
63. Holz GG. Epac: A new cAMP-binding protein in support of glucagon-like peptide-1 receptor-mediated signal transduction in the pancreatic beta-cell. *Diabetes* 2004 Jan; 53(1):5–13.
64. Kemp DM, Habener JF. Insulinotropic hormone glucagon-like peptide 1 (GLP-1) activation of insulin gene promoter inhibited by p38 mitogen-activated protein kinase. *Endocrinology* 2001 Mar; 142(3):1179–1187.
65. Li Y, Cao X, Li LX, Brubaker PL, Edlund H, Drucker DJ. Beta-cell Pdx1 expression is essential for the glucoregulatory, proliferative, and cytoprotective actions of glucagon-like peptide-1. *Diabetes* 2005 Feb; 54(2):482–491.
66. Buteau J, Roduit R, Susini S, Prentki M. Glucagon-like peptide-1 promotes DNA synthesis, activates phosphatidylinositol 3-kinase and increases transcription factor pancreatic and duodenal homeobox gene 1 (PDX-1) DNA binding activity in beta (INS-1)-cells. *Diabetologia* 1999 Jul; 42(7):856–864.
67. Holz GH, Kuhtreiber WM, Habener JF. Induction of glucose competence in pancreatic beta cells by glucagon-like peptide-1(7-37). *Trans Assoc Am Physicians* 1992; 105:260–267.
68. Gromada J, Holst JJ, Rorsman P. Cellular regulation of islet hormone secretion by the incretin hormone glucagon-like peptide 1. *Pflugers Arch* 1998 Apr; 435(5):583–594.
69. Flamez D, Van Breusegem A, Scrocchi LA, Quartier E, Pipeleers D, Drucker DJ et al. Mouse pancreatic beta-cells exhibit preserved glucose competence after disruption of the glucagon-like peptide-1 receptor gene. *Diabetes* 1998 Apr; 47(4):646–652.
70. Egan JM, Bulotta A, Hui H, Perfetti R. GLP-1 receptor agonists are growth and differentiation factors for pancreatic islet beta cells. *Diabetes Metab Res Rev* 2003 Mar; 19(2):115–123.

71. Xu G, Stoffers DA, Habener JF, Bonner-Weir S. Exendin-4 stimulates both beta-cell replication and neogenesis, resulting in increased beta-cell mass and improved glucose tolerance in diabetic rats. *Diabetes* 1999 Dec; 48(12):2270–2276.

72. Stoffers DA, Kieffer TJ, Hussain MA, Drucker DJ, Bonner-Weir S, Habener JF et al. Insulinotropic glucagon-like peptide 1 agonists stimulate expression of homeodomain protein IDX-1 and increase islet size in mouse pancreas. *Diabetes* 2000 May; 49(5):741–748.

73. Zhou J, Wang X, Pineyro MA, Egan JM. Glucagon-like peptide 1 and exendin-4 convert pancreatic AR42 J cells into glucagon- and insulin-producing cells. *Diabetes* 1999 Dec; 48(12):2358–2366.

74. Buteau J, El-Assaad W, Rhodes CJ, Rosenberg L, Joly E, Prentki M. Glucagon-like peptide-1 prevents beta cell glucolipotoxicity. *Diabetologia* 2004 May; 47(5):806–815.

75. Brubaker PL, Drucker DJ. Minireview: Glucagon-like peptides regulate cell proliferation and apoptosis in the pancreas, gut, and central nervous system. *Endocrinology* 2004 Jun; 145(6):2653–2659.

76. Sinclair EM, Drucker DJ. Proglucagon-derived peptides: Mechanisms of action and therapeutic potential. *Physiology (Bethesda)* 2005 Oct; 20:357–365.

77. Orskov C, Holst JJ, Nielsen OV. Effect of truncated glucagon-like peptide-1 [proglucagon-(78-107) amide] on endocrine secretion from pig pancreas, antrum, and nonantral stomach. *Endocrinology* 1988; 123(4):2009–2013.

78. Ishihara H, Maechler P, Gjinovci A, Herrera PL, Wollheim CB. Islet beta-cell secretion determines glucagon release from neighbouring alpha-cells. *Nat Cell Biol* 2003 Apr; 5(4):330–335.

79. Wettergren A, Schjoldager B, Mortensen PE, Myhre J, Christiansen J, Holst JJ. Truncated GLP-1 (proglucagon 78-107-amide) inhibits gastric and pancreatic functions in man. *Dig Dis Sci* 1993; 38(4):665–673.

80. Nauck MA, Niedereichholz U, Ettler R, Holst JJ, Orskov C, Ritzel R et al. Glucagon-like peptide 1 inhibition of gastric emptying outweighs its insulinotropic effects in healthy humans. *Am J Physiol* 1997 Nov; 273(5, pt. 1):E981–E988.

81. Nauck MA, Niedereichholz U, Ettler R, Holst JJ, Orskov C, Ritzel R, Schmiegel WH. Glucagon-like peptide 1 inhibition of gastric emptying outweighs its insulinotropic effects in healthy humans. *Am J Physiol* 1997; 273(5 Pt 1):E981–E988.

82. Layer P, Holst JJ, Grandt D, Goebell H. Ileal release of glucagon-like peptide-1 (GLP-1): Association with inhibition of gastric acid secretion in humans. *Dig Dis Sci* 1995; 40(5):1074–1082.

83. Schirra J, Nicolaus M, Roggel R, Katschinski M, Storr M, Woerle HJ et al. Endogenous glucagon-like peptide 1 controls endocrine pancreatic secretion and antro-pyloro-duodenal motility in humans. *Gut* 2006 Feb; 55(2):243–251.

84. Nishizawa M, Nakabayashi H, Uchida K, Nakagawa A, Niijima A. The hepatic vagal nerve is receptive to incretin hormone glucagon-like peptide-1, but not to glucose-dependent insulinotropic polypeptide, in the portal vein. *J Auton Nerv Syst* 1996; 61(2):149–154.

85. Nakabayashi H, Nishizawa M, Nakagawa A, Takeda R, Niijima A. Vagal hepatopancreatic reflex effect evoked by intraportal appearance of tGLP-1. *Am J Physiol* 1996 Nov; 271(5, pt. 1): E808–E813.

86. Balkan B, Li X. Portal GLP-1 administration in rats augments the insulin response to glucose via neuronal mechanisms. *Am J Physiol Regul Integr Comp Physiol* 2000 Oct; 279(4):R1449–R1454.

87. Wettergren A, Wojdemann M, Holst JJ. Glucagon-like peptide-1 inhibits gastropancreatic function by inhibiting central parasympathetic outflow. *Am J Physiol* 1998 Nov; 275(5, pt. 1):G984–G992.

88. Imeryuz N, Yegen BC, Bozkurt A, Coskun T, Villanueva-Penacarrillo ML, Ulusoy NB. Glucagon-like peptide-1 inhibits gastric emptying via vagal afferent-mediated central mechanisms. *Am J Physiol* 1997 Oct; 273(4, pt. 1):G920–G927.

89. Read N, French S, Cunningham K. The role of the gut in regulation food intake in man. *Nutr Rev* 1994; 52(1):1–10.

90. Flint A, Raben A, Astrup A, Holst JJ. Glucagon-like peptide 1 promotes satiety and suppresses energy intake in humans. *J Clin Invest* 1998 Feb 1; 101(3):515–520.

91. Gutzwiller JP, Ke B, Drewe J, Hildebrand P, Ketterer S, Handschin D et al. Glucagon-like peptide-1: A potent regulator of food intake in humans. *Gut* 1999 Jan; 44(1):81–86.

92. Naslund E, Barkeling B, King N, Gutniak M, Blundell JE, Holst JJ et al. Energy intake and appetite are suppressed by glucagon-like peptide-1 (GLP-1) in obese men. *Int J Obes Relat Metab Disord* 1999 Mar; 23(3):304–311.

93. Gutzwiller JP, Drewe J, Goke B, Schmidt H, Rohrer B, Lareida J et al. Glucagon-like peptide-1 promotes satiety and reduces food intake in patients with diabetes mellitus type 2. *Am J Physiol* 1999 May; 276(5, pt. 2):R1541–R1544.
94. Verdich C, Flint A, Gutzwiller JP, Naslund E, Beglinger C, Hellstrom PM et al. A meta-analysis of the effect of glucagon-like peptide-1 (7-36) amide on ad libitum energy intake in humans. *J Clin Endocrinol Metab* 2001 Sep; 86(9):4382–4389.
95. Turton MD, O'Shea D, Gunn I, Beak SA, Edwards CM, Meeran K et al. A role for glucagon-like peptide-1 in the central regulation of feeding [see comments]. *Nature* 1996 Jan 4; 379(6560):69–72.
96. Tang-Christensen M, Larsen PJ, Goke R, Fink-Jensen A, Jessop DS, Moller M et al. Central administration of GLP-1-(7-36) amide inhibits food and water intake in rats. *Am J Physiol* 1996 Oct; 271(4, pt. 2):R848–R856.
97. Rinaman L. Interoceptive stress activates glucagon-like peptide-1 neurons that project to the hypothalamus. *Am J Physiol* 1999 Aug; 277(2, pt. 2):R582–R590.
98. Rinaman L. A functional role for central glucagon-like peptide-1 receptors in lithium chloride-induced anorexia. *Am J Physiol* 1999 Nov; 277(5, pt. 2):R1537–R1540.
99. Lachey JL, D'Alessio DA, Rinaman L, Elmquist JK, Drucker DJ, Seeley RJ. The role of central GLP-1 in mediating the effects of visceral illness: Differential effects in rats and mice. *Endocrinology* 2004 Sep 30.
100. Scrocchi LA, Brown TJ, MaClusky N, Brubaker PL, Auerbach AB, Joyner AL et al. Glucose intolerance but normal satiety in mice with a null mutation in the glucagon-like peptide 1 receptor gene. *Nat Med* 1996; 2(11):1254–1258.
101. Gros R, You X, Baggio LL, Kabir MG, Sadi AM, Mungrue IN et al. Cardiac function in mice lacking the glucagon-like peptide-1 receptor. *Endocrinology* 2003 Jun; 144(6):2242–2252.
102. Bose AK, Mocanu MM, Mensah KN, Brand CL, Carr RD, Yellon DM. GLP-1 protects schemic and reperfused myocardium via PI3Kinase and p42/p44 MAPK signalling pathways. *Diabetes* 2004; 53(suppl 2):A1. [Ref Type: Abstract.]
103. Nikolaidis LA, Mankad S, Sokos GG, Miske G, Shah A, Elahi D et al. Effects of glucagon-like peptide-1 in patients with acute myocardial infarction and left ventricular dysfunction after successful reperfusion. *Circulation* 2004 Mar 2; 109(8):962–965.
104. Nikolaidis LA, Elahi D, Hentosz T, Doverspike A, Huerbin R, Zourelias L et al. Recombinant glucagon-like peptide-1 increases myocardial glucose uptake and improves left ventricular performance in conscious dogs with pacing-induced dilated cardiomyopathy. *Circulation* 2004 Aug 24; 110(8):955–961.
105. Nystrom T, Gutniak MK, Zhang Q, Zhang F, Holst JJ, Ahren B et al. Effects of glucagon-like peptide-1 on endothelial function in type 2 diabetes patients with stable coronary artery disease. *Am J Physiol Endocrinol Metab* 2004 Dec; 287(6):E1209–E1215.
106. Yamamoto H, Lee CE, Marcus JN, Williams TD, Overton JM, Lopez ME et al. Glucagon-like peptide-1 receptor stimulation increases blood pressure and heart rate and activates autonomic regulatory neurons. *J Clin Invest* 2002 Jul; 110(1):43–52.
107. Yamamoto H, Kishi T, Lee CE, Choi BJ, Fang H, Hollenberg AN et al. Glucagon-like peptide-1-responsive catecholamine neurons in the area postrema link peripheral glucagon-like peptide-1 with central autonomic control sites. *J Neurosci* 2003 Apr 1; 23(7):2939–2946.
108. Zander M, Madsbad S, Madsen JL, Holst JJ. Effect of 6-week course of glucagon-like peptide 1 on glycaemic control, insulin sensitivity, and beta-cell function in type 2 diabetes: a parallel-group study. *Lancet* 2002 Mar 9; 359(9309):824–830.
109. Perry T, Haughey NJ, Mattson MP, Egan JM, Greig NH. Protection and reversal of excitotoxic neuronal damage by glucagon-like peptide-1 and exendin-4. *J Pharmacol Exp Ther* 2002 Sep; 302(3):881–888.
110. During MJ, Cao L, Zuzga DS, Francis JS, Fitzsimons HL, Jiao X et al. Glucagon-like peptide-1 receptor is involved in learning and neuroprotection. *Nat Med* 2003 Sep; 9(9):1173–1179.
111. Perry TA, Greig NH. A new Alzheimer's disease interventive strategy: GLP-1. *Curr Drug Targets* 2004 Aug; 5(6):565–571.
112. Richter G, Feddersen O, Wagner U, Barth P, Goke R, Goke B. GLP-1 stimulates secretion of macromolecules from airways and relaxes pulmonary artery. *Am J Physiol* 1993 Oct; 265(4, pt. 1): L374–L381.
113. Drucker DJ, Erlich P, Asa SL, Brubaker PL. Induction of intestinal epithelial proliferation by glucagon-like peptide 2. *Proc Natl Acad Sci USA* 1996 Jul 23; 93(15):7911–7916.

114. Cheeseman CI, O'Neill D. Basolateral D-glucose transport activity along the crypt-villus axis in rat jejunum and upregulation induced by gastric inhibitory peptide and glucagon-like peptide-2. *Exp Physiol* 1998 Sep; 83(5):605–616.

115. Drucker DJ. Glucagon-like peptides: Regulators of cell proliferation, differentiation, and apoptosis. *Mol Endocrinol* 2003 Feb; 17(2):161–171.

116. Guan X, Stoll B, Lu X, Tappenden KA, Holst JJ, Hartmann B et al. GLP-2-mediated up-regulation of intestinal blood flow and glucose uptake is nitric oxide-dependent in TPN-fed piglets 1. *Gastroenterology* 2003 Aug; 125(1):136–147.

117. Nagell CF, Wettergren A, Pedersen JF, Mortensen D, Holst JJ. Glucagon-like peptide-2 inhibits antral emptying in man, but is not as potent as glucagon-like peptide-1. *Scand J Gastroenterol* 2004 Apr; 39(4):353–358.

118. Wojdemann M, Wettergren A, Hartmann B, Hilsted L, Holst JJ. Inhibition of sham feeding-stimulated human gastric acid secretion by glucagon-like peptide-2. *J Clin Endocrinol Metab* 1999 Jul; 84(7):2513–2517.

119. Henriksen DB, Alexandersen P, Bjarnason NH, Vilsboll T, Hartmann B, Henriksen EE et al. Role of gastrointestinal hormones in postprandial reduction of bone resorption. *J Bone Miner Res* 2003 Dec; 18(12):2180–2189.

120. Henriksen DB, Alexandersen P, Byrjalsen I, Hartmann B, Bone HG, Christiansen C et al. Reduction of nocturnal rise in bone resorption by subcutaneous GLP-2. *Bone* 2004 Feb; 34(1):140–147.

121. Kreymann B, Williams G, Ghatei MA, Bloom SR. Glucagon-like peptide-1 7-36: A physiological incretin in man. *Lancet* 1987 Dec 5; 2(8571):1300–1304.

122. Nauck MA, Kleine N, Orskov C, Holst JJ, Willms B, Creutzfeldt W. Normalization of fasting hyperglycaemia by exogenous glucagon-like peptide 1 (7-36 amide) in type 2 (non-insulin-dependent) diabetic patients. *Diabetologia* 1993; 36(8):741–744.

123. Hvidberg A, Nielsen MT, Hilsted J, Orskov C, Holst JJ. Effect of glucagon-like peptide-1 (proglucagon 78-107amide) on hepatic glucose production in healthy man. *Metabolism* 1994; 43(1):104–108.

124. Creutzfeldt WO, Kleine N, Willms B, Orskov C, Holst JJ, Nauck MA. Glucagonostatic actions and reduction of fasting hyperglycemia by exogenous glucagon-like peptide I(7-36) amide in type I diabetic patients. *Diabetes Care* 1996; 19(6):580–586.

125. D'Alessio DA, Kahn SE, Leusner CR, Ensinck JW. Glucagon-like peptide 1 enhances glucose tolerance both by stimulation of insulin release and by increasing insulin-independent glucose disposal. *J Clin Invest* 1994; 93(5):2263–2266.

126. Toft-Nielsen M, Madsbad S, Holst JJ. The effect of glucagon-like peptide I (GLP-I) on glucose elimination in healthy subjects depends on the pancreatic glucoregulatory hormones. *Diabetes* 1996; 45(5):552–556.

127. Orskov L, Holst JJ, Moller J, Orskov C, Moller N, Alberti KG et al. GLP-1 does not acutely affect insulin sensitivity in healthy man. *Diabetologia* 1996; 39(10):1227–1232.

128. Vella A, Shah P, Reed AS, Adkins AS, Basu R, Rizza RA. Lack of effect of exendin-4 and glucagon-like peptide-1-(7,36)-amide on insulin action in non-diabetic humans. *Diabetologia* 2002 Oct; 45(10):1410–1415.

129. Ahren B, Larsson H, Holst JJ. Effects of glucagon-like peptide-1 on islet function and insulin sensitivity in noninsulin-dependent diabetes mellitus. *J Clin Endocrinol Metab* 1997 Feb; 82(2):473–478.

130. Vella A, Shah P, Basu R, Basu A, Holst JJ, Rizza RA. Effect of glucagon-like peptide 1(7-36) amide on glucose effectiveness and insulin action in people with type 2 diabetes. *Diabetes* 2000 Apr; 49(4):611–617.

131. Meneilly GS, Greig N, Tildesley H, Habener JF, Egan JM, Elahi D. Effects of 3 months of continuous subcutaneous administration of glucagon-like peptide 1 in elderly patients with type 2 diabetes. *Diabetes Care* 2003 Oct; 26(10):2835–2841.

132. Meneilly GS, McIntosh CH, Pederson RA, Habener JF, Gingerich R, Egan JM et al. Effect of glucagon-like peptide 1 on non-insulin-mediated glucose uptake in the elderly patient with diabetes. *Diabetes Care* 2001 Nov; 24(11):1951–1956.

133. Egan JM, Meneilly GS, Habener JF, Elahi D. Glucagon-like peptide-1 augments insulin-mediated glucose uptake in the obese state. *J Clin Endocrinol Metab* 2002 Aug; 87(8):3768–3773.

134. Meneilly GS, McIntosh CH, Pederson RA, Habener JF, Ehlers MR, Egan JM et al. Effect of glucagon-like peptide 1 (7-36 amide) on insulin-mediated glucose uptake in patients with type 1 diabetes. *Diabetes Care* 2003 Mar; 26(3):837–842.

135. Merida E, Delgado E, Molina LM, Villanueva-Penacarrillo ML, Valverde I. Presence of glucagon and glucagon-like peptide-1-(7-36)amide receptors in solubilized membranes of human adipose tissue. *J Clin Endocrinol Metab* 1993; 77(6):1654–1657.

136. Valverde I, Merida E, Delgado E, Trapote MA, Villanueva-Penacarrillo ML. Presence and characterization of glucagon-like peptide-1(7-36) amide receptors in solubilized membranes of rat adipose tissue. *Endocrinology* 1993; 132(1):75–79.

137. Oben J, Morgan L, Fletcher J, Marks V. Effect of the entero-pancreatic hormones, gastric inhibitory polypeptide and glucagon-like polypeptide-1(7-36) amide, on fatty acid synthesis in explants of rat adipose tissue. *J Endocrinol* 1991; 130(2):267–272.

138. Wang Y, Kole HK, Montrose-Rafizadeh C, Perfetti R, Bernier M, Egan JM. Regulation of glucose transporters and hexose uptake in 3T3-L1 adipocytes: Glucagon-like peptide-1 and insulin interactions. *J Mol Endocrinol* 1997 Dec; 19(3):241–248.

139. Egan JM, Montrose-Rafizadeh C, Wang Y, Bernier M, Roth J. Glucagon-like peptide-1(7-36) amide (GLP-1) enhances insulin-stimulated glucose metabolism in 3T3-L1 adipocytes: One of several potential extrapancreatic sites of GLP-1 action. *Endocrinology* 1994; 135(5):2070–2075.

140. Montrose-Rafizadeh C, Yang H, Wang Y, Roth J, Montrose MH, Adams LG. Novel signal transduction and peptide specificity of glucagon-like peptide receptor in 3T3-L1 adipocytes. *J Cell Physiol* 1997 Sep; 172(3):275–283.

141. Bertin E, Arner P, Bolinder J, Hagstrom-Toft E. Action of glucagon and glucagon-like peptide-1-(7-36) amide on lipolysis in human subcutaneous adipose tissue and skeletal muscle in vivo. *J Clin Endocrinol Metab* 2001 Mar; 86(3):1229–1234.

142. Delgado E, Luque MA, Alcantara A, Trapote MA, Clemente F, Galera C et al. Glucagon-like peptide-1 binding to rat skeletal muscle. *Peptides* 1995; 16(2):225–229.

143. Luque MA, Gonzalez N, Marquez L, Acitores A, Redondo A, Morales M et al. Glucagon-like peptide-1 (GLP-1) and glucose metabolism in human myocytes. *J Endocrinol* 2002 Jun; 173(3):465–473.

144. Yang H, Egan JM, Wang Y, Moyes CD, Roth J, Montrose MH et al. GLP-1 action in L6 myotubes is via a receptor different from the pancreatic GLP-1 receptor. *Am J Physiol* 1998 Sep; 275(3, pt. 1): C675–C683.

145. Gonzalez N, Acitores A, Sancho V, Valverde I, Villanueva-Penacarrillo ML. Effect of GLP-1 on glucose transport and its cell signalling in human myocytes. *Regul Pept* 2005 Mar 30; 126(3):203–211.

146. Furnsinn C, Ebner K, Waldhausl W. Failure of GLP-1(7-36)amide to affect glycogenesis in rat skeletal muscle. *Diabetologia* 1995; 38(7):864–867.

147. Fung LC, Chisholm C, Greenberg GR. Glucagon-like peptide-1-(7-36) amide and peptide YY mediate intraduodenal fat-induced inhibition of acid secretion in dogs. *Endocrinology* 1998 Jan; 139(1):189–194.

148. Daniel EE, Anvari M, Fox-Threlkeld JE, McDonald TJ. Local, exendin-(9-39)-insensitive, site of action of GLP-1 in canine ileum. *Am J Physiol Gastrointest Liver Physiol* 2002 Sep; 283(3): G595–G602.

149. Nishizawa M, Nakabayashi H, Kawai K, Ito T, Kawakami S, Nakagawa A et al. The hepatic vagal reception of intraportal GLP-1 is via receptor different from the pancreatic GLP-1 receptor. *J Auton Nerv Syst* 2000 Apr 12; 80(1–2):14–21.

150. Blackmore PF, Mojsov S, Exton JH, Habener JF. Absence of insulinotropic glucagon-like peptide-I(7-37) receptors on isolated rat liver hepatocytes. *FEBS Lett* 1991; 283(1):7–10.

151. Villanueva-Penacarrillo ML, Delgado E, Trapote MA, Alcantara A, Clemente F, Luque MA et al. Glucagon-like peptide-1 binding to rat hepatic membranes. *J Endocrinol* 1995 Jul; 146(1):183–189.

152. Trapote MA, Clemente F, Galera C, Morales M, Alcantara AI, Lopez Delgado MI et al. Inositolphosphoglycans are possible mediators of the glucagon- like peptide 1 (7-36)amide action in the liver. *J Endocrinol Invest* 1996; 19(2):114–118.

153. Redondo A, Trigo MV, Acitores A, Valverde I, Villanueva-Penacarrillo ML. Cell signalling of the GLP-1 action in rat liver. *Mol Cell Endocrinol* 2003 Jun 30; 204(1–2):43–50.

154. Ikezawa Y, Yamatani K, Ohnuma H, Daimon M, Manaka H, Sasaki H. Glucagon-like peptide-1 inhibits glucagon-induced glycogenolysis in perivenous hepatocytes specifically. *Regul Pept* 2003 Mar 28; 111(1–3):207–210.

155. Idris I, Patiag D, Gray S, Donnelly R. Exendin-4 increases insulin sensitivity via a PI-3-kinase-dependent mechanism: contrasting effects of GLP-1. *Biochem Pharmacol* 2002 Mar 1; 63(5): 993–996.

156. Burcelin R, Da Costa A, Drucker D, Thorens B. Glucose competence of the hepatoportal vein sensor requires the presence of an activated glucagon-like peptide-1 receptor. *Diabetes* 2001 Aug; 50(8):1720–1728.

157. Nishizawa M, Moore MC, Shiota M, Gustavson SM, Snead WL, Neal DW et al. Effect of intraportal glucagon-like peptide-1 on glucose metabolism in conscious dogs. *Am J Physiol Endocrinol Metab* 2003 May; 284(5):E1027–E1036.

158. Dardevet D, Moore MC, Neal D, DiCostanzo CA, Snead W, Cherrington AD. Insulin-independent effects of GLP-1 on canine liver glucose metabolism: Duration of infusion and involvement of hepatoportal region. *Am J Physiol Endocrinol Metab* 2004 Jul; 287(1):E75–E81.

159. Ionut V, Hucking K, Liberty IF, Bergman RN. Synergistic effect of portal glucose and glucagon-like peptide-1 to lower systemic glucose and stimulate counter-regulatory hormones. *Diabetologia* 2005 May; 48(5):967–975.

160. Toft-Nielsen MB, Damholt MB, Madsbad S, Hilsted LM, Hughes TE, Michelsen BK et al. Determinants of the impaired secretion of glucagon-like peptide-1 in type 2 diabetic patients. *J Clin Endocrinol Metab* 2001 Aug; 86(8):3717–3723.

161. Naslund E, Gryback P, Backman L, Jacobsson H, Holst JJ, Theodorsson E et al. Distal small bowel hormones: Correlation with fasting antroduodenal motility and gastric emptying. *Dig Dis Sci* 1998 May; 43(5):945–952.

162. Gebhard B, Holst JJ, Biegelmayer C, Miholic J. Postprandial GLP-1, norepinephrine, and reactive hypoglycemia in dumping syndrome. *Dig Dis Sci* 2001 Sep; 46(9):1915–1923.

163. Toft-Nielsen M, Madsbad S, Holst JJ. Exaggerated secretion of glucagon-like peptide-1 (GLP-1) could cause reactive hypoglycaemia. *Diabetologia* 1998 Oct; 41(10):1180–1186.

164. Patti ME, McMahon G, Mun EC, Bitton A, Holst JJ, Goldsmith J et al. Severe hypoglycaemia post-gastric bypass requiring partial pancreatectomy: Evidence for inappropriate insulin secretion and pancreatic islet hyperplasia. *Diabetologia* 2005 Sep 30.

165. Pedersen NB, Jonsson L, Holst JJ. Necrolytic migratory erythema and glucagon cell tumour of the pancreas: The glucagonoma syndrome—report of two cases. *Acta Derm Venereol* 1976; 56(5):391–395.

166. Holst JJ, Orskov C. The incretin approach for diabetes treatment: Modulation of islet hormone release by GLP-1 agonism. *Diabetes* 2004 Dec; 53(suppl 3):S197–S204.

167. Nauck MA, Holst JJ, Willms B. Glucagon-like peptide 1 and its potential in the treatment of non-insulin-dependent diabetes mellitus. *Horm Metab Res* 1997 Sep; 29(9):411–416.

168. Zander M, Madsbad S, Madsen JL, Holst JJ. GLP-1 treatment for 6 weeks improves glycemic control, insulin sensitivity and β-cell function in type 2 diabetic patients. *Diabetes.* (In press 2001.)

169. Goke R, Fehmann HC, Linn T, Schmidt H, Krause M, Eng J et al. Exendin-4 is a high potency agonist and truncated exendin-(9-39)-amide an antagonist at the glucagon-like peptide 1-(7-36)-amide receptor of insulin-secreting beta-cells. *J Biol Chem* 1993; 268(26):19650–19655.

170. Edwards CM, Stanley SA, Davis R, Brynes AE, Frost GS, Seal LJ et al. Exendin-4 reduces fasting and postprandial glucose and decreases energy intake in healthy volunteers. *Am J Physiol Endocrinol Metab* 2001 Jul; 281(1):E155–E161.

171. Holst JJ, Deacon CF. Inhibition of the activity of dipeptidyl-peptidase IV as a treatment for type 2 diabetes. *Diabetes* 1998 Nov; 47(11):1663–1670.

172. Ahren B, Gomis R, Standl E, Mills D, Schweizer A. Twelve- and 52-week efficacy of the dipeptidyl peptidase IV inhibitor LAF237 in metformin-treated patients with type 2 diabetes. *Diabetes Care* 2004 Dec; 27(12):2874–2880.

173. Ahren B, Pacini G, Foley JE, Schweizer A. Improved meal-related beta-cell function and insulin sensitivity by the dipeptidyl peptidase-IV inhibitor vildagliptin in metformin-treated patients with type 2 diabetes over 1 year. *Diabetes Care* 2005 Aug; 28(8):1936–1940.

174. Jeppesen PB, Hartmann B, Thulesen J, Graff J, Lohmann J, Hansen BS et al. Glucagon-like peptide 2 improves nutrient absorption and nutritional status in short-bowel patients with no colon. *Gastroenterology* 2001 Mar; 120(4):806–815.

175. Jeppesen PB, Sanguinetti EL, Buchman A, Howard L, Scolapio JS, Ziegler TR et al. Teduglutide (ALX-0600), a dipeptidyl peptidase IV resistant glucagon-like peptide 2 analogue, improves intestinal function in short bowel syndrome patients. *Gut* 2005 Sep; 54(9):1224–1231.

176. Drucker DJ. Glucagon-like peptides: Regulators of cell proliferation, differentiation, and apoptosis. *Mol Endocrinol* 2003 Feb; 17(2):161–171.

14 The Relationship Between the Insulin Receptor Substrates and Metabolic Disease

Morris F. White

CONTENTS

INTRODUCTION

Although the regulation of plasma glucose is a dominant response associated with insulin action, glucose homeostasis depends on the integration of insulin signals in many tissues and cells—hepatocytes, muscle, adipose, hypothalamic neurons, pancreatic β-cells, and others (1–7). Understanding how insulin action is coordinated and modulated in these tissues by heterologous signaling cascades is a challenging scientific question of clinical importance.

Unlike classical feedback regulation—illustrated by corticotrophin-releasing hormone (CRH) and adrenocorticotropic hormone (ACTH) for cortisol, or gonadotrophin-releasing hormone and gonadotrophins for sex steroids—a well-defined linear feedback mechanism controlling insulin action has never emerged. By contrast, tissue-specific insulin responses are attenuated by circulating nutrients—glucose, amino acids, free fatty acids, and ketones—and proinflammatory cytokines produced in excess during chronic physiologic and inflammatory stress (8). Even compensatory hyperinsulinemia exacerbates the insulin resistance and promotes a cohort of systemic disorders—includ-

From: *Contemporary Endocrinology: The Metabolic Syndrome: Epidemiology, Clinical Treatment, and Underlying Mechanisms*
Edited by: B.C. Hansen and G.A. Bray © Humana Press, Totowa, NJ

ing dyslipidemia, hypertension, cardiovascular disease, and female infertility (9,10). Many laboratories including ours are using mouse genetics to reveal how dysregulated insulin signals in specific tissues can lead to systemic insulin resistance and β-cell failure that progresses to type 2 diabetes (11–14). Understanding the effects of tissue-specific insulin resistance is revealing the principal targets responsible for metabolic disease and its progression to diabetes (15).

THE MAMMALIAN INSULIN/IGF1 RECEPTOR TYROSINE KINASES

The mammalian insulin signaling system includes three well-defined ligands—insulin, insulin-like growth factor-1 (IGF1), and insulin-like growth factor-2 (IGF2)—that regulate the activity of the canonical insulin receptor (IR), the IGF1 receptor (IGF1R), and the IR-related receptor (IRR); however, IRR appears to have a limited role in testicular development that is revealed only upon deletion of both the IR and the IGF1R (16). Thus, central and peripheral insulin and IGF actions are mediated entirely by the IR and IGF1R (Fig. 14.1).

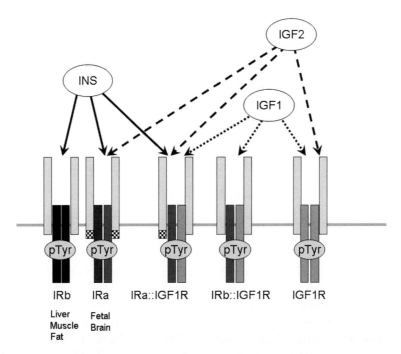

Figure 14.1. The insulin/insulin-like growth factor family. The insulin/IGF family consists of three hormones: insulin, insulin-like growth factor-1 (IGF1), and insulin-like growth factor-2 (IGF2). These peptide ligands bind as indicated in the figure to five distinct receptor isoforms that generate cytoplasmic signals: two insulin receptor isoforms, IRa and IRb; the insulin-like growth factor receptor, IGF1r; and two hybrid receptors, IRa::IGF1r and IRb::IGF1r. IGF2 also binds to the mannose-6-phosphate receptor, which mediates its endocytosis and degradation. The insulin receptor is the primary target for insulin throughout development and life. The IGF1 receptor is the primary target for IGF1. IGF2 binds to the insulin receptor primarily during embryonic development, and binds the IGF1 receptor throughout life. IGF2 also binds to the mannose-6-phosphate receptor, which targets the IGF2 for degradation instead of signaling. Activation of the insulin receptor or the IGF1 receptor mediate signals primarily via the cytoplasmic proteins IRS1 and IRS2, which mediate somatic cell growth and metabolism.

Two insulin receptor (IR) isoforms—IRb or IRa—bind insulin with high or moderate affinity, respectively (Fig. 14.1). The IRa is produced during tissue-specific inclusion of exon-11 in the receptor mRNA; exon-11 encodes 12 amino acids at the end of the α-subunit that promotes IGF2 binding but reduces insulin binding affinity (17,18). IRb lacks exon-11, which increases the affinity, specifically for insulin, while reducing significantly the interaction with IGF2 (Fig. 14.1). IRb predominates in classical insulin-sensitive target tissues, including adult liver, muscle, and adipose tissues; IRa predominates in fetal tissues, the adult central nervous system, and hematopoietic cells (19–22). The IGF1R binds IGF1 and IGF2 at physiological levels, whereas insulin binds to the IGF1R with 50–100-fold less affinity.

The selectivity for insulin or insulin-like growth factor signaling can be complicated owing to post-translational assembly of hybrids between the IGF1R and the IR isoforms (23). Hybrid receptors composed of an αβ-dimer of the IGF1R and IRa (IGF1R::IRb) selectively bind IGF1, whereas IGF1R::IRa binds all three ligands with similar affinities (Fig. 14.1) (24). The physiological significance of tissue-specific alternative splicing of insulin receptors and the assembly of receptor hybrids needs to be resolved in novel genetic models. Hybrids could play significant roles in pancreatic β-cells and muscle, where both insulin and IGF1 receptors are expressed. The selectivity introduced by the receptor hybrids could modulate the consequences of chronic hyperinsulinemia.

INSULIN/IGF SIGNALING: THE BASICS

Insulin resistance is common among mammals and people: Its close association with obesity, advancing age, and physical inactivity is well documented in industrialized nations; and the consequences of insulin resistance are readily studied in laboratory animals (25). Although insulin receptor polymorphisms provide important insight into receptor function, they fail to uncover a general cause of insulin resistance (26). Moreover, the reductions in the number of functional insulin receptors owing to neutralizing antibodies or other inhibitory molecules are unusual causes of extreme systemic insulin resistance (27,28).

Ordinary insulin resistance associated with metabolic disease and type 2 diabetes arises from dysregulation of the insulin/IGF signaling cascades—including impaired coordination of effector proteins and transcription factors (10). Increased insulin secretion frequently compensates for moderate insulin resistance. Type 2 diabetes develops when sufficient insulin is no longer secreted quickly enough to sustain an adequate insulin response (29). Recent work suggests that heterologous signaling cascades, activated by nutrient excess or proinflammatory cytokines, contribute, at least in part, to peripheral insulin resistance (30). Understanding the molecular basis of insulin signaling provides a good foundation to discover ways to prevent insulin resistance and its progression to type 2 diabetes.

The receptors for insulin or IGF1, like the receptors for other growth factors and cytokines, are composed of an extracellular ligand-binding domain that regulates the activity of an intracellular tyrosine kinase (29,31,32). Most receptor tyrosine kinases are activated by ligand-induced dimerization that promotes tyrosine autophosphorylation of the kinase activation-loop (A-loop), and other sites that recruit cellular substrates (33). However, insulin receptors reside in the plasma membrane as inactive covalent dimers. Insulin binding increases flexibility of the A-loop to allow ATP to enter the

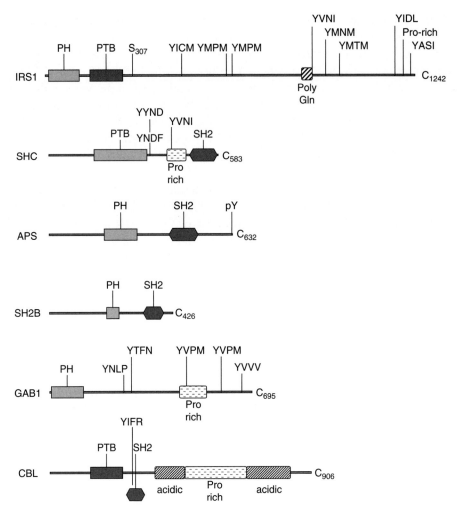

Figure 14.2. Comparison of IRS1 to other signaling scaffolds. A comparison (drawn to scale) of important sequence features of IRS1, including the relative position of the pleckstrin homology (PH) and phosphotyrosine binding (PTB) domains, serine-307, the poly Gln motif, and some potential tyrosine phosphorylation sites. Important motifs in SHC, APS, SH2B, GAB1, and CBL are also shown for comparison.

catalytic site, which promotes phosphorylation of the A-loop to stabilize the active conformation and recruit substrates for phosphorylation (14,29,34,35). Consequently, the principal insulin receptor and IGF1 receptor substrates—the IRS-proteins—are phosphorylated on multiple tyrosine residues during insulin stimulation (Fig. 14.2). Most, if not all, insulin signals are produced or modulated through tyrosine phosphorylation of IRS1, or its homologs IRS2, IRS3, or IRS4, or other scaffold proteins—SHC, CBL, APS, and SH2B, GAB1, GAB2, DOCK1, and DOCK2 (36–42). Although the role of each of these substrates merits attention, work with transgenic mice suggests that many insulin responses associated with somatic growth and nutrient homeostasis are mediated through IRS1 or IRS2—the others play compensatory or modulatory roles (29).

IRS1 and IRS2 are composed of an NH_2-terminal pleckstrin homology (PH) and phosphotyrosine-binding (PTB) domains, followed by a tail of tyrosine and Ser/Thr-phosphorylation sites. The PTB domain binds directly to the phosphorylated NPXY-motif in the activated receptors for insulin, IGF1 or interleukin-4 (IL4); the PH domain also couples IRS-proteins to activated receptors—but the mechanism is unknown (43). IRS2 contains a third region that binds to the activated β-subunit that might explain the dominant role of IRS2 in certain tissues and cells (44,45). IRS1 and IRS2 also contain at least one *kinase interaction motif* (KIM) that binds to the NH_2-terminal JUN kinase (JNK) (46). Other MAP kinases might interact at this site, and other protein interaction motifs are likely to be identified in the future (47).

The tyrosine phosphorylation sites bind common effectors—including enzymes (phosphoinositide 3-kinase, the phosphatase SHP2, or the tyrosine kinase fyn) or adapters (GRB2, NCK, CRK, SHB, and others)—that generate downstream signals. The production of PI-3,4,5-P_3 by PI 3-kinase recruits the Ser/Thr-kinases Pdk1 and Akt to the plasma membrane where Akt is activated by Pdk1-mediated phosphorylation (Fig. 14.3) (48). Akt phosphorylates and regulates many proteins—GSK3β (glycogen synthesis), the BAD·BCL2 heterodimer (apoptosis inhibition), and FOXO transcriptional regulators (gene expression) (Fig. 14.3) (48). Akt also phosphorylates tuberin (TSC2), which inhibits its GAP activity toward the small G-protein RHEB, so RHEB·GTP can accumulate and activate mTOR (Fig. 14.3) (49–51). The strength and duration of these insulin signals are modulated through protein and phospholipid phosphatases, or direct modulation of IRS-protein function by Ser/Thr-phosphorylation (52–55). Depending on the tissue site, dysregulation of these heterologous signaling mechanisms can progress to glucose intolerance, dysregulated lipid metabolism, and other life-threatening metabolic disorders including pancreatic β-cell failure, which causes diabetes.

IRS2 SIGNALING REVEALS THE LINK BETWEEN PERIPHERAL INSULIN ACTION AND PANCREATIC β-CELL FUNCTION

Mice lacking the gene for IRS1 or IRS2 are insulin resistant, with impaired peripheral glucose utilization (56–58). However, IRS1$^{-/-}$ mice never progress to diabetes owing to lifelong compensatory hyperinsulinemia (56). By contrast, metabolic dysregulation is severe in IRS2$^{-/-}$ mice owing to excessive gluconeogenesis, decreased hepatic glycogen synthesis, and unsuppressed plasma free fatty acid/glycerol levels during the hyperinsulinemia (58). IRS2$^{-/-}$ mice progress steadily toward diabetes owing to insufficient compensatory insulin secretion.

Although peripheral insulin resistance is an important component of type 2 diabetes, β-cell failure that prevents compensatory insulin secretion is an essential part of the disorder. The molecular pathophysiology of type 2 diabetes is complex, but dysregulated IRS2 signaling might emerge as a common basis to link peripheral insulin resistance to β-cell failure (29). Increased expression of IRS2 in β-cells promotes compensatory insulin secretion in obese mice and prevents β-cell destruction induced by streptozotocin—a drug that induces type 1 diabetes; IRS2 also improves the survival and function of islet transplants in mice (59). Drugs that increase IRS2 synthesis might be useful treatments for diabetes. For example, expression of the IRS2 gene in β-cells is increased by agonists that stimulate adenosine 3′,5′-monophosphate (cAMP)

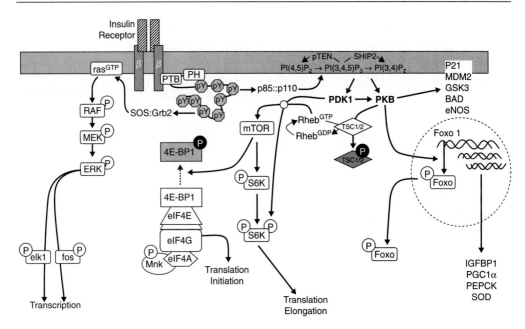

Figure 14.3. Activation of intracellular signaling pathways by insulin. There are two main limbs that propagate the signal generated through the IRS-proteins: the PI 3-kinase and the Grb2/Sos→ras cascade. Activation of the receptors for insulin and IGF1 results in tyrosine phosphorylation of the IRS-proteins, which bind PI 3-kinase and GRB2/SOS. The GRB2/SOS complex promotes GDP/GTP exchange on p21^{ras}, which activates the ras→ raf→ MEK→ ERK1/2 cascade. The activated ERK stimulates transcriptional activity by direct phosphorylation of elk1 and by phosphorylation of fos through p90^{rsk}. The activation of PI 3-kinase by IRS-protein recruitment produces PI 3,4P$_2$ and PI 3,4,5P$_3$ (antagonized by the action of PTEN or SHIP2), which recruit PDK1 and PKB to the plasma membrane, where PKB is activated by PDK-mediated phosphorylation. The mTOR kinase is activated by Rheb^{GTP}, which accumulates upon inhibition of the GAP activity of the TSC1::TSC2 complex by PKB-mediated phosphorylation. The p70^{s6k} is primed—for activation by PDK1—through mTOR-mediated phosphorylation. PKB phosphorylates many substrates, including P21, MDM2, GSK3, and eNOS. PKB-mediated BAD phosphorylation inhibits apoptosis, and phosphorylation of the forkhead proteins results in their sequestration in the cytoplasm, in effect inhibiting their transcriptional activity and reducing the expression of many genes including IGFBP1, PGC1α, PEPCK, and SOD. Insulin stimulates protein synthesis by altering the intrinsic activity or binding properties of key translation initiation and elongation factors (eIFs and eEFs, respectively), including eIF2B, eIF4E, eEF1, eEF2, and the S6 ribosomal protein (174). In particular, phosphorylation of 4E-BP1 releases eIF4E to form an active complex promoting translation initiation. IRS1: insulin receptor substrate 1; PH: pleckstrin homology domain; PTB: phosphotyrosine binding domain; PTEN and SHIP2: phospholipid phosphatases; PKB: protein kinase B; GAP: guanosine triphosphatase associated protein; GRB-2: factor receptor binding protein 2; SOS: son-of-sevenless; GSK3: glycogen synthase kinase 3; MAPKK: MAPK kinase; PDK: PI-dependent protein kinase; PKC: protein kinase C; TSC: tuberous sclerosis complex.

production—including glucagon-like peptide-1 or glucose itself—through pathways that activate the transcription factor CREB (60).

The insulin/IGF1→IRS2 pathway has a major role in β-cell development and survival, especially during compensation for peripheral insulin resistance (61). The progeny of intercrossed mice heterozygous for null alleles of IGF1R and IRS2 reveal that IGF1 receptors promote β-cell development and survival through the IRS2 signaling pathway

(61). However, the critical cellular site for this interaction is not known, as targeted deletion of the IGF1R in β-cells has no effect on β-cell growth (62,63). Thus, the effect of IGF1 on IRS2-medited β-cell growth/survival might not be β-cell autonomous, but might be more closely related to the growth and differentiation of precursors that are essential for lifelong regeneration.

Many factors are required for proper β-cell function, including the homeodomain transcription factor PDX1. PDX1 mutations cause autosomal forms of early-onset diabetes (MODY), because Pdx1 regulates downstream genes needed for β-cell growth and function (Fig. 14.4) (64,65). Thus, it is informative that PDX1 is reduced in IRS2$^{-/-}$ islets, and PDX1 haploinsufficiency further diminishes the function of β-cells lacking IRS2 (66,67). By comparison, transgenic PDX1 expressed in IRS2$^{-/-}$ mice restores β-cell function and normalizes glucose tolerance in the insulin-resistant IRS2$^{-/-}$ mice (66). Importantly, transgenic IRS2 in wild-type or IRS2$^{-/-}$ islets increases PDX1 levels, revealing a direct link between the IRS2 signaling cascades and the function of a transcription factor that is required for β-cell function (Fig. 14.4) (59).

Genetic manipulation of other signaling elements downstream of IRS2 can also restore metabolic regulation in IRS2$^{-/-}$ mice. Foxo1 is a transcription factor that plays a role in many tissues and cells (68). Foxo1 is normally located in the nucleus, but upon activation of the IRS2→PI3K→Akt cascade, Foxo1 is phosphorylated and excluded from the nucleus. The reduction of nuclear Foxo1 significantly alters cellular gene

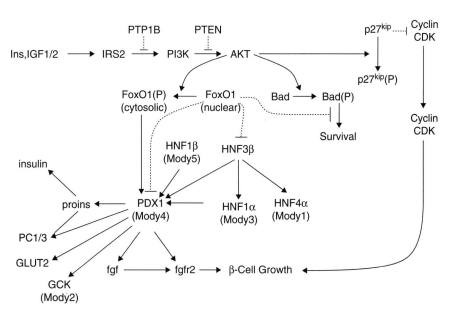

Figure 14.4. A potential pathway linking IRS2 signaling to the expression and function of the homeodomain transcription factor PDX1. The diagram shows the relation between the MODY genes, especially PDX1, and the IRS2-branch of the insulin signaling pathway (66). Drugs that promote IRS2 signaling are expected to promote PDK1 function in β-cells, including the phosphorylation of BAD and FOXO1, which will promote β-cell growth, function, and survival. Induction of PDX1 promotes the expression of gene products that enhance glucose sensing and insulin secretion. Activation of the cAMP → CREB cascade induces IRS2 expression in β-cells, revealing a mechanism that promotes β-cell growth, function, and survival.

expression of effector molecules, or indirectly through neuronal inputs, is an active area of investigation (93).

Mouse genetic models provide recent insights into the regulation of hepatic insulin action. Unexpectedly, acute suppression of hepatic insulin receptors does not dramatically dysregulate fasting glucose production, suggesting that other mechanisms, including neuronal inputs, can provide sufficient metabolic regulation (94,95). Even genetic deletion of the hepatic insulin receptors—the LIRKO mouse—does not seriously disturb fasting glucose levels—although hyperglycemia develops after meals.

Cell-based experiments suggest that IRS2 is an important regulatory point for the PI 3-kinase→Akt cascade in hepatocytes (96,97). IRS2 is the major effector of both the metabolic and growth-promoting actions of insulin in immortalized hepatocytes (96). Moreover, IRS2 signaling is essential for the suppression of gluconeogenesis and apoptosis in neonatal hepatocytes (98,99). IRS2 is highly regulated through feedback and counter-regulatory cascades, which contribute to its importance for hepatic metabolism. During nutrient deprivation, hepatic IRS2 expression is upregulated by nuclear FoxO1 and phosphorylated CREB (97,100). By contrast, sterol regulatory element binding proteins (SREBP)—transcriptional regulators of lipid synthesis—suppress IRS2 expression, at least in part by interfering with FoxO1 binding to the *IRS2* promoter (97). Thus, dysregulation of IRS2 signaling by chronic nutrient excess might explain, at least in part, the relation between obesity and dysregulated hepatic metabolism.

Transient suppression of hepatic IRS1 or IRS2 by more than 70% has only modest effects upon murine nutrient metabolism (101). Genetic deletion of IRS2 in murine hepatocytes (LKO-mice) causes mild hyperinsulinemia and glucose intolerance by 5 weeks of age, which can be difficult to detect (14,102). By contrast, deleting IRS2 from hepatocytes of mice lacking systemic IRS1 causes severe hyperglycemia immediately after birth, which persists during their abbreviated lives (14). Without hepatic IRS2, the mice can respond to compensatory β-cell insulin secretion, and glucose homeostasis is nearly normal; however, mice lacking IRS1 everywhere and lacking hepatic IRS2 are unresponsive to compensatory hyperinsulinemia or exogenous insulin injections, and develop hyperglycemia and diabetes by 5 weeks of age. We conclude provisionally that IRS1 and IRS2 mediate the effects of insulin upon hepatic glucose homeostasis. Moreover, these severely insulin-resistant hepatocytes do not accumulate lipid, which is similar to the complete loss of insulin signaling in type 1 diabetes subjects.

Regardless, dysregulated insulin signaling is associated with hepatic lipid accumulation, which frequently presages type 2 diabetes. Hepatic metabolism is coordinated through many interacting transcription factors and co-regulators, which are coupled to extracellular signals through glucagon-stimulated cAMP-mediated pathways and the insulin-regulated PI3-kinase→Akt cascade (1). Recent work suggests that glucose and lipid metabolism might be differentially sensitive to insulin signaling in hepatocytes because nuclear transcription factors that induce gluconeogenesis (FOXO1) or fatty acid oxidation (FOXA2) can be coupled differently to the insulin signaling cascade (89). Hepatic gluconeogenesis is attenuated when FOXO1 is excluded from the nucleus upon AKT-mediated serine phosphorylation (7); a similar mechanism might exclude FOXA2 from the nucleus to reduce fatty acid oxidation (103). However, FOXA2 phosphorylation appears to be more sensitive to insulin signaling owing to its tighter coupling to IRS1- and IRS2-mediated signals. The greater insulin sensitivity of AKT→FOXA2 signaling compared to AKT→FOXO1 signaling is attributed to differential coupling to

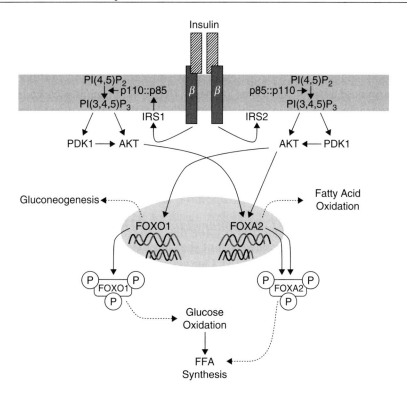

Figure 14.6. A diagram showing the putative specificity between IRS1 and IRS2 signaling in hepatic regulation of gene expression through the phosphorylation and cytosolic translocation of FOXO1 and FOXA2. Nuclear FOXO1 largely mediates gluconeogenesis, whereas nuclear FOXA2 promotes fatty acid oxidation and inhibits synthesis. Since FOXA2 might be targeted for phosphorylation through IRS1 and IRS2 signaling, it might be coupled more tightly than FOXO1 to insulin stimulation under certain conditions. This imbalanced coupling can result in the characteristic gluconeogenesis and fatty acid synthesis that occurs in type 2 diabetes. (See Color Plate following p. 372.)

IRS1 and IRS2 (Fig. 14.6). This imbalanced signaling makes it easier to exclude FOXA2 than FOXO1 from the nucleus of hepatocytes, leading to steatosis on the one hand and uncontrolled gluconeogenesis on the other—especially under conditions of compensatory hyperinsulinemia.

THE MOLECULAR BASIS OF INSULIN RESISTANCE

Introduction

Insulin resistance is a common pathological state that is associated with many health disorders—obesity, hypertension, chronic infection, dysregulated female reproduction, and kidney and cardiovascular diseases (104). Genetic mutations are obvious sources of lifelong insulin resistance, but they are usually associated with rare metabolic disorders. Environmental and physiological stress appears to cause insulin resistance through heterologous signaling cascades (3). Recent studies reveal a variety of factors secreted from adipose tissue that inhibit insulin signaling—FFAs, tumor necrosis factor-alpha (TNFα), and resistin—or factors that promote insulin signaling—adipocyte comple-

central nutrient homeostasis (12,173). Moreover, the effects of GLP1 or exendin-4 upon IRS2 expression suggest a rational mechanism to explain their strong effects upon β-cell function. The identification of other compounds that increase IRS2 expression in β-cells or other tissues could be important treatments for diabetes and related metabolic disorders.

REFERENCES

1. Puigserver P, Rodgers JT. Foxa2: A novel transcriptional regulator of insulin sensitivity. *Nat Med* 2006 Jan; 12(1):38–39.
2. Rodgers JT, Lerin C, Haas W, Gygi SP, Spiegelman BM, Puigserver P. Nutrient control of glucose homeostasis through a complex of PGC-1alpha and SIRT1. *Nature* 2005 Mar 3; 434(7029):113–118.
3. De LC, Olefsky JM. Stressed out about obesity and insulin resistance. *Nat Med* 2006 Jan; 12(1):41–42.
4. Seeley RJ, Tschop M. How diabetes went to our heads. *Nat Med* 2006 Jan; 12(1):47–49.
5. Pocai A, Muse ED, Rossetti L. Did a muscle fuel gauge conquer the brain? *Nat Med* 2006 Jan; 12(1):50–51.
6. Horvath TL, Bruning JC. Developmental programming of the hypothalamus: A matter of fat. *Nat Med* 2006 Jan; 12(1):52–53.
7. Matsumoto M, Accili D. All roads lead to FoxO. *Cell Metab* 2005 Apr; 1(4):215–216.
8. Hotamisligil GS. Inflammatory pathways and insulin action. *Int J Obes Relat Metab Disord* 2003 Dec; 27(suppl 3):S53–S55.
9. Reaven G, Tsao PS. Insulin resistance and compensatory hyperinsulinemia: The key player between cigarette smoking and cardiovascular disease? *J Am Coll Cardiol* 2003 Mar 19; 41(6):1044–1047.
10. DeFronzo RA, Ferrannini E. Regulation of intermediary metabolism during fasting and feeding. In: *Endocrinology*, 4 ed., DeGroot LJ, Jameson JL (eds.), W.B. Saunders, Philadelphia, 2001, pp. 737–755.
11. Hirosumi J, Tuncman G, Chang L, Gorgun CZ, Uysal KT, Maeda K et al. A central role for JNK in obesity and insulin resistance. *Nature* 2002 Nov 21; 420(6913):333–336.
12. Lin X, Taguchi A, Park S, Kushner JA, Li F, Li Y et al. Dysregulation of insulin receptor substrate 2 in beta cells and brain causes obesity and diabetes. *J Clin Invest* 2004 Oct; 114(7):908–916.
13. Kitamura Y, Accili D. New insights into the integrated physiology of insulin action. *Rev Endocr Metab Disord* 2004 May; 5(2):143–149.
14. Dong X, Park S, Lin X, Copps K, Yi X, White MF. IRS1 and IRS2 signaling is essential for hepatic glucose homeostasis and systemic growth. *J Clin Invest* 2006 Jan; 116(1):101–114.
15. Nandi A, Kitamura Y, Kahn CR, Accili D. Mouse models of insulin resistance. *Physiol Rev* 2004 Apr; 84(2):623–647.
16. Nef S, Verma-Kurvari S, Merenmies J, Vassalli JD, Efstratiadis A, Accili D et al. Testis determination requires insulin receptor family function in mice. *Nature* 2003 Nov 20; 426(6964):291–295.
17. Frasca F, Pandini G, Scalia P, Sciacca L, Mineo R, Costantino A et al. Insulin receptor isoform A: A newly recognized, high-affinity insulin-like growth factor II receptor in fetal and cancer cells. *Mol Cell Biol* 1999; 19(5):3278–3288.
18. Sciacca L, Prisco M, Wu A, Belfiore A, Vigneri R, Baserga R. Signaling differences from the A and B isoforms of the insulin receptor (IR) in 32D cells in the presence or absence of IR substrate-1. *Endocrinology* 2003 Jun; 144(6):2650–2658.
19. Mosthaf L, Grako K, Dull TJ, Coussens L, Ullrich A, McClain DA. Functionally distinct insulin receptors generated by tissue-specific alternative splicing. *EMBO J* 1990 Aug; 9(8):2409–2413.
20. Moller DE, Yokota A, Caro JF, Flier JS. Tissue-specific expression of two alternatively spliced insulin receptor mRNAs in man. *Mol Endocrinol* 1989; 3:1263–1269.
21. Goldstein BJ, Kahn CR. Analysis of mRNA heterogeneity by ribonuclease H mapping: Application to the insulin receptor. *Biochem Biophys Res Commun* 1989; 159:664–669.
22. Seino S, Bell GI. Alternative splicing of human insulin receptor messenger RNA. *Biochem Biophys Res Commun* 1989; 159:312–316.
23. Louvi A, Accili D, Efstratiadis A. Growth-promoting interaction of IGF-II with the insulin receptor during mouse embryonic development. *Dev Biol* 1997 Sep 1; 189(1):33–48.

24. Pandini G, Frasca F, Mineo R, Sciacca L, Vigneri R, Belfiore A. Insulin/insulin-like growth factor I hybrid receptors have different biological characteristics depending on the insulin receptor isoform involved. *J Biol Chem* 2002 Oct 18; 277(42):39684–39695.

25. Roth J. Diabetes and obesity. *Diab Met Rev* 1998; 13(1):1–2.

26. Taylor SI. Lilly lecture: Molecular mechanisms of insulin resistance-Lessons from patients with mutations in the insulin receptor gene. *Diabetes* 1992; 41:1473–1490.

27. Flier JS, Kahn CR, Roth J, Bar RS. Antibodies that impair insulin receptor binding in an unusual diabetic syndrome with severe insulin resistance. *Science* 1975; 190:63–65.

28. Maddux BA, Sbraccia P, Kumakura S, Sasson S, Youngren J, Fisher A et al. Membrane glycoprotein PC-1 in the insulin resistance of non-insulin dependent diabetes mellitus. *Nature* 1995; 373(6513):448–451.

29. White MF. Insulin signaling in health and disease. *Science* 2003 Dec 5; 302(5651):1710–1711.

30. Evans JL, Goldfine ID, Maddux BA, Grodsky GM. Are oxidative stress-activated signaling pathways mediators of insulin resistance and beta-cell dysfunction? *Diabetes* 2003 Jan; 52(1):1–8.

31. Ullrich A, Bell JR, Chen EY, Herrera R, Petruzzelli LM, Dull TJ et al. Human insulin receptor and its relationship to the tyrosine kinase family of oncogenes. *Nature* 1985; 313:756–761.

32. Ebina Y, Ellis L, Jarnagin K, Edery M, Graf L, Clauser E et al. The human insulin receptor cDNA: The structural basis for hormone activated transmembrane signalling. *Cell* 1985; 40:747–758.

33. Schlessinger J. Cell signaling by receptor tyrosine kinases. *Cell* 2000 Oct 13; 103(2):211–225.

34. Myers MG, Jr., White MF. The new elements in insulin signaling: Insulin receptor substrate-1 and proteins with SH2 domains. *Diabetes* 1993; 42:643–650.

35. White MF, Kahn CR. The insulin signaling system. *J Biol Chem* 1994; 269(1):1–4.

36. Yenush L, White MF. The IRS-signaling system during insulin and cytokine action. *Bio Essays* 1997; 19(5):491–500.

37. Pawson T, Scott JD. Signaling through scaffold, anchoring, and adaptor proteins. *Science* 1997 Dec 19; 278(5346):2075–2080.

38. Kotani K, Wilden P, Pillay TS. SH2-Balpha is an insulin-receptor adapter protein and substrate that interacts with the activation loop of the insulin-receptor kinase. *Biochem J* 1998 Oct 1; 335(pt. 1):103–109.

39. Lock P, Casagranda F, Dunn AR. Independent SH2-binding sites mediate interaction of Dok-related protein with RasGTPase-activating protein and Nck. *J Biol Chem* 1999 Aug 6; 274(32):22775–22784.

40. Noguchi T, Matozaki T, Inagaki K, Tsuda M, Fukunaga K, Kitamura Y et al. Tyrosine phosphorylation of p62(Dok) induced by cell adhesion and insulin: Possible role in cell migration. *EMBO J* 1999 Apr 1; 18(7):1748–1760.

41. Chiang SH, Baumann CA, Kanzaki M, Thurmond DC, Watson RT, Neudauer CL et al. Insulin-stimulated GLUT4 translocation requires the CAP-dependent activation of TC10. *Nature* 2001 Apr 19; 410(6831):944–948.

42. Baumann CA, Ribon V, Kanzaki M, Thurmond DC, Mora S, Shigematsu S et al. CAP defines a second signalling pathway required for insulin-stimulated glucose transport. *Nature* 2000 Sep 14; 407(6801):202–207.

43. Burks DJ, Wang J, Towery H, Ishibashi O, Lowe D, Riedel H et al. IRS pleckstrin homology domains bind to acidic motifs in proteins. *J Biol Chem* 1998 Nov 20; 273(47):31061–31067.

44. Sawka-Verhelle D, Baron V, Mothe I, Filloux C, White MF, Van Obberghen E. Tyr624 and Tyr628 in insulin receptor substrate-2 mediate its association with the insulin receptor. *J Biol Chem* 1997; 272(26):16414–16420.

45. Sawka-Verhelle D, Tartare-Deckert S, White MF, Van Obberghen E. Insulin receptor substrate-2 binds to the insulin receptor through its phosphotyrosine-binding domain and through a newly identified domain comprising amino acids 591–786. *J Biol Chem* 1996; 271(11):5980–5983.

46. Lee YH, Giraud J, Davis RJ, White MF. c-Jun N-terminal kinase (JNK) mediates feedback inhibition of the insulin signaling cascade. *J Biol Chem* 2003 Jan 31; 278(5):2896–2902.

47. Barr RK, Boehm I, Attwood PV, Watt PM, Bogoyevitch MA. The critical features and the mechanism of inhibition of a kinase interaction motif-based peptide inhibitor of JNK. *J Biol Chem* 2004 Aug 27; 279(35):36327–36338.

48. Lawlor MA, Alessi DR. PKB/Akt: A key mediator of cell proliferation, survival and insulin responses? *J Cell Sci* 2001 Aug; 114(pt. 16):2903–2910.

49. Inoki K, Li Y, Xu T, Guan KL. Rheb GTPase is a direct target of TSC2 GAP activity and regulates mTOR signaling. *Genes Dev* 2003 Aug 1; 17(15):1829–1834.
50. Fisher TL, White MF. Signaling pathways: The benefits of good communication. *Curr Biol* 2004 Dec 14; 14(23):R1005–R1007.
51. Astrinidis A, Henske EP. Tuberous sclerosis complex: Linking growth and energy signaling pathways with human disease. *Oncogene* 2005 Nov 14; 24(50):7475–7481.
52. Rosen ED, Spiegelman BM. Tumor necrosis factor-alpha as a mediator of the insulin resistance of obesity. *Curr Opin Endocrinol Diab* 1999; 6(2):170–176.
53. Chen H, Wertheimer SJ, Lin CH, Katz SL, Amrein KE, Burn P et al. Protein-tyrosine phosphatases PTP1B and syp are modulators of insulin-stimulated translocation of GLUT4 in transfected rat adipose cells. *J Biol Chem* 1997 Mar 21; 272(12):8026–8031.
54. Elchebly M, Payette P, Michaliszyn E, Cromlish W, Collins S, Loy AL et al. Increased insulin sensitivity and obesity resistance in mice lacking the protein tyrosine phosphatase-1B gene [see comments]. *Science* 1999 Mar 5; 283(5407):1544–1548.
55. Zick Y. Role of Ser/Thr kinases in the uncoupling of insulin signaling. *Int J Obes Relat Metab Disord* 2003 Dec; 27(suppl 3):S56–S60.
56. Withers DJ, Gutierrez JS, Towery H, Burks DJ, Ren JM, Previs S et al. Disruption of IRS-2 causes type 2 diabetes in mice. *Nature* 1998; 391(6670):900–904.
57. Kubota N, Tobe K, Terauchi Y, Eto K, Yamauchi T, Suzuki R et al. Disruption of insulin receptor substrate 2 causes type 2 diabetes because of liver insulin resistance and lack of compensatory beta-cell hyperplasia. *Diabetes* 2000 Nov; 49(11):1880–1889.
58. Previs SF, Withers DJ, Ren JM, White MF, Shulman GI. Contrasting effects of IRS-1 vs. IRS-2 gene disruption on carbohydrate and lipid metabolism in vivo. *J Biol Chem* 2000 Sep 19; 275(50): 38990–38994.
59. Hennige AM, Burks DJ, Ozcan U, Kulkarni RN, Ye J, Park S et al. Upregulation of insulin receptor substrate-2 in pancreatic beta cells prevents diabetes. *J Clin Invest* 2003 Nov; 112(10):1521–1532.
60. Park S, Dong X, Fisher TL, Dunn S, Omer AK, Weir G et al. Exendin-4 uses irs2 signaling to mediate pancreatic beta cell growth and function. *J Biol Chem* 2006 Jan 13; 281(2):1159–1168.
61. Withers DJ, Burks DJ, Towery HH, Altamuro SL, Flint CL, White MF. IRS-2 coordinates Igf-1 receptor-mediated beta-cell development and peripheral insulin signalling. *Nat Genet* 1999 Sep; 23(1):32–40.
62. Xuan S, Kitamura T, Nakae J, Politi K, Kido Y, Fisher PE et al. Defective insulin secretion in pancreatic beta cells lacking type 1 IGF receptor. *J Clin Invest* 2002 Oct; 110(7):1011–1019.
63. Kulkarni RN, Holzenberger M, Shih DQ, Ozcan U, Stoffel M, Magnuson MA et al. Beta-cell-specific deletion of the Igf1 receptor leads to hyperinsulinemia and glucose intolerance but does not alter beta-cell mass. *Nat Genet* 2002 May; 31(1):111–115.
64. Jonsson J, Carlsson L, Edlund T, Edlund H. Insulin-promoter-factor 1 is required for pancreas development in mice. *Nature* 1994; 371(6498):606–609.
65. Stoffers DA, Zinkin NT, Stanojevic V, Clarke WL, Habener JF. Pancreatic agenesis attributable to a single nucleotide deletion in the human IPF1 gene coding sequence. *Nat Genet* 1997; 15(1):106–110.
66. Kushner JA, Ye J, Schubert M, Burks DJ, Dow MA, Flint CL et al. Pdx1 restores beta cell function in IRS2 knockout mice. *J Clin Invest* 2002 May; 109(9):1193–1201.
67. Kitamura T, Nakae J, Kitamura Y, Kido Y, Biggs WH, III, Wright CV et al. The forkhead transcription factor Foxo1 links insulin signaling to Pdx1 regulation of pancreatic beta cell growth. *J Clin Invest* 2002 Dec; 110(12):1839–1847.
68. Accili D, Arden KC. FoxOs at the crossroads of cellular metabolism, differentiation, and transformation. *Cell* 2004 May 14; 117(4):421–426.
69. Uchida T, Nakamura T, Hashimoto N, Matsuda T, Kotani K, Sakaue H et al. Deletion of Cdkn1b ameliorates hyperglycemia by maintaining compensatory hyperinsulinemia in diabetic mice. *Nat Med* 2005 Feb; 11(2):175–182.
70. Parsons R. Human cancer, PTEN and the PI-3 kinase pathway. *Semin Cell Dev Biol* 2004 Apr; 15(2):171–176.
71. Kushner JA, Simpson L, Wartschow LM, Guo S, Rankin MM, Parsons R et al. Pten regulation of islet growth and glucose homeostasis. *J Biol Chem* 2005 Sep; 16.
72. Butler AA, Cone RD. Knockout studies defining different roles for melanocortin receptors in energy homeostasis. *Ann N Y Acad Sci* 2003 Jun; 994:240–245.

73. Farooqi IS, Keogh JM, Yeo GS, Lank EJ, Cheetham T, O'Rahilly S. Clinical spectrum of obesity and mutations in the melanocortin 4 receptor gene. *N Engl J Med* 2003 Mar 20; 348(12): 1085–1095.

74. Schwartz MW, Woods SC, Porte D Jr, Seeley RJ, Baskin DG. Central nervous system control of food intake. *Nature* 2000 Apr 6; 404(6778):661–671.

75. Qi Y, Takahashi N, Hileman SM, Patel HR, Berg AH, Pajvani UB et al. Adiponectin acts in the brain to decrease body weight. *Nat Med* 2004 May; 10(5):524–529.

76. Myers MG Jr. Leptin receptor signaling and the regulation of mammalian physiology. *Recent Prog Horm Res* 2004; 59:287–304.

77. Huszar D, Lynch CA, Fairchild-Huntress V, Dunmore JH, Fang Q, Berkemeier LR et al. Targeted disruption of the melanocortin-4 receptor results in obesity in mice. *Cell* 1997; 88:131–141.

78. Obici S, Feng Z, Tan J, Liu L, Karkanias G, Rossetti L. Central melanocortin receptors regulate insulin action. *J Clin Invest* 2001 Oct; 108(7):1079–1085.

79. Challis BG, Pritchard LE, Creemers JW, Delplanque J, Keogh JM, Luan J et al. A missense mutation disrupting a dibasic prohormone processing site in pro-opiomelanocortin (POMC) increases susceptibility to early-onset obesity through a novel molecular mechanism. *Hum Mol Genet* 2002 Aug 15; 11(17):1997–2004.

80. Yamauchi T, Kamon J, Ito Y, Tsuchida A, Yokomizo T, Kita S et al. Cloning of adiponectin receptors that mediate antidiabetic metabolic effects. *Nature* 2003 Jun 12; 423(6941):762–769.

81. Combs TP, Berg AH, Rajala MW, Klebanov S, Iyengar P, Jimenez-Chillaron JC et al. Sexual differentiation, pregnancy, calorie restriction, and aging affect the adipocyte-specific secretory protein adiponectin. *Diabetes* 2003 Feb; 52(2):268–276.

82. Spranger J, Kroke A, Mohlig M, Bergmann MM, Ristow M, Boeing H et al. Adiponectin and protection against type 2 diabetes mellitus. *Lancet* 2003 Jan 18; 361(9353):226–228.

83. Schwartz MW, Porte D Jr. Diabetes, obesity, and the brain. *Science* 2005 Jan 21; 307(5708): 375–379.

84. Woods SC, Lotter EC, McKay LD, Porte D Jr. Chronic intracerebroventricular infusion of insulin reduces food intake and body weight of baboons. *Nature* 1979 Nov 29; 282(5738):503–505.

85. Schwartz M, Figlewicz DP, Baskin DG, Woods SC, Porte D. Insulin in the brain: A hormonal regulator of energy balance. *Endocr Rev* 1992;13:387–414.

86. Schwartz MW, Baskin DG, Kaiyala KJ, Woods SC. Model of the regulation of energy balance and adiposity by the central nervous system. Am J Clin Nutr 1999;69:584–596.

87. Bruning JC, Gautam D, Burks DJ, Gillette J, Schubert M, Orban PC et al. Role of brain insulin receptor in control of body weight and reproduction. *Science* 2000 Sep 22; 289(5487):2122–2125.

88. Burks DJ, de Mora JF, Schubert M, Withers DJ, Myers MG, Towery HH et al. IRS-2 pathways integrate female reproduction and energy homeostasis. *Nature* 2000 Sep 21; 407(6802):377–382.

89. Wolfrum C, Asilmaz E, Luca E, Friedman JM, Stoffel M. Foxa2 regulates lipid metabolism and ketogenesis in the liver during fasting and in diabetes. *Nature* 2004 Dec 23; 432(7020):1027–1032.

90. Montminy M, Koo SH. Diabetes: Outfoxing insulin resistance? *Nature* 2004 Dec 23; 432(7020):958–959.

91. Pocai A, Lam TK, Gutierrez-Juarez R, Obici S, Schwartz GJ, Bryan J et al. Hypothalamic K(ATP) channels control hepatic glucose production. *Nature* 2005 Apr 21; 434(7036):1026–1031.

92. Gribble FM. Metabolism: A higher power for insulin. *Nature* 2005 Apr 21; 434(7036):965–966.

93. Barrett EJ. Insulin's effect on glucose production: Direct or indirect? *J Clin Invest* 2003 Feb; 111(4):434–435.

94. Buettner C, Patel R, Muse ED, Bhanot S, Monia BP, McKay R et al. Severe impairment in liver insulin signaling fails to alter hepatic insulin action in conscious mice. *J Clin Invest* 2005 May; 115(5):1306–1313.

95. Gelling RW, Morton GJ, Morrison CD, Niswender KD, Myers MG, Jr., Rhodes CJ et al. Insulin action in the brain contributes to glucose lowering during insulin treatment of diabetes. *Cell Metab* 2006 Jan; 3(1):67–73.

96. Rother KI, Imai Y, Caruso M, Beguinot F, Formisano P, Accili D. Evidence that IRS-2 phosphorylation is required for insulin action in hepatocytes. *J Biol Chem* 1998 Jul 10; 273(28):17491–17497.

97. Ide T, Shimano H, Yahagi N, Matsuzaka T, Nakakuki M, Yamamoto T et al. SREBPs suppress IRS-2-mediated insulin signalling in the liver. *Nat Cell Biol* 2004 Apr; 6(4):351–357.

98. Valverde AM, Fabregat I, Burks DJ, White MF, Benito M. IRS-2 mediates the antiapoptotic effect of insulin in neonatal hepatocytes. *Hepatology* 2004 Dec; 40(6):1285–1294.

99. Valverde AM, Burks DJ, Fabregat I, Fisher TL, Carretero J, White MF et al. Molecular mechanisms of insulin resistance in IRS-2-deficient hepatocytes. *Diabetes* 2003 Sep; 52(9):2239–2248.

100. Jhala US, Canettieri G, Screaton RA, Kulkarni RN, Krajewski S, Reed J et al. cAMP promotes pancreatic beta-cell survival via CREB-mediated induction of IRS2. *Genes Dev* 2003 Jul 1; 17(13):1575–1580.

101. Taniguchi CM, Ueki K, Kahn CR. Complementary roles of IRS-1 and IRS-2 in the hepatic regulation of metabolism. *J Clin Invest* 2005 Mar; 115(3):718–727.

102. Simmgen M, Knauf C, Lopez M, Choudhury AI, Charalambous M, Cantley J et al. Liver-specific deletion of insulin receptor substrate 2 does not impair hepatic glucose and lipid metabolism in mice. *Diabetologia* 2006 Jan 11; 1–10.

103. Matsumoto M, Accili D. The tangled path to glucose production. *Nat Med* 2006 Jan; 12(1):33–34.

104. Stumvoll M, Goldstein BJ, van Haeften TW. Type 2 diabetes: Principles of pathogenesis and therapy. *Lancet* 2005 Apr 9; 365(9467):1333–1346.

105. Nawrocki AR, Scherer PE. The delicate balance between fat and muscle: Adipokines in metabolic disease and musculoskeletal inflammation. *Curr Opin Pharmacol* 2004 Jun; 4(3):281–289.

106. Steppan CM, Wang J, Whiteman EL, Birnbaum MJ, Lazar MA. Activation of SOCS-3 by resistin. *Mol Cell Biol* 2005 Feb; 25(4):1569–1575.

107. Schmitz-Peiffer C, Whitehead JP. IRS-1 regulation in health and disease. *IUBMB Life* 2003 Jul; 55(7):367–374.

108. White MF, Myers MG. The molecular basis of insulin action. In: *Endocrinology*, 4 ed., DeGroot LJ, Jameson JL (eds.), W.B. Saunders, Philadelphia, 2001, pp. 712–727.

109. Ozcan U, Cao Q, Yilmaz E, Lee AH, Iwakoshi NN, Ozdelen E et al. Endoplasmic reticulum stress links obesity, insulin action, and type 2 diabetes. *Science* 2004 Oct 15; 306(5695):457–461.

110. Hotamisligil GS. The role of TNFalpha and TNF receptors in obesity and insulin resistance. *J Intern Med* 1999 Jun; 245(6):621–625.

111. Hotamisligil GS, Shargill NS, Spiegelman BM. Adipose expression of tumor necrosis factor-α: Direct role in obesity-linked insulin resistance. *Science* 1993; 259:87–91.

112. Hotamisligil GS, Spiegelman BM. Adipose expression of TNFα: Direct role in obesity-linked insulin resistance. *Science* 1999; 259:87–91.

113. Hotamisligil GS, Arner P, Caro JF, Atkinson RL, Spiegelman BM. Increased adipose tissue expression of tumor necrosis factor-α in human obesity and insulin resistance. *J Clin Invest* 1995; 95:2409–2415.

114. Weisberg SP, McCann D, Desai M, Rosenbaum M, Leibel RL, Ferrante AW Jr. Obesity is associated with macrophage accumulation in adipose tissue. *J Clin Invest* 2003 Dec; 112(12):1796–1808.

115. Uysal KT, Wiesbrock SM, Hotamisligil GS. Functional analysis of tumor necrosis factor (TNF) receptors in TNF-alpha-mediated insulin resistance in genetic obesity. *Endocrinology* 1998; 139(12):4832–4838.

116. Uysal KT, Wiesbrock SM, Marino MW, Hotamisligil GS. Protection from obesity-induced insulin resistance in mice lacking TNF-α function. *Nature* 1997 Oct 9; 389:610–614.

117. Hotamisligil GS. Mechanisms of TNF-alpha-induced insulin resistance. *Exp Clin Endocrinol Diabetes* 1999; 107(2):119–125. [Ref Type: Abstract.]

118. Aguirre V, Uchida T, Yenush L, Davis R, White MF. The c-Jun NH(2)-terminal kinase promotes insulin resistance during association with insulin receptor substrate-1 and phosphorylation of Ser(307). *J Biol Chem* 2000 Mar 24; 275(12):9047–9054.

119. De Fea K, Roth RA. Protein kinase C modulation of insulin receptor substrate-1 tyrosine phosphorylation requires serine 612. *Biochemistry* 1997 Oct 21; 36(42):12939–12947.

120. Begum N, Sandu OA, Ito M, Lohmann SM, Smolenski A. Active Rho kinase (ROK-alpha) associates with insulin receptor substrate-1 and inhibits insulin signaling in vascular smooth muscle cells. *J Biol Chem* 2002 Feb 22; 277(8):6214–6222.

121. Eldar-Finkelman H, Krebs EG. Phosphorylation of insulin receptor substrate 1 by glycogen synthase kinase 3 impairs insulin action. *Proc Natl Acad Sci USA* 1997; 94:9660–9604.

122. Staubs PA, Nelson JG, Reichart DR, Olefsky JM. Platelet-derived growth factor inhibits insulin stimulation of insulin receptor substrate-1 associated phosphatidylinositol 3-kinase in 3T3-L1 adipocytes without affecting glucose transport. *J Biol Chem* 1998; 273(39):25139–25147.

123. Hemi R, Paz K, Wertheim N, Karasik A, Zick Y, Kanety H. Transactivation of ErbB2 and ErbB3 by tumor necrosis factor-alpha and anisomycin leads to impaired insulin signaling through serine/threonine phosphorylation of IRS proteins. *J Biol Chem* 2002 Mar 15; 277(11):8961–8969.

124. Egawa K, Nakashima N, Sharma PM, Maegawa H, Nagai Y, Kashiwagi A et al. Persistent activation of phosphatidylinositol 3-kinase causes insulin resistance due to accelerated insulin-induced insulin receptor substrate-1 degradation in 3T3-L1 adipocytes. *Endocrinology* 2000 Jun; 141(6): 1930–1935.
125. Ravichandran LV, Chen H, Li Y, Quon MJ. Phosphorylation of PTP1B at Ser(50) by Akt impairs its ability to dephosphorylate the insulin receptor. *Mol Endocrinol* 2001 Oct; 15(10):1768–1780.
126. Liu YF, Paz K, Herschkovitz A, Alt A, Tennenbaum T, Sampson SR et al. Insulin stimulates PKCzeta-mediated phosphorylation of insulin receptor substrate-1 (IRS-1): A self-attenuated mechanism to negatively regulate the function of IRS proteins. *J Biol Chem* 2001 Apr 27; 276(17):14459–14465.
127. Ozes ON, Akca H, Mayo LD, Gustin JA, Maehama T, Dixon JE et al. A phosphatidylinositol 3-kinase/Akt/mTOR pathway mediates and PTEN antagonizes tumor necrosis factor inhibition of insulin signaling through insulin receptor substrate-1. *Proc Natl Acad Sci USA* 2001 Apr 3; 98:4640–4645.
128. Greene MW, Morrice N, Garofalo RS, Roth RA. Modulation of human insulin receptor substrate-1 tyrosine phosphorylation by protein kinase Cdelta. *Biochem J* 2004 Feb 15; 378(Pt 1):105–116.
129. Jiang G, Dallas-Yang Q, Liu F, Moller DE, Zhang BB. Salicylic acid reverses phorbol 12-myristate-13-acetate (PMA)- and tumor necrosis factor alpha (TNFalpha)-induced insulin receptor substrate 1 (IRS1) serine 307 phosphorylation and insulin resistance in human embryonic kidney 293 (HEK293) cells. *J Biol Chem* 2003 Jan 3; 278(1):180–186.
130. Mauvais-Jarvis F, Ueki K, Fruman DA, Hirshman MF, Sakamoto K, Goodyear LJ et al. Reduced expression of the murine p85alpha subunit of phosphoinositide 3-kinase improves insulin signaling and ameliorates diabetes. *J Clin Invest* 2002 Jan 1; 109(1):141–149.
131. Ueki K, Yballe CM, Brachmann SM, Vicent D, Watt JM, Kahn CR et al. Increased insulin sensitivity in mice lacking p85beta subunit of phosphoinositide 3-kinase. *Proc Natl Acad Sci USA* 2002 Jan 8; 99(1):419–424.
132. Ueki K, Fruman DA, Brachmann SM, Tseng YH, Cantley LC, Kahn CR. Molecular balance between the regulatory and catalytic subunits of phosphoinositide 3-kinase regulates cell signaling and survival. *Mol Cell Biol* 2002 Feb 1; 22(3):965–977.
133. Ueki K, Fruman DA, Yballe CM, Fasshauer M, Klein J, Asano T et al. Positive and negative roles of p85 alpha and p85 beta regulatory subunits of phosphoinositide 3-kinase in insulin signaling. *J Biol Chem* 2003 Nov 28; 278(48):48453–48466.
134. Greene MW, Garofalo RS. Positive and negative regulatory role of insulin receptor substrate 1 and 2 (IRS-1 and IRS-2) serine/threonine phosphorylation. *Biochemistry* 2002 Jun 4; 41(22):7082–7091.
135. Yu C, Chen Y, Cline GW, Zhang D, Zong H, Wang Y et al. Mechanism by which fatty acids inhibit insulin activation of insulin receptor substrate-1 (IRS-1)-associated phosphatidylinositol 3-kinase activity in muscle. *J Biol Chem* 2002 Dec 27; 277(52):50230–50236.
136. Gao Z, Hwang D, Bataille F, Lefevre M, York D, Quon MJ et al. Serine phosphorylation of insulin receptor substrate 1 by inhibitor kappa B kinase complex. *J Biol Chem* 2002 Dec 13; 277(50):48115–48121.
137. Gao Z, Zuberi A, Quon MJ, Dong Z, Ye J. Aspirin inhibits serine phosphorylation of insulin receptor substrate 1 in tumor-necrosis-factor-treated cells through targeting multiple serine kinases. *J Biol Chem* 2003; 278(27):24944–24950.
138. Gual P, Gremeaux T, Gonzalez T, Marchand-Brustel Y, Tanti JF. MAP kinases and mTOR mediate insulin-induced phosphorylation of insulin receptor substrate-1 on serine residues 307, 612 and 632. *Diabetologia* 2003 Nov; 46(11):1532–1542.
139. Rui L, Aguirre V, Kim JK, Shulman GI, Lee A, Corbould A et al. Insulin/IGF-1 and TNF-alpha stimulate phosphorylation of IRS-1 at inhibitory Ser307 via distinct pathways. *J Clin Invest* 2001 Jan; 107(2):181–189.
140. Zick Y. Ser/Thr phosphorylation of IRS proteins: A molecular basis for insulin resistance. *Sci STKE* 2005 Jan 25; 2005(268):e4.
141. Jaeschke A, Hartkamp J, Saitoh M, Roworth W, Nobukuni T, Hodges A et al. Tuberous sclerosis complex tumor suppressor-mediated S6 kinase inhibition by phosphatidylinositide-3-OH kinase is mTOR independent. *J Cell Biol* 2002 Oct 28; 159(2):217–224.

142. Shah OJ, Wang Z, Hunter T. Inappropriate activation of the TSC/Rheb/mTOR/S6K cassette induces IRS1/2 depletion, insulin resistance, and cell survival deficiencies. *Curr Biol* 2004 Sep 21; 14(18):1650–1656.

143. Um SH, Frigerio F, Watanabe M, Picard F, Joaquin M, Sticker M et al. Absence of S6K1 protects against age- and diet-induced obesity while enhancing insulin sensitivity. *Nature* 2004 Sep 9; 431(7005):200–205.

144. Kim JK, Kim YJ, Fillmore JJ, Chen Y, Moore I, Lee J et al. Prevention of fat-induced insulin resistance by salicylate. *J Clin Invest* 2001 Aug; 108(3):437–446.

145. Yuan M, Konstantopoulos N, Lee J, Hansen L, Li ZW, Karin M et al. Reversal of obesity- and diet-induced insulin resistance with salicylates or targeted disruption of Ikkbeta. *Science* 2001 Aug 31; 293(5535):1673–1677.

146. Hundal RS, Petersen KF, Mayerson AB, Randhawa PS, Inzucchi S, Shoelson SE et al. Mechanism by which high-dose aspirin improves glucose metabolism in type 2 diabetes. *J Clin Invest* 2002 May; 109(10):1321–1326.

147. Mothe I, Van Obberghen E. Phosphorylation of insulin receptor substrate-1 on multiple serine residues, 612, 632, 662, and 731, modulates insulin action. *J Biol Chem* 1996 May 10; 271(19): 11222–11227.

148. Jakobsen SN, Hardie DG, Morrice N, Tornqvist HE. 5′-AMP-activated protein kinase phosphorylates IRS-1 on Ser-789 in mouse C2C12 myotubes in response to 5-aminoimidazole-4-carboxamide riboside. *J Biol Chem* 2001 Dec 14; 276(50):46912–46916.

149. Rondinone CM, Reilly RM, Clampit JE, Haasch DL, inventors. Methods of identifying kinases and uses thereof. DN/20050037987, 2005 Feb 17.

150. Rui L, Yuan M, Frantz D, Shoelson S, White MF. SOCS-1 and SOCS-3 block insulin signaling by ubiquitin-mediated degradation of IRS1 and IRS2. *J Biol Chem* 2002 Nov 1; 277(44): 42394–42398.

151. Rui L, Fisher TL, Thomas J, White MF. Regulation of insulin/insulin-like growth factor-1 signaling by proteasome-mediated degradation of insulin receptor substrate-2. *J Biol Chem* 2001 Oct 26; 276(43):40362–40367.

152. Krebs DL, Hilton DJ. A new role for SOCS in insulin action: Suppressor of cytokine signaling. *Sci STKE* 2003 Feb 11; 2003(169):E6.

153. Cope GA, Deshaies RJ. COP9 signalosome: A multifunctional regulator of SCF and other cullin-based ubiquitin ligases. *Cell* 2003 Sep 19; 114(6):663–671.

154. Deshaies RJ. SCF and Cullin/Ring H2-based ubiquitin ligases. *Annu Rev Cell Dev Biol* 1999; 15:435–467.

155. Li Y, Kumar KG, Tang W, Spiegelman VS, Fuchs SY. Negative regulation of prolactin receptor stability and signaling mediated by SCF(beta-TrCP) E3 ubiquitin ligase. *Mol Cell Biol* 2004 May; 24(9):4038–4048.

156. Haruta T, Uno T, Kawahara J, Takano A, Egawa K, Sharma PM et al. A rapamycin-sensitive pathway down-regulates insulin signaling via phosphorylation and proteasomal degradation of insulin receptor substrate-1. *Mol Endocrinol* 2000 Jun; 14(6):783–794.

157. Takano A, Usui I, Haruta T, Kawahara J, Uno T, Iwata M et al. Mammalian target of rapamycin pathway regulates insulin signaling via subcellular redistribution of insulin receptor substrate 1 and integrates nutritional signals and metabolic signals of insulin. *Mol Cell Biol* 2001 Aug; 21(15):5050–5062.

158. Carlson CJ, White MF, Rondinone CM. Mammalian target of rapamycin regulates IRS-1 serine 307 phosphorylation. *Biochem Biophys Res Commun* 2004 Apr 2; 316(2):533–539.

159. Hartley D, Cooper GM. Role of mTOR in the degradation of IRS-1: Regulation of PP2A activity. *J Cell Biochem* 2002; 85(2):304–314.

160. Li Y, Corradetti MN, Inoki K, Guan KL. TSC2: Filling the GAP in the mTOR signaling pathway. *Trends Biochem Sci* 2004 Jan; 29(1):32–38.

161. Harrington LS, Findlay GM, Gray A, Tolkacheva T, Wigfield S, Rebholz H et al. The TSC1-2 tumor suppressor controls insulin-PI3K signaling via regulation of IRS proteins. *J Cell Biol* 2004 Jul 19; 166(2):213–223.

162. Drucker DJ. The biology of incretin hormones. *Cell Metab* 2006 Mar; 3(3):153-165.

163. Brubaker PL, Drucker DJ. Glucagon-like peptides regulate cell proliferation and apoptosis in the pancreas, gut and central nervous system. *Endocrinology* 2004 Mar 24; 145(6):2653-2659.

164. De Leon DD, Deng S, Madani R, Ahima RS, Drucker DJ, Stoffers DA. Role of endogenous gluca-gon-like peptide-1 in islet regeneration after partial pancreatectomy. *Diabetes* 2003 Feb; 52(2): 365–371.
165. Habener JF, Kemp DM. Insulinotropic glucagon-like peptides. In: *Diabetes Mellitus: A Fundamental and Clinical Text,* 3rd ed., LeRoith D, Taylon SI, Olefsky JM (eds.), Lippincott Williams and Wilkins, Philadelphia, 2004, pp. 99–113.
166. Buteau J, Foisy S, Rhodes CJ, Carpenter L, Biden TJ, Prentki M. Protein kinase Czeta activation mediates glucagon-like peptide-1-induced pancreatic beta-cell proliferation. *Diabetes* 2001 Oct; 50(10):2237–2243.
167. Buteau J, Roduit R, Susini S, Prentki M. Glucagon-like peptide-1 promotes DNA synthesis, activates phosphatidylinositol 3-kinase and increases transcription factor pancreatic and duodenal homeobox gene 1 (PDX-1) DNA binding activity in beta (INS-1)-cells. *Diabetologia* 1999 Jul; 42(7):856–864.
168. Idris I, Patiag D, Gray S, Donnelly R. Exendin-4 increases insulin sensitivity via a PI-3-kinase-dependent mechanism: Contrasting effects of GLP-1. *Biochem Pharmacol* 2002 Mar 1; 63(5): 993–996.
169. Hui H, Nourparvar A, Zhao X, Perfetti R. Glucagon-like peptide-1 inhibits apoptosis of insulin-secret-ing cells via a cyclic 5′-adenosine monophosphate-dependent protein kinase A- and a phosphati-dylinositol 3-kinase-dependent pathway. *Endocrinology* 2003 Apr; 144(4):1444–1455.
170. Drucker DJ. Glucagon-like peptides: Regulators of cell proliferation, differentiation, and apoptosis. *Mol Endocrinol* 2003 Feb; 17(2):161–171.
171. Li Y, Hansotia T, Yusta B, Ris F, Halban PA, Drucker DJ. Glucagon-like peptide-1 receptor signaling modulates beta cell apoptosis. *J Biol Chem* 2003 Jan 3; 278(1):471–478.
172. Giraud J, Leshan R, Lee YH, White MF. Nutrient-dependent and insulin-stimulated phosphorylation of insulin receptor substrate-1 on serine 302 correlates with increased insulin signaling. *J Biol Chem* 2004 Jan 30; 279(5):3447–3454.
173. Kitamura T, Nakae J, Biggs J, White MF, Arden KC, Accili D. The transcription factor FKHR pro-motes beta cell survival in IRS-2 knockout mice. *VIII International Symposium on Insulin Receptors and Insulin Action*, 2001 May 5; 85.
174. Rhoads RE. Signal transduction pathways that regulate eukaryotic protein synthesis. *J Biol Chem* 1999 Oct 22; 274(43):30337–30340.

15   Insulin Resistance and Inhibitors of the Insulin Receptor Tyrosine Kinase

Jack F. Youngren

CONTENTS

INSULIN RESISTANCE

Tissue resistance to insulin is a clinically significant phenomenon that predisposes an individual to numerous health risks beyond the well-established role it plays in the pathogenesis of type 2 diabetes mellitus (T2D). Quantification of whole-body insulin resistance in humans typically involves determining the ability of insulin to stimulate glucose uptake into muscle. The hyperinsulinemic, euglycemic clamp procedure provides a measurement of muscle insulin sensitivity, as this tissue accounts for 75% of glucose disposal under these conditions (1). The decrement in glucose disposal in an insulin-resistant state such as obesity is entirely due to reduced muscle glucose uptake (1). However, insulin resistance can occur in any insulin target tissue, and will produce a phenotype distinct for the biological characteristics of that tissue (2).

As in vivo determination of insulin sensitivity of an individual is reflective of muscle glucose disposal, this chapter will focus on the studies of insulin signaling in this tissue. In humans, insulin-stimulated muscle glucose disposal varies widely across the normal population, and the insulin-resistant state represents individuals in the lower end of a normal distribution, rather than a discrete condition. In vivo, muscle insulin sensitivity is regulated on a long-term basis by factors such as obesity, and is altered in a more rapid manner by changes in dietary habits and physical activity (3). Though more difficult to quantify, there is evidence for genetic or intrinsic differences in muscle insulin sensitivity as well (4). In any individual, therefore, the degree of insulin sensitivity is determined by numerous factors, both genetic and environmental. Despite advances in the understanding of cellular alterations that can inhibit the biological response to

From: *Contemporary Endocrinology: The Metabolic Syndrome: Epidemiology, Clinical Treatment, and Underlying Mechanisms*
Edited by: B.C. Hansen and G.A. Bray © Humana Press, Totowa, NJ

insulin, the challenge remains to determine the mechanisms contributing significantly to insulin resistance in an individual who is subject to this range of physiological factors.

INSULIN SIGNALING PATHWAY

As the components of the intracellular signaling pathway of insulin action have been elucidated over the past 15 years, the potential sites for cellular modulation of insulin responsiveness have increased dramatically. As described recently, the insulin signaling system (Fig. 15.1) consists of a complex integrated network of second messenger proteins (5). The divergence of insulin signaling into separate pathways that regulate distinct biological effects has been well described. However, it has also been long recognized that each of these second messenger pathways are also employed in mediating the intracellular effects of a variety of other hormones. The extent to which activities of these separate pathways interrelate to produce a specific and coordinated cellular response to insulin is only recently being appreciated (5).

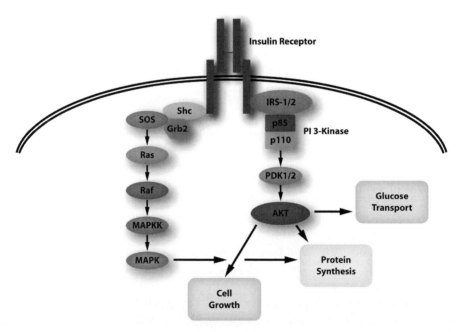

Figure 15.1. The insulin signaling pathway. The binding of insulin to its receptor leads to autophosphorylation of the β-subunits and the tyrosine phosphorylation of insulin receptor substrates (IRS) and other signaling intermediates such as Shc. Phosphorylated IRS proteins serve as docking proteins for other second messengers. Binding of the SH2 domains of PI 3-kinase (PI3K) to phosphotyrosines on IRS-1 activates this enzyme, thus increasing the intracellular concentration of phosphatidylinositol phosphoplipids. This in turn activates phosphatidylinositol phosphate-dependent kinase-1 (PDK-1), which subsequently activates AKT/PKB. The net effect of this pathway is to produce a translocation of the glucose transporter (GLUT4) from cytoplasmic vesicles to the cell membrane to facilitate glucose transport. Insulin stimulation of proliferation and protein synthesis can also be mediated by this pathway, although the Ras/Raf pathway is more closely associated with the mitogenic effects of insulin. (Reproduced with permission from Youngren JF. Regulation of insulin receptor function. Cell Mol Life Sci 2007; 64(7–8): 873–91.)

While distinct mechanisms for altering the function of second messenger proteins have been demonstrated, the significance of many of these effectors in human insulin-resistant states remains to be determined. It is likely that different lifestyle factors such as diet and physical activity patterns impact insulin signaling in different manners. It is also likely that the cellular mechanisms involved in impaired insulin signaling are not consistent across different tissues. Therefore, evidence in support of one mechanism for the development of insulin resistance does not imply that other cellular alterations do not also impact the insulin signaling pathway.

The cellular response to insulin is mediated through the insulin receptor (IR), one of a family of receptor tyrosine kinases (RTK). The IR protein consists of two identical extracellular α-subunits that bind insulin, and two identical transmembrane β-subunits that have intracellular tyrosine kinase activity (Fig. 15.2). When insulin binds to the α-subunit of the receptor, the β-subunit tyrosine kinase is activated, resulting in autophos-

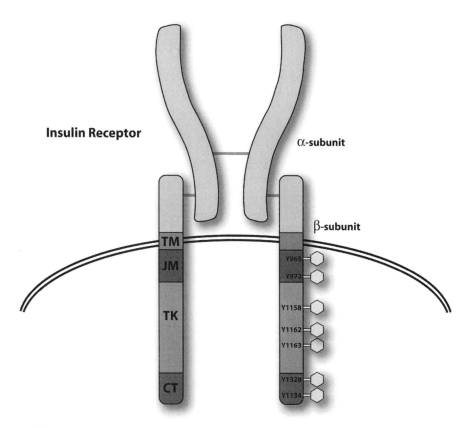

Figure 15.2. Schematic structure of the insulin receptor. The intracellular β-subunit of the IR contains several functionally distinct domains. The IR is anchored to the plasma membrane by the transmembrane domain (TM). The juxtamembrane domain (JM) contains two tyrosine residues that are autophosphorylated in response to insulin binding. Of these, tyrosine 972 is instrumental in binding the PTB domains of IRS proteins and SHC. The tyrosine kinase domain (TK) contains the enzymatic active site of the molecule, as well as the ATP binding site and three key tyrosines (1158, 1162, and 1163) that must be phosphorylated to produce full kinase activity of the IR. Tyrosines in the C-terminus (CT) region are not critical for receptor activation, but are thought to participate in the mitogenic effects of IR signaling. (Reproduced with permission from Youngren JF. Regulation of insulin receptor function. Cell Mol Life Sci 2007; 64(7–8): 873–91.)

phorylation of β-subunit tyrosine residues (6). After autophosphorylation, the activated receptor phosphorylates tyrosine residues on endogenous substrates, such as the insulin receptor substrates, IRS-1 and IRS-2, as well as Shc (Src homology collagen) and APS (adaptor protein with a PH and SH2 domain) (5). These phosphorylated substrates then serve as docking molecules that bind to and activate cellular kinases, initiating the divergent signaling pathways that mediate cellular insulin action. As described elsewhere, the network of second messenger proteins involved in insulin signaling is vast and interactive. Still, the general scheme is that the stimulation of glucose transport and most other metabolic effects of insulin are regulated by the phosphatidylinositol 3-kinase (PI3K) pathway, which is activated when the regulatory subunit of PI3K binds to phosphotyrosine residues on IRS-1. Cell growth and protein synthesis are more closely associated with the Ras/MAPK pathways, which are activated primarily by Shc phosphorylation (reviewed in ref. 7). The ultimate effector system for regulating glucose disposal is the translocation of GLUT4-containing vesicles to the plasma membrane to increase the rate of cellular glucose transport (6).

Insulin-resistant states are accompanied by a decrement in the ability of insulin to initiate these phosphorylation cascades that regulate the activity of insulin second messengers (8,9). Reductions in the enzymatic activity and phosphorylation state of kinases and substrates in these signaling pathways are observed in muscle biopsies from insulin-resistant subjects (10). However, the site(s) of the initial perturbation in signal transduction remain(s) unclear. A reduction in signal transduction upstream from an individual pathway constituent makes it difficult to evaluate whether the signaling molecule is itself functioning normally.

THE INSULIN RECEPTOR

Given its singular role in mediating the cellular response to insulin, a loss of function of the IR would produce the specific resistance to insulin observed in diabetes and related conditions. Employing Cre-loxP technology, which allows for the generation of transgenic mice with tissue-specific blockade of individual gene transcription, investigators have been able to study the effects of ablation of IR in liver, muscle, white adipose, pancreatic β-cell, vascular endothelium, and neurons (11–17). Although the exact phenotype of these different IR knockout models varies depending on the tissue affected, all aspects of the metabolic syndrome can be recreated by a loss of IR expression in these target tissues (reviewed in ref. 2). Transgenic mice that overexpress dominant negative, kinase-deficient insulin receptors exclusively in skeletal and cardiac muscle (18,19) provide a better model for the phenotype to be expected from impaired IR signaling than do IR knockouts. This targeted expression of mutant, inactive receptors produces substantial impairments in insulin-stimulated muscle insulin receptor tyrosine kinase activity, as well as diminished activation of downstream signaling intermediates IRS-1 and PI 3-kinase. These transgenic mice develop obesity, hyperinsulinemia, glucose intolerance, and hypertriglyceridemia (20).

Some insight into the impact that acute modulation of IR signaling capacity would produce in vivo is supplied from studies of small molecules that either inhibit or potentiate IR function. Haluska and co-workers (21) developed a small molecule inhibitor of both the IGF-1R and the IR that demonstrated anti-cancer properties in vivo. In testing the acute metabolic effects of this compound, they found that administrating a single dose produced a significant increase in fasting blood glucose and a subsequent elevation in both glucose and insulin response to an oral glucose tolerance test (21). While these data indicate that acute modulation of the tyrosine kinase activity of the IR can impair glucose homeostasis, there is no way to determine the tissue impacted by IR inhibition or whether the effects observed result from effects beyond the expected inhibition of the IR.

The IR-sensitizing compound TLK16998 can increase insulin-stimulated IR autophosphorylation but does not stimulate the receptor in the absence of insulin (22). As this compound reverses certain models of impaired IR function in insulin resistance (23), its in vivo effects provide information on the biological impact of modulating IR signaling capacity. Single-dose administration lowered blood glucose levels in two models of insulin-resistant diabetes, the obese db/db mouse and the high-fat-fed, streptozotocin-treated mouse (22). In addition, a single dose of TLK16998 in rats ameliorated the impairment in oral glucose tolerance induced by treatment with the protease inhibitor indinavir (24). Together, these data suggest that impairments in skeletal muscle insulin receptor tyrosine kinase activity are sufficient to produce a physiological state very similar to that of the majority of insulin-resistant, nondiabetic humans and that modulation of IR autophosphorylation and tyrosine kinase activity (up or down) induced by insulin significantly impacts whole-body glucose homeostasis.

Insulin Receptor Gene and Processing

The IR gene was originally identified in the mid-1980s (25,26). The highly homologous insulin-like growth-factor-1 receptor (IGF-1R) was cloned shortly thereafter (27), and the full sequence and structure of each gene was soon described (28,29). The IR gene consists of 22 exons and 21 introns spanning 150 kb of chromosome 19 (29). The IR gene product is synthesized as a prepro-receptor, from which a 30-amino-acid signal peptide is cleaved. The pro-receptor is then processed further, undergoing glycosylation, folding, and dimerization. In the golgi apparatus, the dimerized amino acid chains are then cleaved into alpha and beta subunits. These peptides are then linked via disulfide bonds to form a heterotetrameric holo-receptor.

The IR is inserted into the plasma membrane such that the α-subunits, which contain the ligand binding domain, are entirely extracellular. The β-subunits span the membrane and contain the tyrosine kinase domain on the intracellular portion of the subunit. Functionally important regions of the IR include the juxtamembrane region, the autoactivation loop, and the C-terminal region (30). Each of these regions contains tyrosine residues that are phosphorylated in response to insulin binding as part of the activation of the IR substrate kinase activity. A basic understanding of the relationship among phosphorylation state, receptor structure, and IR enzymatic activity is helpful when examining the roles that post-translational modifications of the IR protein and direct IR inhibitors can play in signaling capacity.

Functional Aspects of IR Structure

To date, the crystal structures of neither the full IR nor IGF-1R have been obtained. However, a significant amount of information has been obtained from electron microscopy studies and from crystal structures of receptor peptide fragments enabling models of IR structure to be developed. Structural models developed from electron microscopy studies are not entirely consistent (31). Although the details of IR structure are beyond

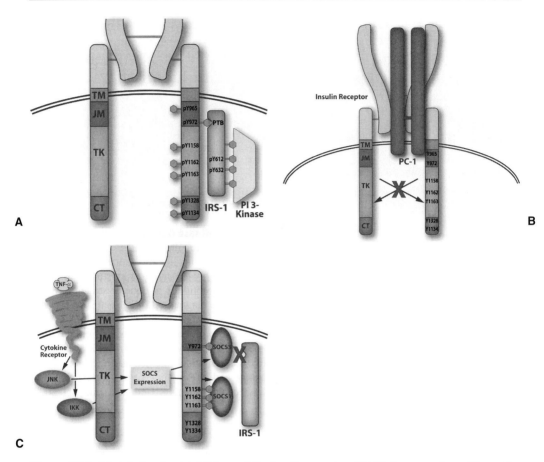

Figure 15.4. Models for direct inhibitors of the insulin receptor. (A) Under normal conditions, the activated IR binds IRS-1 through an interaction between phosphotyrosine 972 (pTyr972) and the SH2 domain of IRS-1. The phosphorylated IRS-1 can then serve as a docking site and activator of PI 3-kinase. (B) Membrane glycoprotein PC-1 has been shown to directly bind to the connecting domain of the IR α-subunit. With the model of IR activation proposed by Ottensmeyer and Yip (128), binding of PC-1 to this region could block the conformational change induced by ligand binding that brings the opposing β-subunits together to allow for *trans*-phosphorylation and activation. (C) The SOCS proteins 1 and 3 bind to phosphotyrosine residues on the activated IR. SOCS-3 interacts with tyrosine 972, which would then interfere with association between the IR and IRS-1, while SOCS-1 interacts with the phosphotyrosines in the activation loop, which would then interfere with IRS-2 binding. As such, these compounds do not block IR activation, but have been shown to decrease phosphorylation of IRS proteins and downstream signal transduction in response to upregulation by cytokines such as TNF-α. (Reproduced with permission from Youngren JF. Regulation of insulin receptor function. Cell Mol Life Sci 2007; 64(7–8): 873–91.)

kinase activity for cellular insulin response has been demonstrated in a variety of IR mutant cell lines with varying capacities of IR tyrosine kinase activity (39). Blocking the ATP binding to the β-subunit results in a complete loss of IR kinase activity (39).

Phosphorylated tyrosine residue 972 serves as a binding site for the PTB domains of IRS proteins, as well as IR substrates Shc and STAT 5B, facilitating the phosphorylation of these substrates on numerous tyrosine moieties (Fig. 15.4A) (40–43). The other primary IRS protein contributing to insulin signaling, IRS-2, is not dependent on tyrosine 972 for phosphorylation by the IR (40). This suggests that specific blockade of tyrosine 972 phosphorylation could impact only IRS-1 mediated signaling.

INSULIN RECEPTOR FUNCTION IN INSULIN RESISTANCE

The mechanisms underlying tissue resistance to insulin have been the focus of considerable investigations since the presence of high insulin levels in type 2 diabetes was first described. Impaired activation of the insulin signaling pathway has been demonstrated in muscle and fat from a variety of human and animal models of insulin resistance (for review see ref. 10). However, the physiological mediators of insulin resistance as well as the sites within the signaling pathway at which they act are still being clarified.

In most models of insulin resistance in humans and animals, investigators have reported a decrease in insulin activation of some components of the insulin signaling pathway. There is no clear consensus as to the exact site along this cascade of kinase and phosphatase reactions at which a reduction in protein phosphorylation or enzyme activity is observed. This is likely due to the facts that different models of insulin resistance likely involve different mechanisms, and discrepant effects on insulin signaling have been reported in different insulin target tissues within the same animal. In some instances, these discrepancies are likely the result of methodological differences. For instance, not all diets employed to study the effects of dietary fat consumption are the same. Also, cellular alterations in response to dietary intervention are not constant across time, so the time points employed can produce contrasting conclusions. The western blotting procedures that are commonly employed to study the protein phosphorylation state are notoriously nonquantitative, making small differences in protein phosphorylation difficult to assess.

IRS-1 is the primary substrate phosphorylated by the IR in target cells, and impaired IRS-1 phosphorylation is reported in the majority of insulin-resistant models (10). However, a decrease in substrate phosphorylation does not necessarily imply impairment in IR tyrosine kinase activity. Mechanisms have been described whereby the phosphorylation state of substrates such as IRS-1 can impair its ability to act as a substrate for the IR (44). Also, not all studies showing decreased IRS-1 tyrosine phosphorylation have demonstrated concurrent reductions in IR autophosphorylation or the tyrosine kinase activity of isolated receptors. However, impaired insulin activation of muscle IR has been reported in nearly every model of human and animal insulin resistance (see below), although there exist an almost equal number of conflicting reports. Whether the existence of contrary findings for nearly all these same conditions reflects methodological differences is not clear. The preponderance of evidence suggests that IR signaling capacity can be modulated by numerous physiological factors, and that several of these alterations represent modifications of the IR protein itself, which can be observed when purified IR is studied outside the cellular environment.

In the next section we will review the physiological states in which impaired IR signaling has been reported in skeletal muscle along with putative mechanisms that have been associated with these alterations. While there are studies of nearly all of these insulin-resistant models that report no association between cellular insulin resistance and impaired IR function, this review will focus instead on published reports demonstrating defects in IR activation in order to understand the mechanisms whereby these processes can contribute to insulin resistance.

Obesity

Obesity is thought to be the primary cause of insulin resistance in western society (45). Many laboratories have reported that IR autophosphorylation and tyrosine kinase activity are reduced in muscle from obese versus lean subjects. This has been demonstrated in IR isolated from muscle and simulated in vitro (46,47), in muscle strips incubated with insulin (48,49), and in IR obtained from muscle biopsies collected following whole-body insulin infusion (50). IR function in muscle biopsies from a heterogeneous population of Pima Indians was studied by employing a highly sensitive, quantitative ELISA to measure in vitro stimulation of IR autophosphorylation. In this population, where increasing obesity is directly related to the development of insulin resistance, a negative correlation was observed between percent body fat and insulin-stimulated IR autophosphorylation (51), suggesting a dose effect of adiposity on muscle IR function. In genetically hyperphagic models of insulin-resistant obesity there is considerable evidence supporting an impaired capacity for skeletal muscle IR activation by insulin (50,52–56).

The negative impact of increasing body fat stores on muscle insulin signaling is likely due to two separate but not mutually exclusive pathways. The adipocyte is now recognized as an endocrine organ. The obese state is associated with an altered hormonal environment that arises from an alteration in the release of cytokines from enlarged adipocytes (57). As described below, fat-derived cytokines can activate cellular pathways that impair cellular insulin signaling (57,58). However, an accumulation of lipids within muscle cells can also directly impair insulin signaling (59). There is evidence that both of these aspects of excess body lipid stores play a role in the impaired IR function observed in human obesity.

The impaired IR signaling observed in human obesity is also not necessarily due entirely to the impact of elevated total fat stores. As discussed below, dietary factors and physical activity patterns, the prime contributors to a positive caloric balance, can independently impact IR signaling. It is likely, however, that the impact of obesity on insulin signaling goes beyond lifestyle differences between lean and obese groups, due to the cellular effects of a surplus of lipids described below. When morbidly obese subjects lost an average of 100 pounds in the one year following gastric bypass surgery, but were still classifiable as obese, there was no reversal in impaired IR function in muscle biopsies (60).

Diet

Several dietary interventions in rodents have been shown to modulate IR function. In addition, data from these studies suggest that the excess caloric intake that produces weight gain impacts IR activity prior to a substantial increase in body fat stores. These results, however, vary with regard to the diet imposed and possibly the rodent strain employed.

When Fisher 344 rats, who are relatively resistant to weight gain, were provided a diet high in fat and refined sugar (HFS), in vitro stimulation of IR autophosphorylation was diminished within two weeks, prior to an increase in total body fat stores (61). A western, or cafeteria, diet, designed to mimic poor eating habits in industrialized societies, led to a downregulation of in vivo stimulation of IR activation in muscle and liver, but only after tissue insulin resistance was first observed and significant weight gain had occurred (62). Other studies showing decreased muscle IR function following a diet high in fat could not differentiate the dietary effects from the resultant development of obesity (56). It is possible that the composition of fatty acids within the diet has a significant impact on the effects on IR function (63). Diets high in fructose also result in significant insulin resistance in rodents. Studies on muscle IR function in response to fructose feeding have shown both reductions in IR phosphorylation (64) and no effect of the diet (65,66).

Human obesity, however, is accompanied by more subtle differences in caloric balance and little if any differences in dietary composition compared to rodent models of diet manipulation or hyperphagia. It is unclear to what extent dietary factors contribute to alterations in IR function in obese humans.

Physical Activity

Regular physical activity improves insulin sensitivity, and a cessation of regular exercise habits leads to a rapid decline in muscle insulin action (3,67). Substantial evidence suggests that regular physical activity increases the signaling capacity of the IR in muscle of humans and rodents, and IR function rapidly declines with a reduction of physical activity or with muscle disuse.

Although muscle insulin sensitivity can be increased during and for up to 24 hours following a single bout of exercise, this effect is independent of alterations in IR activity (68). Rather, an upregulation of IR signaling capacity is part of a multifaceted adaptation to repeated contractile activity, including increased expression of GLUT4, that together enhances the capacity for muscle glucose transport (67). Participation in a moderately intense exercise training program for seven days enhanced insulin stimulation of muscle IR autophosphorylation in vitro (69). In rodents, there are reports that IR function is increased by standard exercise training regimens (70,71) and through spontaneous physical activity induced by providing access to a running wheel (72). In the latter case, when physical activity is curtailed by locking the running wheel, muscle IR function returns to control levels within approximately 2 days (72). In more severe models of reduced muscle activity, IR function is dramatically impaired following limb immobilization or muscle denervation (74,75).

Diabetes

Decreased muscle IR function in patients with type 2 diabetes has been reported in isolated IR stimulated in vitro (46,47,76–78) and in muscle biopsies obtained following in vivo insulin infusion (50,79–81). As with obesity, diabetes does not exist in a vacuum. Insulin resistance precedes the development of type 2 diabetes, and whatever the causes of insulin resistance in the individual it is likely that impaired IR function was observable prior to the progression to postprandial and fasting hyperglycemia. It is likely, however, that the elevation of glucose has a major impact on IR signaling, and a disruption of IR signal transduction is likely worsened by the negative impact of chronic elevations in glucose that characterize the diabetic state (see below).

Inherited Insulin Resistance

Despite the fact that the insulin resistance underlying the development of diabetes may be due to a variety of lifestyle rather than genetic factors, taken as a group, the offspring of patients with type 2 diabetes are insulin resistant compared to the average

tyrosine phosphatases (PTPs). Several PTPs have been identified as contributing to IR dephosphorylation in cells. LAR, SHP-2, and PTP-1B were identified as the primary PTPs in skeletal muscle (104). SHP-2 is believed to interact with the IR via binding of one of its SH2 domains to phosphotyrosine 1158, and this interaction facilitates phosphorylation of IRS-1 (105). SHP-2 therefore contributes positively to cellular insulin action (106). Evidence for the role of LAR and PTP-1B in downregulating IR function comes from their altered expression in insulin target tissues and the demonstration that altered expression of these enzymes can alter insulin signal transduction (106).

Insulin stimulation of cells results in an association between PTP-1B and the IR, and the phosphorylation of PTP-1B on tyrosine residues 66, 152, and 153 (107). This interaction is dependent on tyrosines 1158, 1162, and 1163 of the IR (107), within the region identified as (one of) the PTP-1B binding sites by co-crystallization studies (108,109). Overexpression of PTP-1B decreases IR autophosphorylation in muscle cells and adipocytes (110,111). However, inhibition of the biological effects of insulin was observed only in muscle (110,111).

The generation of transgenic mice provided definitive data on the role of PTP-1B in modulating IR function and insulin sensitivity in vivo. Mice heterozygous or homozygous for a knockout of PTP-1B demonstrate significantly greater tissue insulin sensitivity and an enhanced IR autophosphorylation (112). Correspondingly, overexpression of PTP-1B in muscle induces tissue insulin resistance in mice associated with a decrement in the capacity for IR autophosphorylation (113).

LAR is a membrane-bound PTP that can be co-immunoprecipitated with the IR (114). Overexpression of LAR in hepatoma cells produces a significant reduction in insulin-stimulated IR autophosphorylation (115), while genetic blockade of LAR expression enhances IR signaling (116). Overexpression of LAR in skeletal muscle of transgenic mice results in an insulin-resistant phenotype. There is no discernable defect in IR autophosphorylation in these animals, however, suggesting that LAR may play a more significant role in regulating IRS-2 phosphorylation in vivo (117). Subsequent studies in cultured cells demonstrated that genetic knockdown of LAR expression paradoxically induced insulin resistance but did not affect IR signaling (118). Thus, there is strong evidence suggesting that the phosphatase LAR is not an important regulator of IR function.

While other phosphatases such as TCPTP and PTPepsilonM have been demonstrated to dephosphorylate the IR (112,119–121), the role of these PTPs in cellular insulin signaling has not been fully established.

Increased expression of PTPs may play a role in the impaired IR function observed in obesity. General PTP activity has been reported to be increased in muscle from obese versus lean subjects (122). However, a reduction in PTP activity has been reported in muscle from both obese subjects and patients with type 2 diabetes (123,124). PTP-1B expression is decreased in skeletal muscle from insulin-resistant subjects (124). Thus while the cellular content of PTPs can undoubtedly regulate IR function, there are no data suggesting that expression of these enzymes is altered in a manner that would contribute to the impaired IR signaling observed in insulin-resistant states.

PC-1

Plasma cell membrane glycoprotein 1 (PC-1) was originally identified as a direct inhibitor of IR tyrosine kinase activity by Maddux et al. (125). In studying fibroblasts from an insulin-resistant diabetic patient, it was discovered that the impaired IR signaling capacity observed in culture was absent in IR purified from these cells. A glycoprotein inhibitor was isolated from the patient's fibroblasts and was identified as PC-1 (also referred to as ectonucleotide pyrophosphatase phosphodiesterase 1, ENPP1) (126). Subsequent investigation revealed that the PC-1 protein was overexpressed at least 10-fold in fibroblasts from this patient compared to controls. The mechanism whereby PC-1 could produce the reduction in IR activity was identified when a direct interaction between PC-1 and the α-subunit of the IR was demonstrated (127). This interaction was dependent on the presence of amino acids 485–599 of the IR connecting domain (127). Binding of PC-1 to this region of the IR could interfere with the conformational change in the β-subunits that permits *trans*-phosphorylation of the opposing subunits in the structural model of Ottensmeyer and co-workers (Fig. 15.4B) (128).

The causal relationship between PC-1 overexpression and impaired IR function has been established both in transfected cells (126,127,129) and in genetically modified rodents (130). An overexpression of PC-1 in liver results in insulin resistance and impaired glucose tolerance (130). Transgenic mice that overexpressed PC-1 in multiple tissues, most notably skeletal muscle, demonstrated impaired glucose tolerance and a reduction in insulin-stimulated muscle glucose uptake (125).

To date, there is evidence for PC-1 overexpression contributing to insulin resistance related to obesity, and perhaps the idiopathic insulin resistance seen in the general nonobese population, as insulin action in these groups is inversely associated with elevated PC-1 content in skeletal muscle and adipose tissue (131). Across a wide range of obesity, increasing body fat content is associated with increasing muscle PC-1 content (132). In that study, PC-1 but not obesity emerged as an independent predictor of reduced insulin sensitivity. Muscle PC-1 content is also inversely related to insulin sensitivity in a nonobese, nondiabetic population (86).

The simple relationship between PC-1 content and insulin action is complicated by the presence of a DNA polymorphism in the gene for PC-1 that is both relatively prevalent and apparently functionally significant. The human PC-1 gene is located on chromosome 6q22-6q23. The polymorphism in exon 4 produces an amino acid change in codon 121 from lysine to glutamine (K121Q). When expressed in cells, the Q allele variant of PC-1 displays a stronger association with the IR, and an increased capacity for IR inhibition (129). While it is not clear what the full physiological impact of expressing the Q allele might be, or how different forms of the protein impact the relationship between total PC-1 content and insulin resistance, studies on allele frequencies suggest that the expression of the Q allele significantly contributes to genetic insulin resistance in some populations. Carriers of the Q allele of the PC-1 gene demonstrate a 25% increase in the risk for developing type 2 diabetes with an earlier onset of disease as well (133,134). In addition, a study of over 6,000 subjects identified a three-allele "at-risk" haplotype involving the Q allele and two other polymorphisms in the PC-1 gene (135). Analysis of all polymorphisms in a variety of individuals and family cohorts suggested that alterations in the PC-1 gene are involved in risk for development of childhood and adult obesity as well as T2D (135). While each polymorphism is associated with obesity risk, only the Q allele independently confers risk for type 2 diabetes. The mechanisms whereby the presence of the additional polymorphisms further increase risk for diabetes is not clear, as the functional consequences of these polymorphisms that map to untranslated regions of the PC-1 gene have not been studied.

SOCS PROTEINS

Two additional proteins have been identified that bind to the IR and interfere with the phosphorylation of IR substrates without blocking the activation of the IR. Suppressors of cytokine signaling (SOCS) proteins, SOCS-1 and SOCS-3, are two of a family of eight proteins that are thought to regulate cellular response to cytokines in a negative feedback manner (136). Studies have indicated that SOCS-1, SOCS-3, and SOCS-6 can bind to the IR in cells (137,138). SOCS-3 binds to phosphorylated tyrosine 972, whereas SOCS-1 interacts with the phosphorylated form of the C-terminus, containing tyrosines 1158, 1162, and 1163, that is essential for interaction of the IR with IRS-2 (Fig. 15.4C). The SOCS proteins therefore interact with the activated IR and do not show evidence of inhibiting IR autophosphorylation (138,139). Insulin-stimulated phosphorylation of IRS-1 and IRS-2 is decreased, however, by overexpression of SOCS-1 and SOCS-3 in cells (138,139). This is likely the result of the presence of either SOCS-1 or -3 directly blocking the ability of IRS to interact with the IR.

As expression of SOCS proteins is increased by cytokines (136), SOCS-1 and SOCS-3 are obvious candidates to mediate the insulin resistance involved in obesity and other conditions associated with a heightened inflammatory state. Treatment of muscle cells with TNF-α increases SOCS-1 and -3 expression (139), and SOCS-1 and SOCS-3 content is elevated in liver from obese insulin-resistant mice (140). Knockdown of SOCS expression in adipocytes prevents much of the impaired phosphorylation of IRS-1 and IRS-2 (139). While the contribution of SOCS to obesity-related insulin resistance has been demonstrated in obese diabetic mice with antisense-mediated knockdown of SOCS-1 or -3 expression (140), the observed impairments of IR autophosphorylation in this model must arise from other mechanisms.

Inhibitors That Induce Post-translational Modification of the IR

While the IR inhibiting proteins described above are strong candidates to contribute to various insulin-resistant states, the observation of impaired function of IR following isolation from the intracellular milieu suggests that in the absence of strong protein–protein interactions maintained through the purification processes, some post-translational modification of the IR protein must regulate IR activity. Evidence exists for modulation of IR activity by serine/threonine phosphorylation and by *O*-linked glycosylation.

PROTEIN KINASE C–MEDIATED SERINE PHOSPHORYLATION

Serine phosphorylation undoubtedly contributes to intracellular modulation of the insulin signaling pathway. Serine phosphorylation sites have been mapped on IRS-1 that inhibit the ability of IRS-1 to serve as a substrate of IR tyrosine kinase activity (141). The modulation of IRS-1 function by serine threonine phosphorylation results from the activation of multiple serine kinase pathways. For example, the cytokine TNF-α has been shown to negatively impact IRS-1 function by phosphorylating serine 307 via the c-jun N-terminal kinase (JNK) (142). Serine 307 is in close proximity to the phosphotyrosine binding site of IRS-1 that is meant to interact with the activated IR. Phosphorylation of this residue then results in a reduced capacity for IRS-1 to serve as a substrate of the IR. In contrast, the mechanisms whereby serine phosphorylation regulates IR function are less well characterized. However, there is strong evidence that

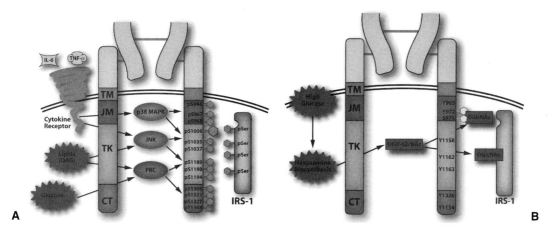

Figure 15.5. Models for inhibition of the insulin receptor by post-translational modification. (A) Phosphorylation of serine threonine residues on the IR β-subunit has been demonstrated via activation of PKC enzymes due to accumulation of lipid intermediates or high levels of glucose. It is likely that structural alterations resulting from these phosphorylations interfere with conformational changes and/or tyrosine phosphorylation of the IR. (B) Serine 976 is a putative site for addition of an O-linked glycosylation with the substrate UDP-N-acetylglucosamine. UDP-N-acetylglucosamine levels are elevated with increasing flux through the hexosamine pathway resulting from hyperglycemia. Glycosylation on this site resulting from increased hexosamine biosynthesis may interfere with IRS-1 binding to IR tyrosine 972 and subsequent phosphorylation. (Reproduced with permission from Youngren JF. Regulation of insulin receptor function. Cell Mol Life Sci 2007; 64(7–8): 873–91.)

serine phosphorylation of the IR contributes to insulin resistance related to obesity as well as the toxicity of glucose on insulin signaling (Fig. 15.5A).

Serine phosphorylation of the IR has been demonstrated in isolated muscle strips (143) and in cultured cells following incubation with phorbol esters (144,145). This mechanism is believed to involve activation of one or more isoforms of protein kinase C (PKC), as expression of either PKCβ1 or β2 is required for this ability of the phorbol esters to downregulate IR signaling (145). Other PKC isoforms (α, δ, θ), when activated by phorbol esters, were able to inhibit IR signaling only when co-expressed with IRS-1 (146).

In studies in cells or with isolated proteins, PKC-mediated phosphorylation of the IR has been demonstrated on serine residues 967/68 of the juxtamembrane region (147), serines 1006, 1035, and 1037 in the catalytic domain (53,148), and serines 1288, 1305/6, 1321, 1327, and threonine 1348 in the C-terminus (147,149–153). It is not clear that each of these phosphorylation sites is involved in the regulation of IR kinase activity (148,154). The downregulation of IR activity by PKCβ1, β2, or θ requires serines 1006, 1035/7, as mutation of the IR at these residues abolishes the PKC effect (144,145). These PKC isoforms, along with PKCδ, directly associate with the IR (155).

An increased PKC activity is thought to play a significant role in several models of human insulin resistance (for reviews see refs. 154 and 156). PKCβ activity is increased in muscle from obese insulin-resistant subjects (157). Pharmacological inhibition of PKC activity can reverse the impaired insulin stimulation glucose transport in muscle strips obtained from obese subjects (48). Increased phosphorylation of the IR on serine

944 has been demonstrated in muscle and liver from obese insulin-resistant rodents (53,158). In humans, serine phosphorylation of muscle IR has been observed in muscle from PCOS patients (101), but not from patients with type 2 diabetes. Serine phosphorylation of the IR has been difficult to demonstrate in IR from human muscle in other models of insulin resistance. However, treatment of purified IR from muscle of obese insulin-resistant subjects and patients with gestational diabetes with phosphatase enzymes to strip away any existing phosphorylation normalizes receptor tyrosine kinase activity (100,157).

This relationship between obesity and increased PKC activity can be explained by the activation of PKC by lipid intermediates within the cell. Obesity and other insulin-resistant states are associated with an accumulation of intramyocellular lipids (IMCL) and it is the activation of PKC enzymes that is thought to mediate the deleterious effects of these intracellular lipids on insulin signaling. Lipid deposition increases the cellular levels of diacylglycerols (DAG), which are known to activate PKC enzymes (154,155). Lipid infusion in humans and rodents increases muscle DAG content and PKC activity coincident with the induction of tissue insulin resistance (159–161). Lipid infusion in rats increases IR serine phosphorylation and reduces insulin-stimulated IR autophosphorylation in a PKC-dependent manner (159).

Beyond the direct and indirect effects on muscle of lipid accumulation, the worsening of insulin resistance as a result of hyperglycemia (or so-called *glucotoxicity*) may also be related to PKC-mediated IR serine phosphorylation (162). Incubation of cells with high glucose levels produces a PKC-mediated inhibition of IR autophosphorylation (163).

CYTOKINE ACTIVATED SERINE KINASES

Lipid accumulation has also been reported to activate stress kinase pathways involving the serine kinases JNK and MAP, which can phosphorylate IRS-1 and impair its capacity to transmit the IR signal (reviewed in ref. 154). These kinases have not been shown to directly inhibit IR activation. However, the decrement in IR autophosphorylation induced by lipid incubation in 3T3-L1 adipocytes was prevented by blocking JNK expression (164).

Serine phosphorylation of the IR in obesity could also arise secondarily to adipocyte secretions via cytokine-mediated pathways. Tumor necrosis factor-α, (TNF-α) and interleukin-6 (IL-6) are both secreted by adipocytes and known to activate serine kinase pathways that could phosphorylate the IR. TNF-α, plasma levels of which are elevated in human and rodent obesity (165,166), produces cellular insulin resistance, which results in increased phosphorylation of IRS-1 on the key regulatory site serine 307 via activation of the serine kinases IKK-β, JNK, p38 MAPK, and/or mTOR (141,167). In muscle cells, TNF-α incubation induces serine phosphorylation of the IR on undisclosed residues coincident with inhibition of insulin-stimulated IR autophosphorylation in a p38 MAPK–dependent manner (167).

Adipocytes produce a substantial proportion of the total circulating IL-6, and levels of this inflammatory cytokine are increased with obesity (166). In cultured muscle cells, IL-6 inhibits insulin-stimulated IR autophosphorylation (168); although it is not known whether the IR is directly serine phosphorylated, IL-6 incubation leads to phosphorylation of IRS-1 on serine 318 in muscle cells (169), an effect likely mediated via JAK/ STAT activation of MAPK pathways.

OTHER MODELS OF POST-TRANSLATIONAL MODIFICATION

In addition to serine/threonine phosphorylation, the activity of the IR could be altered by other mechanisms that modify the molecule. It has long been recognized that flux of a surplus of glucose through the hexosamine biosynthetic pathway produces insulin resistance (8). The end product of this pathway is UDP-N-acetylglucosamine (UDP-GlcNAc), which serves as a substrate for the enzyme O-linked N-acetylglucosamine transferase (OGT). OGT O-glycosylates proteins by adding a GlcNAc moiety to the hydroxyl groups of serine/threonine residues. O-linked beta-N-acetylglucosamine represents a post-translational modification known to modify the function of numerous proteins in a manner more similar to phosphorylation than simple glycosylation (170).

In pancreatic RIN β-cells, glucosamine induces O-glycosylation of both the IR and IRS-1 with a coincident decrease in insulin-stimulated IR autophosphorylation (171). Treatment of cells with an inhibitor of OGT reversed the decrement in IR function. Although the exact site of glycosylation was not determined, one potential O-glycosylation site on the IR is at serine 976 adjacent to the key autophosphorylation site, tyrosine 972, on the juxtamembrane region (Fig. 15.5B). It is possible that O-glycosylation at this site would sterically inhibit phosphorylation of tyr 972 on the IR following insulin biding and thereby interfere with binding and phosphorylation of IR substrates. In support of this model, IR from glucosamine-treated cells demonstrated a decrease in phosphorylated tyr 974 (equivalent on the rodent IR to tyr 972 on the human IR), although it is not clear whether this represented a specific effect of O-glycosylation on this residue, or whether autophosphorylation was diminished at other sites as well (171).

It is tempting then to suggest a role for O-GlcNAc modification of IR function to explain the impaired IR function associated with glucose toxicity. Elevated levels of O-GlcNAc have been observed in tissues from animals with experimental diabetes. However, O-GlcNAc-modified IR has not been observed in vivo. While muscle does express OGT mRNA, the levels are significantly lower than in the pancreas (172), where O-GlcNAc modification has been induced in vitro.

REFERENCES

1. DeFronzo RA. Lilly lecture 1987. The triumvirate: Beta-cell, muscle, liver—a collusion responsible for NIDDM. *Diabetes* 1988; 37(6):667–687.
2. Biddinger SB, Kahn CR. From mice to men: Insights into the insulin resistance syndromes. *Annu Rev Physiol* 2006; 68:123–158.
3. Barnard RJ, Youngren JF. Regulation of glucose transport in skeletal muscle. *FASEB J* 1992; 6(14):3238–3244.
4. Groop LC. Insulin resistance: The fundamental trigger of type 2 diabetes. *Diabetes Obes Metab* 1999; 1(suppl 1):S1–S7.
5. Taniguchi CM, Emanuelli B, Kahn CR. Critical nodes in signalling pathways: Insights into insulin action. *Nat Rev Mol Cell Biol* 2006; 7(2):85–96.
6. Kahn CR, White MF. The insulin receptor and the molecular mechanism of insulin action. *J Clin Invest* 1988; 82(4):1151–1156.
7. Avruch J. Insulin signal transduction through protein kinase cascades. *Mol Cell Biochem* 1998; 182(1–2):31–48.
8. Pirola L, Johnston AM, Van Obberghen E. Modulation of insulin action. *Diabetologia* 2004; 47(2):170–184.
9. White MF. Insulin signaling in health and disease. *Science* 2003; 302(5651):1710–1711.

10. Sesti G, Federici M, Hribal ML, Lauro D, Sbraccia P, Lauro R. Defects of the insulin receptor sub-strate (IRS) system in human metabolic disorders. *FASEB J* 2001; 15(12):2099–2111.
11. Bluher M, Michael MD, Peroni OD, Ueki K, Carter N, Kahn BB et al. Adipose tissue selective insulin receptor knockout protects against obesity and obesity-related glucose intolerance. *Dev Cell* 2002; 3(1):25–38.
12. Bruning JC, Michael MD, Winnay JN, Hayashi T, Horsch D, Accili D et al. A muscle-specific insulin receptor knockout exhibits features of the metabolic syndrome of NIDDM without altering glucose tolerance. *Mol Cell* 1998; 2(5):559–569.
13. Bruning JC, Gautam D, Burks DJ, Gillette J, Schubert M, Orban PC et al. Role of brain insulin receptor in control of body weight and reproduction. *Science* 2000; 289(5487):2122–2125.
14. Kim JK, Michael MD, Previs SF, Peroni OD, Mauvais-Jarvis F, Neschen S et al. Redistribution of substrates to adipose tissue promotes obesity in mice with selective insulin resistance in muscle. *J Clin Invest* 2000; 105(12):1791–1797.
15. Kulkarni RN, Bruning JC, Winnay JN, Postic C, Magnuson MA, Kahn CR. Tissue-specific knockout of the insulin receptor in pancreatic beta cells creates an insulin secretory defect similar to that in type 2 diabetes. *Cell* 1999; 96(3):329–339.
16. Michael MD, Kulkarni RN, Postic C, Previs SF, Shulman GI, Magnuson MA et al. Loss of insulin signaling in hepatocytes leads to severe insulin resistance and progressive hepatic dysfunction. *Mol Cell* 2000; 6(1):87–97.
17. Vicent D, Ilany J, Kondo T, Naruse K, Fisher SJ, Kisanuki YY et al. The role of endothelial insulin signaling in the regulation of vascular tone and insulin resistance. *J Clin Invest* 2003; 111(9):1373–1380.
18. Chang PY, Benecke H, Marchand-Brustel Y, Lawitts J, Moller DE. Expression of a dominant-negative mutant human insulin receptor in the muscle of transgenic mice. *J Biol Chem* 1994; 269(23):16034–16040.
19. Chang PY, Goodyear LJ, Benecke H, Markuns JS, Moller DE. Impaired insulin signaling in skeletal muscles from transgenic mice expressing kinase-deficient insulin receptors. *J Biol Chem* 1995; 270(21):12593–12600.
20. Moller DE, Chang PY, Yaspelkis BB, III, Flier JS, Wallberg-Henriksson H, Ivy JL. Transgenic mice with muscle-specific insulin resistance develop increased adiposity, impaired glucose tolerance, and dyslipidemia. *Endocrinology* 1996; 137(6):2397–2405.
21. Haluska P, Carboni JM, Loegering DA, Lee FY, Wittman M, Saulnier MG et al. In vitro and in vivo antitumor effects of the dual insulin-like growth factor-I/insulin receptor inhibitor, BMS-554417. *Cancer Res* 2006; 66(1):362–371.
22. Manchem VP, Goldfine ID, Kohanski RA, Cristobal CP, Lum RT, Schow SR et al. A novel small molecule that directly sensitizes the insulin receptor in vitro and in vivo. *Diabetes* 2001; 50(4):824–830.
23. Li M, Youngren JF, Manchem VP, Kozlowski M, Zhang BB, Maddux BA et al. Small molecule insulin receptor activators potentiate insulin action in insulin-resistant cells. *Diabetes* 2001; 50(10):2323–2328.
24. Cheng M, Chen S, Schow SR, Manchem VP, Spevak WR, Cristobal CP et al. In vitro and in vivo prevention of HIV protease inhibitor-induced insulin resistance by a novel small molecule insulin receptor activator. *J Cell Biochem* 2004; 92(6):1234–1245.
25. Ebina Y, Ellis L, Jarnagin K, Edery M, Graf L, Clauser E et al. The human insulin receptor cDNA: The structural basis for hormone-activated transmembrane signalling. *Cell* 1985; 40(4):747–758.
26. Ullrich A, Bell JR, Chen EY, Herrera R, Petruzzelli LM, Dull TJ et al. Human insulin receptor and its relationship to the tyrosine kinase family of oncogenes. *Nature* 1985; 313(6005):756–761.
27. Ullrich A, Gray A, Tam AW, Yang-Feng T, Tsubokawa M, Collins C et al. Insulin-like growth factor I receptor primary structure: Comparison with insulin receptor suggests structural determinants that define functional specificity. *EMBO J* 1986; 5(10):2503–2512.
28. Abbott AM, Bueno R, Pedrini MT, Murray JM, Smith RJ. Insulin-like growth factor I receptor gene structure. *J Biol Chem* 1992; 267(15):10759–10763.
29. Seino S, Seino M, Nishi S, Bell GI. Structure of the human insulin receptor gene and characterization of its promoter. *Proc Natl Acad Sci USA* 1989; 86(1):114–118.
30. Hubbard SR, Till JH. Protein tyrosine kinase structure and function. *Annu Rev Biochem* 2000; 69:373–398.

31. De Meyts P, Whittaker J. Structural biology of insulin and IGF1 receptors: Implications for drug design. *Nat Rev Drug Discov* 2002; 1(10):769–783.
32. Cann AD, Kohanski RA. Cis-autophosphorylation of juxtamembrane tyrosines in the insulin receptor kinase domain. *Biochemistry* 1997; 36(25):7681–7689.
33. White MF, Kahn CR. The insulin signaling system. *J Biol Chem* 1994; 269(1):1–4.
34. Yonezawa K, Ando A, Kaburagi Y, Yamamoto-Honda R, Kitamura T, Hara K et al. Signal transduction pathways from insulin receptors to Ras. Analysis by mutant insulin receptors. *J Biol Chem* 1994; 269(6):4634–4640.
35. Kaburagi Y, Momomura K, Yamamoto-Honda R, Tobe K, Tamori Y, Sakura H et al. Site-directed mutagenesis of the juxtamembrane domain of the human insulin receptor. *J Biol Chem* 1993; 268(22):16610–16622.
36. Smith JE, Sheng ZF, Kallen RG. Effects of tyrosine–phenylalanine mutations on auto- and trans-phosphorylation reactions catalyzed by the insulin receptor beta-subunit cytoplasmic domain. *DNA Cell Biol* 1994; 13(6):593–604.
37. Hubbard SR. Crystal structure of the activated insulin receptor tyrosine kinase in complex with peptide substrate and ATP analog. *EMBO J* 1997; 16(18):5572–5581.
38. Ablooglu AJ, Kohanski RA. Activation of the insulin receptor's kinase domain changes the rate-determining step of substrate phosphorylation. *Biochemistry* 2001; 40(2):504–513.
39. Wilden PA, Kahn CR. The level of insulin receptor tyrosine kinase activity modulates the activities of phosphatidylinositol 3-kinase, microtubule-associated protein, and S6 kinases. *Mol Endocrinol* 1994; 8(5):558–567.
40. Chaika OV, Chaika N, Volle DJ, Hayashi H, Ebina Y, Wang LM et al. Mutation of tyrosine 960 within the insulin receptor juxtamembrane domain impairs glucose transport but does not inhibit ligand-mediated phosphorylation of insulin receptor substrate-2 in 3T3-L1 adipocytes. *J Biol Chem* 1999; 274(17):12075–12080.
41. Sawka-Verhelle D, Filloux C, Tartare-Deckert S, Mothe I, Van Obberghen E. Identification of Stat 5B as a substrate of the insulin receptor. *Eur J Biochem* 1997; 250(2):411–417.
42. Kaburagi Y, Yamamoto-Honda R, Tobe K, Ueki K, Yachi M, Akanuma Y et al. The role of the NPXY motif in the insulin receptor in tyrosine phosphorylation of insulin receptor substrate-1 and Shc. *Endocrinology* 1995; 136(8):3437–3443.
43. Gustafson TA, He W, Craparo A, Schaub CD, O'Neill TJ. Phosphotyrosine-dependent interaction of SHC and insulin receptor substrate 1 with the NPEY motif of the insulin receptor via a novel non-SH2 domain. *Mol Cell Biol* 1995; 15(5):2500–2508.
44. Zick Y. Insulin resistance: A phosphorylation-based uncoupling of insulin signaling. *Trends Cell Biol* 2001; 11(11):437–441.
45. Zimmet P, Alberti KG, Shaw J. Global and societal implications of the diabetes epidemic. *Nature* 2001; 414(6865):782–787.
46. Arner P, Pollare T, Lithell H, Livingston JN. Defective insulin receptor tyrosine kinase in human skeletal muscle in obesity and type 2 (non-insulin-dependent) diabetes mellitus. *Diabetologia* 1987; 30(6):437–440.
47. Caro JF, Sinha MK, Raju SM, Ittoop O, Pories WJ, Flickinger EG et al. Insulin receptor kinase in human skeletal muscle from obese subjects with and without noninsulin dependent diabetes. *J Clin Invest* 1987; 79(5):1330–1337.
48. Cortright RN, Azevedo JL, Jr., Zhou Q, Sinha M, Pories WJ, Itani SI et al. Protein kinase C modulates insulin action in human skeletal muscle. *Am J Physiol Endocrinol Metab* 2000; 278(3):E553–E562.
49. Goodyear LJ, Giorgino F, Sherman LA, Carey J, Smith RJ, Dohm GL. Insulin receptor phosphorylation, insulin receptor substrate-1 phosphorylation, and phosphatidylinositol 3-kinase activity are decreased in intact skeletal muscle strips from obese subjects. *J Clin Invest* 1995; 95(5):2195–2204.
50. Cusi K, Maezono K, Osman A, Pendergrass M, Patti ME, Pratipanawatr T et al. Insulin resistance differentially affects the PI 3-kinase- and MAP kinase-mediated signaling in human muscle. *J Clin Invest* 2000; 105(3):311–320.
51. Youngren JF, Goldfine ID, Pratley RE. Decreased muscle insulin receptor kinase correlates with insulin resistance in normoglycemic Pima Indians. *Am J Physiol* 1997; 273(2 Pt 1):E276–E283.
52. Friedman JE, Ishizuka T, Liu S, Farrell CJ, Bedol D, Koletsky RJ et al. Reduced insulin receptor signaling in the obese spontaneously hypertensive Koletsky rat. *Am J Physiol* 1997; 273(5 Pt 1): E1014–E1023.

53. Coba MP, Munoz MC, Dominici FP, Toblli JE, Pena C, Bartke A et al. Increased in vivo phosphory-lation of insulin receptor at serine 994 in the liver of obese insulin-resistant Zucker rats. *J Endocrinol* 2004; 182(3):433–444.

54. Christ CY, Hunt D, Hancock J, Garcia-Macedo R, Mandarino LJ, Ivy JL. Exercise training improves muscle insulin resistance but not insulin receptor signaling in obese Zucker rats. *J Appl Physiol* 2002; 92(2):736–744.

55. Yuan M, Konstantopoulos N, Lee J, Hansen L, Li ZW, Karin M et al. Reversal of obesity- and diet-induced insulin resistance with salicylates or targeted disruption of Ikkbeta. *Science* 2001; 293(5535):1673–1677.

56. Uysal KT, Wiesbrock SM, Marino MW, Hotamisligil GS. Protection from obesity-induced insulin resistance in mice lacking TNF-alpha function. *Nature* 1997; 389(6651):610–614.

57. Arner P. Insulin resistance in type 2 diabetes: Role of the adipokines. *Curr Mol Med* 2005; 5(3):333–339.

58. Tomas E, Kelly M, Xiang X, Tsao TS, Keller C, Keller P et al. Metabolic and hormonal interactions between muscle and adipose tissue. *Proc Nutr Soc* 2004; 63(2):381–385.

59. Petersen KF, Shulman GI. Etiology of insulin resistance. *Am J Med* 2006; 119(5 suppl 1):S10–S16.

60. Pender C, Goldfine ID, Tanner CJ, Pories WJ, MacDonald KG, Havel PJ et al. Muscle insulin recep-tor concentrations in obese patients post bariatric surgery: Relationship to hyperinsulinemia. *Int J Obes Relat Metab Disord* 2004; 28(3):363–369.

61. Youngren JF, Paik J, Barnard RJ. Impaired insulin-receptor autophosphorylation is an early defect in fat-fed, insulin-resistant rats. *J Appl Physiol* 2001; 91(5):2240–2247.

62. Prada PO, Zecchin HG, Gasparetti AL, Torsoni MA, Ueno M, Hirata AE et al. Western diet modulates insulin signaling, c-Jun N-terminal kinase activity, and insulin receptor substrate-1ser307 phosphory-lation in a tissue-specific fashion. *Endocrinology* 2005; 146(3):1576–1587.

63. Taouis M, Dagou C, Ster C, Durand G, Pinault M, Delarue J. N-3 polyunsaturated fatty acids prevent the defect of insulin receptor signaling in muscle. *Am J Physiol Endocrinol Metab* 2002; 282(3): E664–E671.

64. Qin B, Nagasaki M, Ren M, Bajotto G, Oshida Y, Sato Y. Cinnamon extract prevents the insulin resistance induced by a high-fructose diet. *Horm Metab Res* 2004; 36(2):119–125.

65. Bezerra RM, Ueno M, Silva MS, Tavares DQ, Carvalho CR, Saad MJ. A high fructose diet affects the early steps of insulin action in muscle and liver of rats. *J Nutr* 2000; 130(6):1531–1535.

66. Hyakukoku M, Higashiura K, Ura N, Murakami H, Yamaguchi K, Wang L et al. Tissue-specific impairment of insulin signaling in vasculature and skeletal muscle of fructose-fed rats. *Hypertens Res* 2003; 26(2):169–176.

67. Goodyear LJ, Kahn BB. Exercise, glucose transport, and insulin sensitivity. *Annu Rev Med* 1998; 49:235–261.

68. Wojtaszewski JF, Nielsen JN, Richter EA. Invited review: Effect of acute exercise on insulin signal-ing and action in humans. *J Appl Physiol* 2002; 93(1):384–392.

69. Youngren JF, Keen S, Kulp JL, Tanner CJ, Houmard JA, Goldfine ID. Enhanced muscle insulin receptor autophosphorylation with short-term aerobic exercise training. *Am J Physiol Endocrinol Metab* 2001; 280(3):E528–E533.

70. Heled Y, Shapiro Y, Shani Y, Moran DS, Langzam L, Braiman L et al. Physical exercise enhances protein kinase C delta activity and insulin receptor tyrosine phosphorylation in diabetes-prone psam-momys obesus. *Metabolism* 2003; 52(8):1028–1033.

71. Chibalin AV, Yu M, Ryder JW, Song XM, Galuska D, Krook A et al. Exercise-induced changes in expression and activity of proteins involved in insulin signal transduction in skeletal muscle: Differ-ential effects on insulin-receptor substrates 1 and 2. *Proc Natl Acad Sci USA* 2000; 97(1):38–43.

72. Kump DS, Booth FW. Alterations in insulin receptor signalling in the rat epitrochlearis muscle upon cessation of voluntary exercise. *J Physiol* 2005; 562(Pt 3):829–838.

73. Hirose M, Kaneki M, Sugita H, Yasuhara S, Martyn JA. Immobilization depresses insulin signaling in skeletal muscle. *Am J Physiol Endocrinol Metab* 2000; 279(6):E1235–E1241.

74. Hirose M, Kaneki M, Sugita H, Yasuhara S, Ibebunjo C, Martyn JA. Long-term denervation impairs insulin receptor substrate-1-mediated insulin signaling in skeletal muscle. *Metabolism* 2001; 50(2):216–222.

75. Bertelli DF, Ueno M, Amaral ME, Toyama MH, Carneiro EM, Marangoni S et al. Reversal of dener-vation-induced insulin resistance by SHIP2 protein synthesis blockade. *Am J Physiol Endocrinol Metab* 2003; 284(4):E679–E687.

76. Maegawa H, Shigeta Y, Egawa K, Kobayashi M. Impaired autophosphorylation of insulin receptors from abdominal skeletal muscles in nonobese subjects with NIDDM. *Diabetes* 1991; 40(7): 815–819.

77. Obermaier-Kusser B, White MF, Pongratz DE, Su Z, Ermel B, Muhlbacher C et al. A defective intramolecular autoactivation cascade may cause the reduced kinase activity of the skeletal muscle insulin receptor from patients with non-insulin-dependent diabetes mellitus. *J Biol Chem* 1989; 264(16):9497–9504.

78. Scheck SH, Barnard RJ, Lawani LO, Youngren JF, Martin DA, Singh R. Effects of NIDDM on the glucose transport system in human skeletal muscle. *Diabetes Res* 1991; 16(3):111–119.

79. Nyomba BL, Ossowski VM, Bogardus C, Mott DM. Insulin-sensitive tyrosine kinase: relationship with in vivo insulin action in humans. *Am J Physiol* 1990; 258(6, pt. 1):E964–E974.

80. Meyer MM, Levin K, Grimmsmann T, Beck-Nielsen H, Klein HH. Insulin signalling in skeletal muscle of subjects with or without Type II-diabetes and first degree relatives of patients with the disease. *Diabetologia* 2002; 45(6):813–822.

81. Nolan JJ, Freidenberg G, Henry R, Reichart D, Olefsky JM. Role of human skeletal muscle insulin receptor kinase in the in vivo insulin resistance of noninsulin-dependent diabetes mellitus and obesity. *J Clin Endocrinol Metab* 1994; 78(2):471–477.

82. Perseghin G, Ghosh S, Gerow K, Shulman GI. Metabolic defects in lean nondiabetic offspring of NIDDM parents: A cross-sectional study. *Diabetes* 1997; 46(6):1001–1009.

83. Kashyap SR, Belfort R, Berria R, Suraamornkul S, Pratipranawatr T, Finlayson J et al. Discordant effects of a chronic physiological increase in plasma FFA on insulin signaling in healthy subjects with or without a family history of type 2 diabetes. *Am J Physiol Endocrinol Metab* 2004; 287(3): E537–E546.

84. Handberg A, Vaag A, Vinten J, Beck-Nielsen H. Decreased tyrosine kinase activity in partially puri-fied insulin receptors from muscle of young, non-obese first degree relatives of patients with type 2 (non-insulin-dependent) diabetes mellitus. *Diabetologia* 1993; 36(7):668–674.

85. Petersen KF, Dufour S, Befroy D, Garcia R, Shulman GI. Impaired mitochondrial activity in the insulin-resistant offspring of patients with type 2 diabetes. *N Engl J Med* 2004; 350(7):664–671.

86. Frittitta L, Youngren J, Vigneri R, Maddux BA, Trischitta V, Goldfine ID. PC-1 content in skeletal muscle of non-obese, non-diabetic subjects: relationship to insulin receptor tyrosine kinase and whole body insulin sensitivity. *Diabetologia* 1996; 39(10):1190–1195.

87. Grasso G, Frittitta L, Anello M, Russo P, Sesti G, Trischitta V. Insulin receptor tyrosine-kinase activ-ity is altered in both muscle and adipose tissue from non-obese normoglycaemic insulin-resistant subjects. *Diabetologia* 1995; 38(1):55–61.

88. Virkamaki A, Korsheninnikova E, Seppala-Lindroos A, Vehkavaara S, Goto T, Halavaara J et al. Intramyocellular lipid is associated with resistance to in vivo insulin actions on glucose uptake, anti-lipolysis, and early insulin signaling pathways in human skeletal muscle. *Diabetes* 2001; 50(10):2337–2343.

89. Jackson S, Bagstaff SM, Lynn S, Yeaman SJ, Turnbull DM, Walker M. Decreased insulin respon-siveness of glucose uptake in cultured human skeletal muscle cells from insulin-resistant nondiabetic relatives of type 2 diabetic families. *Diabetes* 2000; 49(7):1169–1177.

90. Krutzfeldt J, Kausch C, Volk A, Klein HH, Rett K, Haring HU et al. Insulin signaling and action in cultured skeletal muscle cells from lean healthy humans with high and low insulin sensitivity. *Dia-betes* 2000; 49(6):992–998.

91. Youngren JF, Goldfine ID, Pratley RE. Insulin receptor autophosphorylation in cultured myoblasts correlates to glucose disposal in Pima Indians. *Am J Physiol* 1999; 276(5, pt. 1):E990–E994.

92. Ciaraldi TP, Abrams L, Nikoulina S, Mudaliar S, Henry RR. Glucose transport in cultured human skeletal muscle cells: Regulation by insulin and glucose in nondiabetic and non-insulin-dependent diabetes mellitus subjects. *J Clin Invest* 1995; 96(6):2820–2827.

93. Gaster M, Petersen I, Hojlund K, Poulsen P, Beck-Nielsen H. The diabetic phenotype is conserved in myotubes established from diabetic subjects: evidence for primary defects in glucose transport and glycogen synthase activity. *Diabetes* 2002; 51(4):921–927.

94. Vollenweider P, Menard B, Nicod P. Insulin resistance, defective insulin receptor substrate 2-associ-ated phosphatidylinositol-3′ kinase activation, and impaired atypical protein kinase C (zeta/lambda) activation in myotubes from obese patients with impaired glucose tolerance. *Diabetes* 2002; 51(4): 1052–1059.

95. Henry RR, Abrams L, Nikoulina S, Ciaraldi TP. Insulin action and glucose metabolism in nondiabetic control and NIDDM subjects: Comparison using human skeletal muscle cell cultures. *Diabetes* 1995; 44(8):936–946.

96. Henry RR, Ciaraldi TP, Abrams-Carter L, Mudaliar S, Park KS, Nikoulina SE. Glycogen synthase activity is reduced in cultured skeletal muscle cells of non-insulin-dependent diabetes mellitus subjects: Biochemical and molecular mechanisms. *J Clin Invest* 1996; 98(5):1231–1236.

97. Pender C, Goldfine ID, Kulp JL, Tanner CJ, Maddux BA, MacDonald KG et al. Analysis of insulin-stimulated insulin receptor activation and glucose transport in cultured skeletal muscle cells from obese subjects. *Metabolism* 2005; 54(5):598–603.

98. Catalano PM, Tyzbir ED, Roman NM, Amini SB, Sims EA. Longitudinal changes in insulin release and insulin resistance in nonobese pregnant women. *Am J Obstet Gynecol* 1991; 165(6, pt. 1):1667–1672.

99. Kautzky-Willer A, Prager R, Waldhausl W, Pacini G, Thomaseth K, Wagner OF et al. Pronounced insulin resistance and inadequate beta-cell secretion characterize lean gestational diabetes during and after pregnancy. *Diabetes Care* 1997; 20(11):1717–1723.

100. Shao J, Catalano PM, Yamashita H, Ruyter I, Smith S, Youngren J et al. Decreased insulin receptor tyrosine kinase activity and plasma cell membrane glycoprotein-1 overexpression in skeletal muscle from obese women with gestational diabetes mellitus (GDM): evidence for increased serine/threonine phosphorylation in pregnancy and GDM. *Diabetes* 2000; 49(4):603–610.

101. Dunaif A, Xia J, Book CB, Schenker E, Tang Z. Excessive insulin receptor serine phosphorylation in cultured fibroblasts and in skeletal muscle: A potential mechanism for insulin resistance in the polycystic ovary syndrome. *J Clin Invest* 1995; 96(2):801–810.

102. Corbould A, Kim YB, Youngren JF, Pender C, Kahn BB, Lee A et al. Insulin resistance in the skeletal muscle of women with PCOS involves intrinsic and acquired defects in insulin signaling. *Am J Physiol Endocrinol Metab* 2005; 288(5):E1047–E1054.

103. Yamaguchi Y, Flier JS, Yokota A, Benecke H, Backer JM, Moller DE. Functional properties of two naturally occurring isoforms of the human insulin receptor in Chinese hamster ovary cells. *Endocrinology* 1991; 129(4):2058–2066.

104. Ahmad F, Goldstein BJ. Purification, identification and subcellular distribution of three predominant protein-tyrosine phosphatase enzymes in skeletal muscle tissue. *Biochim Biophys Acta* 1995; 1248(1):57–69.

105. Kharitonenkov A, Schnekenburger J, Chen Z, Knyazev P, Ali S, Zwick E et al. Adapter function of protein-tyrosine phosphatase 1D in insulin receptor/insulin receptor substrate-1 interaction. *J Biol Chem* 1995; 270(49):29189–29193.

106. Cheng A, Dube N, Gu F, Tremblay ML. Coordinated action of protein tyrosine phosphatases in insulin signal transduction. *Eur J Biochem* 2002; 269(4):1050–1059.

107. Bandyopadhyay D, Kusari A, Kenner KA, Liu F, Chernoff J, Gustafson TA et al. Protein-tyrosine phosphatase 1B complexes with the insulin receptor in vivo and is tyrosine-phosphorylated in the presence of insulin. *J Biol Chem* 1997; 272(3):1639–1645.

108. Salmeen A, Andersen JN, Myers MP, Tonks NK, Barford D. Molecular basis for the dephosphorylation of the activation segment of the insulin receptor by protein tyrosine phosphatase 1B. *Mol Cell* 2000; 6(6):1401–1412.

109. Li S, Depetris RS, Barford D, Chernoff J, Hubbard SR. Crystal structure of a complex between protein tyrosine phosphatase 1B and the insulin receptor tyrosine kinase. *Structure (Camb)* 2005; 13(11): 1643–1651.

110. Venable CL, Frevert EU, Kim YB, Fischer BM, Kamatkar S, Neel BG et al. Overexpression of protein-tyrosine phosphatase-1B in adipocytes inhibits insulin-stimulated phosphoinositide 3-kinase activity without altering glucose transport or Akt/Protein kinase B activation. *J Biol Chem* 2000; 275(24):18318–18326.

111. Egawa K, Maegawa H, Shimizu S, Morino K, Nishio Y, Bryer-Ash M et al. Protein-tyrosine phosphatase-1B negatively regulates insulin signaling in l6 myocytes and Fao hepatoma cells. *J Biol Chem* 2001; 276(13):10207–10211.

112. Elchebly M, Payette P, Michaliszyn E, Cromlish W, Collins S, Loy AL et al. Increased insulin sensitivity and obesity resistance in mice lacking the protein tyrosine phosphatase-1B gene. *Science* 1999; 283(5407):1544–1548.

113. Zabolotny JM, Haj FG, Kim YB, Kim HJ, Shulman GI, Kim JK et al. Transgenic overexpression of protein-tyrosine phosphatase 1B in muscle causes insulin resistance, but overexpression with leuko-

cyte antigen-related phosphatase does not additively impair insulin action. *J Biol Chem* 2004; 279(23):24844–24851.

114. Ahmad F, Goldstein BJ. Functional association between the insulin receptor and the transmembrane protein-tyrosine phosphatase LAR in intact cells. *J Biol Chem* 1997; 272(1):448–457.

115. Li PM, Zhang WR, Goldstein BJ. Suppression of insulin receptor activation by overexpression of the protein-tyrosine phosphatase LAR in hepatoma cells. *Cell Signal* 1996; 8(7):467–473.

116. Kulas DT, Zhang WR, Goldstein BJ, Furlanetto RW, Mooney RA. Insulin receptor signaling is augmented by antisense inhibition of the protein tyrosine phosphatase LAR. *J Biol Chem* 1995; 270(6):2435–2438.

117. Zabolotny JM, Kim YB, Peroni OD, Kim JK, Pani MA, Boss O et al. Overexpression of the LAR (leukocyte antigen-related) protein-tyrosine phosphatase in muscle causes insulin resistance. *Proc Natl Acad Sci USA* 2001; 98(9):5187–5192.

118. Mander A, Hodgkinson CP, Sale GJ. Knock-down of LAR protein tyrosine phosphatase induces insulin resistance. *FEBS Lett* 2005; 579(14):3024–3028.

119. Galic S, Klingler-Hoffmann M, Fodero-Tavoletti MT, Puryer MA, Meng TC, Tonks NK et al. Regulation of insulin receptor signaling by the protein tyrosine phosphatase TCPTP. *Mol Cell Biol* 2003; 23(6):2096–2108.

120. Galic S, Hauser C, Kahn BB, Haj FG, Neel BG, Tonks NK et al. Coordinated regulation of insulin signaling by the protein tyrosine phosphatases PTP1B and TCPTP. *Mol Cell Biol* 2005; 25(2):819–829.

121. Nakagawa Y, Aoki N, Aoyama K, Shimizu H, Shimano H, Yamada N et al. Receptor-type protein tyrosine phosphatase epsilon (PTPepsilonM) is a negative regulator of insulin signaling in primary hepatocytes and liver. *Zoolog Sci* 2005; 22(2):169–175.

122. Ahmad F, Azevedo JL, Cortright R, Dohm GL, Goldstein BJ. Alterations in skeletal muscle protein-tyrosine phosphatase activity and expression in insulin-resistant human obesity and diabetes. *J Clin Invest* 1997; 100(2):449–458.

123. Worm D, Vinten J, Staehr P, Henriksen JE, Handberg A, Beck-Nielsen H. Altered basal and insulin-stimulated phosphotyrosine phosphatase (PTPase) activity in skeletal muscle from NIDDM patients compared with control subjects. *Diabetologia* 1996; 39(10):1208–1214.

124. Kusari J, Kenner KA, Suh KI, Hill DE, Henry RR. Skeletal muscle protein tyrosine phosphatase activity and tyrosine phosphatase 1B protein content are associated with insulin action and resistance. *J Clin Invest* 1994; 93(3):1156–1162.

125. Maddux BA, Chang YN, Accili D, McGuinness OP, Youngren JF, Goldfine ID. Overexpression of the insulin receptor inhibitor PC-1/ENPP1 induces insulin resistance and hyperglycemia. *Am J Physiol Endocrinol Metab* 2006; 290(4):E746–E749.

126. Maddux BA, Sbraccia P, Kumakura S, Sasson S, Youngren J, Fisher A et al. Membrane glycoprotein PC-1 and insulin resistance in non-insulin-dependent diabetes mellitus. *Nature* 1995; 373(6513): 448–451.

127. Maddux BA, Goldfine ID. Membrane glycoprotein PC-1 inhibition of insulin receptor function occurs via direct interaction with the receptor alpha-subunit. *Diabetes* 2000; 49(1):13–19.

128. Ottensmeyer FP, Beniac DR, Luo RZ, Yip CC. Mechanism of transmembrane signaling: Insulin binding and the insulin receptor. *Biochemistry* 2000; 39(40):12103–12112.

129. Costanzo BV, Trischitta V, Di Paola R, Spampinato D, Pizzuti A, Vigneri R et al. The Q allele variant (GLN121) of membrane glycoprotein PC-1 interacts with the insulin receptor and inhibits insulin signaling more effectively than the common K allele variant (LYS121). *Diabetes* 2001; 50(4):831–836.

130. Dong H, Maddux BA, Altomonte J, Meseck M, Accili D, Terkeltaub R et al. Increased hepatic levels of the insulin receptor inhibitor, PC-1/NPP1, induce insulin resistance and glucose intolerance. *Diabetes* 2005; 54(2):367–372.

131. Goldfine ID, Maddux BA, Youngren JF, Frittitta L, Trischitta V, Dohm GL. Membrane glycoprotein PC-1 and insulin resistance. *Mol Cell Biochem* 1998; 182(1–2):177–184.

132. Youngren JF, Maddux BA, Sasson S, Sbraccia P, Tapscott EB, Swanson MS et al. Skeletal muscle content of membrane glycoprotein PC-1 in obesity. Relationship to muscle glucose transport. *Diabetes* 1996; 45(10):1324–1328.

133. Abate N, Chandalia M, Satija P, Adams-Huet B, Grundy SM, Sandeep S et al. ENPP1/PC-1 K121Q polymorphism and genetic susceptibility to type 2 diabetes. *Diabetes* 2005; 54(4):1207–1213.

134. Bacci S, Ludovico O, Prudente S, Zhang YY, Di Paola R, Mangiacotti D et al. The K121Q polymorphism of the ENPP1/PC-1 gene is associated with insulin resistance/atherogenic phenotypes, including earlier onset of type 2 diabetes and myocardial infarction. *Diabetes* 2005; 54(10):3021–3025.

135. Meyre D, Bouatia-Naji N, Tounian A, Samson C, Lecoeur C, Vatin V et al. Variants of ENPP1 are associated with childhood and adult obesity and increase the risk of glucose intolerance and type 2 diabetes. *Nat Genet* 2005; 37(8):863–867.

136. Yasukawa H, Sasaki A, Yoshimura A. Negative regulation of cytokine signaling pathways. *Annu Rev Immunol* 2000; 18:143–164.

137. Emanuelli B, Peraldi P, Filloux C, Sawka-Verhelle D, Hilton D, Van Obberghen E. SOCS-3 is an insulin-induced negative regulator of insulin signaling. *J Biol Chem* 2000; 275(21):15985–15991.

138. Mooney RA, Senn J, Cameron S, Inamdar N, Boivin LM, Shang Y et al. Suppressors of cytokine signaling-1 and -6 associate with and inhibit the insulin receptor: A potential mechanism for cytokine-mediated insulin resistance. *J Biol Chem* 2001; 276(28):25889–25893.

139. Ueki K, Kondo T, Kahn CR. Suppressor of cytokine signaling 1 (SOCS-1) and SOCS-3 cause insulin resistance through inhibition of tyrosine phosphorylation of insulin receptor substrate proteins by discrete mechanisms. *Mol Cell Biol* 2004; 24(12):5434–5446.

140. Ueki K, Kadowaki T, Kahn CR. Role of suppressors of cytokine signaling SOCS-1 and SOCS-3 in hepatic steatosis and the metabolic syndrome. *Hepatol Res* 2005;185–192.

141. Gual P, Marchand-Brustel Y, Tanti JF. Positive and negative regulation of insulin signaling through IRS-1 phosphorylation. *Biochimie* 2005; 87(1):99–109.

142. Aguirre V, Werner ED, Giraud J, Lee YH, Shoelson SE, White MF. Phosphorylation of Ser307 in insulin receptor substrate-1 blocks interactions with the insulin receptor and inhibits insulin action. *J Biol Chem* 2002; 277(2):1531–1537.

143. Lin Y, Itani SI, Kurowski TG, Dean DJ, Luo Z, Yaney GC et al. Inhibition of insulin signaling and glycogen synthesis by phorbol dibutyrate in rat skeletal muscle. *Am J Physiol Endocrinol Metab* 2001; 281(1):E8–E15.

144. Strack V, Hennige AM, Krutzfeldt J, Bossenmaier B, Klein HH, Kellerer M et al. Serine residues 994 and 1023/25 are important for insulin receptor kinase inhibition by protein kinase C isoforms beta2 and theta. *Diabetologia* 2000; 43(4):443–449.

145. Bossenmaier B, Mosthaf L, Mischak H, Ullrich A, Haring HU. Protein kinase C isoforms beta 1 and beta 2 inhibit the tyrosine kinase activity of the insulin receptor. *Diabetologia* 1997; 40(7):863–866.

146. Kellerer M, Mushack J, Seffer E, Mischak H, Ullrich A, Haring HU. Protein kinase C isoforms alpha, delta and theta require insulin receptor substrate-1 to inhibit the tyrosine kinase activity of the insulin receptor in human kidney embryonic cells (HEK 293 cells). *Diabetologia* 1998; 41(7):833–838.

147. Feener EP, Backer JM, King GL, Wilden PA, Sun XJ, Kahn CR et al. Insulin stimulates serine and tyrosine phosphorylation in the juxtamembrane region of the insulin receptor. *J Biol Chem* 1993; 268(15):11256–11264.

148. Liu F, Roth RA. Identification of serines-1035/1037 in the kinase domain of the insulin receptor as protein kinase C alpha mediated phosphorylation sites. *FEBS Lett* 1994; 352(3):389–392.

149. Al Hasani H, Eisermann B, Tennagels N, Magg C, Passlack W, Koenen M et al. Identification of Ser-1275 and Ser-1309 as autophosphorylation sites of the insulin receptor. *FEBS Lett* 1997; 400(1):65–70.

150. Bossenmaier B, Strack V, Stoyanov B, Krutzfeldt J, Beck A, Lehmann R et al. Serine residues 1177/78/82 of the insulin receptor are required for substrate phosphorylation but not autophosphorylation. *Diabetes* 2000; 49(6):889–895.

151. Chin JE, Dickens M, Tavare JM, Roth RA. Overexpression of protein kinase C isoenzymes alpha, beta I, gamma, and epsilon in cells overexpressing the insulin receptor: Effects on receptor phosphorylation and signaling. *J Biol Chem* 1993; 268(9):6338–6347.

152. Koshio O, Akanuma Y, Kasuga M. Identification of a phosphorylation site of the rat insulin receptor catalyzed by protein kinase C in an intact cell. *FEBS Lett* 1989; 254(1–2):22–24.

153. Ahn J, Donner DB, Rosen OM. Interaction of the human insulin receptor tyrosine kinase from the baculovirus expression system with protein kinase C in a cell-free system. *J Biol Chem* 1993; 268(10):7571–7576.

154. Schmitz-Peiffer C. Protein kinase C and lipid-induced insulin resistance in skeletal muscle. *Ann N Y Acad Sci* 2002; 967:146–157.

155. Pillay TS, Xiao S, Keranen L, Olefsky JM. Regulation of the insulin receptor by protein kinase C isoenzymes: Preferential interaction with beta isoenzymes and interaction with the catalytic domain of betaII. *Cell Signal* 2004; 16(1):97–104.

156. Hulver MW, Dohm GL. The molecular mechanism linking muscle fat accumulation to insulin resistance. *Proc Nutr Soc* 2004; 63(2):375–380.

157. Itani SI, Zhou Q, Pories WJ, MacDonald KG, Dohm GL. Involvement of protein kinase C in human skeletal muscle insulin resistance and obesity. *Diabetes* 2000; 49(8):1353–1358.

158. Zhou Q, Dolan PL, Dohm GL. Dephosphorylation increases insulin-stimulated receptor kinase activity in skeletal muscle of obese Zucker rats. *Mol Cell Biochem* 1999; 194(1–2):209–216.

159. Reynoso R, Salgado LM, Calderon V. High levels of palmitic acid lead to insulin resistance due to changes in the level of phosphorylation of the insulin receptor and insulin receptor substrate-1. *Mol Cell Biochem* 2003; 246(1–2):155–162.

160. Itani SI, Ruderman NB, Schmieder F, Boden G. Lipid-induced insulin resistance in human muscle is associated with changes in diacylglycerol, protein kinase C, and IkappaB-alpha. *Diabetes* 2002; 51(7):2005–2011.

161. Griffin ME, Marcucci MJ, Cline GW, Bell K, Barucci N, Lee D et al. Free fatty acid-induced insulin resistance is associated with activation of protein kinase C theta and alterations in the insulin signaling cascade. *Diabetes* 1999; 48(6):1270–1274.

162. Kellerer M, Haring HU. Pathogenesis of insulin resistance: modulation of the insulin signal at receptor level. *Diabetes Res Clin Pract* 1995; 28(suppl):S173–S177.

163. Kroder G, Bossenmaier B, Kellerer M, Capp E, Stoyanov B, Muhlhofer A et al. Tumor necrosis factor-alpha- and hyperglycemia-induced insulin resistance: Evidence for different mechanisms and different effects on insulin signaling. *J Clin Invest* 1996; 97(6):1471–1477.

164. Nguyen MT, Satoh H, Favelyukis S, Babendure JL, Imamura T, Sbodio JI et al. JNK and tumor necrosis factor-alpha mediate free fatty acid-induced insulin resistance in 3T3-L1 adipocytes. *J Biol Chem* 2005; 280(42):35361–35371.

165. Hotamisligil GS, Shargill NS, Spiegelman BM. Adipose expression of tumor necrosis factor-alpha: Direct role in obesity-linked insulin resistance. *Science* 1993; 259(5091):87–91.

166. Kern PA, Ranganathan S, Li C, Wood L, Ranganathan G. Adipose tissue tumor necrosis factor and interleukin-6 expression in human obesity and insulin resistance. *Am J Physiol Endocrinol Metab* 2001; 280(5):E745–E751.

167. de Alvaro C, Teruel T, Hernandez R, Lorenzo M. Tumor necrosis factor alpha produces insulin resistance in skeletal muscle by activation of inhibitor kappaB kinase in a p38 MAPK-dependent manner. *J Biol Chem* 2004; 279(17):17070–17078.

168. Tzeng TF, Liu IM, Cheng JT. Activation of opioid mu-receptors by loperamide to improve interleukin-6-induced inhibition of insulin signals in myoblast C2C12 cells. *Diabetologia* 2005; 48(7):1386–1392.

169. Weigert C, Hennige AM, Lehmann R, Brodbeck K, Baumgartner F, Schauble M et al. Direct crosstalk of interleukin-6 and insulin signal transduction via insulin receptor substrate-1 in skeletal muscle cells. *J Biol Chem* 2006; 281(11):7060–7067.

170. Wells L, Hart GW. O-GlcNAc turns twenty: Functional implications for post-translational modification of nuclear and cytosolic proteins with a sugar. *FEBS Lett* 2003; 546(1):154–158.

171. D'Alessandris C, Andreozzi F, Federici M, Cardellini M, Brunetti A, Ranalli M et al. Increased O-glycosylation of insulin signaling proteins results in their impaired activation and enhanced susceptibility to apoptosis in pancreatic beta-cells. *FASEB J* 2004; 18(9):959–961.

172. Lubas WA, Frank DW, Krause M, Hanover JA. O-Linked GlcNAc transferase is a conserved nucleocytoplasmic protein containing tetratricopeptide repeats. *J Biol Chem* 1997; 272(14):9316–9324.

16

Fat Feeding and Muscle Fat Deposition Eliciting Insulin Resistance
An Update

E.W. Kraegen, G.J. Cooney, Jiming M. Ye, and Stuart M. Furler

CONTENTS

INTRODUCTION

Skeletal muscle insulin resistance, defined as a reduced ability of insulin to stimulate tissue utilization and storage of glucose, is an early and major perturbation in the metabolic syndrome. Clinical conditions under the umbrella of the metabolic syndrome include obesity, type 2 diabetes, dyslipidemia, and hypertension, and are known to be influenced by lifestyle factors such as diet and activity. The metabolic syndrome is reaching alarming proportions in many societies. This chapter considers the increasingly compelling evidence that links insulin resistance with the situation when fatty acid supply exceeds energy demand in muscle, resulting in an accumulation of lipid in this tissue. This chapter is an update of a similar-titled chapter written some five years ago (1), and we highlight how knowledge has progressed since 2000. Considered are

From: *Contemporary Endocrinology: The Metabolic Syndrome: Epidemiology, Clinical Treatment, and Underlying Mechanisms*
Edited by: B.C. Hansen and G.A. Bray © Humana Press, Totowa, NJ

evidence for the association between fatty acid metabolism and muscle insulin resistance, possible causal links whereby increased muscle lipid accumulation could result in impaired insulin signalling and insulin resistance, and therapeutic options for ameliorating insulin resistance based on a "lipid-lowering" approach. We also consider how a scenario of excess fatty acid supply to muscle stands in relation to other emerging theories of factors contributing to muscle insulin resistance in obesity and similar states.

We have previously proposed a "lipid supply hypothesis of insulin resistance": *An oversupply and/or accumulation of lipid in muscle and liver leads to changes in metabolism at the level of substrate competition, enzyme regulation, intracellular signaling, and/or gene transcription that account for the insulin resistance seen in states such as the metabolic syndrome and type 2 diabetes*. This was a refinement from studies of around 15 years ago showing that triglyceride accumulates in muscle of high-fat-fed rats, coincident with insulin resistance (2,3). Since that time, the relevance of lipid accumulation to insulin resistance in humans has been demonstrated, and, at the other end of the spectrum, basic animal and cell-based studies have indicated very plausible mechanisms whereby lipid accumulation could generate insulin resistance.

OVERVIEW OF LIPID METABOLISM AND INSULIN RESISTANCE

Muscle lipid accumulation will occur over a period when the total supply of lipid to muscle from all sources (systemic fatty acids, VLDL-triglyceride, gut-derived chylomicrons) exceeds the rate of muscle fatty acid oxidation over that period. The relative contribution of the sources of excess lipid supply to muscle in insulin-resistant states is not known in quantitative terms, and a combination of factors may be involved, combined with the possibility of impaired fatty acid oxidation. In fact it now seems quite likely that mitochondrial dysfunction and/or an impaired capacity for oxidative metabolism (4,5) may be a significant factor in the accumulation of cytosolic lipid in obesity and type 2 diabetes. Rates of muscle lipid supply and utilization also vary considerably according to skeletal muscle type, but red oxidative muscle, with high levels of intramyocellular lipid (6), seems also most prone to dietary-fat-induced insulin resistance (7).

Figure 16.1 sets the scene for many of the metabolic interactions to be discussed in this review. Muscle lipid accumulation is evident as increased levels either of stored muscle triglyceride or of the metabolically active forms of lipid, such as the long-chain acyl CoAs (LCACoAs), diacylglycerols (DAGs), or ceramides. This lipid excess may influence metabolism acutely by changing substrate availability or by altering key enzyme activities by allosteric regulation. Excessive mitochondrial FFA oxidation may impair glucose oxidation via the classic glucose–fatty acid cycle (8). On the other hand, a reduction in the mitochondrial transfer of LCACoAs, perhaps by negative regulation of carnitine palmitoyl transferase (CPT-1) by malonyl CoA (9), may lead to accumulation of cytosolic LCACoAs and subsequent insulin resistance (9–11). Changes in specific fatty acid levels or increased diacylglycerols (DAGs) or ceramides may alter insulin signaling pathways via activation of pathways containing serine kinases (PKCs, JNK, or IKKβ) (12,13) and/or may change gene expression. Finally, adipose tissue secretagogues, derived either from adipocytes themselves or from infiltrating macrophages (14,15), such as TNF-α (16,17), interleukin-6 (18), resistin (19), adiponectin

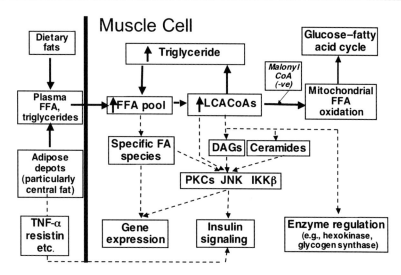

Figure 16.1. Some of the interactions, discussed in the text, whereby an increased muscle uptake of fatty acids, derived from circulating fatty acids or triglycerides, may lead to increased muscle lipid accumulation and insulin resistance.

(20), visfatin (21), or the recently described retinol binding protein 4 (22), may also act in muscle to alter lipid metabolism and/or influence insulin action either positively or negatively. These will be considered in more detail in a later section; suffice it to say that the concept that obesity leads to an inflammation-like state that causes insulin resistance has emerged as a complementary theory to the lipid supply hypothesis for muscle insulin resistance.

ACUTE FATTY ACID ELEVATION CAN CAUSE MUSCLE INSULIN RESISTANCE

Several pieces of evidence strongly suggest that excess fatty acid availability to muscle tissue can directly result in reduced insulin action. First, in vitro incubation of excised muscle strips or muscle cells with excess fatty acids leads to impaired insulin-stimulated glucose uptake (23,24). Second, it is clear that acute in vivo elevation of fatty acids, such as can be generated by triglyceride/heparin infusion, can cause whole-body, muscle, and liver insulin resistance (25–29). The effect in muscle takes several hours to occur (e.g., see refs. 25–27) and is particularly associated with a reduction in insulin-mediated muscle glycogen synthesis (30–34). Thus the effects of increased in vivo FFA availability on insulin signaling and/or on glycogen synthesis appear to take a number of hours to develop. This lack of a short-term effect confounded studies in the late eighties that tried to link fatty acid availability to muscle insulin resistance (35–37). With the benefit of hindsight, these older studies were too short to show the insulin resistance. In addition, they stressed that mechanisms are likely to extend beyond the classic glucose–fatty acid cycle described by Randle, which predicts a short-term reduction in muscle glucose oxidation accompanying fatty acid elevation (8). We have found that there is a significant elevation of muscle triglyceride and total LCACoAs after 3–5 h of triglyceride/heparin infusion when insulin resistance develops (26), similar to that seen when muscle insulin resistance is induced chronically in rats over several weeks by a high-fat diet (10,38). Defects in insulin signaling have been found both with acute FFA elevation and with high-fat feeding (27–29,39,40). Given the strong probability that excess fatty acid availability causes insulin resistance during lipid infusion, we consider it highly likely that excess fatty acid accumulation causes insulin resistance (rather than the theoretically possible converse of insulin resistance causing muscle lipid accumulation). In support, when muscle lipid oxidation is chronically inhibited pharmacologically by etomoxir in rats, cytosolic lipid accumulation and muscle insulin resistance increases (41). Compelling evidence also comes from studies where the early rate-limiting steps controlling muscle fatty acid uptake are manipulated by genetic means. Two such studies demonstrate that muscle triglyceride is enhanced and insulin resistance develops when muscle lipoprotein lipase is overexpressed in mice (42,43). Conversely mouse knockouts of the muscle fatty acid transport protein FATP1 are protected against cytosolic lipid accumulation and insulin resistance in response to a high-fat diet (44). The situation in which another fatty acid transporter CD36 is overexpressed is more complex but also supportive in that muscle triglyceride levels are lowered and insulin sensitivity is enhanced (45); in this model increased fatty acid oxidation may dominate possibly via a link between CD36 and mitochondrial fatty acid transfer (46). These models are quoted here since they represent a direct attempt to manipulate muscle fatty acid fluxes; however, there are other mouse models where gene manipulation of adipose or liver targets have indirectly led to reduced fatty acid availability to muscle and demonstrable protection from insulin resistance associated with obesity or a high-fat diet. Examples include knockouts of hormone-sensitive lipase in adipose tissue (47) and liver VLDL receptor (48). In summary, although it is unlikely to be the only mediator of muscle insulin resistance in obesity and similar states, there is strong evidence that an excess supply of fatty acids per se is a major player. Possible mechanisms (Fig. 16.1) include but go beyond the classic Randle cycle and are considered in more detail later.

MUSCLE TRIGLYCERIDE CONTENT AND INSULIN RESISTANCE

Animal Studies

Rodent feeding studies in the eighties and early nineties established a clear association between muscle triglyceride accumulation and insulin resistance. Rats on high-fat diets develop insulin resistance in a few days, first in the liver (3), and muscle insulin resistance then follows as triglyceride accumulates in this tissue (2,3). Supporting this association, changes in dietary fat subtype (e.g., by increasing omega-3 fats) lessened both insulin resistance and muscle triglyceride accumulation (2,49,50). The muscle lipid–insulin resistance association is now well-established in many animal models (e.g., refs. 17,51,52). Also strengthening the association is the finding that various metabolic manipulations of chronically high-fat-fed rats that lessen muscle lipid accumulation, such as prior exercise, overnight fasting, acutely reducing food fat content (10), or PPAR agonist drug treatment (53,54), also significantly improve insulin sensitivity. It is likely that insulin resistance due to high-fat feeding is even more extreme in liver than in muscle, as demonstrated in time course studies in dogs (55), a study that also shows the strong relationship to increased visceral obesity. In our various rodent high-fat-diet studies, we mostly use high-fat diets that are isocaloric with controlled, high-carbohydrate diets; this suggests that the association of muscle lipids and insulin resistance is related to a relative macronutrient availability rather than to excess energy intake per se, although overnutrition will exacerbate the problem. In summary, based on animal studies, there is a compelling case that a high-fat dietary intake extended for more than a few days will cause muscle lipid accumulation and insulin resistance, with both being readily reversible when the source of lipid oversupply is removed or there is an accelerated rate of muscle lipid utilization.

Human Studies

It is now clear that muscle lipid accumulation is also likely to be a cause of insulin resistance in humans. Studies with careful muscle biopsy on an overweight male Pima Indian group (56) reported a significant association of muscle triglyceride content with insulin resistance. Another muscle biopsy study on middle-aged nondiabetic women showed a negative correlation of intramuscular triglyceride with insulin-mediated activation of glycogen synthase (57). Since the late 1990s, there has been increasing use of either histological staining techniques or noninvasive procedures such as computed tomography (CT) imaging (58,59) or proton magnetic resonance spectroscopy (MRS) methodology (60,61) to quantify and distinguish intramyocellular (IMCL) and extramyocellular (EMCL) lipid content in human studies. These techniques have built up a strong negative association between IMCL and insulin sensitivity in groups of overweight subjects with and without type 2 diabetes (58,59,62), in lean nondiabetic offspring of T2D patients (63–65), or in normal-weight healthy subjects (63–66). More recently, our group reported that in a group of normal-weight to mildly obese subjects, muscle triglyceride is an independent predictor of whole-body insulin sensitivity along with plasma triglycerides and central or total adiposity (67). In addition, we have found that HIV protease inhibitor–related lipodystrophy is associated with increased IMCL and impaired insulin action (Fig. 16.2) (68). This human condition as well as that of the rodent, "fatless" mouse (69), are examples of inadequate capacity for peripheral fat storage, resulting in a spillover of lipids into muscle and liver, in turn leading to insulin resistance in these tissues.

While we believe that it is now established that muscle oversupply of lipid leads to insulin resistance, there remain some confounding aspects. First, the situation appears more complex in considerably obese individuals; while we observed a strong negative correlation between insulin sensitivity and soleus muscle IMCL in subjects with total body fat (measured by DXA) of <470, no such relationship existed for subjects >470 g fat/kg fat free mass (70), suggesting other factors may also become important in determining insulin sensitivity in more extreme obesity. Second, it has been reported that with exercise training there is both an enhanced storage of muscle triglyceride and enhanced insulin sensitivity (71) (reviewed in ref. 72). Interestingly, in a study where T2D subjects were exercise trained for eight weeks, insulin sensitivity improved and muscle IMTG was reduced to normal healthy levels; however, insulin sensitivity remained below the normal range (73). The issue needs further investigation, perhaps using the MRS technique. Third, some have suggested that there may be differing compartmentalization of triglyceride in the myocyte in trained athletes (60,74) or that cyclical muscle lipid depletion/repletion in athletes somehow protects against insulin resistance (71). At this stage, none of these issues have been resolved.

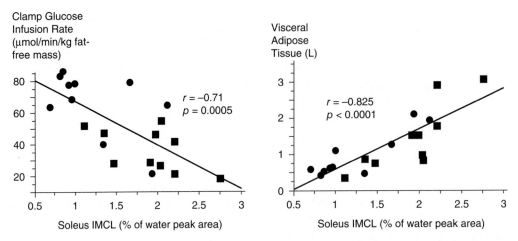

Figure 16.2. Soleus muscle intramyocellular lipid (IMCL) content as determined by proton magnetic resonance spectroscopy is highly negatively correlated to whole-body insulin sensitivity as assessed by euglycemic hyperinsulinemic clamp (left panel), and is positively correlated to visceral adipose tissue volume (right panel). Subjects are HIV-positive subjects with (squares) and without peripheral lipodystrophy (circles). (From ref. 68.)

This problem is less confronting if muscle triglyceride is not the culprit causing insulin resistance. If we take the likely view that the steps causing insulin resistance emanate from cytosolic accumulation of metabolically active forms of lipid such as LCACoAs, DAGs, or ceramides (Fig. 16.1), then it is possible with the enhancement in oxidative capacity of muscle of exercise-trained subjects, or in type 1 versus type 2 muscle fiber types, that accumulation of cytosolic lipid metabolites other than triglycerides may be negatively related to the ability of the muscle to utilize fatty acids, rather than simply being increased in parallel with triglycerides. Certainly the oxidative capacity of skeletal muscle is closely related to insulin sensitivity in human studies (75). The ability of an eight-week moderate exercise training program to reduce muscle DAG and ceramide content concomitant with a significant improvement in glucose tolerance was recently demonstrated in a group of obese subjects (76). This suggests a possible mechanism for the enhancement of insulin sensitivity with exercise training, as elaborated in the next section.

FATTY ACID METABOLITES AND INSULIN ACTION IN MUSCLE

Long-Chain Acyl CoAs

The first step in the metabolism of fatty acids in any tissue is the activation of the fatty acid to its LCACoA derivative by the enzyme acyl CoA synthase. The LCACoAs can then be transported into the mitochondria via the action of acyl carnitine transferase and oxidized in the beta-oxidation pathway. Alternatively, the LCACoAs may be esterified to mono- and diglyceride and stored as triglyceride or incorporated into phospholipid in membranes (for review, see ref. 77). The concentration of LCACoAs is increased by fasting (78) and decreased by insulin (10), and is therefore an indication of the extent of fat metabolism in a tissue. LCACoA levels are increased in muscle from fat-fed insulin-resistant rats, and there is a close link between insulin resistance and increased

LCACOAs in muscle of these animals (79). Amelioration of fat-diet-induced insulin resistance by one of several acute diet or exercise manipulations (10), or by rosiglitazone (53), was closely related to the ability of insulin to suppress muscle LCACoAs. Furthermore, as discussed, muscle LCACoA elevation accompanies insulin resistance generated by acute lipid emulsion infusion in rats (26,28). Our initial human studies suggested an association between total muscle LCACoAs in human muscle obtained during knee surgery and previously determined insulin sensitivity (80). Over the last five years, a number of studies in both animals and humans have strengthened the relationship between LCACoAs and insulin resistance in muscle. In several studies where rodents have been protected against high-fat-diet-induced insulin resistance by gene manipulation of adipose tissue (81) or by altering fat subtype (50), there has been a reduction in muscle LCACoA content accompanying enhanced insulin sensitivity. Similarly in T2D patients where a sustained fall in plasma FFA levels was achieved by administration of the anti-lipolytic agent acipimox, there was a close association between enhanced muscle insulin sensitivity and reduction in LCACoA levels (82). In a study of weight loss in obese subjects, Houmard et al. (83) reported that a fall in some individual muscle LCACoAs (16 : 0, 18 : 0, 18 : 2), but not total LCACoAs, accompanied enhanced insulin sensitivity. It is thus possible that the composition of LCACoAs, as well as total content, may contribute to altered insulin action, as also supported by recent studies involving desaturases (84,85). These issues need further clarification.

What, then, are the possible mechanisms whereby LCACoAs could influence insulin action? LCACoAs have been shown to directly modify the activity of key enzymes of glucose metabolism in liver such as glycogen synthase (86), glucokinase (87), glucose-6-phosphatase (88), and acetyl CoA carboxylase (89). Modification of enzyme activity could also occur in muscle, and we have demonstrated that LCACoAs at concentrations in the physiological range can reduce the activity of hexokinase in rat and human skeletal muscle (90). This inhibition was additive to the well-described inhibition of hexokinase by glucose-6-phosphate. It is therefore quite feasible that some of the inhibitory effects of lipid oversupply on glucose metabolism are direct interactions with the glucose metabolic pathway. In addition, it was recently reported that LCACoAs could inhibit the phosphorylation and activation of AMP-activated protein kinase (AMPK), thus potentially providing a mechanism whereby the energy-sensing AMPK/malonyl CoA network could respond to a lipid excess in muscle (91). Suppression of AMPK activity has been associated with many insulin-resistant states (92), although its causal role, if any, is not clear.

DAGs and Ceramides

Intracellular lipid species may modulate the activity of the insulin signaling cascade. There is clear evidence that DAG-activated members of the protein kinase C family of serine/threonine kinases (PKC theta and PKC epsilon) are translocated and activated in muscle of fat-fed, insulin-resistant rats (93). Shulman's group has reported that mice with a PKC-theta knockout are protected against lipid-induced insulin resistance (94), adding strong support for the importance of this isoform in impairing insulin action. PKC epsilon can be also activated in the presence of increased LCACoA levels (and presumably DAG levels) in the muscle of glucose-infused, insulin-resistant rats (95). Individual fatty acid species may also have specific effects with palmitate, oleate, and linoleate having differential effects on IRS-1 and PKB phosphorylation in a cell line derived from murine muscle (96). Ceramide production may mediate some of the effects of palmitate on insulin signaling, and direct addition of ceramides to muscle cells mimics effects on glycogen synthesis of adding palmitate (96). In contrast to the DAG/ PKC link that interferes with insulin signaling by causing serine phosphorylation of IRS-1 (28), it is controversial as to whether ceramides affect early stages of insulin signaling such as IRS-1 or PI3 kinase; rather the majority view is that ceramides act downstream to inhibit phosphorylation and activation of PKB/Akt (12,13). Two recent clinical studies provide strong support for the involvement of ceramides in muscle insulin resistance (97,98).

A number of questions remain. First, for example, are individual fatty acid metabolites acting principally as signaling molecules or is it mainly a bulk effect that impairs insulin action? Second, what are the relative roles of the alleged culprits LCACoAs, DAGs, and ceramides? Ceramides are formed from saturated fatty acids that do produce substantial insulin resistance, although other dietary fats (with the exception of omega-3β) are "not far behind" in producing deleterious effect (2). It is our current view that DAG accumulation can be particularly deleterious, and DAGs were the only lipid metabolite to be significantly elevated in the rat glucose infusion model at the time of onset of muscle insulin resistance (99). However, further work is needed to clarify whether this can be applied to other insulin resistance studies.

FFAs and Gene Expression

Another way in which the fatty acid composition and content of the diet may alter lipid and glucose metabolism is by regulation of gene expression (reviewed in ref. 100). The discovery of nuclear hormone receptors, which are regulated directly by fatty acids or fatty acid metabolites, provides at least one mechanism for these effects, although not all the actions of fatty acids on gene expression are direct (101). The most widely studied of the fatty acid–activated nuclear hormone receptors are the peroxisome proliferator–activated receptors (PPARs), and in particular PPARα and PPARγ, which are important for fat oxidation in the liver (102) and adipose tissue proliferation (103) respectively. The observation that several hours of fatty acid elevation is enough to alter specific gene expression (104) clearly demonstrates that fatty acid–mediated gene regulation may be a major mechanism by which increased lipid availability influences insulin action. Increased fatty acid availability appears to influence expression of key proteins in muscle lipid metabolism such as CD36 (105,106) and lipoprotein lipase (107). Other studies suggest that high-fat feeding in humans (108) or rodents (108,109) or 48 h lipid infusion in humans (110) alters expression of proteins such as PGC1 and others associated with mitochondrial function. It will be important to clarify this area as it has bearing on whether the mitochondrial dysfunction now believed to be associated with obesity and T2D (4,5) is likely to be a primary or an acquired defect.

Muscle Membrane Composition

A significant correlation has also been demonstrated between the fatty acid composition of muscle membranes and insulin action at a tissue and whole-body level in humans and animals (111–113). Possibilities linking muscle membrane composition to insulin action are changing membrane fluidity, which could affect insulin and other membrane receptor action (114), release of different diacylglycerol molecules after phospholipase activity with altered modulatory effects on cellular processes such as PKC activity

(115), and altered cellular energy expenditure influencing accumulation of intracellular triglyceride (114).

ADIPOSE BODY DEPOTS AND FFA FLUXES TO MUSCLE

While dietary changes, either increasing or reducing lipid, can readily alter muscle lipid accumulation in rodents, the situation in humans seems more complex. A number of studies have suggested that peripheral insulin sensitivity is not easily altered in humans by short-term dietary changes (115). A possible explanation, consistent with the muscle lipid supply hypothesis of insulin resistance, is that chronic levels of intra-myocellular lipid in humans are much harder to vary by dietary means than in rodents. Even when there is significant weight loss in obese subjects, it is not clear whether elevated muscle lipids significantly decline, with reports suggesting (59) and refuting this (116). This apparent species difference is sobering for those performing rodent studies, given the ease of reversing high-fat-diet-induced insulin resistance in the rat (10). Nevertheless while factors determining muscle lipid accumulation in humans and rodents may differ, their accumulation may have very similar implications for potency of insulin action. It may be that where genetic factors are involved, as in many human (and animal) insulin-resistant states, muscle lipid accumulation and/or insulin resistance may be harder to manipulate simply by dietary changes. Sorting this out will require a better knowledge of mechanistic links between muscle lipids and insulin action in the two species.

Two areas of difference whereby lipid accumulation may differ in humans and rodents is, first, the greater dependence on adipose stores in humans for overall lipid supply, and second, the possibly greater influence that modulation of fatty acid utilization may have in humans. There may be a link between increased fatty acid supply from fat depots in humans, particularly associated with increased visceral adiposity, and lipid accumulation in muscle. A number of studies have shown strong correlations between visceral adiposity and insulin resistance (117–120) and newer studies have gone on to show close relationships between visceral adiposity and IMCL (see Fig. 16.2) (70,121,122). The greater insulin sensitivity of women compared to men is also in accord with a gender difference in visceral fat (123), which again suggests that visceral fat may be a specific determinant of insulin resistance. Nevertheless careful studies of fatty acid turnover in obese humans have not supported the conjecture that visceral fat is the likely source of an increased fatty acid supply to peripheral tissues such as muscle (124), although it may contribute in this way to liver fatty acid supply (55,125). Other properties of visceral fat, such as its relatively high expression levels and presumably export of adipokines (126), might contribute to muscle insulin resistance. Further detailed discussion of visceral fat and whether it is causally related to insulin resistance is beyond the scope of this chapter, but the reader is referred to two recent articles that summarize evidence for opposing points of view (127,128).

At the moment it is not clear in quantitative terms how much increased FFA uptake into muscle and reduced utilization of fatty acids each contribute to muscle triglyceride accumulation. A glucose oversupply to muscle may contribute to the reduced utilization of fatty acids. Increased glucose availability and oxidation can inhibit lipid oxidation (129), producing a *glucose-fatty acid cycle in reverse* (130). Some possible mechanisms for this have been proposed and recently reviewed (131). In principle, these mechanisms propose that various factors may lead to a high level of muscle malonyl CoA, which in turn inhibits CPT-1 and mitochondrial transfer of LCACoAs. In support of this concept, we have found that in a rat model of chronic glucose infusion (to produce 3-fold normal basal glucose turnover), muscle becomes insulin resistant and malonyl CoA increases, presumably inhibiting fatty acid oxidation (95,99,132). As discussed already in this chapter, mitochondrial dysfunction resulting in reduced rates of fat oxidation may also contribute to cytosolic lipid accumulation in at least some states of muscle insulin resistance (4,5,108–110,133). Any tendency to increase cytosolic lipids in muscle cells via a reduction in the ability to utilize lipids for energy is exacerbated by what appears to be an adaptation of muscle to more efficiently take up fatty acids in states where there is a high availability of lipids. This could occur either via a high dietary content of fat or from prevailing obesity. Using fatty acid tracers, we have directly demonstrated the increased efficiency of fatty acid uptake into muscle of rats adapted to a high-fat diet (105,134), and supportive findings of increased expression of fatty acid transporters have been reported in human muscle in vitro (106,135). This adaptation makes sense in that it may enhance utilization of the dominant available energy fuel, but it may also contribute to accumulation of cytosolic muscle lipids and insulin resistance.

There is increasing interest in the postprandial state, and it is recognized that with western society dietary habits there is a considerable period of each day spent in a postprandial state. Normal regulation of fatty acid metabolism in this state may be crucial in controlling the daily average lipid supply to liver, muscle, and other tissues (136). It has been suggested that a disruption of the normal role of insulin in the post-prandial period may underlie many of the lipid abnormalities associated with insulin resistance (137). Increased expression of muscle lipoprotein lipase (107) may result in higher uptakes of fatty acids from VLDL triglycerides accompanying high dietary intakes of fat. Additionally we have preliminary tracer data suggesting that the ratio of LPL activity in muscle to that in adipose tissue may be inappropriately high in the fed state in insulin-resistant rats on high-fat diets (138). Thus, there may be multiple metabolic causes of increased cytosolic lipid accumulation in muscle in insulin-resistant states and further work will be needed to clarify this.

CYTOKINES AND INFLAMMATORY PATHWAYS: AN ADDITIONAL COMPONENT OF MUSCLE INSULIN RESISTANCE IN OBESITY AND TYPE 2 DIABETES

Over the last five years, several important publications have provided evidence for a role of inflammatory signaling pathways in obesity and lipid-induced insulin resistance. Initial studies using the lipid infusion model of insulin resistance in rats showed that treatment with high doses of the anti-inflammatory agent salicylate could alleviate insulin resistance by inhibiting the activity of IKK-β, a kinase involved in activating the transcription factor NFκB (139). In the same study, mice lacking the gene for IKK-β did not develop insulin resistance when infused with lipid and exhibited improved insulin signaling in muscle. Subsequent studies demonstrated that salicylates could attenuate insulin resistance in genetic and dietary animal models of obesity (140). Other studies in humans have supported the idea that inflammatory pathways are involved in disrupting insulin signaling and contributing to insulin resistance. Itani et al. (141) observed insulin resistance and activation of the NFkB pathway after acute lipid infusion and Hundal et al. (142) demonstrated improved insulin action in a group of type 2 diabetic subjects treated with high-dose aspirin for two weeks.

More evidence for a role of stress and inflammatory pathways in obesity-induced insulin resistance came from studies demonstrating that tissues from dietary and genetically obese mice have higher activities of the stress-activated c-Jun NH_2 terminal kinases (JNKs) (143). Furthermore, dietary and genetically obese mice deficient in a particular isoform of this enzyme, JNK1, had improved glucose homeostasis and improved insulin signaling in liver, suggesting a significant role for JNK in the pathogenesis of obesity-induced insulin resistance. Other studies have confirmed that over-feeding of rats produces increased JNK activity in muscle and liver—which is associated with increased phosphorylation of the inhibitory Ser-307 site of IRS-1 and substantial insulin resistance in these tissues (52).

The data linking obesity-induced inflammation to insulin resistance also suggests that cytokine and adipokine production from macrophages within adipose tissue as well as adipocytes in adipose tissue could be the signal for increased activation of IKK-β and JNK in liver and muscle (144). The summation of all these data suggests that in obesity, excess lipids and altered cytokine/adipokine levels activate stress pathways in liver and muscle. The increased activity of serine kinases like IKK-β and JNK impinge on the insulin signaling machinery via serine phosphorylation and inactivation of IRS proteins either directly or by activating other serine kinases (PKCs). At the current time, the evidence for acute physiological increases in fatty acid availability elevating inflammatory pathways in muscle tissue is not as strong as for established obesity, but there seems little doubt that activation of stress and inflammatory pathways are involved in the genesis and/or maintenance of insulin resistance in muscle even if the precise mechanisms for these effects are not completely defined.

PHARMACOLOGICAL MANIPULATION OF MUSCLE LIPID ACCUMULATION

We are now in an exciting phase where a number of possibilities are being followed that offer promise to reduce the cytosolic lipid load in muscle. These are expected to complement lifestyle-related approaches such as diet and exercise. These approaches can be categorized in two broad areas: by reducing the systemic supply of fatty acids to muscle and by increasing the utilization of fatty acids by muscle. One key factor with implications for both these areas has been the increased focus on the AMPK/ malonyl CoA network, a key player in the sensing and regulation of energy metabolism in muscle, liver, and other tissues. The multiple actions of AMPK have been recently reviewed elsewhere (131,145), but in the context of this chapter its most relevant actions are to enhance fatty acid oxidation. This occurs principally via reducing malonyl CoA synthesis by phosphorylating and inhibiting acetyl CoA carboxylase (ACC), plus enhancing malonyl CoA degradation by malonyl CoA decarboxylase. Lowering malonyl CoA will lessen inhibition of CPT-1, a rate-limiting enzyme for mitochondrial transfer and oxidation of LCACoAs. Some of the pharmacological approaches being followed are described next.

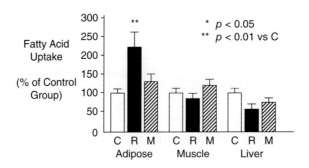

Figure 16.3. Fatty acid uptake in vivo into adipose tissue, muscle, and liver during an acute lipid infusion in control (C), rosiglitazone-pretreated (R), and metformin-pretreated (M) rats. Rosiglitazone pretreatment helps protect muscle and liver from deleterious effects of the lipid load by partitioning fatty acid uptake in favor of adipose tissue. **$p < 0.01$; *$p < 0.05$ versus C. (From ref. 151.)

PPARγ Agonists

PPARγ are effective insulin sensitizers (see recent reviews, refs. 146 and 147). PPARγ is a nuclear receptor principally (but not only) expressed in adipose tissue (148). Its activation by compounds such as the thiazolidinediones (TZDs) has been shown to have a key role in adipogenesis by increasing the gene expression of a number of key enzymes and/or transport proteins involved in adipose tissue metabolism. In addition to its role in adipose tissue proliferation, PPARγ activation can lead to a coordinated enhancement of gene expression resulting in enhanced net adipose tissue uptake of lipids. Evidence suggests that the TZDs might principally affect muscle metabolism "from a distance" by acting in adipose tissue to favor retention of lipid (Fig. 16.3) (149–151).

TZDs lower lipid accumulation in muscle of insulin-resistant rats. The TZD rosiglitazone, while enhancing insulin-mediated muscle glucose uptake and glycogen synthesis, also significantly reduces muscle triglyceride and DAG levels (53), and corrects some biochemical effects (e.g., chronic PKC activation; see ref. 152) that are associated with muscle lipid accumulation and insulin resistance in the high-fat-fed rat (93). While the "modulation of lipid supply" hypothesis seems most plausible for TZD action in vivo, there are other possibilities. For example, there may be local direct actions in muscle (153,154), and gene disruption of PPARγ1 in muscle may have functional effects (reviewed in ref. 155), although it is generally believed that adipose tissue is the major target (e.g., "fatless" mice, or mice without adipose PPARγ (156), do not respond to TZDs). However, TZDs may modulate a "signal" from adipose tissue, such as TNF-α (103), resistin (19), or adiponectin (20), which otherwise could influence insulin sensitivity. In particular, its substantial activation of adiponectin, now established as an activator of AMPK in liver and possibly muscle, may be a significant contributor to TZD insulin sensitization and lipid reduction in these tissues. Mice lacking adiponectin have impaired insulin sensitization by TZDs (20). In summary, it is clear that PPARγ agonists have a powerful effect on reducing systemic fatty acid supply and increasing muscle and liver insulin sensitivity at the expense of some increased weight gain via increased adiposity and fluid retention. Thus, although these agents are not perfect, additional vasoprotective, anti-inflammatory, and tumor-suppressing actions of the

PPARγ agonists elucidated over the last five years (146,147,157) have generally augured well for the therapeutic benefits of this class of compounds.

PPARα Agonists

PPARα is strongly expressed in liver, and in line with this the liver seems to be the principal target of action of PPARα agonists (e.g., fibrates, WY-14653). PPARα activation leads to, inter alia, expression of genes involved in beta oxidation of fatty acids, and it could be argued that reducing lipid by "burning it off" is more desirable than sequestering it in adipose tissue, as is likely with the PPARγ agonists. PPARα is also expressed in muscle, but its effects there are not clear at this stage. Because several of the lipid-lowering agents act with mutually distinct mechanisms and/or on differing principal tissue targets, it is possible that combined therapy will prove to have desirable synergistic effects. The expectation is that compounds with additional PPARα activity will show less tendency to weight gain than PPARδ activity alone (54,158), but further experience with their application to humans is needed. Compounds with combined PPARα and PPARγ action have had desirable metabolic effects in rodent models (e.g., refs. 159–161), but unfortunately a number of combined agonists have not progressed into clinical use because of undesirable side effects (162). The hope is that future compounds may prove to be suitable for human use.

Other compounds under development include PPARδ agonists, AMPK activators, and ACC inhibitors. These are generally aimed at increasing fat oxidation, although each has been implicated in multiple metabolic effects:

- *PPARδ*, recently reviewed (163), is expressed in many tissues, including muscle, where it has been implicated in regulation of fatty acid oxidation and energy homeostasis (164,165); its activation by an agonist GW501516 can reduce weight gain in high-fat-fed mice (164). PPARδ is expressed at much higher levels in muscle than PPARα, and interestingly, its expression increases in states such as prolonged fasting (166) and exercise training (165) when the need for fat oxidation increases. GW501516 also had dramatic effects to correct dyslipidemia in obese monkeys (167) and its overall effects on lipid metabolism are likely to be complex.
- We recently reported that AICAR, a commonly used *AMPK activator*, could enhance insulin sensitivity in muscle and liver of high-fat-fed rats (168), and it now appears that the anti-diabetic drug metformin acts as an AMPK activator in muscle and liver (e.g., refs. 151,169–172). This in fact may be the major pathway for metformin action in liver, in that AMPK activation was necessary for the glucose-lowering action of metformin (173). Both adipokines leptin and adiponectin can also act to activate AMPK (145), and it is likely that at least some of the actions of PPARγ agonists on the liver and possibly muscle are mediated indirectly via adiponectin elevation.
- Finally, supported by the lean phenotype that accompanies ACC knockout in mice (174), chemical *ACC inhibitors* are showing promise to enhance fat oxidation (175). Specific inhibition of ACC isoforms in liver by antisense oligonucleotides appears to effectively enhance liver fat oxidation, reducing ectopic lipid accumulation in that organ (176). We are, however, unaware of similar studies in muscle.

In summary, various rodent knockouts and preclinical pharmacological studies support the concept that chemically enhanced fat oxidation will be beneficial in ameliorating ectopic lipid accumulation and attendant insulin resistance. However, the long-term consequences of such approaches, particularly in the human context, have not been studied in any great detail at this time, and we await such studies with interest.

CONCLUSION

There are a number of potential mechanisms by which fatty acids might influence glucose metabolism and insulin action. Total muscle lipid availability (from systemic and intracellular sources) as well as specific fatty acids may act to regulate enzymes of fat and glucose metabolism and enzymes that alter insulin signaling pathways. The added action of fatty acids to bind specific nuclear receptors and transcription factors provides another direct mechanism whereby different dietary lipids could influence metabolism. Finally, the principles described here are fundamental to understanding metabolic effects of various lipid-lowering agents, particularly in relation to improving insulin sensitivity in insulin-resistant states.

REFERENCES

1. Kraegen EW, Cooney GJ, Ye JM, Furler SM. Fat feeding and muscle fat deposition eliciting insulin resistance. In: *Insulin Resistance and Insulin Resistance Syndrome,* Hansen B, Shafrir E (eds.), Taylor & Francis, London, 2002, pp. 195–209.
2. Storlien LH, Jenkins AB, Chisholm DJ, Pascoe WS, Khouri S, Kraegen EW. Influence of dietary fat composition on development of insulin resistance in rats. *Diabetes* 1991; 40:280–289.
3. Kraegen EW, Clark PW, Jenkins AB, Daley EA, Chisholm DJ, Storlien LH. Development of muscle insulin resistance after liver insulin resistance in high-fat-fed rats. *Diabetes* 1991; 40:1397–1403.
4. Petersen KF, Dufour S, Befroy D, Garcia R, Shulman GI. Impaired mitochondrial activity in the insulin-resistant offspring of patients with type 2 diabetes. *N Engl J Med* 2004; 350:664–671.
5. Kelley DE, He J, Menshikova EV, Ritov VB. Dysfunction of mitochondria in human skeletal muscle in type 2 diabetes. *Diabetes* 2002; 51:2944–2950.
6. Hwang JH, Pan JW, Heydari S, Hetherington HP, Stein DT. Regional differences in intramyocellular lipids in humans observed by in vivo H-1-MR spectroscopic imaging. *J Appl Physiol* 2001; 90:1267–1274.
7. Kraegen EW, James DE, Storlien LH, Burleigh KM, Chisholm DJ. In vivo insulin resistance in individual peripheral tissues of the high fat fed rat: Assessment by euglycaemic clamp plus deoxyglucose administration. *Diabetologia* 1986; 29:192–198.
8. Randle PJ, Garland PB, Hales CN, Newsholme EA. The glucose fatty-acid cycle: Its role in insulin sensitivity and the metabolic disturbances of diabetes mellitus. *Lancet* 1963; i:785–789.
9. Ruderman NB, Saha AK, Vavvas D, Witters LA. Malonyl-CoA, fuel sensing, and insulin resistance. *Am J Physiol* 1999; 39:E1–E18.
10. Oakes ND, Bell KS, Furler SM, Camilleri S, Saha AK, Ruderman NB, Chisholm DJ, Kraegen EW. Diet-induced muscle insulin resistance in rats is ameliorated by acute dietary lipid withdrawal or a single bout of exercise: Parallel relationship between insulin stimulation of glucose uptake and suppression of long-chain fatty acyl-CoA. *Diabetes* 1997; 46:2022–2028.
11. Prentki M, Corkey BE. Are the beta-cell signalling molecules malonyl-CoA and cytosolic long-chain acyl-CoA implicated in multiple tissue defects of obesity and NIDDM? *Diabetes* 1996; 45:273–283.
12. Schmitz-Peiffer C. Signalling aspects of insulin resistance in skeletal muscle: mechanisms induced by lipid oversupply. *Cell Signal* 2000; 12:583–594.
13. Summers SA. Ceramides in insulin resistance and lipotoxicity. *Prog Lipid Res* 2006; 45:42–72.
14. Weisberg SP, McCann D, Desai M, Rosenbaum M, Leibel RL, Ferrante AW Jr. Obesity is associated with macrophage accumulation in adipose tissue. *J Clin Invest* 2003; 112:1796–1808.
15. Xu H, Barnes GT, Yang Q, Tan G, Yang D, Chou CJ, Sole J, Nichols A, Ross JS, Tartaglia LA, Chen H. Chronic inflammation in fat plays a crucial role in the development of obesity-related insulin resistance. *J Clin Invest* 2003; 112:1821–1830.

16. Hotamisligil GS, Spiegelman BM. Tumor necrosis factor alpha: A key component of the obesity-diabetes link. *Diabetes* 1994; 43:1271–1278.
17. Shimabukuro M, Koyama K, Chen GX, Wang MY, Trieu F, Lee Y, Newgard CB, Unger RH. Direct antidiabetic effect of leptin through triglyceride depletion of tissues. *Proc Nat Acad Sci* 1997; 94:4637–4641.
18. Fernandez-Real JM, Broch M, Vendrell J, Gutierrez C, Casamitjana R, Pugeat M, Richart C, Ricart W. Interleukin-6 gene polymorphism and insulin sensitivity. *Diabetes* 2000; 49:517–520.
19. Steppan CM, Bailey ST, Bhat S, Brown EJ, Banerjee RR, Wright CM, Patel HR, Ahima RS, Lazar MA. The hormone resistin links obesity to diabetes. *Nature* 2001; 409:307–312.
20. Kadowaki T, Yamauchi T. Adiponectin and adiponectin receptors. *Endocr Rev* 2005; 26:439–451.
21. Fukuhara A, Matsuda M, Nishizawa M, Segawa K, Tanaka M, Kishimoto K, Matsuki Y, Murakami M, Ichisaka T, Murakami H, Watanabe E, Takagi T, Akiyoshi M, Ohtsubo T, Kihara S, Yamashita S, Makishima M, Funahashi T, Yamanaka S, Hiramatsu R, Matsuzawa Y, Shimomura I. Visfatin: A protein secreted by visceral fat that mimics the effects of insulin. *Science* 2005; 307:426–430.
22. Yang Q, Graham TE, Mody N, Preitner F, Peroni OD, Zabolotny JM, Kotani K, Quadro L, Kahn BB. Serum retinol binding protein 4 contributes to insulin resistance in obesity and type 2 diabetes. *Nature* 2005; 436:356–362.
23. Thompson AL, Lim-Fraser MY-C, Kraegen EW, Cooney GJ. Effects of individual fatty acids on glucose uptake and glycogen synthesis in soleus muscle in vitro. *Am J Physiol* 2000; 279: E577–E584.
24. Sinha S, Perdomo G, Brown NF, O'Doherty RM. Fatty acid-induced insulin resistance in L6 myotubes is prevented by inhibition of activation and nuclear localization of nuclear factor kappa B. *J Biol Chem* 2004; 279:41294–41301.
25. Boden G. Role of fatty acids in the pathogenesis of insulin resistance and NIDDM. *Diabetes* 1997; 46:3–10.
26. Chalkley S, Hettiarachchi M, Chisholm DJ, Kraegen EW. Five hour fatty acid elevation increases muscle lipids and impairs glycogen synthesis in the rat. *Metabolism* 1998; 47:1121–1126.
27. Griffin ME, Marcucci MJ, Cline GW, Bell K, Barucci N, Lee D, Goodyear LJ, Kraegen EW, White MF, Shulman GI. Free fatty acid-induced insulin resistance is associated with activation of protein kinase C theta and alterations in the insulin signaling cascade. *Diabetes* 1999; 48:1270–1274.
28. Yu C, Chen Y, Zong H, Wang Y, Bergeron R, Kim JK, Cline GW, Cushman SW, Cooney GJ, Atcheson B, White MW, Kraegen EW, Shulman GI. Mechanism by which fatty acids inhibit insulin activation of IRS-1 associated phosphatidylinositol 3-kinase activity in muscle. *J Biol Chem* 2002; 277:50230–50236.
29. Belfort R, Mandarino L, Kashyap S, Wirfel K, Pratipanawatr T, Berria R, Defronzo RA, Cusi K. Dose-response effect of elevated plasma free fatty acid on insulin signaling. *Diabetes* 2005; 54:1640–1648.
30. Boden G, Jadali F, White J, Liang Y, Mozzoli M, Chen X, Coleman E, Smith C. Effects of fat on insulin stimulated carbohydrate metabolism in normal men. *J Clin Invest* 1991; 88:960–966.
31. Boden G, Chen XH, Ruiz J, White JV, Rossetti L. Mechanisms of fatty acid induced inhibition of glucose uptake. *J Clin Invest* 1994; 93:2438–2446.
32. Kelley DE, Mokan M, Simoneau JA, Mandarino LJ. Interaction between glucose and free fatty acid metabolism in human skeletal muscle. *J Clin Invest* 1993; 92:91–98.
33. Kim JK, Youn JH. Prolonged suppression of glucose metabolism causes insulin resistance in rat skeletal muscle. *Am J Physiol* 1997; 272:E288–E296.
34. Jucker BM, Rennings AJM, Cline GW, Shulman GI. C-13 and P-31 NMR studies on the effects of increased plasma free fatty acids on intramuscular glucose metabolism in the awake rat. *J Biol Chem* 1997; 272:10464–10473.
35. Bevilacqua S, Buzzigoli G, Bonadonna R, Brandi LS, Oleggini M, Boni C, Geloni M, Ferrannini E. Operation of Randle's cycle in patients with NIDDM. *Diabetes* 1990; 39:383–389.
36. Wolfe BM, Klein S, Peters EJ, Schmidt BF, Wolfe RR. Effect of elevated free fatty acids on glucose oxidation in normal humans. *Metabolism* 1988; 37:323–329.
37. Jenkins AB, Storlien LH, Chisholm DJ, Kraegen EW. Effects of nonesterified fatty acid availability on tissue-specific glucose utilization in rats in vivo. *J Clin Invest* 1988; 82:293–299.
38. Chen MT, Kaufman LN, Spennetta T, Shrago E. Effects of high fat-feeding to rats on the interrelationship of body weight, plasma insulin, and fatty acyl-coenzyme-A esters in liver and skeletal muscle. *Metabolism* 1992; 41:564–569.

39. Zierath JB, Houseknecht KL, Gnudi L, Kahn BB. High-fat feeding impairs insulin-stimulated GLUT4 recruitment via an early insulin-signaling defect. *Diabetes* 1997; 46:215–223.
40. Frangioudakis G, Ye JM, Cooney GJ. Both saturated and n-6 polyunsaturated fat diets reduce phosphorylation of insulin receptor substrate-1 and protein kinase B in muscle during the initial stages of in vivo insulin stimulation. *Endocrinology* 2005; 146:5596–5603.
41. Dobbins RL, Szczepaniak LS, Bentley B, Esser V, Myhill J, McGarry JD. Prolonged inhibition of muscle carnitine palmitoyltransferase-1 promotes intramyocellular lipid accumulation and insulin resistance in rats. *Diabetes* 2001; 50:123–130.
42. Kim JK, Fillmore JJ, Chen Y, Yu CL, Moore IK, Pypaert M, Lutz EP, Kako Y, Velez-Carrasco W, Goldberg IJ, Breslow JL, Shulman GI. Tissue-specific overexpression of lipoprotein lipase causes tissue-specific insulin resistance. *Proc Natl Acad Sci USA* 2001; 98:7522–7527.
43. Ferreira L, Pulawa LK, Jensen DR, Eckel RH. Overexpressing human lipoprotein lipase in mouse skeletal muscle is associated with insulin resistance. *Diabetes* 2001; 50:1064–1068.
44. Kim JK, Gimeno RE, Higashimori T, Kim HJ, Choi H, Punreddy S, Mozell RL, Tan G, Stricker-Krongrad A, Hirsch DJ, Fillmore JJ, Liu ZX, Dong J, Cline G, Stahl A, Lodish HF, Shulman GI. Inactivation of fatty acid transport protein 1 prevents fat-induced insulin resistance in skeletal muscle. *J Clin Invest* 2004; 113:756–763.
45. Ibrahimi A, Bonen A, Blinn WD, Hajri T, Li X, Zhong K, Cameron R, Abumrad NA. Muscle-specific overexpression of FAT/CD36 enhances fatty acid oxidation by contracting muscle, reduces plasma triglycerides and fatty acids, and increases plasma glucose and insulin. *J Biol Chem* 1999; 274:26761–26766.
46. Campbell SE, Tandon NN, Woldegiorgis G, Luiken JJ, Glatz JF, Bonen A. A novel function for fatty acid translocase (FAT)/CD36: involvement in long chain fatty acid transfer into the mitochondria. *J Biol Chem* 2004; 279: 36235–36241.
47. Park SY, Kim HJ, Wang S, Higashimori T, Dong J, Kim YJ, Cline G, Li H, Prentki M, Shulman GI, Mitchell GA, Kim JK. Hormone-sensitive lipase knockout mice have increased hepatic insulin sensitivity and are protected from short-term diet-induced insulin resistance in skeletal muscle and heart. *Am J Physiol Endocrinol Metab* 2005; 289:E30–39.
48. Goudriaan JR, Tacken PJ, Dahlmans VE, Gijbels MJ, van Dijk KW, Havekes LM, Jong MC. Protection from obesity in mice lacking the VLDL receptor. *Arterioscler Thromb Vasc Biol* 2001; 21:1488–1493.
49. Storlien LH, Kraegen EW, Chisholm DJ, Ford GL, Bruce DG, Pascoe WS. Fish oil prevents insulin resistance induced by high-fat feeding in rats. *Science* 1987; 237:885–888.
50. Neschen S, Moore I, Regittnig W, Yu CL, Wang YL, Pypaert M, Petersen KF, Shulman GI. Contrasting effects of fish oil and safflower oil on hepatic peroxisomal and tissue lipid content. *Amer J Physiol* 2002; 282:E395–E401.
51. Russell JC, Shillabeer G, Bartana J, Lau DCW, Richardson M, Wenzel LM, Graham SE, Dolphin PJ. Development of insulin resistance in the jcr-La-Cp rat: Role of triacylglycerols and effects of Medica 16. *Diabetes* 1998; 47:770–778.
52. Prada PO, Zecchin HG, Gasparetti AL, Torsoni MA, Ueno M, Hirata AE, Corezola do Amaral ME, Hoer NF, Boschero AC, Saad MJ. Western diet modulates insulin signaling, c-Jun N-terminal kinase activity, and insulin receptor substrate-1ser307 phosphorylation in a tissue-specific fashion. *Endocrinology* 2005; 146:1576–1587.
53. Oakes ND, Camilleri S, Furler SM, Chisholm DJ, Kraegen EW. The insulin sensitizer, BRL 49653, reduces systemic fatty acid supply and utilization and tissue lipid availability in the rat. *Metabolism* 1997; 46:935–942.
54. Ye JM, Doyle PJ, Iglesias MA, Watson DG, Cooney GJ, Kraegen EW. Peroxisome proliferator-activated receptor (PPAR)-alpha activation lowers muscle lipids and improves insulin sensitivity in high fat-fed rats: Comparison with PPAR-gamma activation. *Diabetes* 2001; 50:411–417.
55. Kim SP, Ellmerer M, Van Citters GW, Bergman RN. Primacy of hepatic insulin resistance in the development of the metabolic syndrome induced by an isocaloric moderate-fat diet in the dog. *Diabetes* 2003; 52:2453–2460.
56. Pan DA, Lillioja S, Kriketos AD, Milner MR, Baur LA, Bogardus C, Jenkins AB, Storlien LH. Skeletal muscle triglyceride levels are inversely related to insulin action. *Diabetes* 1997; 46:983–988.
57. Phillips DIW, Caddy S, Ilic V, Fielding BA, Frayn KN, Borthwick AC, Taylor R. Intramuscular triglyceride and muscle insulin sensitivity: Evidence for a relationship in nondiabetic subjects. *Metabolism* 1996; 45:947–950.

58. Goodpaster BH, He J, Watkins S, Kelley DE. Skeletal muscle lipid content and insulin resistance: Evidence for a paradox in endurance-trained athletes. *J Clin Endoc Metab* 2001; 86:5755–5761.

59. Goodpaster BH, Theriault R, Watkins SC, Kelley DE. Intramuscular lipid content is increased in obesity and decreased by weight loss. *Metabolism* 2000; 49:467–472.

60. Boesch C, Slotboom J, Hoppeler H, Kreis R. In vivo determination of intra-myocellular lipids in human muscle by means of localized H-1-MR-spectroscopy. *Magn Reson Med* 1997; 37:484–493.

61. Szczepaniak LS, Babcock EE, Schick F, Dobbins RL, Garg A, Burns DK, McGarry JD, Stein DT. Measurement of intracellular triglyceride stores by H spectroscopy: Validation in vivo. *Am J Physiol* 1999; 276:E977–E989.

62. Levin K, Schroeder HD, Alford FP, Beck-Nielsen H. Morphometric documentation of abnormal intramyocellular fat storage and reduced glycogen in obese patients with Type II diabetes. *Diabetologia* 2001; 44:824–833.

63. Krssak M, Petersen KF, Dresner A, DiPietro L, Vogel SM, Rothman DL, Shulman GI, Roden M. Intramyocellular lipid concentrations are correlated with insulin sensitivity in humans: An H-1 NMR spectroscopy study. *Diabetologia* 1999; 42:113–116.

64. Jacob S, Machann J, Rett K, Brechtel K, Volk A, Renn A, Maerker E, Matthaei S, Schick F, Claussen C-D, Haring H-U. Association of increased intramyocellular lipid content with insulin resistance in lean nondiabetic offspring of Type 2 diabetic subjects. *Diabetes* 1999; 48:1113–1119.

65. Perseghin G, Scifo P, De Cobelli F, Pagliato E, Battezzatic A, Arcelloni C, Vanzulli A, Testolin G, Pozza G, Del Maschio A, Luzi L. Intramyocellular triglyceride content is a determinant of in vivo insulin resistance in humans: An H-1-C-13 nuclear magnetic resonance spectroscopy assessment in offspring of type 2 diabetic parents. *Diabetes* 1999; 48:1600–1606.

66. Virkamaki A, Korsheninnikova E, Seppala-Lindroos A, Vehkavaara S, Goto T, Halavaara J, Hakkinen AM, Yki-Jarvinen H. Intramyocellular lipid is associated with resistance to in vivo insulin actions on glucose uptake, antilipolysis, and early insulin signaling pathways in human skeletal muscle. *Diabetes* 2001; 50:2337–2343.

67. Kriketos AD, Furler SM, Gan SK, Poynten AM, Chisholm DJ, Campbell LV. Multiple indexes of lipid availability are independently related to whole body insulin action in healthy humans. *J Clin Endocrinol Metab* 2003; 88:793–798.

68. Gan SK, Samaras K, Thompson CH, Kraegen EW, Carr A, Cooper DA, Chisholm DJ. Altered myocellular and abdominal fat partitioning predict disturbance in insulin action in HIV protease inhibitor-related lipodystrophy. 2002; *Diabetes* 51: 3163–3169.

69. Gavrilova O, Marcus-Samuels B, Graham D, Kim JK, Shulman GI, Castle AL, Vinson C, Eckhaus M, Reitman ML. Surgical implantation of adipose tissue reverses diabetes in lipoatrophic mice. *J Clin Invest* 2000; 105:271–278.

70. Gan SK, Kriketos AD, Poynten AM, Furler SM, Thompson CH, Kraegen EW, Campbell LV, Chisholm DJ. Insulin action, regional fat, and myocyte lipid: altered relationships with increased adiposity. *Obes Res* 2003; 11:1295–1305.

71. Kelley DE, Mandarino LJ. Fuel selection in human skeletal muscle in insulin resistance: A reexamination. *Diabetes* 2000; 49:677–683.

72. Kiens B. Skeletal muscle lipid metabolism in exercise and insulin resistance. *Physiol Rev* 2006; 86:205–243.

73. Bruce CR, Kriketos AD, Cooney GJ, Hawley JA. Disassociation of muscle triglyceride content and insulin sensitivity after exercise training in patients with Type 2 diabetes. *Diabetologia* 2004; 47:23–30.

74. Vock R, Weibel ER, Hoppeler H, Ordway G, Weber JM, Taylor CR. Design of the oxygen and substrate pathways: V. Structural basis of vascular substrate supply to muscle cells. *J Exp Biol* 1996; 199:1675–1688.

75. Bruce CR, Anderson MJ, Carey AL, Newman DG, Bonen A, Kriketos AD, Cooney GJ, Hawley JA. Muscle oxidative capacity is a better predictor of insulin sensitivity than lipid status. *J Clin Endocrinol Metab* 2003; 88:5444–5451.

76. Bruce CR, Thrush AB, Mertz VA, Bezaire V, Chabowski A, Heigenhauser GJ, Dyck DJ. Endurance training in obese humans improves glucose tolerance, mitochondrial fatty acid oxidation and alters muscle lipid content. *Am J Physiol Endocrinol Metab* 2006; in press.

77. Faergeman NJ, Knudsen J. Role of long-chain fatty acyl-CoA esters in the regulation of metabolism and cell signalling. *Biochem J* 1997; 323:1–12.

78. Carroll JE, Villadiego A, Morse DP. Fatty acid oxidation intermediates and the effect of fasting on oxidation in red and white skeletal muscle. *Muscle & Nerve* 1983; 6:367–373.
79. Oakes ND, Cooney GJ, Camilleri S, Chisholm DJ, Kraegen EW. Mechanisms of liver and muscle insulin resistance induced by chronic high-fat feeding. *Diabetes* 1997; 46:1768–1774.
80. Ellis BA, Poynten A, Lowy AJ, Furler SM, Chisholm DJ, Kraegen EW, Cooney GJ. Long-chain acyl-CoA esters as indicators of lipid metabolism and insulin sensitivity in rat and human muscle. *Am J Physiol* 2000; 279:E554–E560.
81. Kim JK, Kim HJ, Park SY, Cederberg A, Westergren R, Nilsson D, Higashimori T, Cho YR, Liu ZX, Dong J, Cline GW, Enerback S, Shulman GI. Adipocyte-specific overexpression of FOXC2 prevents diet-induced increases in intramuscular fatty acyl CoA and insulin resistance. *Diabetes* 2005; 54:1657–1663.
82. Bajaj M, Suraamornkul S, Romanelli A, Cline GW, Mandarino LJ, Shulman GI, DeFronzo RA. Effect of a sustained reduction in plasma free fatty acid concentration on intramuscular long-chain fatty Acyl-CoAs and insulin action in type 2 diabetic patients. *Diabetes* 2005; 54:3148–3153.
83. Houmard JA, Tanner CJ, Yu CL, Cunningham PG, Pories WJ, MacDonald KG, Shulman GI. Effect of weight loss on insulin sensitivity and intramuscular long-chain fatty Acyl-CoAs in morbidly obese subjects. *Diabetes* 2002; 51:2959–2963.
84. Vessby B, Gustafsson IB, Tengblad S, Boberg M, Andersson A. Desaturation and elongation of Fatty acids and insulin action. *Ann NY Acad Sci* 2002; 967:183–195.
85. Voss MD, Beha A, Tennagels N, Tschank G, Herling AW, Quint M, Gerl M, Metz-Weidmann C, Haun G, Korn M. Gene expression profiling in skeletal muscle of Zucker diabetic fatty rats: Implications for a role of stearoyl-CoA desaturase 1 in insulin resistance. *Diabetologia* 2005; 48:2622–2630.
86. Wititsuwannakul D, Kim K-H. Mechanism of palmityl coenzyme A inhibition of liver glycogen synthase. *J Biol Chem* 1977; 252:7812–7817.
87. Tippett PS, Neet KE. An allosteric model for the inhibition of glucokinase by long acyl coenzyme A. *J Biol Chem* 1982; 257:12846–12852.
88. Fulceri R, Gamberucci A, Scott HM, Giunti R, Burchell A, Benedetti A. Fatty acyl-CoA esters inhibit glucose-6-phosphatase in rat liver microsomes. *Biochem J* 1995; 307:391–397.
89. Nikawa J-I, Tanabe T, Ogiwara H, Shiba T, Numa S. Inhibitory effects of long-chain acyl coenzyme A analogues on liver acetyl coenzyme A carboxylase. *FEBS Lett* 1979; 102:223–226.
90. Thompson AL, Cooney GJ. Acyl-CoA inhibition of hexokinase in rat and human skeletal muscle is a potential mechanism of lipid-induced insulin resistance. *Diabetes* 2000; 49:1761–1765.
91. Taylor EB, Ellingson WJ, Lamb JD, Chesser DG, Winder WW. Long-chain acyl-CoA esters inhibit phosphorylation of AMP-activated protein kinase at threonine-172 by LKB1/STRAD/MO25. *Am J Physiol* 2005; 288:E1055–1061.
92. Ruderman NB, Saha AK, Kraegen EW. Minireview: Malonyl CoA, AMP-activated protein kinase, and adiposity. *Endocrinology* 2003; 144:5166–5171.
93. Schmitz-Peiffer C, Browne CL, Oakes ND, Watkinson A, Chisholm DJ, Kraegen EW, Biden TJ. Alterations in the expression and cellular localization of protein kinase C isozymes epsilon and theta are associated with insulin resistance in skeletal muscle of the high-fat-fed rat. *Diabetes* 1997; 46:169–178.
94. Kim JK, Fillmore JJ, Sunshine MJ, Albrecht B, Higashimori T, Kim DW, Liu ZX, Soos TJ, Cline GW, O'Brien WR, Littman DR, Shulman GI. PKC-theta knockout mice are protected from fat-induced insulin resistance. *J Clin Invest* 2004; 114:823–827.
95. Laybutt DR, Schmitz-Peiffer C, Saha AK, Ruderman NB, Biden TJ, Kraegen EW. Muscle lipid accumulation and protein kinase C activation in the insulin-resistant chronically glucose-infused rat. *Am J Physiol* 1999; 277:E1070–E1076.
96. Schmitz-Peiffer C, Craig DL, Biden TJ. Ceramide generation is sufficient to account for the inhibition of the insulin-stimulated PKB pathway in C2C12 skeletal muscle cells pretreated with palmitate. *J Biol Chem* 1999; 274:24202–24210.
97. Adams JM II, Pratipanawatr T, Berria R, Wang E, DeFronzo RA, Sullards MC, Mandarino LJ. Ceramide content is increased in skeletal muscle from obese insulin-resistant humans. *Diabetes* 2004; 53:25–31.
98. Straczkowski M, Kowalska I, Nikolajuk A, Dzienis-Straczkowska S, Kinalska I, Baranowski M, Zendzian-Piotrowska M, Brzezinska Z, Gorski J. Relationship between insulin sensitivity and sphingomyelin signaling pathway in human skeletal muscle. *Diabetes* 2004; 53:1215–1221.

99. Kraegen EW, Saha AK, Preston E, Wilks D, Hoy AJ, Cooney GJ, Ruderman NB. Increased malonyl-CoA and diacylglycerol content and reduced AMPK activity accompany insulin resistance induced by glucose infusion in muscle and liver of rats. *Am J Physiol 2006;* 290:E471–479.

100. Jump DB. Fatty acid regulation of gene transcription. *Crit Rev Clin Lab Sci* 2004; 41:41–78.

101. Duplus E, Glorian M, Forest C. Fatty acid regulation of gene transcription. *J Biol Chem* 2000; 275:30749–30752.

102. Lemberger T, Desvergne B, Wahli W. Peroxisome proliferator-activated receptors: A nuclear receptor signaling pathway in lipid physiology. *Annu Rev Cell Dev Biol* 1996; 12:335–363.

103. Spiegelman BM. PPAR-gamma: Adipogenic regulator and thiazolidinedione receptor. *Diabetes* 1998; 47:507–514.

104. Fabris R, Nisoli E, Lombardi AM, Tonello C, Serra R, Granzotto M, Cusin I, Bohner-Jeanrenaud F, Federspil G, Carruba MO, Vettor R. Preferential channeling of energy fuels toward fat rather than muscle during high free fatty acid availability in rats. *Diabetes* 2001; 50:601–608.

105. Hegarty BD, Cooney GJ, Kraegen EW, Furler SM. Increased efficiency of fatty acid uptake contributes to lipid accumulation in skeletal muscle of high fat-fed insulin-resistant rats. *Diabetes* 2002; 51:1477–1484.

106. Bonen A, Parolin ML, Steinberg GR, Calles-Escandon J, Tandon NN, Glatz JF, Luiken JJ, Heigenhauser GJ, Dyck DJ. Triacylglycerol accumulation in human obesity and type 2 diabetes is associated with increased rates of skeletal muscle fatty acid transport and increased sarcolemmal FAT/CD36. *Faseb J* 2004; 18:1144–1146.

107. de Fourmestraux V, Neubauer H, Poussin C, Farmer P, Falquet L, Burcelin R, Delorenzi M, Thorens B. Transcript profiling suggests that differential metabolic adaptation of mice to a high fat diet is associated with changes in liver to muscle lipid fluxes. *J Biol Chem* 2004; 279:50743–50753.

108. Sparks LM, Xie H, Koza RA, Mynatt R, Hulver MW, Bray GA, Smith SR. A high-fat diet coordinately downregulates genes required for mitochondrial oxidative phosphorylation in skeletal muscle. *Diabetes* 2005; 54:1926–1933.

109. Sreekumar R, Unnikrishnan J, Fu A, Nygren J, Short KR, Schimke J, Barazzoni R, Nair KS. Impact of high-fat diet and antioxidant supplement on mitochondrial functions and gene transcripts in rat muscle. *Am J Physiol* 2002; 282:E1055–1061.

110. Richardson DK, Kashyap S, Bajaj M, Cusi K, Mandarino SJ, Finlayson J, DeFronzo RA, Jenkinson CP, Mandarino LJ. Lipid infusion decreases the expression of nuclear encoded mitochondrial genes and increases the expression of extracellular matrix genes in human skeletal muscle. *J Biol Chem* 2005; 280:10290–10297.

111. Pan DA, Hulbert AJ, Storlien LH. Dietary fats, membrane phospholipids and obesity. *J Nutr* 1994; 124:1555–1565.

112. Borkman M, Storlien LH, Pan DA, Jenkins AB, Chisholm DJ, Campbell LV. The relation between insulin sensitivity and the fatty acid composition of skeletal-muscle phospholipids. *N Engl J Med* 1993; 328:238–244.

113. Haugaard SB, Madsbad S, Hoy CE, Vaag A. Dietary intervention increases n-3 long-chain polyunsaturated fatty acids in skeletal muscle membrane phospholipids of obese subjects: Implications for insulin sensitivity. *Clin Endocrinol (Oxf)* 2006; 64:169–78.

114. Storlien LH, Kriketos AD, Calvert GD, Baur LA, Jenkins AB. Fatty acids, triglycerides and syndromes of insulin resistance. *Prostagland Leuk Essent Fatty Acids* 1997; 57:379–385.

115. Storlien LH, Baur LA, Kriketos AD, Pan DA, Cooney GJ, Jenkins AB, Calvert GD, Campbell LV. Dietary fats and insulin action. *Diabetologia* 1996; 39:621–631.

116. Malenfant P, Tremblay A, Doucet E, Imbeault P, Simoneau JA, Joanisse DR. Elevated intramyocellular lipid concentration in obese subjects is not reduced after diet and exercise training. *Am J Physiol* 2001; 280:E632–E639.

117. Carey DG, Jenkins AB, Campbell LV, Freund J, Chisholm DJ. Abdominal fat and insulin resistance in normal and overweight women: Direct measurements reveal a strong relationship in subjects at both low and high risk of NIDDM. *Diabetes* 1996; 45:633–638.

118. Park KS, Rhee BD, Lee K-U, Kim SY, Lee HK, Koh C-S, Min HK. Intra-abdominal fat is associated with decreased insulin sensitivity in healthy young men. *Metabolism* 1991; 40:600–603.

119. Ross R, Fortier L, Hudson R. Separate associations between visceral and subcutaneous adipose tissue distribution, insulin and glucose levels in obese women. *Diabetes Care* 1996; 19:1404–1411.

120. Simoneau J-A, Colberg SR, Thaete FL, Kelley DE. Skeletal muscle glycolytic and oxidative enzyme capacities are determinants of insulin sensitivity and muscle composition in obese women. *FASEB J* 1995; 9:273–278.
121. Gan SK, Samaras K, Thompson C, Kraegen EW, Carr A, Cooper D, Chisholm DJ. Correlations between intramyocellular lipid, visceral fat and insulin sensitivity: A study of HIV positive subjects with and without peripheral lipodystrophy. *Diabetes* 2001; 50(suppl 2):A315–316.
122. Weiss R, Dufour S, Taksali SE, Tamborlane WV, Petersen KF, Bonadonna RC, Boselli L, Barbetta G, Allen K, Rife F, Savoye M, Dziura J, Sherwin R, Shulman GI, Caprio S. Prediabetes in obese youth: a syndrome of impaired glucose tolerance, severe insulin resistance, and altered myocellular and abdominal fat partitioning. *Lancet* 2003; 362:951–957.
123. Carey DGP, Campbell LV, Chisholm DJ. Is visceral fat (intra-abdominal and hepatic) a major determinant of gender differences in insulin resistance and dyslipidemia? *Diabetes* 1996; 45(suppl):110A.
124. Nielsen S, Guo Z, Johnson CM, Hensrud DD, Jensen MD. Splanchnic lipolysis in human obesity. *J Clin Invest* 2004; 113:1582–1588.
125. Barzilai N, She L, Liu BQ, Vuguin P, Cohen P, Wang JL, Rossetti L. Surgical removal of visceral fat reverses hepatic insulin resistance. *Diabetes* 1999; 48:94–98.
126. Einstein FH, Atzmon G, Yang XM, Ma XH, Rincon M, Rudin E, Muzumdar R, Barzilai N. Differential responses of visceral and subcutaneous fat depots to nutrients. *Diabetes* 2005; 54:672–678.
127. Lebovitz HE, Banerji MA. Point: visceral adiposity is causally related to insulin resistance. *Diabetes Care* 2005; 28:2322–2325.
128. Miles JM, Jensen MD. Counterpoint: Visceral adiposity is not causally related to insulin resistance. *Diabetes Care* 2005; 28:2326–2328.
129. Sidossis LS, Stuart CA, Shulman GI, Lopaschuk GD, Wolfe RR. Glucose plus insulin regulate fat oxidation by controlling the rate of fatty acid entry into the mitochondria. *J Clin Invest* 1996; 98:2244–2250.
130. Wolfe RR. Metabolic interactions between glucose and fatty acids in humans. *Amer J Clin Nutr* 1998; 67:S519–S526.
131. Ruderman N, Prentki M. AMP kinase and malonyl-CoA: Targets for therapy of the metabolic syndrome. *Nat Rev Drug Discov* 2004; 3:340–351.
132. Laybutt DR, Chisholm DJ, Kraegen EW. Specific adaptations in muscle and adipose tissue in response to chronic systemic glucose oversupply in rats. *Am. J Physiol* 1997; 36:E1–E9.
133. Kim JY, Hickner RC, Cortright RL, Dohm GL, Houmard JA. Lipid oxidation is reduced in obese human skeletal muscle. *Am J Physiol Endocrinol Metab* 2000; 279:E1039–1044.
134. Hegarty BD, Furler SM, Oakes ND, Kraegen EW, Cooney GJ. Peroxisome proliferator-activated receptor (PPAR) activation induces tissue-specific effects on fatty acid uptake and metabolism in vivo: A study using the novel PPARalpha/gamma agonist tesaglitazar. *Endocrinology* 2004; 145:3158–3164.
135. Cameron-Smith D, Burke LM, Angus DJ, Tunstall RJ, Cox GR, Bonen A, Hawley JA, Hargreaves M. A short-term, high-fat diet up-regulates lipid metabolism and gene expression in human skeletal muscle. *Am J Clin Nutr* 2003; 77:313–318.
136. Evans K, Clark ML, Frayn KN. Effects of an oral and intravenous fat load on adipose tissue and forearm lipid metabolism. *Am J Physiol* 1999; 276:E241–248.
137. Frayn KN. Non-esterified fatty acid metabolism and postprandial lipaemia. *Atherosclerosis* 1998; 141(suppl 1):S41–416.
138. Furler SM, Wilks DL, Preston E, Frangioudakis G, Cooney GJ, Kraegen EW. A diet high in saturated fat blunts the tissue-specific adaptation of lipoprotein lipase activity to feeding in rats. *Diabetologia* 2005; 48:A237–A237.
139. Kim JK, Kim YJ, Fillmore JJ, Chen Y, Moore I, Lee J, Yuan M, Li ZW, Karin M, Perret P, Shoelson SE, Shulman GI. Prevention of fat-induced insulin resistance by salicylate. *J Clin Invest* 2001; 108:437–446.
140. Yuan M, Konstantopoulos N, Lee J, Hansen L, Li ZW, Karin M, Shoelson SE. Reversal of obesity- and diet-induced insulin resistance with salicylates or targeted disruption of Ikkβ. *Science* 2001; 293:1673–1677.
141. Itani SI, Ruderman NB, Schmieder F, Boden G. Lipid-induced insulin resistance in human muscle is associated with changes in diacylglycerol, protein kinase C and IkB-alpha. *Diabetes* 2002; 51:2005–2011.

142. Hundal RS, Petersen KF, Mayerson AB, Randhawa PS, Inzucchi S, Shoelson SE, Shulman GI. Mechanism by which high-dose aspirin improves glucose metabolism in type 2 diabetes. *J Clin Invest* 2002; 109:1321–1326.

143. Hirosumi J, Tuncman G, Chang L, Gorgun CZ, Uysal KT, Maeda K, Karin M, Hotamisligil GS. A central role for JNK in obesity and insulin resistance. *Nature* 2002; 420:333–336.

144. Hotamisligil GS. Role of endoplasmic reticulum stress and c-Jun NH2-terminal kinase pathways in inflammation and origin of obesity and diabetes. *Diabetes* 2005; 54(suppl 2):S73–78.

145. Kahn BB, Alquier T, Carling D, Hardie DG. AMP-activated protein kinase: ancient energy gauge provides clues to modern understanding of metabolism. *Cell Metab* 2005; 1:15–25.

146. Staels B, Fruchart JC. Therapeutic roles of peroxisome proliferator-activated receptor agonists. *Diabetes* 2005; 54:2460–2470.

147. Lehrke M, Lazar MA. The many faces of PPARgamma. *Cell* 2005; 123:993–999.

148. Lehmann JM, Moore LB, Smitholiver TA, Wilkison WO, Willson TM, Kliewer SA. An antidiabetic thiazolidinedione is a high affinity ligand for peroxisome proliferator-activated receptor gamma (PPAR-gamma). *J Biol Chem* 1995; 270:12953–12956.

149. Oakes ND, Kennedy CJ, Jenkins AB, Laybutt DR, Chisholm DJ, Kraegen EW. A new antidiabetic agent, BRL 49653, reduces lipid availability and improves insulin action and glucoregulation in the rat. *Diabetes* 1994; 43:1203–1210.

150. Oakes ND, Thalen PG, Jacinto SM, Ljung B. Thiazolidinediones increase plasma-adipose tissue FFA exchange capacity and enhance insulin-mediated control of systemic FFA availability. *Diabetes* 2001; 50:1158–1165.

151. Ye JM, Dzamko N, Cleasby ME, Hegarty BD, Furler SM, Cooney GJ, Kraegen EW. Direct demonstration of lipid sequestration as a mechanism by which rosiglitazone prevents fatty-acid-induced insulin resistance in the rat: Comparison with metformin. *Diabetologia* 2004; 47:1306–1313.

152. Schmitz-Peiffer C, Oakes ND, Browne CL, Kraegen EW, Biden TJ. Reversal of chronic alterations of skeletal muscle protein kinase C from fat-fed rats by BRL-49653. *Am J Physiol* 1997; 273: E915–E921.

153. Bahr M, Spelleken M, Bock M, Vonholtey M, Kiehn R, Eckel J. Acute and chronic effects of Troglitazone (CS-045) on isolated rat ventricular cardiomyocytes. *Diabetologia* 1996; 39:766–774.

154. Park KS, Ciaraldi TP, Abramscarter L, Mudaliar S, Nikoulina SE, Henry RR. Troglitazone regulation of glucose metabolism in human skeletal muscle cultures from obese Type II diabetic subjects. *J Clin Endocrinol Metab* 1998; 83:1636–1643.

155. Kintscher U, Law RE. PPARgamma-mediated insulin sensitization: The importance of fat versus muscle. *Am J Physiol 2005;* 288:E287–291.

156. He W, Barak Y, Hevener A, Olson P, Liao D, Le J, Nelson M, Ong E, Olefsky JM, Evans RM. Adipose-specific peroxisome proliferator-activated receptor {gamma} knockout causes insulin resistance in fat and liver but not in muscle. *Proc Natl Acad Sci USA* 2003.

157. Argmann CA, Cock TA, Auwerx J. Peroxisome proliferator-activated receptor gamma: the more the merrier? *Eur J Clin Invest* 2005; 35:82–92; discussion at 80.

158. Guerre-Millo M, Gervois P, Raspe E, Madsen L, Poulain P, Derudas B, Herbert JM, Winegar DA, Willson TM, Fruchart JC, Berge RK, Staels B. Peroxisome proliferator-activated receptor alpha activators improve insulin sensitivity and reduce adiposity. *J Biol Chem* 2000; 275:16638–16642.

159. Murakami K, Tobe K, Ide T, Mochizuki T, Ohashi M, Akanuma Y, Yazaki Y, Kadowaki T. A novel insulin sensitizer acts as a coligand for peroxisome proliferator-activated receptor-alpha (PPAR-alpha) and PPAR-gamma: Effect of PPARalpha activation on abnormal lipid metabolism in liver of Zucker Fatty rats. *Diabetes* 1998; 47:1841–1847.

160. Hegarty BD, Furler SM, Oakes ND, Kraegen EW, Cooney GJ. Peroxisome proliferator-activated receptor (PPAR) activation induces tissue-specific effects on fatty acid uptake and metabolism in vivo: A study using the novel PPARalpha/gamma agonist tesaglitazar. *Endocrinology* 2004; 145:3158–3164.

161. Ye JM, Iglesias MA, Watson DG, Ellis B, Wood L, Jensen PB, Sorensen RV, Larsen PJ, Cooney GJ, Wassermann K, Kraegen EW. PPARalpha/gamma ragaglitazar eliminates fatty liver and enhances insulin action in fat-fed rats in the absence of hepatomegaly. Am J Physiol 2003; 284: E531–540.

162. Smyth S, Heron A. Diabetes and obesity: The twin epidemics. *Nat Med* 2006; 12:75–80.

163. Barish GD, Narkar VA, Evans RM. PPAR delta: A dagger in the heart of the metabolic syndrome. *J Clin Invest* 2006; 116:590–597.

164. Tanaka T, Yamamoto J, Iwasaki S, Asaba H, Hamura H, Ikeda Y, Watanabe M, Magoori K, Ioka RX, Tachibana K, Watanabe Y, Uchiyama Y, Sumi K, Iguchi H, Ito S, Doi T, Hamakubo T, Naito M, Auwerx J, Yanagisawa M, Kodama T, Sakai J. Activation of peroxisome proliferator-activated receptor delta induces fatty acid beta-oxidation in skeletal muscle and attenuates metabolic syndrome. *Proc Natl Acad Sci USA* 2003; 100:15924–15929.

165. Luquet S, Lopez-Soriano J, Holst D, Fredenrich A, Melki J, Rassoulzadegan M, Grimaldi PA. Peroxisome proliferator-activated receptor delta controls muscle development and oxidative capability. *Faseb J* 2003; 17:2299–2301.

166. Holst D, Luquet S, Nogueira V, Kristiansen K, Leverve X, Grimaldi PA. Nutritional regulation and role of peroxisome proliferator-activated receptor delta in fatty acid catabolism in skeletal muscle. *Biochim Biophys Acta* 2003; 1633:43–50.

167. Oliver WR Jr, Shenk JL, Snaith MR, Russell CS, Plunket KD, Bodkin NL, Lewis MC, Winegar DA, Sznaidman ML, Lambert MH, Xu HE, Sternbach DD, Kliewer SA, Hansen BC, Willson TM. A selective peroxisome proliferator-activated receptor delta agonist promotes reverse cholesterol transport. *Proc Natl Acad Sci USA* 2001; 98:5306–5311.

168. Iglesias MA, Ye JM, Frangioudakis G, Saha A, Tomas E, Ruderman NB, Cooney GJ, Kraegen EW. AICAR administration causes an apparent enhancement of muscle and liver insulin action in insulin resistant high-fat fed rats. *Diabetes* 2002; 51:2886–2894.

169. Zhou G, Myers R, Li Y, Chen Y, Shen X, Fenyk-Melody J, Wu M, Ventre J, Doebber T, Fujii N, Musi N, Hirshman MF, Goodyear LJ, Moller DE. Role of AMP-activated protein kinase in mechanism of metformin action. *J Clin Invest* 2001; 108:1167–1174.

170. Musi N, Hirshman MF, Nygren J, Svanfeldt M, Bavenholm P, Rooyackers O, Zhou G, Williamson JM, Ljunqvist O, Efendic S, Moller DE, Thorell A, Goodyear LJ. Metformin increases AMP-activated protein kinase activity in skeletal muscle of subjects with type 2 diabetes. *Diabetes* 2002; 51:2074–2081.

171. Liu Y, Wan Q, Guan Q, Gao L, Zhao J. High-fat diet feeding impairs both the expression and activity of AMPKa in rats' skeletal muscle. *Biochem Biophys Res Commun* 2006; 339:701–707.

172. Collier CA, Bruce CR, Smith AC, Lopaschuk G, Dyck DJ. Metformin counters the insulin-induced suppression of fatty acid oxidation and stimulation of triacylglycerol storage in rodent skeletal muscle. *Am J Physiol* 2006; in press.

173. Shaw RJ, Lamia KA, Vasquez D, Koo SH, Bardeesy N, Depinho RA, Montminy M, Cantley LC. The kinase LKB1 mediates glucose homeostasis in liver and therapeutic effects of metformin. *Science* 2005; 310:1642–1646.

174. Abu-Elheiga L, Matzuk MM, Abo-Hashema KA, Wakil SJ. Continuous fatty acid oxidation and reduced fat storage in mice lacking acetyl-CoA carboxylase 2. *Science* 2001; 291:2613–2616.

175. Harwood HJ Jr, Petras SF, Shelly LD, Zaccaro LM, Perry DA, Makowski MR, Hargrove DM, Martin KA, Tracey WR, Chapman JG, Magee WP, Dalvie DK, Soliman VF, Martin WH, Mularski CJ, Eisenbeis SA. Isozyme-nonselective N-substituted bipiperidylcarboxamide acetyl-CoA carboxylase inhibitors reduce tissue malonyl-CoA concentrations, inhibit fatty acid synthesis, and increase fatty acid oxidation in cultured cells and in experimental animals. *J Biol Chem* 2003; 278:37099–37111.

176. Savage DB, Choi CS, Samuel VT, Liu ZX, Zhang D, Wang A, Zhang XM, Cline GW, Yu XX, Geisler JG, Bhanot S, Monia BP, Shulman GI. Reversal of diet-induced hepatic steatosis and hepatic insulin resistance by antisense oligonucleotide inhibitors of acetyl-CoA carboxylases 1 and 2. *J Clin Invest* 2006; 116(3):817–824.

17 Alterations in Atypical Protein Kinase C Activation in Insulin Resistance Syndromes

Robert V. Farese

CONTENTS

INTRODUCTORY OVERVIEW

The metabolic syndrome with associated obesity is not only a frequent precursor for type 2 diabetes mellitus, but, in its own right, contributes importantly to the development of cardiovascular disease. Hyperlipidemic and hypertensive components of the metabolic syndrome are particularly important pathogenetic factors for development of cardiovascular disease; so is the presence of inflammatory factors in vessel walls. In

From: *Contemporary Endocrinology: The Metabolic Syndrome: Epidemiology, Clinical Treatment, and Underlying Mechanisms*
Edited by: B.C. Hansen and G.A. Bray © Humana Press, Totowa, NJ

type 2 diabetes, these problems are compounded by the development of hyperglycemia, another cardiovascular risk factor.

A common denominator in the metabolic syndrome, obesity, and type 2 diabetes is systemic insulin resistance. Although not all obese subjects are insulin resistant, most, if not all, subjects who have the metabolic syndrome or type 2 diabetes will be found to manifest significant insulin resistance if studied in depth with euglycemic-hyperinsulinemic clamp methods. Moreover, the hyperinsulinemia that results from systemic insulin resistance may cause or contribute importantly to the development of hyperlipidemia, hypertension, inflammation, and other derangements that underlie the cardiovascular disease that is present in these disorders.

Defects in insulin signaling mechanisms are consistently seen in muscles of human and experimental animals that have either type 2 diabetes or obesity. These defects involve the activation of two key signaling factors, atypical protein kinase C (aPKC) and protein kinase B (PKB/Akt). Moreover, similar defects in insulin signaling to these factors are also seen in muscles of rodents consuming a high-fat diet, an experimental surrogate for obesity. Disordered lipid metabolism appears to play a key role in the development of skeletal muscle insulin resistance.

Unlike defects in insulin signaling in muscles of both obese and diabetic animals, defects in insulin signaling in the liver are consistently observed in diabetic animals, but not in high-fat-fed or obese animals. Sparing of hepatic insulin signaling mechanisms is undoubtedly important for maintaining relatively normal glucose metabolism in simple obesity.

Insulin signaling defects in diabetic liver differ from those seen in diabetic muscle. Most notably, whereas aPKC activation is uniformly impaired in diabetic muscle, it is consistently conserved in diabetic liver; this is particularly important, as aPKC contributes importantly to insulin-induced increases in sterol response element binding protein-1c (SREBP-1c), which controls the expression of an array of enzymes engaged in lipid synthesis. Conserved aPKC activation in liver most likely contributes to insulin-dependent increases in hepatic lipid synthesis and production of lipids that lead to hepatosteatosis, hypertriglyceridemia, and reciprocal decreases in HDL-lipoproteins. The pro-inflammatory factor NFkB also functions downstream of aPKC.

In contrast to conserved aPKC activation, PKB activation is consistently impaired in diabetic liver; this is important, as PKB regulates hepatic glucose output. Thus, in type 2 diabetes, there are two major insulin signaling problems in the liver that contribute to the development of cardiovascular disease: (1) impaired PKB and subsequent hyperglycemia; and (2) conserved aPKC and resultant hyperlipidemia, and possibly activation of inflammatory factors that are dependent on NFkB increases. This bifurcation of insulin signaling and differential activation of aPKC and PKB in liver provides a reasonable explanation for a heretofore poorly understood paradox: Hepatic outputs of both glucose and lipid are increased in an "insulin-resistant" diabetic liver.

GENERAL ASPECTS OF INSULIN SIGNALING

During the past decade, it has become increasingly clear that metabolic effects of insulin on glucose and lipid metabolism are mediated through downstream effectors of phosphatidylinositol (PI) 3-kinase (3K), namely aPKC and PKB (Fig. 17.1). PI3K is activated by insulin receptor substrates (IRSs), chiefly IRS-1 and/or IRS-2, which are

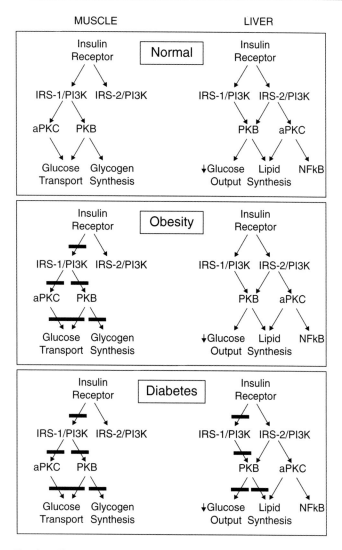

Figure 17.1. Insulin signaling in muscle (left) and liver (right) in normal conditions (top), simple obesity (middle), and overt diabetes (bottom).

In skeletal muscle, IRS-1, via PI3K, controls aPKC and PKB activation. Insulin signaling to IRS-1, PI3K, aPKC, and PKB is impaired in simple obesity and diabetes. In addition, the activation of aPKC by PIP_3 is impaired in simple obesity and diabetes.

In liver, IRS-2, via PI3K, controls aPKC activation. In contrast, both IRS-1 and IRS-2, via PI3K, control PKB activation. The expression of sterol regulatory element binding protein 1-c (SREBP-1c), which transactivates many genes active in fat synthesis, including fatty acid synthase (FAS), is controlled by aPKC and PKB. Increases in lipid synthesis lead to increases in secretion of VLDL-triglycerides. PKB, and possibly other undefined factors, but not aPKC, increase glycogen synthesis and diminish glucose production and release. In simple obesity, insulin signaling is grossly intact in the liver. With the onset of diabetes, IRS-1 signaling to PI3K and PKB is diminished, but IRS-2 signaling to PI3K and aPKC is better or fully conserved. Thus, in hyperinsulinemic states of simple obesity and type 2 diabetes, increased IRS-2 signaling to aPKC leads to increases in SREBP-1c expression, lipid synthesis, and VLDL-triglyceride secretion. In diabetes, diminishing signaling to IRS-1 and PKB leads to increases in hepatic glucose output.

phosphorylated on tyrosine residues by the insulin receptor. In turn, PI3K increases the conversion of PI-4.5-$(PO_4)_2$ (PIP_2) to PI-3, 4, 5-$(PO_4)_3$ (PIP_3), which, in conjunction with 3-phosphoinositide-dependent protein kinase-1 (PDK1), partially activates aPKC and PKB by phosphorylating specific threonine residues in the aPKC and PKB "activation loop." PKB is further activated by phosphorylation of serine residues by PDK2. On the other hand, aPKC is further activated by PIP_3-induced increases in autophosphorylation of specific threonine residues, and conformational changes involving molecular unfolding and exposure of the substrate binding site in the catalytic domain, which is otherwise restrained by a pseudosubstrate sequence in the regulatory domain (1). Interestingly, in human vastus lateralis muscle, the phosphorylation of the activation loop site by PDK1 appears to be largely constitutive, and subsequent activating effects of PIP_3 appear to be more important.

Both aPKC (2–6) and PKB (7–10) are important for increasing glucose transport through insulin-sensitive glucose transporters, namely GLUT4, and to a lesser extent GLUT1, in muscle and adipose tissue. However, the liver readily takes up glucose through the GLUT2 glucose transporter, which is not regulated by insulin. In compelling support of a role for aPKC in glucose transport, we have recently found (unpublished observations) that knockdown of aPKC in cultured 3T3/L1 adipocytes and L6 myotubes by silence/interfering RNA, or muscle-specific knockout of aPKC by gene targeting methods in mice, blocks insulin-stimulated glucose transport.

Although glucose transport is rate-limiting for glucose utilization in muscle and adipose tissue, and although skeletal muscle is a major organ for glucose disposal during glucose loading (e.g., following carbohydrate-rich meals), the liver, particularly in the fasting state, is the major determinant for blood glucose levels. Indeed, abolition of insulin-stimulated glucose transport by specific depletion of muscle aPKC does not cause fasting hyperglycemia in the absence of a defect in insulin secretion.

PKB, rather than aPKC, appears to be particularly important for stimulating glycogen synthesis and promoting glucose utilization and storage in liver, muscle, and adipose tissue (11), and diminishing gluconeogenesis (12) and glucose release (13) by the liver. Nevertheless, aPKC, as well as PKB, is required for glucose transport effects of insulin, and, indeed, at least some defects in glucose disposal (e.g., as observed at higher insulin concentrations in clamp studies (see below) in obese and diabetic subjects) appear to be better explained by a defect in aPKC, rather than PKB, activation in muscle.

In contrast to hepatic glucose regulation, insulin effects on lipid synthesis in liver have been postulated to be controlled largely through activation of aPKC, which increases the expression of SREBP-1c (14), which regulates the expression of genes that promote lipid synthesis. Whether PKB participates in the activation of SREBP-1c is debated (14,15). However, in diabetic liver, wherein PKB activation is markedly diminished and aPKC activation is conserved, aPKC activation may be the major mechanism for insulin-dependent increases in hepatic lipid synthesis.

TISSUE-SPECIFIC DIFFERENCES IN UPSTREAM ACTIVATORS OF aPKC AND PKB

Although aPKC and PKB operate downstream of IRS and PI3K, there are considerable differences in upstream factors controlling aPKC and PKB activation in various tissues (Fig. 17.1). In muscle, both aPKC and PKB operate largely downstream of IRS-

1-dependent PI3K, as judged by findings in IRS-1 knockout mice (16). However, this dual activation does not necessarily mean that levels of activated aPKC and PKB in muscle fluctuate in parallel in different physiological and pathophysiological states. Indeed, PKB activation is maximally activated at lower insulin concentrations and lower levels of IRS-1-dependent PI3K activation than those required for full aPKC activation (submitted for publication), and pathological factors can alter aPKC responsiveness without altering PKB responsiveness.

In contrast to muscle, in livers of IRS-1 knockout mice, whereas insulin activation of PKB is markedly diminished, insulin activation of aPKC is intact. (16). On the other hand, the activation of aPKC, as well as PKB, is diminished in IRS-2-deficient mouse hepatocytes (17). It may therefore be surmised that, in mouse liver, aPKC activation is largely dependent on IRS-2 rather than IRS-1, and PKB activation is dependent on both IRS-2 and IRS-1.

Different from muscle and liver, in white (16) and brown (18) mouse adipocytes, aPKC activation is dependent on both IRS-1 and IRS-2, whereas PKB activation is not inhibited by loss of either IRS-2 or IRS-1. Thus, in mouse adipocytes, it appears that aPKC activation is dependent on both IRS-2 and IRS-1, whereas requirements for PKB activation can be satisfied by activation of either IRS-1 or IRS-2, possibly along with other factors (e.g., IRS-3) that are capable of activating PI3K. Interestingly, insulin-stimulated glucose transport follows the same pattern as aPKC activation in white and brown adipocytes deficient in IRS-1 or IRS-2 (18,19).

In white and brown adipocytes, insulin-induced activation and plasma membrane localization of aPKC within specific lipid raft microdomains is dependent, not only on IRS-1 and IRS-2, but also on Cbl (20) and Cbl-dependent PI3K (21). Cbl is also required for activation of Crk, C3G, and TC10, independently of PI3K (20). Thus, Cbl appears to coordinate PI3K-dependent and PI3K-independent pathways that are needed for insulin-stimulated glucose transport in adipocytes. However, it is uncertain whether Cbl and Cbl-dependent (or analagous) factors are operative in skeletal muscle (21).

INSULIN SIGNALING DEFECTS IN MUSCLE AND ADIPOSE TISSUE IN TYPE 2 DIABETES

The insulin activation of aPKC is consistently defective in muscles of nonobese type 2 Goto-Kakizaki (GK) diabetic rats (22), ob/ob obese diabetic mice (see ref. 30), and obese type 2 diabetic monkeys (23) and humans (24–26). Defective aPKC activation has also been observed in adipocytes of type 2 diabetic GK rats (27) and ob/ob diabetic mice (unpublished).

Defects in muscle aPKC activation in diabetic states are at least partly due to impaired activation of IRS-1-dependent PI3K. In addition, there is poor responsiveness of aPKC to the PI3K lipid product, PIP_3 (23,25), and this may be as important, or, in some cases, more important, than changes in IRS-1-dependent PI3K activity. (See Fig. 17.1.)

Different from aPKC, the phosphorylation and enzymatic activation of muscle PKB has been found to be intact in some glucose-insulin clamp studies of diabetic human subjects and animals (22–28). Given the presence of concomitant defects in IRS-1-dependent PI3K activation, the seemingly normal activation of PKB in diabetic muscle has been an enigma. Moreover, in other clamp studies, PKB activation has been found to be defective in diabetic muscle (29). Fortunately, recent information (accepted for publication in *Diabetologia*) obtained from euglycemic-hyperinsulinemic clamps, performed at both maximal and half-maximal insulin concentrations, seems to have resolved the issue of a dichotomy between aPKC and PKB activation in diabetic muscle. Thus, in normal human muscle, PKB activation is near maximal when insulin-stimulated glucose disposal is only half-maximal, at a plasma insulin level of approximately 100 μU/ml insulin; on the other hand, aPKC activation and glucose disposal run parallel courses and approach maximal at plasma insulin levels at approximately 400 μU/ml. Further, in diabetic subjects, PKB activation is impaired at the lower submaximal, but not at the higher maximal, insulin level. In contrast, aPKC activation is impaired at both lower and higher insulin concentrations.

In interpreting the above-described data, it should be recalled that there are *spare receptors* that mediate insulin responses; that is, in normal conditions, maximal downstream responses are elicited when only a relatively small fraction of insulin receptors are occupied. Accordingly, a defect in receptor activation, as known to occur in type 2 diabetic muscle, can be abrogated at higher insulin levels, thus restoring distal responses that are otherwise intact; this scenario seems to fit the pattern of PKB activation in diabetic muscle. However, if post-receptor signaling factors are themselves compromised, a defect would be apparent at all levels of insulin receptor occupancy; this scenario seems to fit the pattern of aPKC activation in diabetic muscle. These findings further imply that the defect in PKB activation in diabetic muscle is due to a defect in upstream signaling factors and may therefore be considered to be *receptor* in type, whereas the defect in aPKC activation is *post-receptor* in type, and probably reflects an alteration in aPKC itself. In keeping with the latter idea, note that there are both diminished levels and impaired responsiveness to PIP_3 in muscles of diabetic subjects (25).

INSULIN SIGNALING DEFECTS IN MUSCLE IN OBESITY

Defective activation of aPKC has been observed (Fig. 17.1), not only in muscles of type 2 diabetic rats, monkeys, and humans, but also in muscles of obese diabetic ob/ob mice (30), obese diabetic db/db mice (31), obese pre-diabetic monkeys (23), obese glucose-intolerant humans (24,25), and obese glucose-tolerant humans (26,32), including those who have polycystic ovary syndrome, which is most likely an advanced manifestation of the metabolic syndrome in females. Of course, in ob/ob and db/db mice, it is not clear if it is the diabetes or the obesity that is responsible for defective aPKC activation. However, in obese glucose-tolerant women (26,32), defective aPKC activation is seen even in the absence of clinically recognizable abnormalities in glucose metabolism, and, in obese glucose-tolerant women with polycystic ovary disease (32), the defect in aPKC activation is comparable in magnitude to that seen in overt type 2 diabetes (25,26). Thus, although hyperglycemia can impair aPKC activation (22), defects in muscle aPKC activation in obesity do not appear to be due to alterations in glucose metabolism.

Along with defects in aPKC activation, defects in muscle IRS-1-dependent PI3K and PKB activation have been found in some studies of obese subjects; on the other hand, statistically significant defects in IRS-1-dependent PI3K and PKB activation are not always seen, for example, in euglycemic-hyperinsulinemic clamp studies of obese glucose-intolerant (25) and obese glucose-tolerant (26,32) humans, conducted and evaluated at maximal insulin levels, wherein only post-receptor type (see above) insulin defects would be apparent. Whether or not receptor-type defects in IRS-1-dependent PI3K and PKB activation would have been evident at lower insulin concentrations (i.e., at partial insulin receptor occupancy) in these clamp studies of obese subjects needs to be reevaluated.

DEFECTIVE ACTIVATION OF aPKC IN MUSCLE BY PIP$_3$ IN INSULIN-RESISTANT STATES

The failure to observe significant defects in IRS-1-dependent PI3K activation in some situations, and the knowledge that the lipid product of PI3K, that is, PIP$_3$, directly activates aPKCs by three distinct mechanisms (1), of which only one involves PDK1 (the activation of which is not impaired in diabetic muscle; see 23,25), prompted us to examine the direct activation of aPKC by PIP$_3$ in aPKCs obtained (by specific immunoprecipitation) from muscles of insulin-resistant animals and humans. Indeed, marked defects in PIP$_3$-dependent activation of aPKCs were found in muscles of obese glucose-intolerant (25) and glucose-tolerant (32) humans, obese pre-diabetic monkeys (23), and type 2 diabetic monkeys (23) and humans (25), regardless of whether IRS-1-dependent PI3K activation was measurably impaired. Thus, it may be surmised that defects in muscle aPKC activation in type 2 diabetes and obesity may be due to either impaired activation of IRS-1-dependent PI3K, or poor responsiveness of aPKCs to PIP$_3$, or both.

Interestingly, defective activation of aPKC by PIP$_3$ has also been found in cultured myocytes and adipocytes of obese humans (33). In addition to defects in aPKC activation, there are defects in insulin-stimulated glucose transport in these cultured myocytes and adipocytes (24,33). It is intriguing that these defects in aPKC activation and insulin-stimulated glucose transport persist in cultured cells that have been passaged several times; accordingly, this could be interpreted to suggest an intrinsic defect. On the other hand, there is considerable information indicating that defects in aPKC responsiveness in most states of obesity and type 2 diabetes are acquired and, fortunately, reversible with therapy.

INSULIN SIGNALING IN MUSCLES OF HIGH-FAT-FED RODENTS

High-fat feeding rapidly induces an insulin-resistant state in rodents that seems to be analogous to diet-dependent obesity. In studies of rodents placed on a western-type moderately high-fat diet (40% of calories), aPKC activation by insulin is defective in muscles of both rats (34) and mice (30,35). In high-fat-fed mice, the defect in aPKC activation is due to both impaired activation of IRS-1-dependent PI3K and diminished aPKC responsiveness to PIP$_3$, and PKB activation is similarly impaired (30,35). In high-fat-fed rats, however, there is no appreciable change in IRS-1-dependent PI3K, IRS-2-dependent PI3K, or PKB activation, and the defect in muscle aPKC activation appears to be due solely to poor aPKC responsiveness to PIP$_3$ (34).

INSULIN SIGNALING IN LIVERS OF DIABETIC RODENTS

In livers of type 2 diabetic GK rats (Fig. 17.1), the activation of IRS-1-dependent PI3K and PKB by insulin is markedly impaired, but, in contrast, the activation of IRS-2-dependent PI3K and aPKC is intact (30 and unpublished observations). This pattern of diminished PKB activation and normal aPKC activation in livers of GK-diabetic rats is virtually the same as that observed in livers of IRS-1 knockout mice (16), and is also seen in livers of ob/ob obese diabetic mice (30). Presumably, compromise of IRS-1 function and maintenance of full or partial, but sufficient, IRS-2 function accounts for the selective loss of PKB and the conservation of aPKC activation in diabetic liver.

INSULIN SIGNALING IN LIVERS OF HIGH-FAT-FED RODENTS AND OBESE MONKEYS

In contrast to the defects seen in diabetic rodents, the activation of both IRS-1-dependent PI3K and IRS-2-dependent PI3K (unpublished observations), as well as both PKB and aPKC (30), is normal in livers of high-fat-fed mice. This does not imply that glucose handling by the liver is normal in high-fat-fed mice, but rather suggests that any such defects are probably more reflective of lipid- or other metabolite-dependent alterations in gluconeogenesis, or glucose storage or release, rather than altered insulin signaling.

As in high-fat-fed rodents, insulin signaling to IRS-1-dependent PI3K, IRS-2-dependent PI3K, aPKC, and PKB in obese insulin-resistant pre-diabetic monkeys is comparable to that seen in lean control monkeys (unpublished observations). Thus, the findings on insulin signaling in both liver and muscle of spontaneously obese monkeys are remarkably similar to findings in high-fat-fed mice.

From the above findings, it appears that insulin signaling in the liver to both aPKC and PKB is conserved in insulin-resistant conditions prior to the development of overt diabetes (i.e., in obesity and the metabolic syndrome). However, further studies in other models of nondiabetic obesity are needed to confirm this postulate.

METABOLIC CONSEQUENCES OF DIVERGENT ALTERATIONS OF INSULIN SIGNALING IN MUSCLE AND LIVER IN OBESITY AND DIABETES

Collectively, the above-described findings suggest that defects in aPKC activation, with or without associated defects in PKB activation, play a key role in the development of skeletal muscle insulin resistance. Moreover, it is worth reemphasizing that poor aPKC activation by IRS-1-dependent PI3K and/or PIP_3 in skeletal muscle is consistently observed in insulin-resistant states, both in early and later phases, and that gross insulin signaling defects in the liver to PKB are readily apparent in diabetic, but probably not in pre-diabetic, states of insulin resistance.

It is particularly interesting that aPKC activation in the liver is conserved in all forms of obesity and diabetes in animals that have been thus far studied. This is particularly important, as aPKCs can mediate insulin-induced increases in expression of hepatic SREBP-1c (14). Thus, conserved aPKC activation in liver provides an explanation for the maintenance of hepatic lipid synthesis, particularly in hyperinsulinemic conditions of obesity and type 2 diabetes. Indeed, increased expression/activation of SREBP-1c has been observed in insulin-resistant hyperinsulinemic lipodystrophic and ob/ob-diabetic mice (36), and we have observed increases in hepatic aPKC activation and SREBP-1c expression/activation in type 2 diabetic hyperinsulinemic GK rats, high-fat-fed mice, and ob/ob mice (unpublished observations). Moreover, dependency of increases in SREBP-1c on aPKC has been documented by liver-specific knockout or inhibition of hepatic aPKC by adenoviral-mediated expression of kinase-inactive aPKC (unpublished observations). Thus, conserved aPKC activation in liver seems to account for increased lipid synthesis and secretion of very-low-density lipoproteins in insulin-resistant hyperinsulinemic states, regardless of whether hepatic PKB activation is impaired.

CROSSTALK BETWEEN LIVER AND MUSCLE

It should be emphasized that the finding that insulin signaling in the liver is grossly normal in obesity and becomes defective only later when diabetes develops should not be construed to mean that the liver is involved only in later, but not in earlier, stages of insulin resistance. To the contrary, there is now considerable reason to believe that alterations in hepatic lipid synthesis contribute most importantly to the development of defects in insulin signaling in skeletal muscle. Indeed, alterations in liver lipid metabolism may in fact be responsible for impaired aPKC activation in muscle. If this proves true, it should also be realized that a defect in insulin signaling in muscle would limit glucose disposal and thereby increase plasma insulin, which in turn would activate IRS-2-dependent PI3K, aPKC, and SREBP-1c in the liver, thus compounding the problem of excessive hepatic lipid synthesis. This would create a vicious cycle in which lipid synthesis in liver begets insulin resistance in muscle, and vice versa.

In keeping with the idea that the lipid synthesis in the liver adversely affects insulin signaling in muscle, we have found that aPKC activation in muscle by both insulin in vivo and PIP_3 in vitro is impaired in situations in which hepatic lipid synthesis is increased, and conversely, paradoxically enhanced by inhibition of aPKC, SREBP-1c, and lipid synthesis in the liver. Oddly enough, in these situations, despite changes in muscle aPKC activation, aPKC activation in the liver is unchanged. Thus, there appears to be a means of communication whereby aPKC activation (by insulin or other experimental means) and subsequent increases in lipid synthesis in liver adversely alter aPKC activation in muscle, but not vice versa. In addition to increasing SREBP-1c expression, aPKC activation in the liver may increase the activity of NFkB, which is pro-inflammatory and has been linked to insulin resistance as well as cardiovascular disease. Whether this communication whereby events in liver downregulate insulin functions in muscle are mediated by lipids, NFkB-dependent cytokines, or other factors remains to be determined.

TREATMENT OF INSULIN SIGNALING DEFECTS

Exercise

Like insulin, exercise acutely activates aPKC activity and stimulates glucose transport in skeletal muscle (37). Unlike insulin, exercise-induced increases in aPKC activity and glucose transport are not mediated by PI3K. We suspect that aPKC is required for exercise-induced increases in glucose transport, but further studies are needed to answer this question.

The mechanism whereby exercise activates muscle aPKC activity is uncertain. One possibility is that exercise activates phospholipase D (PLD) and increases the production of phosphatidic acid (PA), which, like PIP_3, can activate aPKC. The mechanism for exercise-induced activation of PLD is unknown, but factors that activate 5′-AMP kinase-activated protein kinase (AMPK; a sensor of 5′-AMP, which indirectly reflects ATP and thus cellular energy levels), which is also activated by exercise, apparently increase PLD activity by mechanisms requiring the activation of proline-rich tyrosine kinase-2 (PYK2) and extracellular signal-regulated kinase (ERK) (37). However, exercise does not activate PYK2, and ERK does not appear to be required for exercise effects on glucose transport. Moreover, the extent to which exercise uses AMPK to activate PLD, aPKC, and glucose transport is controversial; indeed, AMPK may not be required for exercise effects on glucose transport (38), and its activation may be a redundant mechanism for activating glucose transport during exercise.

Exercise provokes increases in both GLUT4 translocation/glucose transport (39) and aPKC (25) activity in muscles of type 2 diabetic subjects that are greater than those of insulin, but less than the maximal increases seen in normal subjects. If in fact aPKC is required for exercise-induced glucose transport, it would be expected that exercise should be able to bypass diabetes-related defects in IRS-1-dependent PI3K to activate aPKC and glucose transport. Nevertheless, defects that limit aPKC responsiveness to PIP_3 would most likely also limit responses to phosphatidic acid or other factors, and thereby limit exercise effects on glucose transport.

Caloric Restriction

Whereas ad-lib feeding leads to obesity and diabetes in monkeys, this outcome can be avoided by caloric restriction and maintenance of an ideal body weight (23). It was therefore of great interest to find that caloric restriction also prevents or greatly diminishes the development of defects in insulin-stimulated aPKC activation in monkey muscle (23). Of further interest, in obese humans, caloric restriction and moderate weight loss improves insulin-stimulated muscle aPKC activity (28). These and other findings suggest that defects in aPKC activation are largely acquired. However, we cannot rule out the possibility that there is an initial genetic partial defect in aPKC activity that may be intensified by obesity.

Thiazolidinediones

The TZD, rosiglitazone, improves diabetes-dependent defects in aPKC activation in rat adipocytes (27), rat muscle (22), human muscle (25) and monkey muscle (unpublished observations). Increases in insulin-stimulated aPKC activity in rat adipocytes (27), rat muscle (22) and monkey muscle are not accompanied by changes in IRS-1-dependent PI3K activation, and, in these cases, other mechanisms appear to be more important; for example, in monkey muscle, rosiglitazone improves aPKC activation by increasing responsiveness to PIP_3 (unpublished observations). On the other hand, in human muscle, rosiglitazone (25) and troglitazone (40) increase IRS-1-dependent PI3K activation. Thus, there are at least two mechanisms whereby TZDs improve muscle aPKC activation.

The mechanism(s) responsible for TZD-induced increases in aPKC activation by insulin is (are) uncertain. However, administration of exogenous adiponectin (AGRP30), an adipocyte-derived circulating protein, increases muscle aPKC responsiveness to PIP_3 (unpublished observations), and both rosiglitazone and adiponectin activate AMPK, which diminishes lipid availability in liver and muscle, and may thereby improve aPKC activity/responsiveness.

Metformin

Metformin, which is well recognized to improve hepatic glucose output in diabetic subjects, also increases insulin-stimulated peripheral glucose disposal, presumably in muscle. Recent findings indicate that metformin activates AMPK in both muscle and liver (41) via LKB1 (42). This is interesting, as AMPK increases aPKC activity and glucose transport (see above). AMPK also diminishes hepatic SREBP-1c expression and lipid synthesis, and stimulates fatty acid β-oxidation. These salutary effects on hepatic and muscle lipid metabolism may in turn improve aPKC activity in diabetic muscle. Indeed, we have found that metformin activates AMPK, PYK2, ERK, and aPKC cultured L6 myotubes, and each of these factors is required for stimulatory effects of metformin on GLUT4 translocation and glucose transport (submitted for publication). Moreover, metformin treatment of type 2 diabetic humans provokes increases in basal and insulin-stimulated aPKC activity in muscle (virtually to normal), largely by increasing aPKC responsiveness to PIP_3, without altering IRS-1-dependent PI3K activation (43).

CONCLUSION

To summarize, muscle aPKC activation by insulin is impaired in all examined insulin-resistant states in rodents, monkeys, and humans. Thus, defective aPKC activation in muscle appears to be an important proximate mechanism for systemic insulin resistance in obesity, the metabolic syndrome, and type 2 diabetes. This defect in muscle aPKC activation in obesity and diabetes is due to both diminished activation of IRS-1/PI3K and poor aPKC responsiveness to the PI3K lipid product, PIP_3. Most likely, defects in muscle aPKC activation in human forms of obesity and type 2 diabetes are acquired, as they can be largely prevented or diminished by caloric restriction and weight control, exercise, or treatment with TZD or metformin. On the other hand, insulin signaling defects to aPKC are maintained in cultured adipocytes and myocytes of obese or diabetic humans, and the reason for this "memory" needs to be elucidated.

Presently, we have no information on insulin signaling in livers of obese or diabetic humans. If, however, insulin signaling defects in human liver are similar to those seen in livers of obese and diabetic rodents and monkeys, it may be surmised that: (1) IRS-1 and PKB activation are compromised in liver and contribute to hyperglycemia in diabetic humans; but, on the other hand, (2) aPKC activation is conserved or increased in response to hyperinsulinemia, thereby contributing to hyperlipidemia in obese and diabetic humans. Accordingly, therapeutic efforts in obesity, the metabolic syndrome, and type 2 diabetes should focus on: (1) improving aPKC and PKB activation in muscle; (2) inhibiting aPKC and aPKC-dependent processes (e.g., SREBP-1c expression and NFkB activation in liver); and (3) improving PKB activation in liver. In addition to treating the hyperglycemia of diabetes, more aggressive treatment of insulin resistance is needed to effectively diminish the prevalence of cardiovascular disease.

REFERENCES

1. Standaert ML, Bandyopadhyay G, Kanoh Y, Sajan MP, Farese RV. Insulin and PIP_3 activate PKC-ζ by mechanisms that are both dependent and independent of phosphorylation of activation loop (T410) and autophosphorylation (T560) sites. *Biochemistry* 2001; 40:249–255.

2. Bandyopadhyay G, Standaert ML, Zhao L, Yu B, Avignon A, Galloway L, Karnam P, Moscat J, Farese RV. Activation of protein kinase C (α, β and ζ) by insulin in 3T3/L1 cells: Transfection studies suggest a role for PKC-ζ in glucose transport. *J Biol Chem* 1997; 272:2551–2558.

3. Bandyopadhyay G, Standaert ML, Galloway L, Moscat J, Farese RV. Evidence for involvement of protein kinase C (PKC)-ζ and noninvolvement of diacylglycerol-sensitive PKCs in insulin-stimulated glucose transport in L6 myotubes. *Endocrinology* 1997; 138:4721–4731.

4. Standaert ML, Galloway L, Karnam P, Bandyopadhyay G, Moscat J, Farese RV. Protein kinase C-ζ as a downstream effector of phosphatidylinositol 3-kinase during insulin stimulation in rat adipocytes: Potential role in glucose transport. *J Biol Chem* 1997; 272:30075–30082.

5. Kotani K, Ogawa W, Matsumoto M, Kitamura T, Sakaue H, Hino Y, Miyake K, Sano W, Akimoto K, Ohno S, Kasuga M. Requirement of atypical protein kinase Cλ for insulin stimulation on glucose uptake but not for Akt activation in 3T3/L1 adipocytes. *Mol Cell Biol* 1998; 18:6971–6982.

6. Bandyopadhyay G, Kanoh Y, Sajan MP, Standaert ML, Farese RV. Effects of adenoviral gene transfer of wild-type, constitutively active, and kinase-defective protein kinase C-λ on insulin-stimulated glucose transport in L6 myotubes. *Endocrinology* 2000; 141:4120–4127.

7. Kohn AD, Summers SA, Birnbaum MJ, Roth RA. Expression of a constitutively active Akt Ser/Thr kinase in 3T3/L1 adipocytes stimulates glucose uptake and glucose transporter 4 translocation. *J Biol Chem* 1996; 271:31372–31378.

8. Tanti J, Grillo S, Gremeaux T, Coffer PJ, Van Obberghen E, Le Marchand-Brustel Y. Potential role of protein kinase B in glucose transporter 4 translocation in adipocytes. *Endocrinology* 1997; 138:2005–2009.

9. Wang Q, Somwar R, Bilan PJ, Liu Z, Jin J, Woodgett JR, Klip A. Protein kinase B/Akt participates in GLUT4 translocation in L6 myoblasts. *Mol Cell Biol* 1999; 19:4008–4018.

10. Hill MM, Clark SF, Tucker DF, Birnbaum MJ, James DE, Macaulay SL. A role for protein kinase Bβ/Akt2 in GLUT4 translocation in adipocytes. *Mol Cell Biol* 1999; 19:7771–7781.

11. Peak M, Rochford JJ, Borthwick AC, Yeaman SJ, Agius L. Signalling pathways involved in the stimulation of glycogen synthesis by insulin in rat hepatocytes. *Diabetologia* 1998; 41:16–25.

12. Daitoku H, Yamagata K, Matsuzaki H, Hatta M, Fukamizu A. Regulation of PGC-1 promotor activity by protein kinase B and the forkhead transcription factor FKHR. *Diabetes* 2003; 52:642–649.

13. Schmoll D, Walker KS, Alessi DR, Grempler R, Burchell A, Guo S, Walther R, Unterman TG. Regulation of glucose-6-phosphatase gene expression by protein kinase B-alpha and the forkhead transcription factor FKHR: Evidence for insulin response unit-dependent and -independent effects of insulin on promotor activity. *J Biol Chem* 2000; 275:36324–36333.

14. Matsumoto M, Ogawa W, Akimoto K, Inoue H, Miyaki K, Furukawa K, Hayashi Y, Iguchi H, Matsuki Y, Hiramatsu R, Shimano H, Yamada N, Ohno S, Kasuga M, Noda T. PKCλ in liver mediates insulin-induced SREBP-1c expression and determines both hepatic lipid content and overall insulin sensitivity. *J Clin Invest* 2003; 100:3164–3172.

15. Fleischmann M, Lynedjian PB. Regulation of sterol regulatory-element binding protein expression in liver: Role of insulin and protein kinase B/Akt. *Biochem J* 2000; 349:13–17.

16. Sajan MP, Standaert ML, Miura A, Kahn RC, Farese RV. Tissue-specific differences in activation of atypical protein kinase C and protein kinase B in muscle, liver and adipocytes of insulin receptor substrate-1 knockout mice. *Molecular Endocrinology* 2004; 18:2513–2521.

17. Valverde AM, Burks DJ, Fabregat I, Fisher TL, Carretero J, White MF, Benito M. Molecular mechanisms of insulin resistance in IRS-2-deficient hepatocytes. *Diabetes* 2003; 52:2239–2248.

18. Miura A, Sajan MP, Standaert ML, Bandyopadhyay G, Kahn CR, Farese RV. Insulin substrates 1 and 2 are required for activation of atypical protein kinase C and Cbl-dependent Phosphatidylinositol 3-kinase during insulin action I immortalized brown adipocytes. *Biochemistry* 2004; 43:15503–15509.

19. Arribas M, Valverde AM, Burks D, Klein J, Farese RV, White MF, Benito M. Essential role of protein kinase C-zeta in the impairment of insulin-induced glucose transport in IRS-2-deficient brown adipocytes. *FEBS Lett* 2003; 536:161–166.

20. Saltiel AR, Pessin JE. Insulin signaling in microdomains of the plasma membrane. *Traffic* 2003; 4:711–716.

21. Chang L, Chiang SH, Saltiel AR. Insulin signaling and the regulation of glucose transport. *Mol Med* 2005 Nov 23 (epub ahead of print).

22. Kanoh Y, Bandyopadhyay G, Sajan MP, Standaert ML, Farese RV. Rosiglitazone, insulin treatment and fasting correct defective activation of protein kinase C-ζ by insulin in vastus lateralis muscles and adipocytes of diabetic rats. *Endocrinology* 2001; 142:1595–1605.

23. Standaert ML, Ortmeyer HK, Hansen BC, Sajan MP, Kanoh Y, Bandyopadhyay G, Farese RV. Skeletal muscle insulin resistance in obesity-associated type 2 diabetes mellitus in monkeys is linked to a defect in insulin activation of protein kinase C-ζ/λ/ι. *Diabetes* 2002; 51:2936–2943.

24. Vollenweider P, Menard B, Nicod P. Insulin resistance, defective IRS-2-associated phosphatidylinositol-3' kinase activation, and impaired atypical protein kinase C (ζ/λ) activation in myotubes from obese patients with impaired glucose tolerance. *Diabetes* 2002; 51:1052–1059.

25. Beeson M, Sajan MP, Dizon M, Kanoh Y, Bandyopadhyay G, Standaert ML, Farese RV. Activation of protein kinase C-ζ by insulin and PI-3,4,5-(PO$_4$)$_3$ is defective in muscle in type 2 diabetes and impaired glucose tolerance. Amelioration by rosiglitazone and exercise *Diabetes* 2003; 52:1926–1934.

26. Kim Y-B, Nikoulina SE, Ciaraldi TP, Henry RR, Kahn BB. Normal insulin-dependent activation of Akt/protein kinase B, with diminished activation of phosphoinositide 3-kinase in muscle in type 2 diabetes. *J Clin Invest* 1999; 104:733–741.

27. Kanoh Y, Bandyopadhyay G, Sajan MP, Standaert ML, Farese RV. Thiazolidinedione treatment enhances insulin effects on protein kinase C-ζ/λ activation and glucose transport in adipocytes of nondiabetic and Goto-Kakizaki type II diabetic rats. *J Biol Chem* 2000; 275:16690–16696.

28. Kim YB, Kotani K, Ciaraldi TP, Henry RR, Kahn BB. Insulin-stimulated PKC C-λ/ζ activity is reduced in skeletal muscle of humans with obesity and type 2 diabetes. *Diabetes* 2003; 52:1935–1942.

29. Karlsson HKR, Zierath JR, Kane S, Krook A, Lienhard GE, Wallberg-Henriksson H. Insulin-stimulated phosphorylation of the Akt substrate AS160 is impaired in skeletal muscle of type 2 diabetic subjects. *Diabetes* 2005; 54:1692–1697.

30. Standaert ML, Sajan MP, Miura A, Kanoh Y, Chen HC, Farese RV Jr, Farese RV. Insulin-induced activation of atypical protein kinase C, but not protein kinase B, is maintained in diabetic (*ob/ob* and Goto-Kakizaki) liver. *J Biol Chem* 2004; 279:24929–24934.

31. Hori H, Sasaoka T, Ishihara H, Wadu T, Murakami S, Ishiki M, Kobayashi M. Association of SH2-containing inositol phosphatase 2 with the insulin resistance of *db/db* mice. *Diabetes* 2002; 51:2387–2394.

32. Beeson M, Sajan MP, Gomez-Daspet J, Luna V, Dizon M, Grebenev D, Powe JL, Lucidi S, Miura A, Kanoh Y, Bandyopadhyay G, Standaert ML, Yeko TR, Farese RV. Defective activation of protein kinase C-ζ by insulin and phosphatidylinositol 3-kinase in obesity and polycystic ovary syndrome. *Metab Synd Rel Disord* 2004; 2:49–56.

33. Sajan MP, Standaert ML, Miura A, Bandyopadhyay G, Vollenweider P, Franklin DM, Lea-Currie R, Farese RV. Impaired activation of protein kinase C-ζ by insulin and phosphatidylinositol-3,4,5-(PO$_4$)$_3$ in cultured adipocytes and myotubes of obese subjects. *J Clin Endo Metab* 2004; 89:3994–3998.

34. Kanoh Y, Sajan MP, Bandyopadhyay G, Miura A, Standaert ML, Farese RV. Defective activation of protein kinase C ζ and λ by insulin and phosphatidylinositol-3,4,5-(PO$_4$)$_3$ in skeletal muscle of rats following high-fat feeding and streptozotocin-induced diabetes. *Endocrinology* 2003; 144:947–954.

35. Chen HC, Rao M, Sajan MP, Standaert ML, Kanoh Y, Miura A, Farese RV Jr, Farese RV. Role of adipocyte-derived factors in enhancing insulin signaling in skeletal muscle and white adipose tissue of mice lacking acyl CoA:diacylglycerol acyltransferase 1. *Diabetes* 2004; 53:1445–1451.

36. Shimomura I, Matsuda M, Hammer RE, Bashmakov Y, Brown MS, Goldstein JL. Decreased IRS-2 and increased SREBP-1c lead to mixed insulin resistance and sensitivity in livers of lipodystrophic and ob/ob mice. *Mol Cell* 2000; 6:77–86.

37. Chen HC, Bandyopadhyay G, Sajan MP, Kanoh Y, Standaert ML, Farese RV, Jr, Farese RV. Activation of the ERK pathway and atypical protein kinase C isoforms in exercise- and AICAR-stimulated glucose transport. *J Biol Chem* 2002; 277:23554–23562.

38. Nielsen JN, Jorgensen SB, Frosig C, Viollet B, Andreelli F, Vaulont S, Kiens B, Richter E.A. Wojtaszewski JFP. A possible role for AMP-activated protein kinase in exercise-induced glucose utilization: Insights from humans and transgenic animals. *Biochem Soc Trans* 2001; 31:186–190.

39. Kennedy J, Hirshman MF, Aronson D, Goodyear LJ, Horton ES. Acute exercise induced GLUT4 translocation in skeletal muscle of normal human subjects and subjects with type 2 diabetes. *Diabetes* 1999; 48:1192–1197.

40. Kim Y-B, Ciaraldi TP, Kong A, Chu N, Henry RR, Kahn B. Troglitazone, but not metformin, restores insulin-stimulated phosphoinositide 3-kinase activity and increases p110β protein levels in skeletal muscle of type 2 diabetic humans. *Diabetes* 2002; 51:443–448.

41. Zhou G, Myers R, Li Y, Chen Y, Shen X, Fenyk-Melody J, Wu M, Ventre J, Doebber T, Fujii N, Musi N, Hirshman MF, Goodyear LJ, Moller DE. Role of AMP-activated protein kinase in mechanism of metformin action. *J Clin Invest* 2001; 108:1167–1174.
42. Shaw RJ, Lamia KA, Vasquez D, Koo S-H, Bardeesy N, DePinho RA, Montminy M, Cantley LC. The kinase LKB1 mediates glucose homeostasis in liver and therapeutic effects of metformin. *Science* 2005; 310:1642–1646.
43. Luna V, Casauban L, Sajan MP, Gomez-Daspet J, Powe JL, Miura A, Rivas J, Standaert ML, Farese RV. Metformin improves atypical protein kinase C activation by insulin and phosphatidylinositol-3,4,5,-(PO$_4$)$_3$ in diabetic muscle. *Diabetologia* 2006; 49:375–382.

18

The Liver, Glucose Homeostasis, and Insulin Action in Type 2 Diabetes Mellitus

Jerry Radziuk and Susan Pye

CONTENTS

INTRODUCTION

Diabetes, and in particular type 2 diabetes (T2DM), is considered clinically unequivocal when fasting hyperglycemia supervenes. However, it has long been clear that this is a final manifestation of a process that has evolved over a long period of time, perhaps even from early fetal development (1). More proximally, fasting hyperglycemia is preceded by impaired glucose tolerance (2). These lesions in turn are foreshadowed by a variety of cellular/biochemical abnormalities (deviations) that can be detected in subjects (or animal models) who are at risk for the development of diabetes. It has been noted that if science had focused on lipid instead of glucose metabolism in addressing the etiology of diabetes, a similar spectrum of deficiencies would have been detected in these pathways (3). Similarly, early lesions in insulin secretion have also been described by a number of investigators (e.g., 4–6). This serves to point out, not the difficulty of the detection of the first step in the development of diabetes, but rather the (network of) linkages that exist between all aspects of metabolism at the systemic level.

From: *Contemporary Endocrinology: The Metabolic Syndrome: Epidemiology, Clinical Treatment, and Underlying Mechanisms*
Edited by: B.C. Hansen and G.A. Bray © Humana Press, Totowa, NJ

These linkages have been, in some sense, expressed in the concept of insulin sensitivity. Insulin plays a crucial role in all aspects of metabolism whether it be carbohydrate, lipid, protein, or finally, energy. Type 2 diabetes is characterized by insensitivity, or resistance, to this hormone. Originally defined as a resistance of glucose metabolism to insulin (7,8), this resistance has been extended to all aspects of metabolism, particularly, perhaps, lipid. Clinically, this has been expressed as the conjunction of an ever-growing number of disorders termed the *insulin resistance syndrome* (*hyperinsulinemic syndrome*, *syndrome X*) (8–14), which, besides insulin resistance, includes type 2 diabetes, obesity, dyslipidemias, atherosclerotic heart disease, disorders of the coagulation system, as well as perhaps disorders in appetite and cognitive function. This linkage has been paralleled at the molecular level, by the series of tissue-specific knockouts of insulin receptors—in the liver, muscle, adipose, nervous, and beta-cell (15–17). All these display a degree of abnormality in glucose metabolism from very mild (15) to florid diabetes (16,17). Insulin action is mediated by a large number (network) of signaling pathways (e.g., 18) and modulated by a large number (network) of influences whether they be metabolic, hormonal (systemic or local), or neural.

Another aspect of these ablations or inactivating mutations, as well as of many others (e.g., GLUT4, PEPCK, GK) (19–22), is that they generally cause some degree of metabolic dysfunction and diabetes-like phenotypes. They are, however, rarely lethal and the mice can be otherwise quite normal. This does suggest a degree of redundancy in the system (which seems like a good safeguard). The word *network* has been used a number of times above. One could easily conclude that this redundancy arises from the structure of the network, with its large number of alternative pathways between most metabolic points. In fact, this could be taken as an argument for the optimality of the network structure of the metabolic system and its regulation. It is simultaneously interesting to note that once the system deviates from "normal," treatments most often aimed at specific metabolic targets, although initially effective in lowering glycemia, nevertheless become less so with time, so that the system proceeds quite inexorably along the new pathway (23–25). Additional treatments are added, eventually with the same effect. This again suggests a systemic structure that is best described as a network and may help to understand why individual treatments may not be as effective as would be predicted from in vitro or animal model observations.

THE BIOLOGY OF DIABETES: FOCUS ON HYPERGLYCEMIA

As pointed out above, hyperglycemia is a central manifestation of type 2 diabetes. It is likely pivotal in the development of its complications. Clearly it can be caused by increases in glucose production, decreases in its removal, or both. Conversely, the increased glycemia would compensate for the fall in the metabolic clearance rate of glucose (MCR) since the product of this fractional removal and the glucose concentration could remain near constant (26). This would not inherently be a problem, except that not all tissues are insulin-dependent (such as the nerves and the mesangial tissues of the kidney). Uptake in such tissues would be proportional to circulating glucose concentrations and hence elevated with a resulting flow down toxic pathways. Toxic pathways (e.g., the hexosamine pathway) (27–32) have, however, also been implicated in the pathogenesis of insulin resistance in insulin-*dependent* tissues such as muscle.

How hyperglycemia can contribute to this process is more problematic. Insulin resistance is characterized by a decrease in clearance of glucose into such tissues so that uptake, even at elevated glucose concentrations, may not be increased. Put another way, any increases in glucose levels, caused only by the impaired clearance, should not result in higher influx of glucose into these target cells (33). *Overproduction* of glucose, however, would result in hyperglycemia over and above that which could arise from the target cell resistance, and hence in an increased entry of glucose into cells and flux down the potentially toxic pathways.

IS GLUCOSE PRODUCTION INCREASED IN TYPE 2 DIABETES?

This is a critical question since an affirmative answer would focus attention on the liver as the locus of potentially primary lesions in the etiology of diabetes. As we have pointed out (32), peripheral insulin resistance could be at least partly accounted for as secondary to the toxic effects of hyperglycemia. The importance of the potential contribution of increased endogenous glucose production (EGP) to hyperglycemia in DM2 has, therefore, motivated a large number of measurements of this rate. We recently presented an overview of EGP measurements (33) in 42 papers. Eighteen of these found an EGP unchanged from controls (e.g., 34–39) and 24 found an increase (e.g., 40–47). A number of potential bases for these variations were identified, including different patient populations, non-steady-state conditions, different tracers and modes of administration, as well as the variety of mathematical models used in the analysis (48–50).

GLUCOSE DYNAMICS IN PATIENTS WITH DIABETES: ANOTHER LOOK

These issues were reexamined in two different groups of diabetic subjects, (1) newly diagnosed/diet-treated, obese, and (2) established (mean 8 y duration), less obese, and compared them to age-, BMI-, and gender-matched control subjects. Our hypotheses were that (1) identical results should be obtained, whatever the experimental approach, if the appropriate mathematical approach for that experiment was used, and (2) that glucose fluxes in DM2 would display greater changes over time than those in controls. Endogenous glucose production (EGP) was calculated using a one-compartment model of glucose (and tracer) kinetics (33,48). Tracer infusions were unprimed or primed with either a fixed or adjusted (to glucose concentration) tracer injection. Our own observations (50) and a reanalysis of previous data (33) showed:

Pathophysiology

- Fasting endogenous glucose production in T2DM varies over the course of a day, decreasing from values 20–50% above control in the early morning to normal by evening. When elevated, it is strongly correlated with glucose levels.
- Since glycemia decreases during the day, the disappearance rates of glucose must be higher than EGP and therefore exceed control rates to an even greater extent, thus allowing increased flux via glucotoxic pathways.
- Metabolic clearance rate of glucose (MCR) is decreased and constant or nearly constant over a period of at least 10 h. It is correlated to glycemia throughout the same period. It therefore contributes to the stable part of the hyperglycemia.

- Although subjects in the three studies were not matched, those with relatively recent onset of diabetes demonstrated both higher endogenous glucose production and higher metabolic clearance rate than those with established diabetes.

Methods

- Assessment of basal (fasting) endogenous glucose production in DM2 is therefore, in general, a non-steady-state problem.
- All methods yield consistent results when an appropriate model and parameters are used (32,33).
- The volume of distribution must be estimated individually to avoid non-steady-state error.

Since higher glycemia is generally associated with both longer duration of diabetes and increased endogenous glucose production (e.g., 2,14), the higher morning endogenous glucose production early in the disease was somewhat surprising. It does suggest, however, that the decreases in metabolic clearance rate are progressive and therefore at least partly secondary to the disease process. Endogenous glucose production may then fall due to its direct suppression by increasing glucose levels (51–53). It should also be noted that, as the metabolic clearance rate decreases, the impact of smaller changes in endogenous glucose production on glycemia becomes greater (32). Summarizing, *(1) glucose production is unequivocally elevated at least during a portion of the 24 h cycle; (2) glucose dynamics evolve in time—both acutely in the course of the day, and chronically with the duration of the disease.*

DIURNAL RHYTHMS AND GLUCOSE METABOLISM

The high morning fasting glycemia in T2DM, which declines during the day to a nadir in the evening, suggests that this may be part of a diurnal cycle in glucose metabolism. It is generally recognized that it is negative feedback loops that maintain the fasting glucose set-point in a narrow range of concentrations. If insulin resistance impairs this finely tuned relationship, the glucose system may revert to more "primitive" diurnal rhythms. This question was posed in a group of subjects with T2DM and a group of matching nondiabetic controls (54). All study participants fasted from 8 A.M. and were monitored for 24 h from 2 P.M. on the first day to 2 P.M. the next, while continuing their fast. Sleep was monitored during the night to ensure that there were no significant periods of sleep apnea, which might alter metabolism.

Glucose Levels and Fluxes

Glucose levels (Fig. 18.1A) initially decreased from 7.2 ± 0.3 mM, plateaued near 6.3 mM, and rose continuously between midnight and 7 A.M., when they peaked at 8.0 ± 0.5 mM, gradually decreasing thereafter to 6.3 ± 0.4 mM. In contrast, age-, weight-, and gender-matched control subjects showed constant glucose levels (4.9 ± 0.2 mM) until the near the end of the study, when a drift to about 4.4 mM occurred.

Using concentrations of concurrently infused [^{13}C-U]glucose, the metabolic clearance rate of glucose was 1.73 ± 0.10 ml/kg-min in control and 1.40 ± 0.14 in diabetic subjects. A gradual rise in endogenous glucose production from 7.8 ± 0.5 to 11.1 ± 0.5 μmol/kg-min over the course of the night (Fig. 18.1B), on the other hand, drove the nocturnal increase in glucose levels and explained the additional morning hyperglycemia in the diabetic subjects. As endogenous glucose production then decreases, glucose

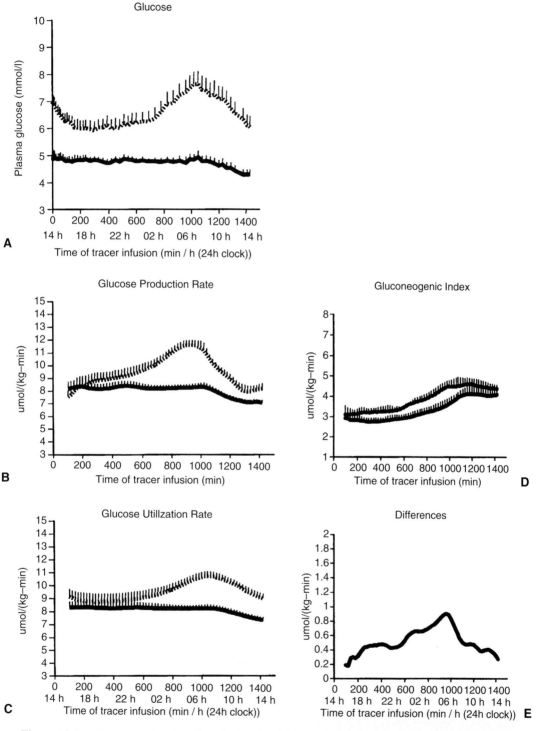

Figure 18.1. (A) Glucose levels in fasted subjects with T2DM (dashed line) and controls (solid line). (B) Endogeneous glucose production and (C) glucose utilization rates for the same subjects. (D) Index of gluconeogenesis calculated from the incorporation of ^{14}C from [^{14}C]lactate into glucose. Both control (lower curve) and diabetic (upper curve) subjects demonstrate a gradual increase in the index with fasting, although this occurs more rapidly in diabetes. Subtraction of the control index from that in diabetes reveals a superimposed excursion in the gluconeogenic index in diabetes (E).

removal (Rd, Fig. 18.1C) supervenes and glycemia also decreases throughout the day. All differences were statistically significant.

A diurnal pattern in endogenous glucose production was also found by Boden (55), but this was during an isoglycemic clamp. These data are consistent with our findings, which, however demonstrate in addition that *endogenous glucose production drives the diurnal pattern in glycemia seen in diabetes.*

Source of Glucose

[^{14}C]lactate was infused simultaneously in these studies to generate an index of gluconeogenesis, from the rate of incorporation of this label into glucose. This index displayed the appropriate increase (56) as fasting progresses, both in control and diabetic subjects. The difference between the diabetic and normal indexes (Fig. 18.1E), moreover, also displayed a nocturnal rise and morning fall, thus paralleling the endogenous glucose production, and strongly suggesting that the nocturnal increase in EGP is due to gluconeogenesis, consistent with previous observations of fasting gluconeogenesis (56–59). Concentrations of lactate, the major glucogenic substrate, are elevated in diabetes, but do not reflect the additional nocturnal rise in endogenous glucose production, indicating that it is not substrate-driven.

Free Fatty Acids and Hormones

Free fatty acids (FFA) likely promote glucogenesis (e.g., 60,61), and a number of hormones (primarily counterregulatory) could drive the process (Fig. 18.2). In the present study, FFA were not different between the two groups, increasing only after 24 h of fasting in both. Leptin directly modulates glucose production (62,63) and can redistribute this flux between gluconeogenesis and glycogenolysis, stimulating the former process (64). Levels in our two groups were variable among individuals with a similar pattern overall, decreasing gradually over 24 h. Glucagon concentrations were higher in T2DM, but did not change significantly during the study, as previously reported (55). Although a suprachiasmatic nucleus-related (SCN) glucagon rhythm was seen in rats (65), it was not related to any periodicity in glucose.

Insulin reflected the hypersecretion (66–70) in T2DM and decreased gradually over the duration of the fast. Importantly, there was no significant change in concentrations in T2DM during the cyclical rise in glucose production/gluconeogenesis.

In our studies, both plasma cortisol and melatonin displayed a cyclicity similar to that in endogenous glucose production. It is not likely that cortisol entrains endogenous glucose production in T2DM, however, for the following reasons: (1) The increase in endogenous glucose production leads that in cortisol by an average of 2 h. (2) Cortisol remains elevated after endogenous glucose production returns to control rates (an increase that might well be separately related to fasting (71)). (3) The same rise in controls does not alter endogenous glucose production, and (4) crosscorrelations between cortisol and endogenous glucose production are poor (54).

Glucocorticoids are implicated in control of glucose metabolism (72) and perhaps in the dawn phenomenon (73). In addition, a significant portion of cortisol production appears to take place in the splanchnic bed, thus targeting the liver (74), and glucocorticoid receptor antagonists reduce endogenous glucose production in diabetic rodent models, or normal dogs (75). A tonic effect of glucocorticoids might thus be anticipated. However, blocking corticosterone synthesis did not affect the morning rise in glucose concentrations seen in humans (76). This is therefore consistent with the above results.

The Hypothalamus and the Suprachiasmatic Nucleus in the Regulation of Endogenous Glucose Production

Diurnal variations in metabolism and blood pressure have been related to the hypothalamic biological clock (77–80). In rodents a rise in plasma glucose concentrations at dusk (the end of the sleep period) has been shown to be due to a rise in endogenous glucose production (81,82). Elegant studies in mice demonstrated that this rise in endogenous glucose production was generated via the SCN/PVN (suprachiasmatic/paraventricular nuclei) pathway inducing a sympathetic stimulation of endogenous glucose production (83). This neural pathway resembles that controlling melatonin secretion: Photic information is conveyed from the retina to the SCN, relayed through the PVN, and a multisynaptic pathway, to the pineal gland, which secretes melatonin (84), providing the rationale for using melatonin as a surrogate measure for suprachiasmatic nucleus activity in our studies. Changes in melatonin concentrations in the present studies are correlated with the changes in endogenous glucose production in diabetic subjects, suggesting the possibility that this flux, too, may be regulated by the biological clock resident in the suprachiasmatic nucleus. Interestingly, however, the nocturnal excursion of melatonin in the diabetic subjects is postponed and attenuated relative to controls (Fig. 18.2), raising the possibility that, unlike the case in rodents, the suprachiasmatic nucleus may be involved in suppressing a cyclical nocturnal increase in EGP, which is then unmasked in diabetes.

It is important to note, however, that (1) the glucose rise in mice is at dusk (dawn in humans) and is shorter lived than the cycle seen in our studies, (2) it occurs in normals, whereas the diurnal cycle observed in our studies took place only in T2DM, and (3) the biological clock–related rise is primarily due to glycogenolysis (85), which is controlled by the sympathetic innervation of the liver (83,86), whereas the changes seen in our studies were due to gluconeogenesis. It is less likely therefore that the cyclical behavior of endogenous glucose production seen here is due to coupling with a hypothalamic biological clock, and it appears that the circadian aspect of the cycles in endogenous glucose production may, to some extent, be fortuitous.

Postprandial Suppression of Endogenous Glucose Production in Normal Controls and Type 2 Diabetic Subjects

Postprandial hyperglycemia, along with fasting hyperglycemia, contributes to HbA1c. Both also, and to some extent independently, contribute to the risk of complications (87,88), particularly cardiovascular disease (89,90). Hepatic insulin resistance has been singled out as the most significant factor contributing to glucose intolerance (67). A suppression of endogenous glucose production to rates that exceed those in normal controls during meals has been shown in T2DM in a large number of studies (67,91–99). Other studies, however, have demonstrated such a decrease in suppression only in more severe diabetes (100) or only at low insulin concentrations (101,102). Because basal endogenous glucose production has often been found to be elevated, when suppression was considered as a fractional or absolute change from this basal rate, it has also been

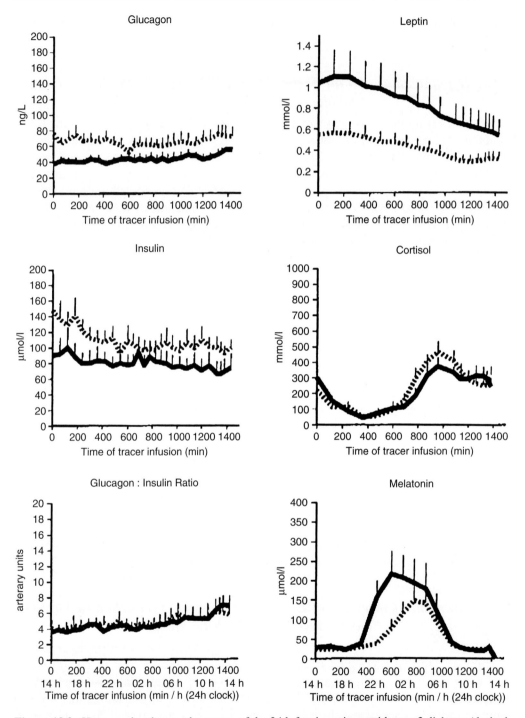

Figure 18.2. Hormone levels over the course of the 24 h fast in patients with type 2 diabetes (dashed lines) and control subjects (solid lines). The panels on the left show the levels of glucagon, insulin, and the glucagon : insulin ratio. The panels on the right show leptin, cortisol, and melatonin concentrations.

found to be normal (91,103–105) both after meals and during simulation of postprandial glucose and hormone profiles. Suppression was also found to be normal in mild diabetes (100) or first-degree relatives of individuals with DM2 (106). Two recent reevaluations (97,99) were based on clamping the specific activity of endogenous glucose. Both demonstrated a rapid (30 min) 50% suppression of endogenous glucose production in both normal and diabetic subjects, followed by a second phase (~150 min) where endogenous glucose production was higher in DM2. As a decrement from basal rates, however, the difference in postprandial endogenous glucose production between the two groups became small.

Analogously to basal endogenous glucose production, the apparent divergence in results above might again be attributed to perspective. We demonstrated (32,33,50, and above) that, in T2DM, basal fasting endogenous glucose production is decreasing continuously throughout the morning. One potentially important viewpoint for postprandial endogenous glucose production in diabetes is, then, *relative to this falling endogenous glucose production.*

To examine this, we compared subjects with T2DM and weight- and gender-matched controls. Each subject, after fasting overnight, underwent two studies where metabolic clearance of glucose and endogenous glucose production were determined using tracer methods. The first study consisted of a 10 h fast. The second study differed, in that a mixed meal was interposed after 4 h of intravenous (iv) tracer ([U-^{13}C]glucose) infusion. The carbohydrate component of the meal consisted of glucose labeled with [6-^{3}H]glucose. Using non-steady-state compartmental analysis of glucose kinetics (107–111), metabolic clearance rate was calculated from the iv tracer. Endogenous glucose concentration was calculated from the difference in total and ingested glucose, and its appearance was calculated using the determined metabolic clearance rate. Preliminary results (112) are summarized below:

1. Glucose levels are higher and metabolic clearance rate (and therefore insulin sensitivity) lower in diabetes compared to control subjects.

2. *Controls*: Basal endogenous glucose production rate was near constant during the 10 h study period (as in 50). Postprandial endogenous glucose production was suppressed to 60% below this basal rate.

3. *Diabetes*: Basal endogenous glucose production fell by ~30% over 10 h. In the meal study, endogenous glucose production fell at the same rate preprandially and then to 50% below pre-meal rates postprandially. However, *relative to the extrapolated (and falling) preprandial rate*, there was only a minor further decrease in endogenous glucose production (~10%).

4. In the diabetic subjects, there was no recovery of endogenous glucose production toward basal 6 h after the meal, perhaps because from the perspective of the extrapolated rate, endogenous glucose production was not suppressed.

Postprandially, endogenous glucose production thus appears to follow different rules in diabetes. Two conclusions might be drawn:

1. In type 2 diabetes, meal-related suppression of endogenous glucose production in diabetes may only be apparent, and simply a continued fall of this rate, in the context of the diurnal cycle of endogenous glucose production expressed on the background of an absorptive increase in glucose, analogous to that in the isoglycemic clamp previously reported (55) in diabetes.

2. This primacy of the dependence of the fall in endogenous glucose production on ambient glycemia may also be a manifestation of a postprandial hepatic insensitivity to insulin, more profound than had been anticipated.

The results may also help to explain the diversity of the literature results, summarized above, since under non-steady-state conditions it is clear that the assumptions made on the constancy of basal endogenous glucose production, and the time at which studies are done, may well contribute to the direction of the results.

HEPATIC INSULIN ACTION AND THE METABOLIC MACHINERY UNDERLYING GLUCOSE METABOLISM IN THE LIVER

The ablation of insulin receptors in the liver (LIRKO) leads to liver dysfunction and a severe insulin resistance (17), resulting in dramatic elevations of blood glucose concentrations, severe glucose intolerance, and the inability of insulin to suppress gluconeogenesis. It also appears that as long as liver insulin sensitivity is preserved, mice are protected from diabetes (113). This is consistent with the finding that the responsiveness of hepatic glucose production to insulin is the major determinant of glucose tolerance (67). This is further consistent with previous findings in the literature (e.g., 114,115) on the importance of liver insulin resistance in the pathogenesis of diabetes, but not others (e.g., 116). Although insulin action can be indirect—via inhibition of protein degradation (117) and the mobilization of substrates for glucose synthesis such as alanine, via the release of free fatty acids, which promote glucose production (118–120), or via hypothalamic neuronal pathways (121,122)—its principal actions are directly on the liver. The latter are further amplified since insulin is secreted directly into the portal vein, and therefore arrives, undiluted, at the liver parenchyma. The primary actions of insulin are therefore most likely on the enzymatic machinery that regulates the production and uptake of glucose by the liver.

The transport of glucose across the hepatic membrane is mediated, at least partly, by the glucose transporter, GLUT2, which is necessary to the equibration of the hepatocyte glucose with the extracellular space (123), and is not rate limiting (124). Regulation of hepatic glucose output and uptake occurs at the level of gluconeogenetic, glycolytic, and glycogen synthetic fluxes. In particular it is primarily localized to the substrate cycles, which comprise these pathways (125). Substrate cycles are an efficient mechanism for increasing the sensitivity of the regulation of flux through such metabolic pathways (126–128). Two nonequilibrium and chemically distinct reactions occurring in opposite directions can yield large changes in the net flux through this cycle with only small changes in either (or both) of the component reactions. The cost of the additional energy dissipation is justified by the ability of such a system to rapidly translate control messages into large alterations in the net flux, thus dramatically increasing sensitivity to external signals. For example, 10% changes in enzyme activity or activation can yield fold changes in flux, even reversing its direction. Moreover, the sensitivity is determined by the rate of cycling and is proportional to the ratio of cycling rate to flux.

These cycles include:

A. Hepatic glucose uptake/output
   (1) Glucose cycle (glucokinase (GK)/glucose-6-phosphatase (G6Pase))
B. Glycogen metabolism
   (2) Glycogen cycle (synthase/phosphorylase)

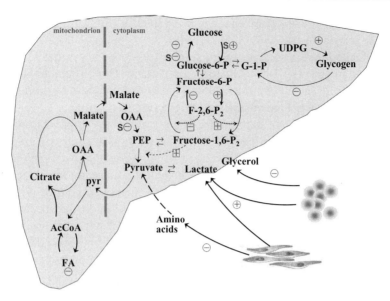

Figure 18.3. Effects of insulin on metabolic pathways in the liver. Inhibitory effects on enzyme activities or substrate concentrations are indicated with (−) and stimulatory effects with (+). Primary effects are indicated by circles and secondary effects by boxes. Effects on new enzyme synthesis are preceded by an "S." (See Color Plate following p. 372.)

C. Glycolysis/gluconeogenesis
 (3) Phosphofructokinase/fructose-1,6-diphosphatase cycle
 (4) Pyruvate/phosphoenolpyruvate cycle (phosphoenolpyruvate carboxykinase (PEPCK)/ pyruvate kinase (PK))

Fluxes through these cycles have been shown to occur continuously. For example, glycogen synthesis occurs during fasting (129) and glycogenolysis during meal absorption (130,131). Glucose uptake (and detritiation of [2-H³] glucose) occurs continuously during net glucose production (e.g., 132). Similarly, although not part of a substrate cycle, gluconeogenesis occurs even when there is no net glucose output (110). Since regulation occurs at the level of these substrate cycles, these are the most likely loci for insulin action. Details of the pathways, components of substrate cycles, and their regulation by insulin are given in (133). The metabolic pathways are excerpted from (133) and summarized in Figure 18.3. The control points at which insulin exerts its effects are specifically indicated.

The complexities of the interactions among fluxes are illustrated by the following considerations, summarized in (134).

Glucogenic Metabolite Fluxes: Glycogenic Substrates and Signals

The somewhat counterintuitive observation was made that in humans, following a meal, approximately half of the hepatic glycogen synthesized arose by the gluconeogenic pathway (135–139). This was also shown in rats (140), and the gluconeogenic flux was found to be necessary to glycogen synthesis since its inhibition resulted in a parallel reduction in glycogen synthesis from glucose (141,142). Lactate appeared to be the major substrate (139). It arose both peripherally and from the splanchnic bed, and a significant portion appeared to arise in the liver itself (110), likely due to hepatic zonation and perivenous production (143,144).

The glucogenic fluxes also contributed signals for glycogen synthesis. This was seen in perfused rat livers (145,146): Glucose (or perhaps G6P originating from it) and glucogenic flux from lactate (or the G6P arising from it) appear to promote glycogen synthesis by different mechanisms; perfusate glucose itself, or the glucose-6-phosphate arising from hepatic uptake of the glucose, did not alone determine the amount of glycogen synthesized—rather it set the range within which such synthesis may take place. On the other hand, the availability of lactate or its uptake by the liver determined the rate of glycogen synthesis within the range set by the glucose concentration (145,146). Glycogen synthesized both from glucogenic substrate and directly from glucose is subject to these signals. Finally, we demonstrated that in rat livers (high therapeutic) metformin inhibits lactate uptake concomitantly with decreases in glycogen synthesis (by both direct and glyconeogenic pathways) (147). This has been confirmed in vivo (148) and in hepatocytes (149). These effects are consistent (134) with the metabolic zonation of the liver (143), which appears to be linked to a large gradient in oxygen tension since O_2 (by way of H_2O_2) may signal a coordinated expression of PEPCK and GK (144).

Hepatic Glucose Uptake and Glycogen Synthesis

Circulating glucose is an equally important substrate for glycogen synthesis with glucogenic metabolites. Glucokinase (GK) activity is stimulated by translocation from nuclear to cytoplasmic sites, a regulatory protein, and (meal-related) metabolic products of fructose and glucose. Insulin and glucagon alter its expression (150–152). G6Pase activity is decreased by carbohydrate feeding (153–155), although meal-related glucogenic substrate may increase both its activity and expression (152,156). Thus, postprandially, GK and G6Pase are regulated in a coordinated fashion (156) that promotes the deposition of glycogen from both glucose and glucogenic substrate. Glucose (157–159), G6P generated by GK (160), and insulin (161–164) stimulate glycogen synthase through an enzyme cascade that also involves the deactivation of phosphorylase, providing a *pull mechanism* for glycogen synthesis and a *switch* that rapidly converts the liver from glycogenolysis to net synthesis under refed conditions (165).

GK and gluconeogenic flux to G6P (with a simultaneous inhibition of G6Pase) also provide substrate (166) and thus contribute to a simultaneous *push* or mass effect. *Although insulin sets up the enzymes in a synthetic mode, both the regulatory and mass effects provided by substrates for glycogen synthesis appear to be necessary for net glycogen synthesis* (167). Glycogen formed during the absorptive period is necessary for subsequent glucose production. Defective glycogen synthesis or breakdown result in inadequate production and hypoglycemia as seen in the glycogen storage diseases (168). Glycogen synthesis is therefore a highly coordinated process where both glucose and glucogenic substrates, particularly lactate, participate as both substrates and signals. Insulin signaling also appears more complex than the alteration of enzyme activity or synthesis.

Links Between Gluconeogenesis and Hepatic Glycogen in Type 2 Diabetes

Liver glucose metabolism in diabetes is abnormal. As already described, a prominent feature is an increase in hepatic glucose production at least for some time during the postabsorptive period (2,33,47,50,169). This increase in hepatic glucose production is at least partly caused by an increase in gluconeogenesis (169–172). Increased glycoge-nolysis may also contribute (173,174). Interestingly, these observations are consistent with an increased glycogen mass, which can be seen in subjects with type 2 diabetes or obesity in several (175,176), but not all, studies (177). Insulin-resistant animal models also show a simultaneously increased lactate uptake by the liver (178), suggest-ing that this could be an important signal/substrate both for gluconeogenesis and gly-cogen synthesis under these circumstances. It could be further speculated that lactate (as well as fatty acids) mobilized from visceral fat (179–181) and immediately available to the liver from the portal vein could thus contribute signals for the abnormal liver metabolism in diabetes. On the other hand, in diabetic rats glycogen was found to be predominantly gluconeogenic in origin (182), suggesting a decreased effectiveness of this flux in promoting overall glycogen synthesis. Lactate has also been considered as a marker for insulin sensitivity (183) and may thus decrease, under some circumstances in T2DM. A number of associations can therefore be postulated but remain unclear. As a consequence, the precise molecular loci of in vivo insulin action and resistance are also uncertain.

Hepatic Action of Insulin in Type 2 Diabetes

The overall effects of insulin on glucose metabolism in the liver are summarized in Figure 18.4.

GLUCOSE PRODUCTION

Systemically, the actions of insulin and metabolite signals at the molecular level translate into a coordinated response to physiological stimuli as already seen above for meals. Insulin has both direct (184–189) and indirect (118–122) effects on the suppres-sion of glucose production. A number of studies demonstrated a decrease in the hepatic sensitivity to insulin (40,45,46,67,120,190,191) in T2DM, although this was again most clearly seen at low concentrations of insulin (68,100). Certainly part of this defect is at the level of direct effects of insulin on the liver (e.g., 189). However, attenuation of the insulin-mediated suppression of peripheral glycolysis and lipolysis will contribute both

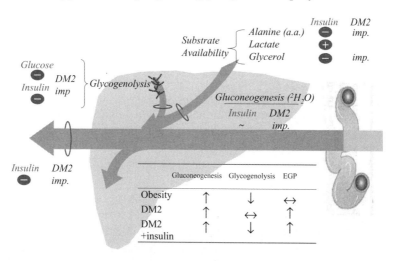

Figure 18.4. Summary of insulin effects on the components of principal glucose fluxes during meal absorption, and their impairment in type 2 diabetes. (See Color Plate following p. 372.)

substrate and stimulus to the process of new glucose formation (192,193). Analogously to the effects of meals, it is not surprising that other studies show normal sensitivity of the suppression of endogenous glucose production to insulin (94,104,194). The variation in results could be due to the different populations studied, the different quantitative expressions (e.g., fractional) of suppression, as well as the precise circumstances of the measurement of insulin sensitivity, for example, during hyperglycemia (isoglycemia in diabetes) or euglycemia (190). In fact, normalization of glycemia with an overnight insulin infusion improved hepatic insulin sensitivity (195).

It is also worthy of note that the early increase in insulin secretion after meal ingestion appears to be critical not only to peripheral glucose uptake (196), but also to the subsequent suppression of endogenous glucose production (197,198).

A good deal of work has also focused on the fractional assignment of insulin effects on glucose production to the component processes, gluconeogenesis and glycogenolysis (e.g., 199). Using the incorporation of deuterated water into gluconeogenetic glucose, it was shown that, during physiological glucose clamps (equivalent to the postprandial insulin excursion), gluconeogenesis decreased to some extent (30–50%) in normal subjects and even less in patients with T2DM (10–20%) (200,201). Glycogenolysis, on the other hand, was reduced almost to zero in both control and diabetic subjects. Similar results were obtained in dogs (202). These data do not appear to be compatible with the multiple sites at which insulin can exert control on the gluconeogenetic process as described above in Figure 18.3, testifying again to the complexity of the system, where the integrated action of the enzymic network may not always be predictable from that of individual enzymes.

Glucose Uptake

The liver is strategically positioned between the gut and the systemic circulation. It has been postulated that one of the consequences of this location is that the liver can take up a large fraction (up to 60%) of newly absorbed nutrients, specifically glucose, after a meal, store it as glycogen, and rerelease it into the systemic circulation postabsorptively, thus buffering the potential impact of meal glucose on peripheral glycemia (92,203,204,205; for review: 110,134).

Measurements of splanchnic glucose uptake in diabetic subjects suggested that this uptake was impaired and a major cause of postprandial (and subsequent) hyperglycemia (204). Very large fractional uptakes were subsequently shown to be unlikely (108,110) and were found to be closer to 3–5% (108,110,206) in normal humans. This, however, translated into an overall splanchnic glucose uptake of ~20 g after an oral glucose load—the equivalent of ~25% of the amount of glucose ingested (108,110,134,206). In type 2 diabetes, some estimates obtained using both splanchnic balance techniques and tracer methods indicated that splanchnic glucose uptake was unchanged (46,93,100,207) or perhaps increased (208). Others came to the opposite conclusion—that splanchnic glucose uptake was decreased (105,190,204,209,210), thus contributing to hyperglycemia. It was suggested that this decrease occurred only in response to oral glucose loading (209), since diabetes appeared to eliminate an apparent enhancement of splanchnic glucose uptake vis-a-vis that administered intravenously.

Whether insulin alone increases splanchnic glucose uptake is not entirely clear. Fractional splanchnic extraction remains near 4% when insulin is increased (209), leaving splanchnic uptake unchanged (211). Comparisons of increasing doses of insulin in normal humans suggest that there is an effect on splanchnic glucose uptake (190) and that this responsiveness is impaired in T2DM.

GLUCOSE–LIPID INTERACTIONS, REGULATION BY INSULIN, AND TYPE 2 DIABETES

It has long been recognized (212) that free fatty acids (FFA) interfere with the action of insulin on glucose metabolism, both in the peripheral tissues and in the liver.

Insulin is also intimately involved in the regulation of lipid metabolism. The regulatory network is equally complex. Moreover, carbohydrate and lipid metabolism are closely and intricately linked (e.g., 133). The following is an illustration of this complexity.

Lipolysis is inhibited by feeding, mediated by increases in insulin concentrations, decreasing the availability of fatty acids for hepatic lipid synthesis (212,213). VLDL synthesis is also decreased by the actions of insulin on apoB synthesis and degradation (213,214). In addition, insulin stimulates de novo lipogenesis by increasing the activity of pyruvate dehydrogenase complex and SREBP-1c-mediated synthetic enzymes. In the established fed state, insulin switches to the stimulation of VLDL synthesis, leading to the export of fat from the liver to adipose tissue (215–217).

Inappropriate lipid metabolism contributes to insulin resistance (213,214). This state is also characterized by increases in circulating FFA, particularly postprandially, due to an attenuated inhibition of lipolysis by insulin (212). FFA are also inefficiently oxidized by muscle. This could then lead to the accumulation of visceral fat that is seen in the insulin-resistance syndrome (218). Visceral fat could in turn provide additional FFA directly to the liver. Thus additional substrate is available for the synthesis of VLDL. At the same time, the lipogenic pathway, which is under the control of SREBP, remains sensitive to insulin, which is now chronically elevated secondary to the resistant state. The sum of these effects is an increase in hepatic FFA, the intracellular triglyceride with which it equilibrates, long-chain fatty acyl CoA (LCFACoA) and malonyl CoA, and lipid production. The LCFACoA and malonyl CoA simultaneously stimulate FA oxidation and esterification. The former process will then enhance gluconeogenesis (e.g., Randle cycle, see 219) and hyperglycemia. As illustrated in Figure 18.5, the gluconeogenic flux increased in this way (or induced by insulin or by non-insulin-responsive PEPCK overexpression) (220,221) can stimulate an increase in glucose substrate for de novo lipogenesis (as can GK overexpression (222), or insulin stimulation of GK expression). This leads to a positive feedback loop that appears to be characteristic of insulin-resistant states.

Normally, increases in gluconeogenesis will be compensated by decreases in glycogenolysis. In DM2, this *autoregulation* is impaired so that both likely contribute to increased endogenous glucose production (223). In addition, FFA interfere with the action of insulin to decrease glycogenolysis, thus also causing the hepatic insulin insensitivity seen. The increased glycogenolytic rate may be maintained since accelerated gluconeogenesis is also reflected in increased glycogen synthesis, resulting in enhanced *glycogen cycling*. Glucose-6-phosphatase activity is also stimulated by FFA, so that these altered fluxes result in a higher rate of endogenous glucose production (e.g., 224).

Supporting evidence for the above sequence was seen when visceral fat excision improved insulin sensitivity in a rat model of insulin resistance (225), and when

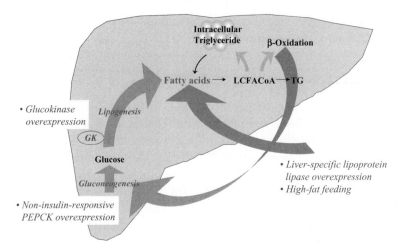

Figure 18.5. Schematic illustrating some of the interactions between glucose and lipid metabolism, and demonstrating that increased glucose production will increase both FFA and liver lipid deposition, which in turn will accelerate gluconeogenesis. (See Color Plate following p. 372.)

overexpression of hepatic lipoprotein lipase (226) caused hepatic insulin resistance. High-fat-fed rats (227) and New Zealand obese mice (228) both demonstrated increased fructose-1,6-bisphosphatase activity and increased endogenous glucose production. A potential cause is decreased fructose-2,6-bisphosphate, since this metabolite regulates the enzyme. This was further suggested by increasing fructose-2,6-bisphosphate levels by enzyme overexpression in KK diabetic mice (229), which decreased endogenous glucose production, as well as normalizing G-6-Pase and GK activity and lowering VLDL secretion. Such observations emphasize the intricate links between glucose and lipid metabolism, but also attenuate the potential causality of impaired fat metabolism in T2DM.

Metabolic Zonation: The Effects of O_2 and Nonalcoholic Steatohepatitis

A further dimension of regulation is added by a metabolic zonation that underlies liver metabolism (143,144). For example, the periportal region is more gluconeogenic and the perivenous region is more glycolytic. This adds another potential dimension to the regulation of hepatic metabolism. It has been conceptually supported by observations such as the modulation by insulin of glucagon-induced glycogenolysis exclusively in perivenous hepatocytes. Metabolic zonation essentially reflects the gradient in oxygen tension in the liver. Both glucose and lipid metabolism are dependent on oxygen availability within the liver. As O_2 is involved in the regulation of enzyme activity and expression, it may also be involved in abnormal reactions. Accumulation of TG increases the availability of FFA. Increased β-oxidation in the presence of partial uncoupling of phosphorylation and oxidation in hepatocytes leads to free radical formation, which, along with the potential intrinsic cytotoxicity of FFA, may lead to accumulation of cytokines and endotoxins, tissue inflammation, and the manifestations of non-alcoholic steatohepatitis (NASH). In addition, both hyperglycemia and hyperinsulinemia have been shown to contribute to the progression to fibrosis in NASH. Inversely, fatty liver disease is strongly associated with insulin resistance, even without the presence of T2DM (230–233).

COMPLEXITY AND THE SYSTEM PERSPECTIVE

We have seen that both carbohydrate and lipid metabolism conform to complex metabolic networks of enzyme and hormonal regulatory reactions. Moreover, the interactions between the two systems add another level of complication, leading to questions of causality and primacy. Does an impairment of glucose metabolism lead to the remaining metabolic abnormalities? Or is it an impairment of lipid metabolism? As pointed out by McGarry, diabetes could equally well have been considered a lipid disorder (3). These questions are, to some extent, paradoxical. Additionally one may consider that the effects of hormones, and insulin in particular, are mediated by intricate systems of signaling proteins. Examples of some of these systems that are involved in liver carbohydrate and lipid metabolism include: the sterol regulatory element binding protein (SREBP) (e.g., 215), FoxO1 transcription factors (234), AMP-activated protein kinase—a master switch in glucose and lipid metabolism (235), peroxisome prolfierator-activated receptor-γ (PPARγ) (236), the CREB-binding protein (237), the Farnesoid X receptor (238), a PGC-1α/SIRT1 complex (239), p38 Mitogen-activated protein kinase (240), as well as, of course, the insulin receptor substrates (IRS 1 and 2) (241). It could be added that metabolic and inflammatory responses are also related via lipid-mediated signals (e.g., 242).

Most of the signaling factors listed above are integrative in nature. That is, they control the coordination of a battery of related enzymes and hence an integrated metabolic response, for example, to a meal or to stress. The complexity of the interrelationships, compensatory or autoregulatory responses, seems to preclude the simple elaboration of causes and effects. It is perhaps preferable to consider the entire metabolic system as an entity (which it is). *Insulin resistance may then be an intrinsic feature of the system as a whole*, rather than being manifested through a specific impaired enzyme reaction or signaling protein.

Theoretical Approaches

A number of approaches have been developed to incorporate the vast amount of structural and experimental data that are available on metabolic pathways and interactions. These tend to aim for isomorphic and comprehensive descriptions of the biochemical systems. They can be described as *bottom-up* since they make conjectures about system behavior based on the detailed structure of the system. The pathway analysis developed by Palsson (243) is primarily structural. Metabolic flux analysis or flux balance analysis adds mass balance around intracellular metabolites to the picture (244). Biochemical systems theory (245) allows a large number of nonlinear interacting components, and metabolic control analysis is aimed at evaluating to what extent the various reactions of the metabolic pathways determine the fluxes and metabolite concentrations (246,247). These have greatly improved understanding of the systems studied.

An alternative approach could be termed *physiological* or *top-down*. It searches for complex system attributes which are manifested as the potential for altered behaviors of the observed system (the patient or animal model), some of which may be characterized as "disease states." In this context, we have made three somewhat unexpected observations in subjects with T2DM, which were described in detail above (and in 54):

1. *Endogenous, primarily liver, glucose production in type 2 diabetes is never in steady state, displaying rather a cyclical (diurnal) temporal pattern. This phasic behavior is restricted to diabetes and is not seen in normal controls. Because of this, it is not convincingly related to the hypothalamic biological clock or the rhythms it controls. Endogenous glucose production then drives the periodic pattern of glycemia, again only in diabetes.

2. *The cyclical behavior of endogenous glucose production is determined by the same pattern in the rate of gluconeogenesis, suggesting that this behavior is more fundamental than simply hormone-induced changes in the relatively labile molecule, glycogen.

3. *The cyclical behavior of endogenous glucose production in T2DM appears to override insulin control during meals, so that postprandial endogenous glucose production tracks the declining basal rate of production much more closely than the discontinuity induced by the meal-generated suppression seen in nondiabetic subjects.

Endogenous glucose production and glycemia thus exist in two stable states: the steady state (normal) and a cyclical state (T2DM). This would in fact be characteristic of the behavior of a nonlinear system and likely testifies to the complex nonlinear nature of metabolism. In response to changes in a critical parameter, or an appropriate perturbation, a transition between the steady and the cyclical state may occur (248), and the patient becomes diabetic. This idea is bolstered by the recent observation (249) that the transition between the nondiabetic and diabetic state occurs with relative abruptness, compatible with its nature as a switch between the two states. The transition to a (limit) cycle in turn provides a conceptual (mathematical) explanation for the rapidity of onset of fasting hyperglycemia observed in reference 249.

The concept is further supported by the existence of a multiplicity of susceptibility factors (e.g., the thrifty genotype/phenotype) that define the parameters predisposing to the switch, coupled with a variety of *environmental* factors that may acutely provoke it.

Such transitions between stable states are characteristic of, and in fact, define *dynamical diseases* (250,251) such as Cheyne-Stokes respiration (252), some cardiac arrhythmias (253), and aplastic anemia (254). Interestingly, the onset of type 1 diabetes has been described as a collective dynamic instability within a complex framework (255) rather than a single etiologic factor.

The hypothesis proposed here is that the metabolic system is intrinsically nonlinear and may exhibit behavior that would characterize type 2 diabetes as a *dynamical disease*. This would imply that the concept of "insulin sensitivity" or "insulin resistance" is embedded in the system behavior and can accommodate an even greater degree of liver insulin resistance in diabetes than might have been anticipated. It seems furthermore that a reservation expressed by the European Association for the Study of Diabetes and the American Diabetes Association (256) and an accompanying editorial implies that, without more evidence, the syndrome should not be classified as a disease entity. Rather it remains a cluster of individual risk factors for cardiovascular disease. The factors that comprise the syndrome are frequently a matter of definition, and therefore vary depending on the criteria used (256). They also tend to increase in number— for example, with the addition of various markers of inflammation (e.g., C-reactive protein (4)) and coagulation factors (e.g., plasminogen activator inhibitor, fibrinogen (256–259)).

The components of the metabolic syndrome often also have an association with insulin resistance (256). This, however, does not imply an etiological role for insulin resistance in this syndrome, since it could be simply another marker for pathological processes arising from a different (e.g., inflammatory, metabolic) cause. This would be compatible with the system perspective proposed since insulin resistance would be only one feature of its altered behavior in diabetes. It would be also compatible with the many interventions (knockouts, diets, etc.) and pathways potentially leading to a diabetic state. In addition, therapeutic interventions alter the course of the disease only temporarily, delaying rather than reversing the disease process (23–25), since only a particular metabolic site, rather than the disease process, is targeted.

REFERENCES

1. Hales CN, Barker DJP, Clark PMS et al. Fetal and infant growth and impaired glucose tolerance at age 64. In *Fetal and Infant Origins of Adult Disease,* Barker DJP (ed.), BMJ Publications, London, 1992, pp. 253–257.
2. DeFronzo RA. The triumvirate—beta-cell, muscle, and liver: A collusion responsible for NIDDM. *Diabetes* 1988; 37:667–687.
3. McGarry JD. What if Minkowski had been ageusic? An alternative angle on diabetes. *Science* 1992; 258:755–770.
4. Efendic S, Grill V, Luft R, Wajngot A. Low insulin response: A marker of prediabetes. *Adv Exp Med Biol* 1988; 246:167–174.
5. Mitrakou A, Kelley D, Mokan M, Veneman T, Pangburn T, Reilly J, Gerich J. Role of reduced suppression of glucose production and diminished early insulin release in impaired glucose tolerance. *N Engl J Med* 1992; 326:22–29.
6. Reaven GM, Shen SW, Silvers A, Farquhar JW. Is there a delay in the plasma insulin response of patients with chemical diabetes mellitus? *Diabetes* 1971; 20:416.
7. Himsworth HP. Diabetes mellitus: Its differentiation into insulin-sensitive and insulin-insensitive types. *Lancet* 1936; 1:127.
8. Ferrannini E, Buzzigoli G, Bonadonna R, Giorico MA, Oleggini M, Graziadei L, Pedrinelli R, Brandt L, Bevilacqua S. Insulin resistance in essential hypertension. *N Engl J Med* 1987; 317:350–357.
9. Bjorntorp P. Abdominal obesity and the development of noninsulin dependent diabetes mellitus. *Diabetes Metab Rev* 1988; 4:615–622.
10. Stout RW. Insulin and atheroma: 20 yr perspective. *Diabetes Care* 1990; 13:631–654.
11. Laws W, Reaven GM. Insulin resistance and coronary heart disease risk factors. *Bailliere's Clin Endocrinol Metab* 1993; 4:1063–1078.
12. Juhan-Vague I, Alessi MC, Vague P. Increased plasma plasminogen activator inhibitor 1 levels: A possible link between insulin resistance and atherothrombosis. *Diabetologia* 1991; 34:457–462.
13. Sanyal AJ, Campbell-Sargent C, Mirshahi F, Rizzo WB, Contos MJ, Sterling RK, Luketic VA, Shiffman ML, Clore JN. Nonalcoholic steatohepatitis: Association of insulin resistance and mitochondrial abnormalities. *Gastroenterology* 2001; 120:1183–192.
14. DeFronzo R, Bonadonna R, Ferrannini E. Pathogenesis of NIDDM: A balanced overview. *Diabetes Care* 1992; 15:318.
15. Bruning JC, Michael MD, Winnay JN, Hayashi T, Horsch D, Accilli D, Goodyear L, Kahn CR. A muscle-specific insulin receptor knockout exhibits features of the metabolic syndrome of NIDDM without altering glucose tolerance. *Mol Cell* 1998; 2:559–569.
16. Kulkarni RN, Bruning JC, Winnay JN, Postic C, Magnuson MA, Kahn CR. Tissue-specific knockout of the insulin receptor in pancreatic beta cells creates an insulin secretory defect similar to that in type 2 diabetes. *Cell* 1999; 96:329–339.
17. Michael MD, Kulkarni RN, Postic C, Previs SF, Shulman GI, Magnuson MA, Kahn CR. Loss of insulin signaling in hepatocytes leads to severe insulin resistance and progressive hepatic dysfunction. *Mol Cell* 2000; 6:87–97.
18. Häring H, Mehnert H. Pathogenesis of type 2 (non-insulin-dependent) diabetes mellitus: Candidates for a signal transmitter defect causing insulin resistance of the skeletal muscle. *Diabetologia* 1993; 36:176–182.

19. Minokoshi Y, Kahn CR, Kahn BB. Tissue-specific ablation of the GLUT4 glucose transporter or the insulin receptor challenges assumptions about insulin action and glucose homeostasis. *J Biol Chem* 2003; 278:33609–33612.
20. She P, Burgess SC, Shiota M, Flakoll P, Donahue EP, Malloy CR, Sherry AD, Magnuson MA. PEPCK knockout mice preserve euglycemia during starvation. *Diabetes* 2003; 52:1649–1654.
21. Froguel P, Vaxillaire M, Sun F. Close linkage of glucosekinase locus on chromosome 7p to early-onset noninsulin dependent diabetes mellitus. *Nature* 1992; 36:162–164.
22. Miller SP, Gulshan RA, Karschina EJ, Bell GI, LaPorte DC, Lange AJ. Characterization of glucokinase mutations associated with maturity-onset diabetes of the young type 2 (MODY-2): Different glucokinase defects lead to a common phenotype. *Diabetes* 1999; 48:1645–1651.
23. UK Prospective Diabetes Study (UKPDS) Group. Effect of intensive blood glucose control with metformin on complications in overweight patients with type 2 diabetes (UKPDS 34). *Lancet* 1998; 352:854–865.
24. UK Prospective Diabetes Study (UKPDS) Group. Intensive blood-glucose control with sulphonyl-urease or insulin compared with conventional treatment and risk of complications in patients with type 2 diabetes (UKPDS 33). *Lancet* 1998; 352:837–853.
25. Diabetes Prevention Program Research Group. Reduction in the incidence of type 2 diabetes with lifestyle intervention or metformin. *N Engl J Med* 2002; 346:393–403.
26. Commerford SR, Bizeau M, McRae H, Jampolis A, Thresher JS, Pagliassotti MJ. Hyperglycemia compensates for diet-induced insulin resistance in liver and skeletal muscle of rats. *Am J Physiol* 2001; 281:R1380–1389.
27. Rossetti L, Giaccari A, DeFronzo RA. Glucose toxicity. *Diabetes Care* 1990; 13:610–630.
28. Baron AD, Zhu JS, Zhu JH et al. Glucosamine induces insulin resistance in vivo by affecting GLUT 4 translocation in skeletal muscle: Implications for glucose toxicity. *J Clin Invest* 1995; 96:2792–2801.
29. Boden G, Ruiz J, Kim CJ, Chen X. Effects of prolonged glucose infusion on insulin secretion, clearance and action in normal subjects. *Amer J Physiol* 1995; 270:E251–258.
30. Rossetti L. Perspective: Hexosamines and nutrient sensing. *Endocrinology* 2000; 141:1922–1925.
31. Beisswenger PJ, Wood ME, Scott KH, Touchette AD, O'Dell RM, Szwergold BS. Alpha-dicarbonyls increase in the postprandial period and reflect degree of hyperglycemia. *Diabetes Care* 2001; 24:726–732.
32. Radziuk J, Pye S. Tracers in the analysis of glucose metabolism in health and diabetes: Basal conditions. Bailliere's Best Practice and Research. *Clin Endocrinol Metab* 2003; 17:323–342.
33. Radziuk J, Pye S. Quantitation of basal endogenous glucose production in type 2 diabetes: Importance of the volume of distribution. *Diabetologia* 2002; 45:1053–1084.
34. Chen IY-D, Jeng C-Y, Hollenbeck CB, Wu M-S, Reaven GM. Relationship between plasma glucose and insulin concentration, glucose production, and glucose disposal in normal subjects and patients with non-insulin-dependent diabetes. *J Clin Invest* 1988; 82:21–25.
35. Hother-Nielsen O, Beck-Nielsen H. On the determination of basal glucose production rate in patients with type 2 (non-insulin dependent) diabetes mellitus using primed-continuous 3-^{3}H-glucose infusion. *Diabetologia* 1990; 33:603–610.
36. Hother-Nielsen O, Beck-Nielsen H. Insulin resistance but normal basal rates of glucose production in patients with newly diagnosed mild diabetes mellitus. *Acta Endocrinol (Copenh)* 1991; 124: 637–645.
37. Beck-Nielsen H, Hother-Nielsen O, Vaag A, Alford F. Pathogenesis of type 2 (non-insulin-dependent) diabetes mellitus: The role of skeletal muscle glucose uptake and hepatic glucose production in the development of hyperglycemia—a critical comment. *Diabetologia* 1994; 37:217–221.
38. Jeng C-Y, Sheu WH-H, Fuh MM-T, Chen IY-D, Reaven GM. Relationship between hepatic glucose production and fasting plasma glucose concentration in patients with NIDDM. *Diabetes* 1994; 43:1440–1444.
39. Rigalleau V, Beylot M, Laville M, Guillot C, Deleris G, Aubertin J, Gin H. Measurement of post-absorptive glucose kinetics in non-insulin-dependent diabetic patients: Methodological aspects. *Eur J Clin Invest* 1996; 26:231–236.
40. Firth RG, Bell PM, Marsh HM, Hansen I, Rizza RA. Postprandial hyperglycemia in patients with non-insulin-dependent diabetes mellitus: Role of hepatic and extra-hepatic tissues. *J Clin Invest* 1986; 77:1525–1532.

41. Baron AD, Schaeffer L, Shragg P, Kolterman OG. Role of hyperglucagonemia in maintenance of increased rates of hepatic glucose output in type II diabetes. *Diabetes* 1987; 36:274–283.
42. Glauber H, Wallace P, Brechtel G. Effects of fasting on plasma glucose and prolonged tracer measurement of hepatic glucose output in NIDDM. *Diabetes* 1987; 36:1187–1194.
43. DeFronzo R. The triumvirate—beta cell, muscle, liver: A collusion responsible for NIDDM. *Diabetes* 1988; 37:667–687.
44. Consoli A, Nurjhan N, Capani F, Gerich J. Predominant role of gluconeogenesis in increased hepatic glucose production in NIDDM. *Diabetes* 1989; 38:550–557.
45. DeFronzo R. Pathogenesis of type 2 (non-insulin-dependent) diabetes mellitus: A balanced overview. *Diabetologia* 1992; 35:389–397.
46. Dineen S, Gerich J, Rizza R. Carbohydrate metabolism in non-insulin-dependent diabetes mellitus. *New Engl J Med* 1992; 327:707–713.
47. Fery F. Role of hepatic glucose production and glucose uptake in the pathogenesis of fasting hyperglycemia in type 2 diabetes: Normalization of glucose kinetics by short-term fasting. *J Clin Endocrinol Metab* 1994; 7:536–542.
48. Steele R. Influences of glucose loading and of injected insulin on hepatic glucose output. *Ann NY Acad Sci* 1959; 82:420–430.
49. Hother-Nielsen O, Beck-Nielsen H. On the determination of basal glucose production rate in patients with type 2 (non-insulin-dependent) diabetes mellitus using primed-continuous 3-^{3}H-glucose infusion. *Diabetologia* 1990; 33:603–610.
50. Radziuk J, Pye S. Production and metabolic clearance of glucose under basal conditions in type 2 diabetes. *Diabetologia* 2001; 44:983–991.
51. Sacca L, Hendler PE, Sherwin RS. Hyperglycemia inhibits glucose production in man independent of changes in glucoregulatory hormones. *J Clin Endocrinol Metab* 1979; 47:1160–1163.
52. Rossetti L, Giaccari A, Barzilai N, Howard K, Sebel G, Hu M. Mechanisms by which hyperglycemia inhibits hepatic glucose production in conscious rats. Implications for the pathophysiology of fasting hyperglycemia in diabetes. *J Clin Invest* 92:1126–1134.
53. Basu A, Caumo A, Bettini F, Gelisio A, Alzaid A, Cobelli C, Rizza RA. Impaired basal glucose effectiveness in NIDDM: Contribution of defects in glucose disappearance and production, measured using an optimized minimal model independent protocol. *Diabetes* 1997; 46:421–432.
54. Radziuk J, Pye S. Diurnal rhythm in endogenous glucose production is a major contributor to fasting hyperglycemia in type 2 diabetes: Suprachiasmatic defect or limit cycle behaviour. *Diabetologia* 2005; 49:1619–1628.
55. Boden G, Chen X, Urbain JL. Evidence for a circadian rhythm of insulin sensitivity in patients with NIDDM caused by cyclic changes in hepatic glucose production. *Diabetes* 1996; 45:1044–1050.
56. Wajngot A, Chandramouli V, Schumann WC, Ekberg K, Jones PK, Efendic S, Landau B. Quantitative contributions of gluconeogenesis to glucose production during fasting in type 2 diabetes mellitus. *Metabolism* 2001; 50:47–52.
57. Consoli A, Nurjhan N, Capani F, Gerich J. Predominant role of gluconeogenesis in increased hepatic glucose production in NIDDM. *Diabetes* 1989; 38:550–557.
58. Boden G, Chen X, Stein TP. Gluconeogenesis in moderately and severely hyperglycemic patients with type 2 diabetes mellitus. *Am J Physiol* 2001; 280:E23–30.
59. Gastaldelli A, Baldi S, Pettiti M, Toschi S, Camastra S, Natali A, Landau B, Ferrannini E. Influence of obesity and type 2 diabetes on gluconeogenesis and glucose output in humans: A quantitative study. *Diabetes* 2000; 49:1367–1373.
60. Lam TKT, Carpentier A, Lewis GF, van de Werve G, Fantus IG, Gaicca A. Mechanisms of the free fatty acid-induced increase in hepatic glucose production. *Am J Physiol Endocrino Metab* 2003; 284: E8683–E873.
61. Boden G, Cheung P, Stein TP, Kresge K, Mozzoli M. FFA cause hepatic insulin resistance by inhibiting insulin suppression of glycogenolysis. *Am J Physiol Endocrinol Metab* 2002; 283: E12–E19.
62. Nemecz M, Preininger K, Englisch R, Furnsinn C, Schneider B, Waldhausl W, Roden M. Acute effects of leptin on hepatic glycogenolysis and gluconeogenesis in perfused rat liver. *Hepatology* 1999; 29:166–172.
63. Anderwald C, Muller G, Koca G, Furnsinn C, Waldhausl W, Roden M. Short-term leptin-dependent inhibition of hepatic gluconeogenesis is mediated by insulin receptor substrate-2. *Mol Endocrinol* 2002; 16:1612–1628.

64. Liu L, Karkanias GB, Morales JC, Hawkins M, Barzilai N, Wang J, Rossetti L. Intracerebroventricular leptin regulates hepatic but not peripheral glucose fluxes. *J Biol Chem* 1998; 273:31160–31167.

65. Ruitger M, la Fleur SE, van Heijningen C, van der Vliet J, Kalsbeek A, Buijs RM. The daily rhythm in plasma glucose concentrations in the rat is modulated by the biological clock and by feeding behavior. *Diabetes* 2003; 52:1709–1715.

66. Paquot N, Scheen AJ, Dirlewanger M, Lefebvre PJ, Tappy L. Hepatic insulin resistance in obese non-diabetic subjects and in type 2 diabetic patients. *Obesity Res* 2002; 10:129–134.

67. Bavenholm PN, Pigon J, Ostenson C-G, Efendic S. Insulin sensitivity of suppression of endogenous glucose production is the single most important determinant of glucose tolerance. *Diabetes* 2001; 50:1449–1454.

68. Staehr P, Hother-Nielsen O, Levin K, Holst JJ, Beck-Nielsen H. Assessment of hepatic insulin action in obese type 2 diabetic patients. *Diabetes* 2001; 50:1363–1370.

69. Boden G, Cheung P, Homko C. Effects of acute insulin excess and deficiency on gluconeogenesis and glycogenolysis in type 1 diabetes. *Diabetes* 2003; 52:133–137.

70. Gastaldelli A, Toschi E, Pettiti M, Frascerra S, Quinones-Galvan A, Sironi A, Natali A, Ferrannini E. Effect of physiological hyperinsulinemia on gluconeogenesis in nondiabetic subjects and in type 2 diabetic patients. *Diabetes* 2001; 50:1807–1812.

71. Dallman MF, Akana SF, Bhatnagar S, Bell ME, Choi S, Chu A, Horsley C, Levin N, Meijer AJ, Soriano LR, Strack AM, Viau V. Starvation: Early signals, sensors and sequelae. *Endocrinology* 1999; 140:4015–4023.

72. Dineen S, Alzaid A, Miles J, Rizza R. Effects of normal nocturnal rise in cortisol on carbohydrate and fat metabolism in IDDM. *Am J Physiol* 1995; 268:E595–E603.

73. Bolli GB, Gerich JE. The "dawn phenomenon": A common occurrence in both insulin-dependent and non-insulin-dependent diabetes mellitus. *New Engl J Med* 1984; 310:746–750.

74. Basu R, Singh RJ, Basu A, Chitilapilly EG, Johnson CM, Toffolo G, Cobelli C, Rizza RA. Splanchnic cortisol production occurs in humans: Evidence for conversion of cortisone to cortisol via the 11-[beta]hydroxysteroid dehydrogenase (11(beta)-HSD) type 1 pathway. *Diabetes* 2004; 53:2051–2059.

75. Jacobson PB, von Geldern TW, Ohman L, Ostrland M, Wang J, Zinker B, Wilcox D, Nguyen PH, Mika A, Fung S, Fey T, Goos-Nilsson A, Grynfarb M, Barkhem T et al. Hepatic glucocorticoid receptor antagonism is sufficient to reduce elevated hepatic glucose output and improve glucose control in animal models of type 2 diabetes. *J Pharmacol Exp Therap* 2005; 314:191–200.

76. Shamoon H, Hendler R, Sherwin RS. Altered responsiveness to cortisol, epinephrine, and glucagon in insulin-infused juvenile-onset diabetics: A mechanism for diabetic instability. *Diabetes* 1980:29:284–291.

77. Van Cauter E, Blackman JD, Roland D, Spire JP, Refetoff S, Polonsky KS. Modulation of glucose regulation and insulin secretion by circadian rhythmicity and sleep. *J Clin Invest* 1991; 88:934–942.

78. LaFleur SE, Kalsbeek A, Wortel J, Buijs RM. A suprachiasmatic nucleus generated rhythm in basal glucose concentrations. *J Neuroendocrinol* 1999; 11:643–652.

79. Goncharuk VD, Van Heerikhuize J, Dai J-P, Swaab D, Buijs RM. Neuropeptide changes in the suprachiasmatic nucleus in primary hypertension indicate functional impairment in the biological clock. *J Comp Neurol* 2001; 431:320–330.

80. Staels B. When the clock stops ticking, metabolic syndrome explodes. *Nature Med* 2006; 12:54–55.

81. LaFleur SE, Kalsbeek A, Wortel J, Fekkes ML, Buijs RM. A daily rhythm in glucose tolerance: A role for the suprachiasmatic nucleus. *Diabetes* 2001; 50:1237–1243.

82. Pocal A, Lam TKT, Gutierrez-Juarez R, Obici S, Schwartz G, Bryan J, Aguilar-Bryan L, Rossetti L. Hypothalamic KATP channels control hepatic glucose production. *Nature* 2005; 434:1026–1031.

83. Kalsbeek A, LaFleur SE, Van Heijningen C, Buijs RM. Suprachiasmatic GABAergic inputs to the paraventricular nucleus control plasma glucose concentrations in the rat via sympathetic innervation of the liver. *J Neurosci* 2004; 24:7604–7613.

84. Moore RY. Neural control of the pineal gland. *Behavioural Brain Res* 1996; 73:125–130.

85. Ishikawa K, Shimazu T. Daily rhythms of glycogen synthase and phosphorylase activities in rat liver: Influence of food and light. *Life Sci* 1976; 19:1873–1878.

86. Chu C, Sindelar DK, Neal DW, Allen EJ, Donahue EP, Cherrington AD. Effect of a selective rise in sinusoidal norephrine on HGP is due to an increase in glycogenolysis. *Am J Physiol Endocrinol Metab* 1998; 274:E162–E171.

87. International Diabetes Federation IGT/IFG Consensus Statement. Report of an Expert Consensus Workshop, 1–4 August 2001, Stoke Poges, UK. Impaired glucose tolerance and impaired fasting glycaemia: The current status on definition and intervention. *Diab Med* 2002; 19:708–723.

88. Schianca GP, Maduli E, Rossi A, Bartoli E, Sainaghi PP. The significance of impaired fasting versus impaired glucose tolerance: Importance of insulin secretion and resistance. *Diabetes Care* 2003; 26:1333–1337.

89. Haffner SM. The importance of hyperglycemia in the nonfasting state to the development of cardiovascular disease. *Endocr Rev* 1998; 19:583–592.

90. Bonora E, Muggeo M. Postprandial blood glucose as a risk factor for cardiovascular disease in type II diabetes: The epidemiological evidence. *Diabetologia* 2001; 44:2107–2114.

91. Firth RG, Bell PM, Marsh HM, Hansen I, Rizza RA. Postprandial hyperglycemia in patients with non-insulin-dependent diabetes mellitus: Role of hepatic and extra-hepatic tissues. *J Clin Invest* 1986; 77:1525–1532.

92. Mitrakou A, Kelley D, Veneman T, Jenssen T, Pangburn T, Reilly J, Gerich J. Contribution of abnormal muscle and liver metabolism to postprandial hyperglycemia in noninsulin-dependent-diabetes mellitus. *Diabetes* 1990; 39:1381–1390.

93. Ferrannini E, Simonson D, Katz L, Reichard G, Bevilacqua S, Barrett E, Olsson M, DeFronzo RA. The disposal of an oral glucose load in patients with non-insulin-dependent diabetes. *Metabolism* 1988; 47:79–85.

94. Alzaid AA, Dinneen SF, Turk DJ, Caumo A, Cobelli C, Rizza RA. Assessment of insulin action and glucose effectiveness in diabetic and nondiabetic humans. *J Clin Invest* 1994; 94:2341–2348.

95. Osei K. The role of splanchnic glucose output in determining glycemic responses after mixed meal in Type 2 diabetic patients and normal subjects. *Pancreas* 1987; 2:386–392.

96. Mevorach M, Giacca A, Aharon Y, Hawkins M, Shamoon H, Rossetti L. Regulation of endogenous glucose production by glucose per se is impaired in type 2 diabetes mellitus. *J Clin Invest* 1998; 102:744–753.

97. Singhal P, Caumo A, Carey PE, Cobelli C, Taylor R. Regulation of endogenous glucose production after a mixed meal in type 2 diabetes. *Am J Physiol Endocrinol Metab* 2002; 283:E275–E283.

98. Brehm ARW, Krssak M, Anderwald C, Bernroider E, Shulman GI, Cobelli C, Hofer A, Nowotny P, Waldhausl W, Roden M. Hepatic glucose metabolism in type 2 diabetes after mixed meal ingestion. *Diabetologia* 2002; 45(suppl 2):A188.

99. Krssak M, Brehm A, Bernroider E, Anderwald C, Nowotny P, Dalla Man C, Cobelli C, Cline GW, Shulman GI, Waldhausl W, Roden M. Alterations in postprandial hepatic glycogen metabolism in type 2 diabetes. *Diabetes* 2004; 53:3048–3056.

100. Fery F, Melot C, Balasse EO. Glucose fluxes and oxidation after an oral glucose load in patients with non-insulin-dependent diabetes mellitus of variable severity. *Metabolism* 1993; 42:522–530.

101. Staehr P, Hother-Nielsen O, Levin K, Holst JJ, Beck-Nielsen H. Assessment of hepatic insulin action in obese type 2 diabetic patients. *Diabetes* 2001; 50:1363–1370.

102. Firth R, Bell P, Rizza R. Insulin action in non-insulin-dependent diabetes mellitus: the relationship between hepatic and extrahepatic insulin resistance and obesity. Metab Clin Exper 1987; 36:1091–1095.

103. Katz H, Homan M, Jensen M, Caumo A, Cobelli C, Rizza R. Assessment of insulin action in NIDDM in the presence of dynamic changes in insulin and glucose concentration. *Diabetes* 1994; 43:289–96.

104. Turk D, Alzaid A, Dinneen S, Nair KS, Rizza R. The effects of non-insulin-dependent diabetes mellitus on the kinetics of onset of insulin action in hepatic and extrahepatic tissues. *J Clin Invest* 1995; 95:755–762.

105. Basu A, Basu R, Shah P, Vella A, Johnson M, Jensen M, Nair KS, Schwenk F, Rizza RA. Type 2 diabetes impairs splanchnic uptake of glucose but does not alter intestinal glucose absorption during enteral glucose feeding: Additional evidence for a defect in hepatic glucokinase activity. *Diabetes* 2001; 50:1351–1362.

106. Nielsen MF, Nyholm B, Caumo A, Chandramouli V, Schumann WC, Cobelli C, Landau BR, Rizza RA, Schmitz O. Prandial glucose effectiveness and fasting gluconeogenesis in insulin-resistant first-degree relatives of patients with type 2 diabetes. *Diabetes* 2000; 49:2135–2141.

107. Radziuk J, Norwich KH, Vranic M. Measurement and validation of non-steady turnover rates with application to the insulin and glucose systems. *Fed Proc* 1974; 33:1855–1864.

108. Radziuk J, McDonald TJ, Rubenstein D, Dupre J. Initial splanchnic extraction of ingested glucose in normal man. *Metabolism* 1978; 27:657–669.

109. Radziuk J. Mathematical basis for the measurement of the rates of glucose appearance and synthesis in vivo. In: *Methods in Diabetes Research: Vol II. Clinical Methods,* Clarke WL, Larner J, Pohl SL (eds.), Wiley, New York, 1986, pp. 143–164.

110. Radziuk J. Tracer methods and the metabolic disposal of a carbohydrate load in man. *Diab/Metab Rev* 1987; 3:231–267.

111. Radziuk J. Assessment methods of carbohydrate metabolism in the liver (glycogenolysis, gluconeo-genesis, and glycogen synthesis). In: *Clinical Research in Diabetes and Obesity: Part I. Methods, Assessment, and Metabolic Regulation,* Draznin B, Rizza R (eds.), Humana Press, Totowa NJ, 1997, pp. 171–201.

112. Radziuk J, Pye S. Endogenous glucose production in type 2 diabetes—basal and postprandial: Role of diurnal rhythms. *J Invest Med* 2004; 52:379–388.

113. Lauro D, Kido Y, Castle AL, Zarnowski MJ, Hayashi H, Ebina Y, Accili D. Impaired glucose toler-ance in mice with a targeted impairment of insulin action in muscle and adipose tissue. *Nat Genet* 1998; 294–298.

114. Gerich JE. Is muscle the major site of insulin resistance in Type 2 (non-insulin-dependent) diabetes mellitus? *Diabetologia* 1991; 34:607–610.

115. Consoli A. Role of liver in pathophysiology of NIDDM. *Diabetes Care* 1992; 15:430–441.

116. Beck-Nielsen H, Hother-Nielsen O, Vaag A, Alford F. Pathogenesis of Type 2 (non-insulin-dependent) diabetes mellitus: The role of skeletal muscle glucose uptake and hepatic glucose production in the development of hyperglycaemia—a critical comment. *Diabetologia* 1994; 37: 217–221.

117. Insulin-mediated reduction of whole body protein breakdown. *J Clin Invest* 1985; 76:2306–2311.

118. Ader M, Bergman R. Peripheral effects of insulin dominate suppression of fasting hepatic glucose production. *Am J Physiol* 1990; 258:E1020–E1032.

119. Sindelar DK et al. The role of fatty acids in mediating the effects of peripheral insulin on hepatic glucose production in the conscious dog. *Diabetes* 1997; 46:187–196.

120. Lewis GF, Sinman B, Groenwoud Y, Vranic M, Giacca A. Hepatic glucose production is regulated both by direct hepatic and extrahepatic effects of insulin in humans. *Diabetes* 1996; 45:454–462

121. Obici S, Feng Z, Karkanias G, Baskin DG, Rossetti L. Decreasing hypothalamic insulin receptors causes hyperphagia and insulin resistance in rats. *Nat Neurosci* 2002; 5:566–572.

122. Obici S, Shang BB, Karkanias G, Rossetti L. Hypothalamic insulin signaling is required for inhibition of glucose production. *Nat Med* 2002; 8:1376–1382.

123. Burcelin R, Munoz MC, Guillam M-T, Thorens B. Liver hyperplasia and paradoxical regulation of glycogen metabolism and glucose-sensitive gene expression in GLUT2-null hepatocytes. *J Biol Chem* 2000; 275:10930–10936.

124. Hetenyi G Jr, Kopstick FX, Retlstorf LJ. The effect of insulin on the distribution of glucose between the blood plasma and the liver in alloxan-diabetic and adrenalectomized rats. *Can J Biochem Physiol* 1963; 41:2431–2439.

125. Pilkis SJ, Claus TH. Hepatic gluconeogenesis/glycolysis: Regulation and structure/function relation-ships of substrate cycle enzymes. *Ann Rev Nutr* 1990; 11:465–515.

126. Newsholme EA, Crabtree B. Substrate cycles in metabolic regulation and heat generation. *Biochem Soc Symp* 1976; 41:61–110.

127. Hers HG. *Biochem Soc Trans* 1976; 4:985–988.

128. Katz J, Rognstad R. *Curr Top Cell Regul* 1976; 10:238–289.

129. Hellerstein MK, Neese RA, Linfoot P, Christiansen M, Turner S, Letscher A. Hepatic gluconeogenic fluxes and glycogen turnover during fasting in humans: A stable isotope study. *J Clin Invest* 1997; 100:1305–1319.

130. David M, Petit W, Laughlin M, Shulman R, King J, Barrett E. Simultaneous synthesis and degrada-tion of rat liver glycogen. *J Clin Invest* 1990; 86:612–617.

131. Shulman GI, Rothman DL, Chung Y, Rossetti L, Petit WA, Barrett EJ, Shulman RG. ^{13}C NMR studies of glycogen turnover in the perfused rat liver. *J Biol Chem* 1988; 263:5027–5029.

132. Zhang Z, Radziuk J. Insulin effects on hepatic glucose production: Extent and pathways. *Diabetologia* 1997; 40(supp 1)979:A249.

133. Radziuk J, Pye S. The liver, insulin action and resistance. In: *Contemporary Endocrinology: Insulin Resistance*, Reaven G, Laws A (eds.), Humana Press, Totowa, NJ, 1999, pp. 197–231.
134. Radziuk J, Pye S. Hepatic glucose uptake, gluconeogenesis and the regulation of glycogen synthesis. *Diab Metab Res Rev* 2001; 17:250–272.
135. Radziuk J. Hepatic glycogen formation by direct uptake of glucose following oral glucose loading in man. *Can J Physiol Pharmacol* 1979; 57:1196–1199.
136. Radziuk J. Glucose and glycogen metabolism following glucose ingestion: A turnover approach. In: *Carbohydrate Metabolism: Quantitative Physiology and Modelling*, Cobelli C, Bergman R (eds.), Wiley, London, 1981, pp. 239–266.
137. Radziuk J. Source of carbon in hepatic glycogen synthesis during absorption of an oral glucose load in humans. *Fed Proc* 1982; 41:88–90.
138. Radziuk J. Hepatic glycogen in humans: I. Direct formation after oral and intravenous glucose or after a 24-hr fast. *Am J Physiol* 1989; 257:E145–157.
139. Radziuk J. Hepatic glycogen in humans: II. Gluconeogenetic formation after oral and intravenous glucose. *Am J Physiol* 1989; 257:E158–169.
140. Hems DA, Whitton PO, Taylor EA. Glycogen synthesis in the perfused liver of the starved rat. *Biochem J* 1972; 129:529–538.
141. Sugden MC, Watts DI, Palmer TN, Myles DD. Direction of carbon flux in starvation and after refeeding: In vitro and in vivo effects of 3-mercaptopicolinate. *Biochem Intern* 1983; 7:329–337.
142. Newgard CB, Moore SV, Foster DW, McGarry JD. Efficient hepatic glycogen synthesis in refeeding rats requires continued carbon flow through the gluconeogenic pathway. *J Biol Chem* 1984; 259:6958–6963.
143. Jungermann K, Thurman RG. Hepatocyte heterogeneity in the metabolism of carbohydrates. *Enzyme* 1992; 46:33–58.
144. Jungermann K, KietzmannT. Role of oxygen in the zonation of carbohydrate metabolism and gene expression in the liver. *Kidney Int* 1997; 51:402–412.
145. Zhang Z, Radziuk J. Effects of lactate on pathways of glycogen formation in the perfused rat liver. *Biochem J* 1991; 280:419–425.
146. Zhang Z, Radziuk J. The coordinated regulation of hepatic glycogen formation in the perfused rat liver by glucose and lactate. *Am J Physiol* 1994; 266:E583–E591.
147. Radziuk J, Zhang Z, Wiernsperger N, Pye S. Effects of metformin on lactate uptake and gluconeogenesis in the perfused rat liver. *Diabetes* 1997; 46:1406–1413.
148. Song S, Andrikopoulos S, Filippis C, Thorburn AW, Khan D, Proietto J. Mechanism of fat-induced hepatic gluconeogenesis: effect of metformin. *Am J Physiol Endocrinol Metab* 2001; 281: E275–E282.
149. Otto M, Breinholt J, Westergaard N. Metformin inhibits glycogen synthesis and gluconeogenesis in cultured rat hepatocytes. *Diab Obes Metab* 2003; 5:189–194.
150. Agius L, Peak M, Newgard CB, Gomez-Foix AM, Guinovart JJ. Evidence for a role of glucose-induced translocation of glucokinase in the control of glycogen synthesis. *J Biol Chem* 1996; 48:30479–33048.
151. Towle HC. Metabolic regulation of gene transcription in mammals. *J Biol Chem* 1995; 270: 23235–23238.
152. Argaud D, Kirby TL, Newgard CB, Lange AJ. Stimulation of glucose-6-phosphatase gene expression by glucose and fructose-2,6-bisphosphate. *J Biol Chem* 1997; 272:12854–12861.
153. Newgard CB, Foster DW, McGarry JD. Evidence for suppression of hepatic glucose-6-phosphatase activity with carbohydrate feeding. *Diabetes* 1984; 33:192–195.
154. Minassian C, Daniele N, Bordet J-C, Zitoun C, Mithieux G. Liver glucose-6-phosphatase activity is inhibited by refeeding in rats. *J Nutr* 1995; 125:2727–2732.
155. Gardner L, Liu Z, Barrett E. The role of glucose-6-phosphatase in the action of insulin on hepatic glucose production in the rat. *Diabetes* 1984; 42:192–195.
156. Mithieux G. New knowledge regarding glucose-6-phosphatase gene and protein and their roles in the regulation of glucose metabolism. *Eur J Endocrinol* 1997; 136:137–145.
157. Hers HG. The control of glycogen metabolism in the liver. *Ann Rev Biochem* 1976; 45:167–189.
158. van de Werve G, Jeanrenaud B. Liver glycogen metabolism: An overview. *Diab/Metab Rev* 1987; 3:47–78.
159. Nutall FQ, Gilboe DP, Gannon MC, Niewohner CB, Tan AWH. Regulation of glycogen synthesis in the liver. *Am J Med* 1988; 85(suppl 5A):77–85.

160. O'Doherty RM, Lehman DL, Seoane J, Gomez-Foix AM, Guinovart JJ, Newgard CB. Differential metabolic effects of adenovirus-mediated glucokinase and hexokinase I overexpression in rat primary hepatocytes. *J Biol Chem* 1997; 271:20524–20530.

161. Ortmeyer H, Bodkin N, Hansen B. Insulin regulates liver glycogen synthase and glycogen phosphorylase activity reciprocally in rhesus monkeys. *Am J Physiol* 1997; 272:E133–E138.

162. Kruszynska YT, Home PD, Albert KGMM. In vivo regulation of liver and skeletal muscle glycogen synthase activity by glucose and insulin. *Diabetes* 1986; 35:662–667.

163. Terrettaz J, Assimacopoulos-Jeannet F, Jeanrenaud B. Inhibition of hepatic glucose production by insulin in vivo in rats: Contribution of glycolysis. *Am J Physiol* 1986; 250:E346–E351.

164. Liu Z, Gardner L, Barrett E. Insulin and glucose suppress hepatic glycogenolysis by distinct enzymatic mechanisms. *Metabolism* 1993; 42:1546–1551.

165. Fernandez-Novell JM, Roca A, Bellido D, Vilaró S, Guinovart JJ. Translocation and aggregation of hepatic glycogen synthase during the fasted to refed transition in rats. *Eur J Biochem* 1996; 238:570–575.

166. Soskin S. The liver and carbohydrate metabolism. *Endocrinology* 1940; 26:297–308.

167. Parkes JL, Grieninger G. Insulin, not glucose, controls hepatocellular glycogen deposition. *J Biol Chem* 1985; 260:8090–8097.

168. Gitzelman R, Spycher MA, Feil G, Muller J, Seilnacht B, Stahl M, Bosshard NU. Liver glycogen synthase deficiency: A rarely diagnosed entity. *Eur J Ped* 1996; 155:561–567.

169. Consoli A. Role of liver in pathophysiology of NIDDM. *Diabetes Care* 1992; 15:430–441.

170. Stumvoll M, Perriello G, Nurjhan N, Bucci A, Welle S, Jansson PA, Dailey G, Bier D, Jenssen T, Gerich J. Glutamine and alanine metabolism in NIDDM. *Diabetes* 1996; 45:863–888.

171. Perriello G, Pampanelli S, Del Sindaco P, Lalli C, Ciofetta M, Volpi E, Santeusanio F, Brunetti P, Bolli GB. Evidence of increased systemic glucose production and gluconeogenesis in early stages of NIDDM. *Diabetes* 1997; 46:1010–1016.

172. Magnusson I, Rothman DL, Katz LD, Shulman RG, Shulman GI. Increased rate of gluconeogenesis in type II diabetes mellitus: A 13C nuclear magnetic resonance study. *J Clin Invest* 1992; 86:489–497.

173. Hellerstein MK. Isotopic studies of carbohydrate metabolism in non-insulin-dependent diabetes mellitus. *Curr Op Endocrinol Diab* 1995; 2:518–529.

174. Magnusson I, Rothman DL, Jucker B, Cline GW, Shulman RG, Shulman GI. Liver glycogen turnover in fed and fasted humans. *Am J Physiol* 1994; 266:E796–803.

175. Clore JN, Post EP, Bailey J, Nestler JE, Blackard WG. Evidence for increased liver glycogen in patients with noninsulin-dependent diabetes mellitus after a 3-day fast. *J Clin Endocrinol Metab* 1992; 74:660–666.

176. Müller C, Assimacopoulos-Jeannet F, Mosimam F, Schneiter Ph, Riou JP, Pachiaudi C, Felber JP, Jequier E, Jeanrenaud B, Tappy L. Endogenous glucose production, gluconeogenesis and liver glycogen concentration in obese non-diabetic patients. *Diabetologia* 1997; 40.

177. Magnusson I, Rothman DL, Katz LD, Shulman RG, Shulman GI. Increased rate of gluconeogenesis in type II diabetes mellitus: A 13C nuclear magnetic resonance study. *J Clin Invest* 1992; 86:489–497.

178. Llado I, Palou A, Pons A. Hepatic glycogen and lactate handling in dietary obese rats. *Ann Nutr Metabol* 1998; 42:181–188.

179. Chen YD, Varasteh BB, Reaven GM. Plasma lactate concentration in obesity and type 2 diabetes. *Diabete et Metabolisme* 1993; 19:348–354.

180. Lovejoy J, Newby FD, Gebhart SS, DiGirolamo M. Insulin resistance in obesity is associated with elevated basal lactate levels and diminished lactate appearance following intravenous glucose and insulin. *Metabolism* 1992; 41:22–27.

181. King JL, DiGirolamo M. Lactate production from glucose and response to insulin in perfused adipocytes from mesenteric and epididymal regions of lean and obese rats. *Obes Res* 1998; 6:69–75.

182. Giaccari A, Rossetti L. Predominant role of gluconeogenesis in the hepatic glycogen repletion of diabetic rats. *J Clin Invest* 1992; 89:36–45.

183. Watanabe RM, Lovejoy J, Steil GM, Digirolamo M, Bergman RN. Insulin sensitivity accounts for glucose and lactate kinetics after intravenous glucose. *Diabetes* 1995; 44:954–962.

184. Madison LL, Mebane D, Lecocq F, Combes B. Physiological significance of the secretion of endogenous insulin into the portal circulation: V. The quantitative importance of the liver in the disposition of glucose loads. *Diabetes* 1963; 12:8–15.

185. Barrett E, Liu Z. Hepatic glucose metabolism and insulin resistance in NIDDM and obesity. *Bailliere's Clin Endocrinol Metab* 1993; 7:875–901.

186. Barrett EJ, Ferrannini E, Gusberg R, Bevilacqua S, DeFronzo RA. Hepatic and extrahepatic splanchnic glucose metabolism in the postabsorptive and glucose fed dog. *Metabolism* 1985; 34:410–420.

187. Maheux P, Chen Y-D, Polonsky K, Reaven G. Evidence that insulin can directly inhibit hepatic glucose production. *Diabetologia* 1997; 40:1300–1306.

188. Cherrington AD, Edgerton D, Sindalar DK. The direct and indirect effects of insulin on hepatic glucose production in vivo. *Diabetologia* 1998; 41:987–996.

189. Lewis GF, Carpentier A, Vranic M, Giacca A. Resistance to insulin's acute direct hepatic effect in suppressing steady-state glucose production in individuals with type 2 diabetes. *Diabetes* 1999; 48:570–576.

190. Basu A, Basu R, Shah P, Vella A, Johnson M, Nair KS, Jensen MD, Schwenk F, Rizza RA. Effects of type 2 diabetes on the ability of insulin and glucose to regulate splanchnic and muscle glucose metabolism: Evidence for a defect in hepatic glucokinase activity. *Diabetes* 2000; 49:272–283.

191. Gastadelli A, Toschi E, Pettiti M, Frascerra S, Quinones-Galvan A, Sironi AM, Natali A, Ferrannini E. Effect of physiological hyperinsulinemia on gluconeogenesis in nondiabetic subjects and in type 2 diabetic patients. *Diabetes* 2001; 50:1807–1812.

192. Rebrin K, Steil GM, Getty L, Bergman RN. Free fatty acid as a link in the regulation of hepatic glucose output by peripheral insulin. *Diabetes* 1995; 44:1038–1045.

193. Vaag A, Alford F, Henriksen FL, Christopher M, Beck-Nielsen H. Multiple defects of both hepatic and peripheral intracellular glucose processing contribute to the hyperglycemia of diabetes. *Diabetologia* 1995; 38:326–336.

194. Pigon J, Giacca A, Ostenson C-G, Lam L, Vranic M, Efendic S. Normal hepatic insulin sensitivity in lean, mild noninsulin-dependent diabetic patients. *J Clin Endocrinol Metab* 1996; 81:3702–3708.

195. Wise SD, Nielsen MF, Cryer PE, Rizza RA. Overnight normalization of glucose concentrations improves hepatic but not extrahepatic insulin action in subjects with type 2 diabetes mellitus. *J Clin Endocrinol Metab* 1998; 83:2461–2469.

196. Radziuk J, Inculet R. The effects of ingested and intravenous glucose on forearm uptake of glucose and glucogenic substrate in normal man. *Diabetes* 1983; 32:977–981.

197. Luzi L, DeFronzo RA. Effect of loss of first-phase secretion on hepatic glucose production and tissue glucose disposal in humans. *Am J Physiol* 1989; 257:E241–246.

198. Del Prato S, Tiengo A. The importance of first-phase insulin secretion: Implications for the therapy of type 2 diabetes mellitus. *Diab/Metab Res Rev* 2001; 17:164–174.

199. Boden G. Gluconeogenesis and glycogenolysis in health and diabetes. *J Invest Med* 2004; 52:375–378.

200. Gastaldelli A, Toschi E, Pettiti M et al. Effect of physiological hyperinsulinemia on gluconeogenesis in nondiabetic subjects and type 2 diabetic patients. *Diabetes* 2001; 50:1807–1812

201. Boden G, Cheung P, Stein TP et al. FFA cause hepatic insulin resistance by inhibiting insulin suppression of glycogenolysis. *Am J Physiol* 2002; 283:E12–19.

202. Edgerton DS, Carin S, Emschwiller M et al. Small increases in insulin inhibit hepatic glucose production solely caused by an effect of glycogen metabolism. *Diabetes* 2001; 50:1872–1882.

203. Perley MJ, Kipnis DM. Plasma insulin response to oral and intravenous glucose: studies in normal and diabetic subjects. *J Clin Invest* 1967; 46:1954–1962.

204. Felig P, Wahren J, Hendler R. Influence of maturity-onset diabetes on splanchnic glucose balance after oral glucose ingestion. *Diabetes* 1978; 27:121–126.

205. Wahren J, Hagenfeldt L, Felig P. Splanchnic and leg exchange of glucose, amino acids, and free fatty acids during exercise in diabetes mellitus. *J Clin Invest* 1975; 55:1303–1314.

206. Ferrannini E, Bjorkman O, Reichard GA, Pilo A, Olsson M, Wahren J, DeFronzo RA. The disposal of an oral glucose load in healthy subjects. *Diabetes* 1985; 34:580–588.

207. Pehling G, Tessari P, Gerich JE, Haymond MW, Service FJ, Rizza RA. Abnormal meal carbohydrate disposition in insulin-dependent diabetes. *J Clin Invest* 1984; 74:985–991.

208. McMahon M, Marsh M, Rizza RA. Effects of basal insulin supplementation on disposition of mixed meal in obese patients with NIDDM. *Diabetes* 1989; 38:291–303.

209. Ferrannini E, Wahren J, Felig P, DeFronzo RA. The role of fractional glucose extraction in the regulation of splanchnic glucose metabolism in normal and diabetic man. *Metabolism* 1980; 29:28–35.

210. Ludvik B, Nolan JJ, Roberts A, Baloga J, Joyce M, Bell JM, Olefsky JM. Evidence for decreased splanchnic glucose uptake after oral glucose administration in non-insulin-dependent diabetes mellitus. *J Clin Invest* 1997; 100:2354–2361.

211. DeFronzo RA, Ferrannini E, Hendler R, Felig P, Wahren J. Regulation of splanchnic and peripheral glucose uptake by insulin and hyperglycemia in man. *Diabetes* 1983; 32:35–45.

212. McGarry JD. Dysregulation of fatty acid metabolism in the etiology of type 2 diabetes. *Diabetes* 2002; 51:7–18.

213. Zammit VA, Waterman IJ, Topping D, McKay G. Insulin stimulation of hepatic triacylglycerol secretion and the etiology of insulin resistance. *J Nutr* 2001; 131:2074–2077.

214. Ginsberg HN, Zhang Y-L, Hernandez-Ono A. Regulation of plasma triglycerides in insulin resistance and diabetes. *Arch Med Res* 2005; 36:232–240.

215. Horton JD, Goldstein JL, Brown MS. SREBPs: Activators of complete program of cholesterol and fatty acid synthesis in the liver. *J Clin Invest* 2002; 109:1125–1131.

216. Foufelle F, Ferre P. New perspectives in the regulation of hepatic glycolytic and lipogenic genes by insulin and glucose: A role for the transcription factor sterol regulatory element binding protein-1c. *Biochem J* 2002; 366:377–391.

217. Hellerstein MK. De novo lipogenesis in humans: metabolic and regulatory aspects. *Eur J Clin Nutr* 1999; 53(suppl 1):S53–S65.

218. Heilbronn L, Smith SR, Ravussin E. Failure of fat cell proliferation, mitochondrial function and fat oxidation results in ectopic fat storage, insulin resistance and type II diabetes mellitus. *Int J Obes* 2004; 28:S12–S21.

219. Randle PJ. Regulatory interactions between lipids and carbohydrates: the glucose fatty acid cycle after 35 years. *Diab Metab Rev* 1998; 14:263–283.

220. Rosella G, Zajac J, Kaczmarczyk S, Andrikopoulos S, Proietto J. Impaired suppression of gluconeogenesis induced by overexpression of a noninsulin-responsive phosphoenolpyruvate carboxykinase gene. *Met Endoc* 1993; 7:1456–1462.

221. Rosella G, Zajac JD, Baker L, Kaczmarczyk SJ, Andrikopoulos S, Adams TE, Proietto J. Impaired glucose tolerance and increased weight gain in transgenic rats overexpressing a non-insulin-responsive phosphoenolpyruvate carboxykinase gene. *Mol Endoc* 1995; 9(10):1396–1404.

222. O'Doherty RM, Lehman DL, Telemaque-Potts S, Newgard CB. Metabolic impact of glucokinase overexpression in liver: Lowering blood glucose in fed rats is accompanied by hyperlipidemia.

223. Boden G, Chen X, Capulong E, Mozzoli M. Effects of free fatty acids on gluconeogenesis and autoregulation of glucose production in type 2 diabetes. *Diabetes* 2001; 50:810–816.

224. Gustafson LA, Neeft M, Reijngoud D-J, Kuipers F, Sauerwein HP, Romijn JA, Herling AW, Burger H-J, Meijer AJ. Fatty acid and amino acid modulation of glucose cycling in isolated rat hepatocytes. *Biochem J* 2001; 358:665–671.

225. Gabriely I, Barzilai N. Surgical removal of visceral adipose tissue: Effects on insulin action. *Curr Diab Repts* 2003; 3:201–206.

226. Kim JK, Fillmore JJ, Chen Y, Yu C, Moore IK, Pypaert M, Lutz EP, Kako Y, Velez-Carrasco W, Goldberg IJ, Breslow JL, Shulman GI. Tissue-specific overexpression of lipoprotein lipase causes tissue-specific insulin resistance. *Proc Natl Acad Sci USA* 2001; 98:7522–7527.

227. Oakes N, Cooney G, Camilleri S, Chisholm D, Kraegen E. Mechanisms of liver and muscle insulin resistance induced by chronic high-fat feeding. *Diabetes* 1997; 46:1768–1774.

228. Andrikopoulos S, Proietto J. The biochemical basis of increased hepatic glucose production in a mouse model of type 2 (non-insulin-dependent) diabetes mellitus. *Diabetologia* 1995; 38:1389–1396.

229. Wu C, Okar DA, Newgard CB, Lange AJ. Increasing fructose 2,6-bisphosphate overcomes hepatic insulin resistance of type 2 diabetes. *Am J Physiol* 2002; 282:E38–E45.

230. Angulo P. Nonalcoholic fatty liver disease. *N Engl J Med* 2002; 346:1221–1231.

231. Robertson G, Leclerq I, Farrell GC. Nonalcoholic steatosis and steatohepatitis: II. Cytochrome P-450 enzymes and oxidative stress. *Am J Physiol Gastrointest Liver Physiol* 2001; 281:G1135–G1139.

232. den Boer M, Voshol PJ, Kuipers F, Havekes LM, Romijn JA. Hepatic steatosis: A mediator of the metabolic syndrome, lessons from animal models. *Arterioscler Thromb Vasc Biol* 2004; 24:644–649.

233. Song S. The role of increased liver triglyceride content: A culprit of diabetic hyperglycemia? *Diab Metab Res Rev* 2002; 18:5–12.

234. Zhang W, Patil S, Chauhan B, Guo S, Powell DR, Le J, Klotsas A, Matika R, Xiao X, Franks R, Heidenreich KA, Sajan MP, Farese RV, Stolz DB, Tso P, Koo SH, Montminy M, Unterman TG. FoxO1 regulates multiple metabolic pathways in the liver: Effects on gluconeogenic, glycolytic, and lipogenic expression. *J Biol Chem* 2006; 281:10105–10117.

235. Hardie DG. AMP-activated protein kinase: a master switch in glucose and lipid metabolism. *Rev Endoc Metab Disord* 2004; 5:119–125.

236. Role of peroxisome prolfierator-activated receptor-γ in the glucose-sensing apparatus of liver and beta cells. *Diabetes* 2004; 53(suppl 1):S60–S65.

237. Zhou XY, Shibusawa N, Naik K, Porras D, Temple K, Ou H, Kaihara K, Roe MW, Brady MJ, Wondisford FE. Insulin regulation of hepatic gluconeogenesis through phosphorylation of CREB-binding protein. *Nature Med* 2004; 10:633–637.

238. Duran-Sandoval D, Caiou B, Percevault F, Hennuyer N, Grefhorst A, van Dijk TH, Gonzalez FJ, Fruchart J-C, Kuipers F, Staels B. The farnesoid X receptor modulates hepatic carbohydrate metabolism during the fasting-refeeding transition. *J Biol Chem* 2005; 280:29971–29979.

239. Rodgers JT, Lerin C, Haas W, Gygl SP, Spiegelman B, Puigserver P. Nutrient control of glucose homeostasis through a complex of PGC-1α and SIRT1. *Nature* 2005; 434:113–118.

240. Cao W, Collins QF, Becker TC, Robidoux J, Lupo EG Jr, Xiong Y, Daniel KW, Floerling L, Collins S. p38 mitogen-activated protein kinase plays a stimulatory role in hepatic gluconeogenesis. *J Biol Chem* 2005; 280:42731–42737.

241. Taniguchi CM, Ueki K, Kahn CR. Complementary roles of IRS-1 and IRS-2 in the hepatic regulation of metabolism. *J Clin Invest* 2005; 115:718–727.

242. Makowski L, Hotamisligil GS. Fatty acid binding proteins: The evolutionary crossroads of inflammatory and metabolic responses. *J Nutr* 2004; 134:2464S–2468S.

243. Schilling CH, Letscher D, Palsson BO. Theory for the systemic definition of metabolic pathways and their use in interpreting metabolic function from a pathway-oriented perspective. *J Theor Biol* 2000; 203:229–248.

244. Schilling CH, Edwards JS, Letscher D, Palsson BO. Combining pathway analysis with flux balance analysis for the comprehensive study of metabolic systems. *Biotechnol Bioeng* 2001; 71:286–306.

245. Savageau MA. Biochemical systems theory: Alternative views of metabolic control. In: *Control of Metabolic Processes*, Cornish-Bowden A, Cardenas ML (eds.), Plenum Press, New York, 1990, p. 69.

246. Hofmeyr JH, Cornish-Bowden A. Quantitative assessment of regulation in metabolic systems. *Eur J Biochem* 1991; 200:2231.

247. Brand MD. Regulation analysis of energy metabolism. *J Exp Biol* 1997; 200:193.

248. Minorsky N. *Nonlinear Oscillations,* Princeton NJ, Van Nostrand, 1962.

249. Ferrannini E, Nannipieri M, Williams K, Gonzales C, Haffner SM, Stern MP. Mode of onset of type 2 diabetes from normal or impaired glucose tolerance. *Diabetes* 2004; 53:160–165.

250. Mackey MC, Glass L. Oscillations and chaos in physiological control systems. *Science* 1977; 197:287–289.

251. Glass L, Mackey MC. Pathological oscillations resulting from instabilities in physiological control systems. *Ann NY Acad Sci* 1979; 316:214–235.

252. Guyton AC, Crowell JW, Moore JW. Basic oscillating mechanism of Cheyne-Stokes breathing. *Am J Physiol* 1956; 187:395–398.

253. Guevara MR, Shrier A, Glass L. Phase-locked rhythms in periodically stimulated heart cell aggregates. *Am J Physiol* 1988; 254:H1–H10.

254. Lasota A, Mackey MC, Wazewska-Czyzewska M. Minimizing therapeutically induced anemia. *J Math Biol* 1981; 13:149–158.

255. Freiesleben De Blasio B, Bak P, Pociot F, Karlsen AE, Nerup J. Onset of type 1 diabetes: A dynamical instability. *Diabetes* 1999; 48:1677–1685.

256. Kahn R, Buse J, Ferrannini E, Stern M. The metabolic syndrome: time for critical appraisal. Joint statement form the American Diabetes Association and the European Association for the study of diabetes. *Diabetologia* 2005; 48:1684–1699.

257. Gale EAM. The myth of the metabolic syndrome. *Diabetologia* 2005; 48:1679–1683.

258. Pietropaolo M, Barinas-Mitchell E, Kuller LH. The heterogeneity of diabetes: unraveling a dispute: is systemic inflammation related to islet autoimmunity? *Diabetes* 2007; 56(5):1189–1197.

259. Yudkin JS. Insulin resistance and the metabolic syndrome-or the pitfalls of epidemiology. *Diabetologia* 2007; 50(8):1576–1586.

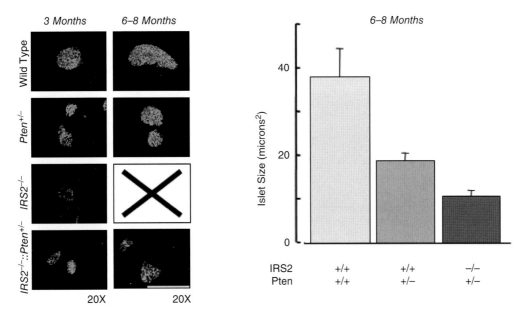

Figure 14.5. Islet histology of *IRS2+/−::Pten+/−* intercross mice. Representative islet histology of pancreas sections from 3-month-old (left panels) and 6–8-month-old (right panels) mice immunostained with antibodies against insulin (green) and glucagon (red) photographed with a 5× or 20× objective. Scale bars: 500 µm. Islet morphometric analysis of *IRS2+/−::Pten+/−* intercross mice at 6–8 months of age. Islet size calculated by mean cross-sectional area of multicelled islets reported as microns $\times 10^3$/islet. Results are expressed as mean ±SEM of at least 5 mice per group. (See discussion on p. 263.)

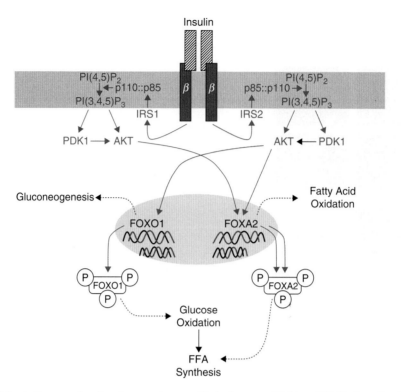

Figure 14.6. A diagram showing the putative specificity between IRS1 and IRS2 signaling in hepatic regulation of gene expression through the phosphorylation and cytosolic translocation of FOXO1 and FOXA2. Nuclear FOXO1 largely mediates gluconeogenesis, whereas nuclear FOXA2 promotes fatty acid oxidation and inhibits synthesis. Since FOXA2 might be targeted for phosphorylation through IRS1 and IRS2 signaling, it might be coupled more tightly than FOXO1 to insulin stimulation under certain conditions. This imbalanced coupling can result in the characteristic gluconeogenesis and fatty acid synthesis that occurs in type 2 diabetes. (See discussion on p. 265.)

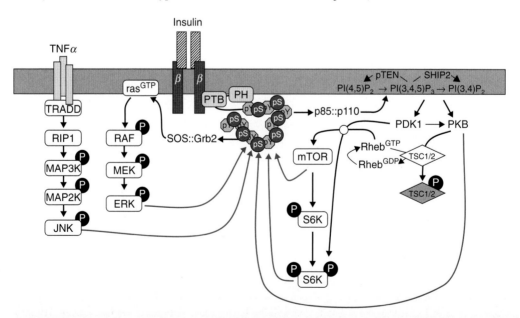

Figure 14.7. Schematic diagram of feedback inhibition of insulin signaling mediated by serine phosphorylation of IRS1. Various kinases in the insulin signaling cascade are implicated in this feedback mechanism, including PKB, mTOR, S6K, and ERK. Other kinases activated by heterologous signals are also involved. (See discussion on p. 266.)

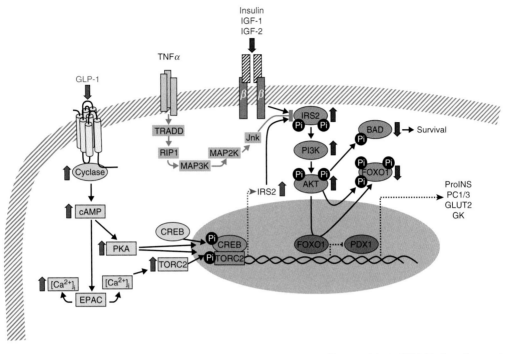

Figure 14.8. A diagram describing the intersection of glucagon-like peptide-1 (GLP1) signaling and insulin/IGF signaling. GLP1 strongly activates the cAMP→CREB signaling cascade in β-cells, which promotes the expression of various genes, including IRS2. Since IRS2 is important for activation of various pathways that promote β-cell function, some of the long-term effects of GLP1 can be mediated through IRS2 expression. IRS-2 function is also a target of proinflammatory cytokines, so IRS2 can integrate many of the conflicting signals that reach β-cell. (See discussion on p. 268.)

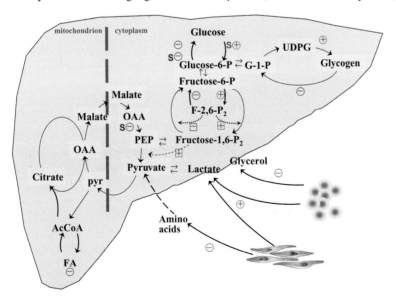

Figure 18.3. Effects of insulin on metabolic pathways in the liver. Inhibitory effects on enzyme activities or substrate concentrations are indicated with (−) and stimulatory effects with (+). Primary effects are indicated by circles and secondary effects by boxes. Effects on new enzyme synthesis are preceded by an "S". (See discussion on p. 353.)

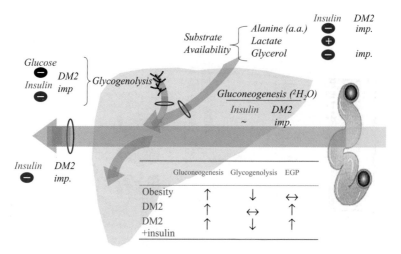

Figure 18.4. Summary of insulin effects on the components of principal glucose fluxes during meal absorption, and their impairment in type 2 diabetes. (See discussion on p. 355.)

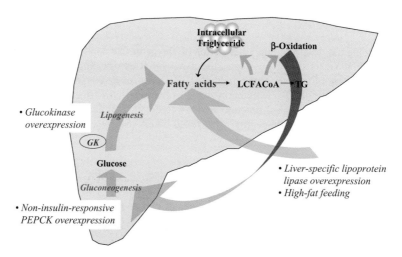

Figure 18.5. Schematic illustrating some of the interactions between glucose and lipid metabolism, and demonstrating that increased glucose production will increase both FFA and liver lipid deposition, which in turn will accelerate gluconeogenesis. (See discussion on p. 357.)

19 Chronomics of the Metabolic Syndrome

Barbara Caleen Hansen

CONTENTS

ABSTRACT

Wars are raging over the definition of the *metabolic syndrome*—and whether it even exists or is a useful concept. Looking closely at the various viewpoints concerning the definition of the syndrome, one comes to the inescapable conclusion that they are *all* right! Although some would equate this defining of the syndrome to the efforts of the six men of Industan (who to learning were much inclined), others would cry, "The Emperor has no clothes!" Still others would see it as Stone Soup, gathering ingredients from hither and yon. Let us hope instead that we have provided Soup for the Soul and rekindled your interest in this, the most prevalent of syndromes.

A LONG LOOK BACK

The best prospective study starts with a long look back. For the metabolic syndrome, a case may be made that the diabetic patient succumbing to heart disease has fully manifested the endpoint(s) of this syndrome. But what are the intermediate points or

From: *Contemporary Endocrinology: The Metabolic Syndrome: Epidemiology, Clinical Treatment, and Underlying Mechanisms*
Edited by: B.C. Hansen and G.A. Bray © Humana Press, Totowa, NJ

features, and how did the patient get there? What was the natural trajectory, and what mechanisms drove the development of this complex disorder? What caused him to get it early—or late—within his expected life span? Were there features in his early stages of progression that had long-range predictive capability? Most importantly, can this ultimate endpoint be postponed or prevented?

DEFINING THE METABOLIC SYNDROME: THE IMPORTANCE OF VIEWPOINT

Today, in 0.18 seconds, Google found 2,020,000 citations to the metabolic syndrome, and 1,320,000 emerged in a search of the insulin-resistance syndrome. The metabolic syndrome is an aging-related cluster of metabolic disorders associated with excess adiposity, and plausibly mechanistically linked. It frequently develops as the *prodrome* to the development of overt type 2 diabetes mellitus (T2DM). Over the years, the metabolic syndrome has had various names. These names and their respective guidelines for diagnosis reflect the viewpoint of each of the writers (1); however, while personal opinions based on experience are often very sincere, they can also be very flawed (2). John Godfrey Saxe (1816–1887) popularized an old Hindu folktale in a poem entitled *The Blind Men and the Elephant*:

> *It was six men of Industan to learning much inclined,*
> *Who went to see the elephant, though all of them were blind,*
> *That each by observation might satisfy his mind.*

The first fell against the side—and found it like a wall, the second—the tusk—like a spear, the third—the trunk—like a snake, the fourth—the leg—like a tree, the fifth—an ear—like a leaf, and the sixth—the tail—like a rope.

We conclude this section by paraphrasing the poem in terms of the metabolic syndrome:

> *Often in scientific wars the disputants we have seen,*
> *Rail on somewhat in ignorance of what each other mean,*
> *And each is partly right, and all are in the wrong;*
> *They prate about a syndrome that none has clearly seen!*

Nevertheless, despite the varied points of view, metabolic syndrome exists, just as an elephant exists. How, then, shall it be defined?

KEY FEATURES OF THE METABOLIC SYNDROME: A REDUCTIONIST APPROACH FOR THE EPIDEMIOLOGIST OR FOR THE CLINICAL PRACTITIONER

Over the past 10 years, medical organizations have drafted a series of definitions for the metabolic syndrome (3–8).

Whether the metabolic syndrome is an obesity syndrome (9), a lipid syndrome (3,8,10), an insulin-resistance syndrome (4,11,12), or a pre-diabetes syndrome (3,6,13), its underlying mechanisms are not yet clear (14). What is clear is that key risk factors for both CVD and diabetes precede the onset of type 2 diabetes (11,12,15,16). In addition, there are specific high-impact risk factors for CVD that are not related to the metabolic syndrome, including smoking and high LDL cholesterol, two factors whose contributions are so strong that they lower the weight of the metabolic syndrome to predict CVD (16).

Consistency has emerged in defining the key features of the syndrome: excess adiposity, disturbed glucose metabolism, dyslipidemia, and hypertension. Each has multiple methods of assessment, and each method has cut points or criteria specific to it that may not be fully congruous with other methods of assessment for the same key feature. In our current approaches to analyzing the metabolic syndrome, we generally identify each component part. In assessing these parts, we attempt to determine what fraction of the variance in one is determined by the level of another. Although some 100+ variables have been associated with the metabolic syndrome, not all of these appear to carry equal weight in defining either progression or risk of endpoints. Few key variables document the metabolic syndrome at its *earliest* time points, while many are important at later time points in this progressive and changing pattern (and therefore *perform* as epidemiologically more predictive features). Furthermore, the complications of diabetes increase in those who also have the features of the metabolic syndrome (17–19).

Absolute cut points of clearly specified variables that are easily measured with high reliability are sought by the epidemiologist in order to classify individuals into groups with or without the metabolic syndrome (15,20–29). Also, clinicians seek clean and clear definitions leading to unambiguous diagnoses (30,31). Yet clinicians must function at the pattern recognition level, assessing the patient as a whole and across time. Has he or she been gaining weight? Showing increases in triglycerides? Becoming less active? In short, is the syndrome progressing?

Our perspective on the metabolic syndrome is that it consists of four major features, and a large number of minor or contributory features of uncertain impact, all of these changing over time. These four features are shown in Table 19.1 and have been identified as (1) excess adiposity/obesity, (2) disturbed glucose metabolism and insulin action, (3) dyslipidemia, and (4) hypertension. In Table 19.1 we provide the varied range of methods of assessing each feature and their currently suggested cut points, and later provide caveats on the relative weighting of these features at different time points in the progression to the diabetes and cardiovascular endpoints.

The simplicity of the current NCEP ATP III definition, as modified in 2005 (8), has its advantages, and its criteria are asterisked in Table 19.1. The NCEP ATP III definition may, however, impose more structure than is necessary, and most surely identifies average cut points and not ones that necessarily reflect specific points in time in the progression to overt diabetes (see the section on chronomics, below). A consensus definition, merging in part the IDF (7) and NCEP ATP III (32) definitions, simplifies for the purpose of clinical expediency the many contributors that may additively result in the aging-related phenomenon we currently term the *metabolic syndrome*.

Preference is given to this "feature" approach, in which key aspects are identified, and multiple methods of assessing those aspects provided, each with guidance as to where values deviate from normal and therefore may be contributing to future disturbances and pathology leading to diabetes and CVD. Within each feature, controlling for one aspect generally accounts for most of the variability in the others within that feature—being collectively likely to reflect the same or a related metabolic disturbance. Evidence from longitudinal analysis as discussed below, however, suggests that two of these aspects (and possibly more) could reasonably be separated into two distinct features each, leading to a total of six major features. In the following discussion, the four

Table 19.1
Features of the Metabolic Syndrome and Methods of Assessing These Features

I.   Excess adiposity/obesity
     a. Body mass index (BMI) >30 kg/m^2 (wider risk range >27 kg/m^2).
     b. Waist circumference ≥94 cm (men) ** or ≥80 cm (women) ** *or* >102 cm (>40
         inches)* (men, U.S.); >88 cm (>35 inches)* (women, U.S.).
     c. Waist-to-hip ratio >0.90 (men) or >0.85 (women).
     d. *Note:* Past obesity (recent weight loss by intent or due to ill health) and family history
         of obesity (one or both parents) should also be considered as adiposity-related risk
         enhancers.
II. Dyslipidemia
     a. Triglycerides ≥150 mg/dl (1.7 mmol/l)* **
     b. HDL cholesterol <40 mg/dl (0.9 mmol/l)* ** (men) and <50 mg/dl (1.1 mmol/l)*
         (women)
     c. Lipid-lowering drug treatment (or on treatment*)
III. Disturbed glucose metabolism and insulin action
     a. Impaired fasting glucose (IFG) (fasting plasma glucose 100–125 mg/dl) (>100 mg/dl,
         >5.6 mmol/l)* ** (or treated for glucose lowering*)
     b. Impaired glucose tolerance (IGT) by
         i.   Oral glucose tolerance test (2 hr glucose >180 mg/dl)
         ii. Intravenous glucose tolerance test (Kgluc <2.5)
     c. Overt diabetes (with or without treatment)
         i.   This is included as it would not be useful to define someone as being cured of
              metabolic syndrome—no longer having it—once their glycemic levels pass a
              certain threshold currently defined as "diabetes."
     d. Hyperinsulinemia
         i.   Fasting insulin levels >75% for the assay
              1. Unfortunately, the assay for insulin has not yet been standardized for direct
                 comparisons across laboratories.
         ii. Insulin resistance (as assessed by the euglycemic hyperinsulinemic clamp
              procedure)
         iii. Insulin resistance as assessed by the HOMA formula or by Quicki (not
              significantly better on an individual basis than fasting insulin level)
         iv. Diminished insulin response to glucose (by either of the glucose tolerance
              methods)
IV. Hypertension
     a. Systolic blood pressure ≥130 mm Hg* ** (Syst or Diast or on antihypertensive drug)*
         or
     b. Diastolic blood pressure ≥85 mm Hg* **
     c. Treatment for hypertension

   Three of five of the asterisked (*) items constitutes the AHA/NHLBI NCEP ATP III revised definition
(8); obesity plus two of the double-asterisked (**) items constitutes the IDF definition (7,32).

basic features are identified, and then we examine the justification for the splitting of
two.
   Concerning excess adiposity, there is no a priori reason that one and only one way to
assess adiposity should be selected. Instead, any of several adiposity indicators works
well, and each is highly correlated with the others. For assessing obesity/excess adiposity
(33,34), it may be minimally important whether one selects the body mass index (BMI),

the waist circumference (thought to reflect visceral/intraabdominal fat (35)), the waist/ hip ratio, or direct measurement of adipose tissue mass by dual X-ray absorptiometry (DXA) or by underwater weighing—each produces an indicator of degree of excess adiposity and each is highly correlated with the others. Preferences for one method of obesity assessment over another will vary with the clinical setting and the availability of various methods. Interestingly, while the presence of obesity appears to be very important for the development of the metabolic syndrome, the *degree* of obesity is much less critical to the likelihood of progressing to the syndrome. Thus some individuals with very high levels of adiposity do not yet manifest the syndrome. This flexible menu of methods used to assess each feature, shown in Table 19.1, is a boon to the clinician (36), but is the bane of the epidemiologist, who wishes to see the same variables always measured in the same way and with the application of strict cut points (37).

In addition to the features in Table 19.1, around which there is some consensus, there are many variables that have been identified as associated with the metabolic syndrome and with its complications (38). Some of these are included in Table 19.2, and some, such as CRP, are candidates for biomarkers of the metabolic syndrome (39–44); however, these lack the broad endorsement of the features included in Table 19.1.

Most importantly, it is our view that the differences in opinions relate largely to the varying degree of understanding and acceptance of the dual concepts of *pattern recognition* and *chronomics*, and lack of this appreciation has led some to question, "Why diagnose it at all?" (2,8,9,31,45,46).

THE COMPLEXITY OF THE METABOLIC SYNDROME: PATTERN RECOGNITION

The complexity of the metabolic syndrome increases with the number of pieces included, and this complexity requires greater flexibility, not more structure and reductionism. With increasing numbers of variables and ranges of progressively changing variables, describing this complexity becomes more challenging. Yet, just as we can recognize a human face in an instant, despite it being made up of a thousand different points, so we can see the metabolic syndrome as a pattern emerging both in the examination of individual subject progression data and in large-scale population or epidemiological data.

Pattern recognition and identification of risk factors by cluster analysis are important approaches for those seeking the mechanistic underpinnings of the metabolic syndrome, but challenging to describe with precision and to quantify.

As scientists/clinical investigators, we often find it necessary to put on blinders, to bring focus to our work, and to ignore at least temporarily the complexity involved in the many cofactors and confounders. Those studying dyslipidemia seldom want to hear about the CNS control of the pancreatic beta-cell. Nor do lipidologists (to site just one group of metabolic syndrome investigators) have significant interest in the fact that beta-cells secrete insulin with a periodicity of 10–12 minutes per cycle, a periodicity that is exaggerated in the early phases of the metabolic syndrome and completely lost in the later phases (prior to the development of overt type 2 diabetes) (47–49).

Defects in the responsiveness of some metabolic pathways are likely to be acquired or secondary and are potentially reversible. Others may have a genetic or aging basis not readily amenable to mitigation.

Table 19.2
Additional Features That May Be Contributory to the Metabolic Syndrome

I.   Markers of vascular and adipose inflammation
     a. CRP
     b. TNFα
     c. Adiponectin
     d. RANTES
     e. MIF
     f. Other acute phase proteins
     g. Von Willebrand Factor
     h. Thrombomodulin
     i. tPA
     j. ICAM-1
     k. VCAM-1
     l. E-selectin
     m. CFN-cellular fibronectin
II. Markers of procoagulation state (increased production of procoagulation factors and
     increased production of inhibitors of fibrinolytic pathways)
     a. Fibrinogen
     b. PAI-1
     c. Factor VII
     d. Factor VIIa
     e. D-dimer
III. Disturbances of microvascular flow
     a. Impaired peripheral vascular flow
     b. Impaired flow-mediated dilation (usually brachial artery)
     c. Impaired endothelial-mediated flow
IV. Aging
V.   Additional dyslipidemia variables
     a. Small dense LDL
     b. LDL/HDL ratio
     c. FFA
     d. ApoB
     e. Apo A-1
     f. Lp(a)
     g. Total cholesterol
VI. Additional glucose/insulin-related variables
     a. Impaired β-cell response to glucose
     b. microalbuminuria

Inter-organ interactions may also add to the complexity. For example, disturbances in hepatic lipid synthesis may contribute to defects in insulin signaling in skeletal muscle (see Farese's discussion in Chapter 17). Tissue specificity of disturbed mechanisms changes across time. Thus, for example, the *non*concordant development of defects in insulin signaling across tissue types must become part of our conceptualization of the metabolic syndrome. Developmental and adaptive changes also are occurring within individuals, bringing forth compensatory responses that may restore a prior state, or normalize certain variables/features, at least temporarily, and thus obscure developing pathophysiology.

How many different physiological processes are involved in the metabolic syndrome as it is currently conceptualized? And how many counterregulatory mechanisms are in play among those processes that may be (temporarily) restoring equilibrium or (temporarily) normalizing a variable? Suppose each process has its own longitudinal trajectory (as we have diagrammed in Fig. 19.1) with flexible crosslinks to other processes. A set of processes may be involved in insulin secretion, insulin action, and glucose homeostasis, with particular involvement of the CNS, pancreas, muscle, adipose tissue, and liver (50). Another set of processes may be involved in producing a dyslipidemic profile, including dietary fat, gastrointestinal function, hepatic function, endothelial enzymes, and macrophages—and these intersect with the insulin/glucose-related processes. The closeness or frequency of these intersections dictates the degree to which a pattern, here labeled a *syndrome*, can be discerned.

Consider further the impact of the above two sets of processes (glucose/insulin/pancreas/muscle and dyslipidemia/liver/insulin) on the cardiovascular system, coronary arteries, blood vessels, blood pressure regulation, baroreceptors, kidneys, electrolyte transport, and free fatty acids, *and the mental gymnastics become daunting.* These *macroprocesses and interactions between organ systems* are seen to create the pattern that is currently recognized as the metabolic syndrome. Finally reverting from the macrosystem level to the microlevel, the *gene*, gene–gene and gene–environment interactions multiply by manyfold the complexity we are attempting to synthesize and diagnose. Nevertheless, the search for patterns in this complexity can lead to the formulation of new hypotheses and provide guidance for future research.

The metabolic syndrome involves complexity at the morphological level, as well as at the physiological functional level. Our concept of the metabolic syndrome is evolving, as we gain a clearer picture of the intersecting processes responsible for one of the most complex of the diseases of aging.

Changes in the state of a person or animal occur over short periods (fasting, exercise), extended periods (feeding, body-weight reduction), and lifetime periods (development of type 2 diabetes or cardiovascular disease). The trajectories and rates of progression of each of these are highly variable both within and across individuals. Some have referred to this as a *chaotic dynamic system*, affected by both initiating events and external conditions. Periodic episodes of imbalance can give way to relative balance and imperfect steady states. The presence or absence of the metabolic syndrome may be measured at one or several time points in this relative steady state, frequently neglecting to look both backward and forward at each variable to observe where this variable was three years ago and where it will be three years from now.

Finding similarities in metabolic syndrome features in *Drosophila*, monkeys, and humans can help to understand these developmental and progressive processes. Pattern recognition across such species and across time adds further to defining their dynamic processes and to hypothesizing or identifying their molecular underpinnings.

THE LONGITUDINAL DEVELOPMENT OF THE METABOLIC SYNDROME

Chronomics, the newest of the "omics," brings attention the fact that the moment of assessment of the criterion variable set included in Table 19.1 is a snapshot of a longitudinal progression. This new "omic" refers both to the changes *within* variables/tissue/cells over time, and to changes *in their interactions or dominance over the integrated system over time*. In the evolution of metabolic syndrome features, the least examined "omic" is the *chronomic factor*. For those seeking initiating events or points for intervention in understanding the progressive process, a chronomic assessment suggests that exact cut points across three to six variables may not be possible—except as statistical constructs. Certainly these cut points have little relevance to an individual patient who will be best served by a pattern recognition approach and an understanding of the progressive nature of the highly associated features of the metabolic syndrome. It is his/her trajectory or chronomic profile that provides the best indicator of an impending or present health problem deserving of intervention. It is important that the progression pattern be understood in order to adjust for minor failure in alignments at a given point in time.

Data from longitudinal studies of both humans and nonhuman primates (51), as these subjects progress from normal young adults through various *phases* in the progression to overt type 2 diabetes, have provided the basis for plotting the trajectory patterns for each of the key variables of the metabolic syndrome that are shown in Figure 19.1. Nonhuman primates, studied longitudinally from normal young adult (Phase 1) through the development of the metabolic syndrome and onward to the manifestation of spontaneous severe type 2 diabetes (Phase 9), help to clarify similar trajectories observed in several studies of human progression to diabetes (52), including those of the long-term studies of the Pima Indians (53) and those of Hispanic Americans (54–56).

It is revealing and noteworthy that each variable has a different pattern across time and phase of progression, and that there are few variables that are truly linearly positively or negatively related, or related to each other through the whole dynamic evolution to the disease endpoint(s)—in this case, diabetes (Fig. 19.1). In fact, the shapes of these trajectories, even within a feature, vary. For example, compare the trajectory of fasting plasma insulin to that of insulin resistance/insulin sensitivity as measured by the gold standard (a euglycemic hyperinsulinemic clamp to measure insulin action on glucose uptake rate (M)).

If one seeks to define the level of a particular variable that best defines risk, or is most predictive, it should be readily apparent that the level immediately before the threshold or cut point on a continuum will always be the best predictor (e.g., glucose of 120 best predicts glucose of 125), but how informative is this?

Thus, lining up the cut points becomes simpler when in close proximity to a diagnostic threshold (prior consensus cut points). It is possible to line up several indicators of impending diabetes: the fasting glucose that is highly predictive of an emerging diagnostic level (e.g., 120 mg/dL predicting 126 mg/dL) with the degree of impaired glucose tolerance (2 h glucose elevation) that most closely associates with fasting glucose level. As one distances oneself in time backward from the threshold criterion variable level (i.e., to a fasting glucose of 85–90 mg/dL), prediction becomes less certain, but gains power if small disturbances in related variables/features are considered; for example, a small increase in triglycerides levels may predict the impending development of the metabolic syndrome. It is the aligning of the threshold levels to bring concordance to a dynamic moving progression that has led to the current relative consensus on a metabolic syndrome definition (10,57). Furthermore, the bias is toward defining it late, in close proximity to the development of T2DM and cardiovascular disease (CVD) (53), so as to improve its use as a risk predictor, ignoring the fact that

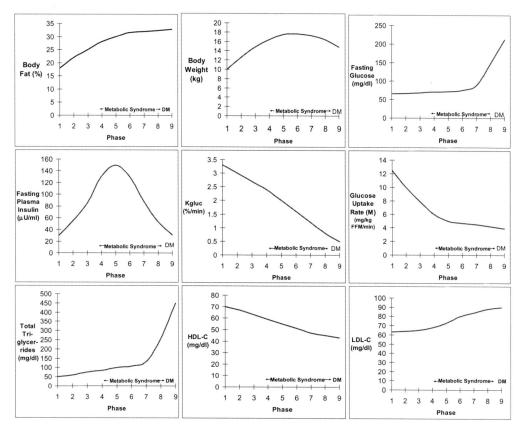

Figure 19.1. The longitudinal trajectories of 9 variables used in defining the presence of the metabolic syndrome (trajectories derived from longitudinal data of nonhuman primates progressing from normal to overtly diabetic): *adiposity* (percent body fat and body weight change in adulthood); *disturbed glucose metabolism/insulin action* (fasting plasma glucose, impaired glucose tolerance [K glucose, the glucose disappearance rate during an intravenous glucose tolerance test], fasting plasma insulin, and glucose uptake rate in response to maximal insulin stimulation—the "glucose clamp"); and *dyslipidemia* (hypertriglyceridemia, lowered HDL-cholesterol, and no change or small increase in LDL cholesterol). Note that *hypertension* is not included in this figure as its longitudinal trajectory does not closely approximate any of these others, and it appears to be more likely a sporadic fellow traveler rather than an integral part of the syndrome.

Phases are defined as: Phase 1—normal lean young adult; Phase 2—normal lean or overweight middle-aged or aging adults; Phase 3—earliest signs of progression deviating from normal; Phase 4—statistically significant increase in fasting insulin and triglycerides and reduction in insulin sensitivity; Phase 5—highest beta-cell responsiveness to glucose, progressive decline in glucose tolerance but not yet IGT; Phase 6—declining acute insulin response to glucose, peak insulin level declining, low insulin sensitivity, further declining glucose tolerance; Phase 7—impaired glucose tolerance or impaired fasting glucose, significantly reduced (from elevated) beta-cell response to glucose and fasting insulin levels (both still above normal levels of Phase 1); Phase 8—overt diabetes meeting the ADA criteria for diagnosis of diabetes mellitus; Phase 9—severe diabetes requiring insulin treatment for maintenance of health and well being.

each variable exists as a continuum and that the criteria defined in Table 19.1 are rather arbitrarily selected thresholds (58).

Thus, the higher the ability of a given level of a factor to predict an endpoint, the closer that criterion is to being part of the endpoint. A plasma triglyceride level of 140 mg/dL predicts developing metabolic syndrome, and a fasting glucose of 120 mg/dL strongly predicts diabetes. In the real world, however, we are not looking to predict with 100% confidence something likely to occur within months, but rather to identify, early in the metabolic syndrome trajectory, those whose progressive collective changes predict untoward outcomes in the future (59,60). Thus, highly predictive abnormal levels are those proximal to the criterion threshold and are less ambiguous (as some would wish) and are less arbitrary. With a longer-range view, prospective predictions of risk estimates become less stable, and it is this uncertainty that makes some uncomfortable with the metabolic syndrome definition.

Concerning our disputes about the definitions and cut points for metabolic syndrome features, it is easy to ignore the fact that some features of this developing and progressive set of disorders dominate the characterization in the *earliest* phases (and thus are furthest away in time from the ultimate consequences of the syndrome (CVD and T2DM), and least precise and least proximal in the prediction of risk); these factors may, however, be the most tractable/reversible or controllable in the earliest stages of disease progression. Other features and their cut points become most powerful as predictors immediately proximal in time to specific endpoints. Thus IFG and IGT strongly predict diabetes, while obesity does not. Yet successful treatment of and mitigation of the disease of obesity prevents IFG and IGT almost completely and is powerful in preventing the development of the metabolic syndrome, when weight loss is sustained.

Returning to the issue of how many features should be identified in the metabolic syndrome, in the preceding discussion we identified four, with the caveat that six may be more appropriate. The disturbances in glucose metabolism are in part independent of the disturbances in insulin action (see Fig. 19.1). Insulin action declines early in the progression, then shows no measurable further deterioration in humans or monkeys. Impaired fasting glucose and impaired glucose tolerance are clearly late events in the progression. Changes in circulating triglycerides should be identified separately from the changes in HDL cholesterol and other lipid fractions (e.g., increased particle density of low-density lipoprotein).

As the metabolic syndrome has emerged as a major risk factor for diabetes and CVD, the clinical management of the metabolic syndrome (61), by diet and lifestyle modifications (62–67), and by pharmaceutical interventions (68–70), including the whole family of peroxisome proliferator–activated receptor (PPAR) agonists, has raised the potential that earlier interventions could prevent its development. Many new molecules are now under development (71–74) to encourage aggressive management of the features and to promote methods to reduce and slow or prevent the progression to overt CVD and diabetes. The power of calorie restriction to mitigate or to prevent these metabolic disorders has frequently been noted (e.g., 75–78).

While knowledge of a single underlying pathological cause would help in verifying the features and their criterion variables and would reinforce estimates of the magnitude of risk, we are not there yet. Surely the identification of the cause of risk factor clustering could lead to a better understanding of the underlying pathology, and perhaps to another renaming of the syndrome.

Understanding the complexity, linking a series of associated but different patterns changing across time, is likely to be a key research objective in moving from the genomic to the proteomic to the physiological system integration essential to understanding the casual mechanisms of the metabolic syndrome.

WHAT IS THE RECIPE FOR THE METABOLIC SYNDROME? WHAT IS IN IT? WHAT IS NOT?

Stone Soup (or as the Scandinavians call it, Nail Soup) also carries messages for what constitutes the metabolic syndrome "soup." As the story goes:

Some travelers arrive at a village carrying nothing but an empty pot. They fill the pot with water, drop in a large stone, and place it over the fire. The curious villagers ask what they are doing, and learn that the travelers are making a wonderful "stone soup," which would be improved by a garnish they are missing. Each villager passes by and adds another ingredient, and finally a delicious and nourishing pot of soup is enjoyed by all.

We are in the stage of adding ingredients to the metabolic syndrome soup pot. Perhaps a recipe will emerge that will explain the sequence and importance of each contributory factor. Delineation and specification of processes and interactions may, after all, emerge to be a catalyst to improving our understanding of what is now blurry.

REFERENCES

1. Nestel P. Metabolic syndrome: Multiple candidate genes, multiple environmental factors—multiple syndromes? *Int J Clin Pract Suppl* 2003; 134:3–9.
2. Kahn R et al. The metabolic syndrome—time for a critical appraisal: Joint statement from the American Diabetes Association and the European Association for the Study of Diabetes. *Diabetes Care* 2005; 28(9):2289–2304.
3. Alberti KG, Zimmet PZ. Definition, diagnosis and classification of diabetes mellitus and its complications: Part 1. Diagnosis and classification of diabetes mellitus provisional report of a WHO consultation. *Diabet Med* 1998; 15(7):539–553.
4. Balkau B, Charles MA. Comment on the provisional report from the WHO consultation: European Group for the Study of Insulin Resistance (EGIR). *Diabet Med* 1999: 16(5):442–443.
5. Executive summary of the Third Report of the National Cholesterol Education Program (NCEP) Expert Panel on Detection, Evaluation, and Treatment of High Blood Cholesterol in Adults (Adult Treatment Panel III). *JAMA* 2001; 285(19):2486–2497.
6. Einhorn D et al. American College of Endocrinology position statement on the insulin resistance syndrome. *Endocr Pract* 2003; 9(3):237–252.
7. Alberti KG, Zimmet P, Shaw J. Metabolic syndrome—a new world-wide definition: A consensus statement from the International Diabetes Federation. *Diabet Med* 2006; 23(5):469–480.
8. Grundy SM et al. Diagnosis and management of the metabolic syndrome: An American Heart Association/National Heart, Lung, and Blood Institute scientific statement. *Circulation* 2005; 112(17):2735–2752.
9. Zimmet P et al. The metabolic syndrome: A global public health problem and a new definition. *J Atheroscler Thromb* 2005; 12(6):295–300.
10. Grundy SM et al. Definition of metabolic syndrome: Report of the National Heart, Lung, and Blood Institute/American Heart Association conference on scientific issues related to definition. *Circulation*, 2004; 109(3):433–438.
11. Cheal KL et al. Relationship to insulin resistance of the Adult Treatment Panel III diagnostic criteria for identification of the metabolic syndrome. *Diabetes* 2004; 53(5):1195–1200.

12. Liao Y et al. Critical evaluation of Adult Treatment Panel III criteria in identifying insulin resistance with dyslipidemia. *Diabetes Care* 2004; 27(4):978–983.

13. Zimmet P, MM Alberti KG, Serrano Rios M. A new International Diabetes Federation worldwide definition of the metabolic syndrome: The rationale and the results. *Rev Esp Cardiol* 2005; 58(12):1371–1376.

14. Meigs JB et al. Body mass index, metabolic syndrome, and risk of type 2 diabetes or cardiovascular disease. *J Clin Endocrinol Metab* 2006; 91(8):2906–2912.

15. Reaven GM. Banting lecture 1988: Role of insulin resistance in human disease. *Diabetes* 1988; 37(12):1595–1607.

16. Wilson PW et al. Metabolic syndrome as a precursor of cardiovascular disease and type 2 diabetes mellitus. *Circulation* 2005; 112(20):3066–3072.

17. Costa LA et al. Aggregation of features of the metabolic syndrome is associated with increased prevalence of chronic complications in Type 2 diabetes. *Diabet Med* 2004; 21(3):252–255.

18. Bonora E et al. The metabolic syndrome is an independent predictor of cardiovascular disease in Type 2 diabetic subjects: Prospective data from the Verona Diabetes Complications Study. *Diabet Med* 2004; 21(1):52–58.

19. Ford ES, Giles WH, Mokdad AH. Increasing prevalence of the metabolic syndrome among U.S. adults. *Diabetes Care* 2004; 27(10):2444–2449.

20. Camus JP. *[Gout, diabetes, hyperlipemia: A metabolic trisyndrome.]* *Rev Rhum Mal Osteoartic* 1966; 33(1):10–14.

21. Crepaldi G, Nosadini R. Diabetic cardiopathy: Is it a real entity? *Diabetes Metab Rev* 1988; 4(3):273–288.

22. DeFronzo RA, Ferrannini E. Insulin resistance: A multifaceted syndrome responsible for NIDDM, obesity, hypertension, dyslipidemia, and atherosclerotic cardiovascular disease. *Diabetes Care* 1991; 14(3):173–194.

23. Eriksson J, Taimela S, Koivisto VA. Exercise and the metabolic syndrome. *Diabetologia* 1997; 40(2):125–135.

24. Kaplan NM. The deadly quartet: Upper-body obesity, glucose intolerance, hypertriglyceridemia, and hypertension. *Arch Intern Med* 1989; 149(7):1514–1520.

25. Scott R et al. Will acarbose improve the metabolic abnormalities of insulin-resistant type 2 diabetes mellitus? *Diab Res Clin Pract* 1999 Mar; 43(3):179–185.

26. Shafrir E. Animal models of syndrome X. *Curr Top Diab Res* 1993; 12:165–181.

27. Zimmet P. The epidemiology of diabetes mellitus and related conditions. In: *The Diabetes Annual/6*, Alberti K, Krall LP (eds.), 1991, Elsevier, Amsterdam.

28. Ford ES. Prevalence of the metabolic syndrome defined by the International Diabetes Federation among adults in the U.S. *Diabetes Care* 2005; 28(11):2745–2749.

29. Ford ES. Rarer than a blue moon: The use of a diagnostic code for the metabolic syndrome in the U.S. *Diabetes Care* 2005; 28(7):1808–1809.

30. Alexander CM. The coming of age of the metabolic syndrome. *Diabetes Care* 2003; 26(11):3180–3181.

31. Grundy SM. Does a diagnosis of metabolic syndrome have value in clinical practice? *Am J Clin Nutr* 2006; 83(6):1248–1251.

32. Gotto AM Jr et al. The metabolic syndrome: A call to action. *Coron Artery Dis* 2006; 17(1):77–80.

33. Bray GA. Obesity is a chronic, relapsing neurochemical disease. *Int J Obes Relat Metab Disord* 2004; 28(1):34–38.

34. Bonnet F et al. Waist circumference and the metabolic syndrome predict the development of elevated albuminuria in non-diabetic subjects: The DESIR Study. *J Hypertens* 2006; 24(6):1157–1163.

35. Carr DB et al. Intra-abdominal fat is a major determinant of the National Cholesterol Education Program Adult Treatment Panel III criteria for the metabolic syndrome. *Diabetes* 2004; 53(8):2087–2094.

36. Deen D. Metabolic syndrome: Time for action. *Am Fam Physician* 2004; 69(12):2875–2882.

37. Ford ES. Risks for all-cause mortality, cardiovascular disease, and diabetes associated with the metabolic syndrome: A summary of the evidence. *Diabetes Care* 2005; 28(7):1769–1778.

38. Grundy SM. Obesity, metabolic syndrome, and cardiovascular disease. *J Clin Endocrinol Metab* 2004; 89(6):2595–2600.

39. Kahn SE et al. Obesity is a major determinant of the association of C-reactive protein levels and the metabolic syndrome in type 2 diabetes. *Diabetes* 2006; 55(8):2357–2364.

40. Wang YY et al. Association between hematological parameters and metabolic syndrome components in a Chinese population. *J Diab Compl* 2004: 18(6):322–327.

41. Corsetti JP et al. Metabolic syndrome best defines the multivariate distribution of blood variables in postinfarction patients. *Atherosclerosis* 2003; 171(2):351–358.

42. Sowers JR. Recommendations for special populations: Diabetes mellitus and the metabolic syndrome. *Am J Hypertens* 2003; 16(11, pt. 2):41S–45S.

43. Chan JC et al. The central roles of obesity-associated dyslipidaemia, endothelial activation and cytokines in the Metabolic Syndrome–an analysis by structural equation modelling. *Int J Obes Relat Metab Disord* 2002; 26(7):994–1008.

44. Herder C et al. Systemic immune mediators and lifestyle changes in the prevention of type 2 diabetes: Results from the Finnish Diabetes Prevention Study. *Diabetes* 2006; 55(8):2340–2346.

45. Schneider JG et al. The metabolic syndrome in women. *Cardiol Rev* 2006; 14(6):286–291.

46. Reaven GM. The metabolic syndrome: Is this diagnosis necessary? *Am J Clin Nutr* 2006; 83(6):1237–1247.

47. Koerker DJ et al. Synchronous sustained oscillations of C-peptide and insulin in the plasma of fasting monkeys. *Endocrinology* 1978; 102:1649–1652.

48. Hansen BC et al. Neural influences on oscillations in basal plasma levels of insulin in monkeys. *Am J Physiol (Endocrinol Metab 1)* 1981; 240:E5–E11.

49. Hansen BC et al. Rapid oscillations in plasma insulin, glucagon, and glucose in obese and normal weight humans. *J Clin Endocrinol Metab* 1982; 54:785–792.

50. Seeley RJ, Tschop M. How diabetes went to our heads. *Nat Med* 2006; 12(1):47–49; discussion at 49.

51. Kaufman D et al. Early appearance of the metabolic syndrome in socially reared bonnet macaques. *J Clin Endocrinol Metab* 2005; 90(1):404–408.

52. Junien C et al. [Nutritional epigenomics of metabolic syndrome.] *Med Sci (Paris)* 2005; 21(spec. no.):44–52.

53. Weyer C et al. The natural history of insulin secretory dysfunction and insulin resistance in the pathogenesis of type 2 diabetes mellitus. *J Clin Invest* 1999; 104(6):787–794.

54. Lorenzo C et al. The metabolic syndrome as predictor of type 2 diabetes: The San Antonio heart study. *Diabetes Care* 2003; 26(11):3153–3159.

55. Lorenzo C et al. Geographic variations of the International Diabetes Federation and the National Cholesterol Education Program–Adult Treatment Panel III definitions of the metabolic syndrome in nondiabetic subjects. *Diabetes Care* 2006; 29(3):685–691.

56. Lorenzo C et al. Trend in the prevalence of the metabolic syndrome and its impact on cardiovascular disease incidence: The San Antonio Heart Study. *Diabetes Care* 2006; 29(3):625–630.

57. Third report of the National Cholesterol Education Program (NCEP) Expert Panel on Detection, Evaluation, and Treatment of High Blood Cholesterol in Adults (Adult Treatment Panel III) final report. *Circulation* 2002; 106(25):3143–3421.

58. Aguilar-Salinas CA et al. Design and validation of a population-based definition of the metabolic syndrome. *Diabetes Care* 2006; 29(11):2420–2426.

59. Ludwig DS, Ebbeling CB. Type 2 diabetes mellitus in children: Primary care and public health considerations. *JAMA* 2001; 286(12):1427–1430.

60. Golley RK et al. Comparison of metabolic syndrome prevalence using six different definitions in overweight pre-pubertal children enrolled in a weight management study. *Int J Obes (Lond)* 2006; 30(5):853–860.

61. Grundy SM et al. Clinical management of metabolic syndrome: Report of the American Heart Association/National Heart, Lung, and Blood Institute/American Diabetes Association conference on scientific issues related to management. *Circulation* 2004; 109(4):551–556.

62. Knowler WC et al. Reduction in the incidence of type 2 diabetes with lifestyle intervention or metformin. *N Engl J Med* 2002; 346(6):393–403.

63. Sacks FM et al. Effects on blood pressure of reduced dietary sodium and the Dietary Approaches to Stop Hypertension (DASH) diet: DASH-Sodium Collaborative Research Group. *N Engl J Med* 2001; 344(1):3–10.

64. Sahyoun NR et al. Whole-grain intake is inversely associated with the metabolic syndrome and mortality in older adults. *Am J Clin Nutr* 2006; 83(1):124–131.

65. Grundy SM, Abate N, Chandalia M. Diet composition and the metabolic syndrome: What is the optimal fat intake? *Am J Med* 2002; 113(suppl 9B):25S–29S.

66. Trichopoulou A et al. Adherence to a Mediterranean diet and survival in a Greek population. *N Engl J Med* 2003; 348(26):2599–2608.

67. Foster GD et al. A randomized trial of a low-carbohydrate diet for obesity. *N Engl J Med* 2003; 348(21):2082–2090.

68. Van Gaal LF et al. Effects of the cannabinoid-1 receptor blocker rimonabant on weight reduction and cardiovascular risk factors in overweight patients: 1-year experience from the RIO-Europe study. *Lancet* 2005; 365(9468):1389–1397.

69. Despres JP, Golay A, Sjostrom L. Effects of rimonabant on metabolic risk factors in overweight patients with dyslipidemia. *N Engl J Med* 2005; 353(20):2121–2134.

70. Pi-Sunyer FX et al. Effect of rimonabant, a cannabinoid-1 receptor blocker, on weight and cardiometabolic risk factors in overweight or obese patients: RIO-North America—a randomized controlled trial. *JAMA* 2006; 295(7):761–775.

71. Nissen SE et al. Effects of a potent and selective PPAR-alpha agonist in patients with atherogenic dyslipidemia or hypercholesterolemia: Two randomized controlled trials. *JAMA* 2007; 297(12): 1362–1373.

72. Sauerberg P et al. Identification and synthesis of a novel selective partial PPARdelta agonist with full efficacy on lipid metabolism in vitro and in vivo. *J Med Chem* 2007; 50(7):1495–1503.

73. Goldstein BJ et al. Effect of tesaglitazar, a dual PPAR alpha/gamma agonist, on glucose and lipid abnormalities in patients with type 2 diabetes: A 12-week dose-ranging trial. *Curr Med Res Opin* 2006; 22(12):2575–2590.

74. Gonzalez IC et al. Design and synthesis of a novel class of dual PPARgamma/delta agonists. *Bioorg Med Chem Lett* 2007; 17(4):1052–1055.

75. Bodkin NL, Hansen BC. Prevention of Syndrome X by long-term dietary restriction (DR) in aged rhesus monkeys. In: *The Gerontologist*, 1995.

76. Ortmeyer HK, Bodkin NL, Hansen BC. Chronic caloric restriction alters glycogen metabolism in rhesus monkeys. *Obes Res* 1994; 2:549–555.

77. DeLany JP et al. Long-term calorie restriction reduces energy expenditure in aging monkeys. *J of Gerontol A Biol Sci Med Sci* 1999; 54:B5–B11.

78. Hansen BC, Bodkin NL, Ortmeyer HK. Calorie restriction in non human primates: Mechanisms of reduced morbidity and mortality. *Toxicol Sci* 1999; 52S:56–60.

Index

Hypertension, 14, 19–20, 88–89, 381
  C-reactive protein in, 173–174
  hyperinsulinemia-related, 79
  insulin in, 88–89
  obesity-related, 38, 94
    insulin in, 88–89
    sympathetic nervous system stimulation
      in, 91–93
    thermogenesis in, 94
  treatment of
    dietary, 61, 98–99
    pharmacological, 99
Hypertriglyceridemia
  C-reactive protein-related, 174–175
  in diabetes mellitus, 205
  epinephrine levels in, 95–97
  in insulin resistance, 205–206
    animal studies of, 310–311
    human studies of, 311–312
  as metabolic syndrome diagnostic
    criterion, 14, 16–17
  postprandial, 17–18
  tumor necrosis factor-α–related, 175
Hypoglycemia, GLP-1-related, 245
Hypothalamus
  in endogenous glucose production, 349
  insulin resistance in, 263

I

IGF-1. *See* Insulin-like growth factor-1
IKK-β, 308, 309, 316, 317
Inflammation
  adipose tissue in, 194–197
  as atherosclerosis risk factor, 168
  dietary reduction of, 44, 45
  in insulin resistance, 21, 316–317
  in insulin signaling, 316–317
  markers of, 378
  resistin in, 42–43
  as risk factor clustering cause, 47
  subclinical, obesity-associated, 41–42
Inflammatory molecules, in adipose tissue, 194–197
Inflammatory signaling, crosstalk with insulin signaling, 127
Insulin
  in apolipoprotein B degradation, 207, 211
  in diabetes mellitus, 355–357
  effect of GLP-1 on, 238–240, 242–245

hepatic effects of, 352–357
in hepatic glucose metabolism, 355–357
as hypertension cause, 88–89
in musculature, physiological mechanisms of, 112–117
renal sodium reabsorption-enhancing effect of, 88–89
secretion of
  GLP-1stimulated, 238–240
  glucose-stimulated, 224
sympathetic nervous system-stimulating activity of, 87–91
  effect of glucose on, 89–90
vasodilatory actions of, 112–115
  capillary recruitment of, 117
  in glucose homeostasis, 115–117
  nitric oxide-dependency of, 113–115
Insulin infusion sensitivity test, 75–76
Insulin/insulin-like growth factor family, 256–57
Insulin-like growth factor-1, 108, 256
  tyrosine kinase activity of, 256–257
Insulin-like growth factor-1 receptors, 283, 287
Insulin-like growth factor-2, 256
Insulin receptor(s), 282–297
  ablation of, 282
  autophosphorylation in, 108, 109, 281–282, 283
    effect of diet on, 288–289
    in muscle cell cultures, 290
    in obesity, 288
    structural aspects of, 284–285
  basic function of, 284
  in diabetes mellitus, 289
  direct inhibitors of, 286
  O-glycosylation in, 297
  hybrid, 257
  insulin binding with, 281–282
  in insulin resistance, 287–291
  isoforms of, 256, 257
  in muscle, 287–291
    effect of physical activity on, 289
  in obesity, 296
  post-translational modification of, 294–297
  protein inhibitors of, 291–294
  serine phosphorylation of, 296
  "spare," 334